TEXTBOOK OF HUMAN HISTOLOGY

VOLUME 2

ORGAN SYSTEMS AND FUNCTIONAL HISTOLOGY

Edited by:
Dr. Neda Nikolovski

ALLIED HEALTH PRESS

Textbook of Human Histology

Volume 2: Organ Systems and Functional Histology

Editor: **Dr. Neda Nikolovski**

Allied Health Press
4164 Lakeshore Road
Burlington ON L7L 1A4
Canada
www.alliedhealthpress.com
Email: orders@arclereducation.com

ISBN: 978-1-77956-777-2

ABOUT THE EDITOR

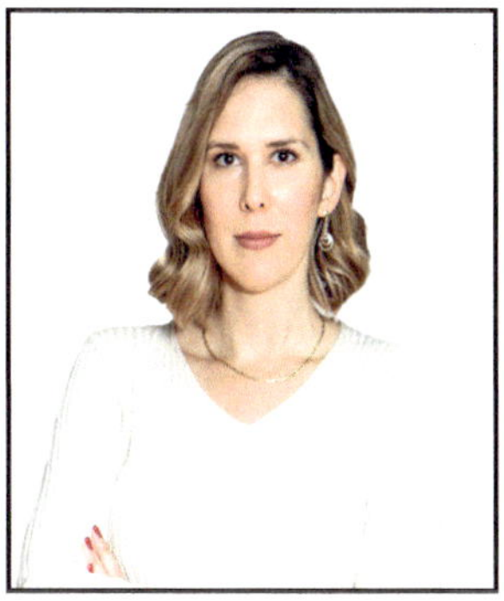

Dr. Neda Nikolovski, a Molecular Biologist and Physiologist holding a PhD in Immunology, has been dedicated to scientific research since 2015 at the Institute for Biological Research, Belgrade University, Belgrade, Serbia. Her primary areas of expertise encompass immunology, autoimmunity, neurodegenerative diseases, multiple sclerosis and its animal models, dendritic cells, and cell-based immunotherapy in autoimmune conditions. She is author of 27 research papers published in esteemed international journals and has contributed her expertise as a reviewer for numerous international publications.

Brief Table of Contents

Chapter Openers

A list of Chapter Outline is presented providing a brief Introduction to what will be covered in the chapter.

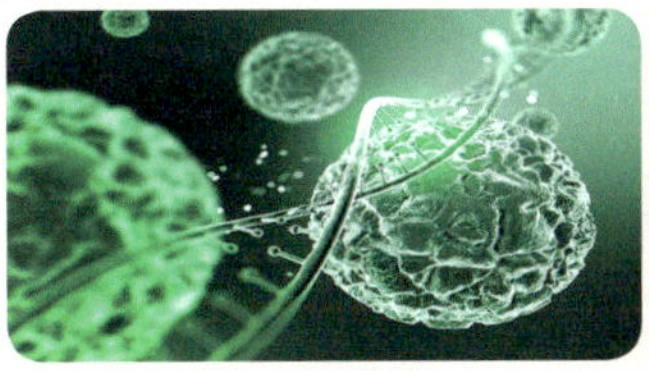

Introduction

Often referred to as the science of life, biology is a broad field of study aimed at comprehending the several kinds of life on Earth, from tiny creatures to sophisticated multicellular entities. Comprising several subfields, including molecular biology, ecology, and evolutionary biology, each of which advances our knowledge of living systems, this field clarifies the mechanisms controlling life events, including development, reproduction, and interaction with the surroundings, which is the central goal of biology. Moreover, biology fills in the void between the natural sciences and medicine by offering a necessary understanding of health, illness, and the interactions between organisms and their environments. Dealing with urgent global issues such as climate change, biodiversity loss, and new diseases depends on an awareness of these complex biological interactions, therefore highlighting the critical part biology plays in modern civilization. Fundamentally, biology explores and tests ideas about the living world using the scientific method. Through methodical observation and experimentation,

LEARNING OBJECTIVES

After studying this chapter, you will be able to:

1. Discuss the scientific method in biology;
2. Explain the cell theory;
3. Discuss the genetics and heredity;
4. Evolution and natural selection;
5. Focus on ecology and ecosystems;
6. Learn about human biology;
7. Evaluate the plant biology;
8. Explain the microbiology;
9. Focus on current trends in biology.

1.1. The Scientific Method in Biology

Learning Outcome

1. Describe the steps of the scientific method;
2. Focus on hypothesis formation;
3. Learn about experimental design.

Learning Outcomes

The beginning of each section of every chapter contains a set of Learning Outcomes that inform students of concepts they should understand. These outcomes help students understand what they should be able to do if they have mastered the material in that section.

Test Your Knowledge

Throughout each chapter, Test Your Knowledge cues you to note which topics have been covered and to self-test your understanding of the material presented.

Test Your Knowledge

1. Explain why correlation does not imply causation in scientific experiments.
2. How does the scientific method help reduce the influence of personal opinions in research?

Chapter Summary

The Summary Section appear at the end of each chapter and summarize main concepts covered throughout the chapter. These points provide key concepts in an engaging and meaningful way.

Summary

The investigation of biological principles highlights the importance of a comprehensive view of life by reflecting the intricate interactions that occur within living systems. The complexity of biology goes beyond individual species or systems, as this essay highlights; it also includes the interactions that mold ecosystems and affect biodiversity. Researchers can conduct in-depth analyses of metabolomic data using sophisticated technologies like MetaboAnalyst, which offer insights into the molecular mechanisms underlying these interactions. As demonstrated by the developments in MetaboAnalyst, for example, the integration of diverse omics data promotes a thorough understanding of metabolic pathways and helps identify important biological markers necessary for research on development and disease (Chong et al., 2018). Additionally, the phenomenon of ecological invasions is a key component of biological research and a vital field of study. The introduction of non-native species into unfamiliar habitats has significant ramifications and calls for multidisciplinary management strategies. Examining the origins and effects of these biological incursions, invasion science has become a crucial field that highlights the need to comprehend ecological dynamics and community interactions. As interest in biological invasions increases, new findings are emerging that put conventional ecological theories and practices to the test. The importance of incorporating various scientific viewpoints is shown by this developing discipline, which also highlights how invasive species shape ecosystems and advances our knowledge of ecological resilience (David et al., 2013). When taken as a whole, these discoveries from invasion science and metabolomics highlight the value of multidisciplinary biology research. Fostering cross-disciplinary collaboration and utilizing technological breakthroughs to improve our comprehension of intricate biological interactions are crucial as we look to the future of biological research. In addition to deepening our understanding of the complexities of life, this method lays the groundwork for tackling urgent environmental issues. Future studies can ensure the continued relevance of biology in a world that is constantly changing by acknowledging the interconnection of biological systems and opening the door to creative solutions that support sustainability and biodiversity conservation. We might imagine a thorough comprehension of life that serves both academia and society at large through ongoing investigation and integration of scientific knowledge.

Knowledge Assessment

The chapter includes material designed to review and reinforce each content. It includes Critical Thinking Questions to help test of your understanding of information presented in the chapter and Short answer Questions to review your understanding of the key concepts presented in the chapter.

Critical Thinking Questions

1. **Who is known as the "Father of Modern Biology"?**
   a. Aristotle
   b. Charles Darwin
   c. Gregor Mendel
   d. Louis Pasteur
2. **What is the basic unit of life?**
   a. Atom
   b. Molecule
   c. Cell
   d. Organism
3. **Which branch of biology studies the interaction of organisms with their environment?**
   a. Genetics
   b. Ecology
   c. Physiology
   d. Botany
4. **Which macromolecule is the main source of energy for living organisms?**
   a. Proteins
   b. Lipids
   c. Carbohydrates
   d. Nucleic acids
5. **DNA is primarily responsible for which function in living organisms?**
   a. Energy production
   b. Protein synthesis
   c. Storing genetic information
   d. Regulating body temperature

Short Answer Questions

1. What is biology, and why is it important to study biology?
2. What are the three main domains of life, and how are they different from one another?
3. Define homeostasis and give an example of how it works in living organisms.
4. What is the cell theory, and why is it fundamental to biology?
5. How do autotrophs and heterotrophs differ in the way they obtain energy?
6. What is the scientific method, and how is it applied in biological research?
7. Discuss how biology helps address global challenges such as climate change, disease, and food security.
8. Explain the levels of biological organization from the smallest unit to the largest. Provide examples at each level.
9. Describe the relationship between structure and function in biology, giving specific examples from cells or organs.
10. How has the discovery of genetics shaped our understanding of inheritance and variation among organisms?

Supplementary Materials

Key Terms: A list of key terms is given for quick reference

KEY TERMS FROM THIS CHAPTER

Annotation enrichment analysis	Biological structure	Cell
Cell theory	Cellular structure	Ecology
Ecosystems	Genetics	Human biology
Microbiology	Natural selection	Organism
Plant biology		

Further Resources: Recommendations for additional readings, websites, and multimedia resources.

References

1. Argelaguet, R., Velten, B., Arnol, D., Dietrich, S., Zenz, T., Marioni, J. C., Buettner, F., et al. (2018). Multi-omics factor analysis—A framework for unsupervised integration of multi-omics data sets. *Molecular Systems Biology, 14*. https://doi.org/10.15252/msb.20178124.
2. Bacher, S., Blackburn, T. M., Essl, F., & Genovesi, P. (2017). *Socio-Economic Impact Classification of Alien Taxa (SEICAT)*. https://core.ac.uk/download/286567949.pdf (accessed on 8th March 2025).
3. Barnett, R., Brace, S., Cucchi, T., & Dobney, K. (2013). *Divergent Evolutionary Processes Associated with Colonization of Offshore Islands*. https://core.ac.uk/download/20664364.pdf (accessed on 8th March 2025).

Detailed Table of Contents

CHAPTER 3

Respiratory System 75

CHAPTER 4

Digestive System (Oral Cavity) 109

CHAPTER 5

CHAPTER 6

CHAPTER 7

CHAPTER 12

Female Reproductive System 387

CHAPTER 13

Endocrine System 423

Index 463

LIST OF FIGURES

PREFACE

Microscopic anatomy of the human body sheds light on the orientation of specialized structures to maintain complicated physiological processes. Under the thin sections of the skin, blood vessels, glands, and other organs, one can view the manner in which cells are arranged into layers, networks, and compartments which facilitate the numerous processes of life. Whether it is the epidermis, with its protective functions, or the alveolar walls in the lung, with their delicate task of gaseous exchange; or any other tissue, each one bears the impress of its destiny, and manifests in some way its own peculiar functions. This pattern tracing, as students move through the various organ systems, provides them with an appreciation of the whole in terms of the interplay between form and function at a scale that is not visible without the aid of a microscope.

The development of improved histological methods has revolutionized concepts of organ structure. New staining techniques enable us to differentiate cell types and extracellular elements with a degree of clarity never before seen, and immunohistochemistry and in situ hybridization provide information on the distribution of proteins and nucleic acids in tissues. Such techniques not only hone diagnostic skills but also lead the way to investigations of developmental biology, regenerative medicine, and pathology. With microscopic observations being combined with molecular understanding, the field remains to bring together the basic science and the clinical realm, providing potent instruments in teaching as well as discovery.

This book, *Textbook of Human Histology: Volume 2,* is a companion text that builds on the discovery started in the first installment by exploring thirteen major organ systems. It is devised to take learners through the histological characteristics of the following systems: the integumentary, the circulatory, the respiratory, the digestive, the urinary, the reproductive, and the endocrine systems. The chapters are each composed of both close-up micrographs and text explanations that aid in the mastery of normal tissue appearance as well as their variations in pathology. Designed either to complement laboratory sessions or to serve as a basis of self-paced learning, this book is intended to offer a clear, unified structure of learning human histology on an organ-system level.

Chapter 1 introduces the integumentary system, which outlines how the skin is organized into layers, along with its appendages and the specialized cells that help provide protection, sensation, and thermoregulation. In Chapter 2, the circulatory system is given attention with the description of the structure of the arteries, veins, and capillaries, and the histology of the heart and lymphatic vessels. In Chapter 3, the respiratory system is discussed, starting with the pseudostratified epithelium of the trachea up to the thin-walled alveoli where gaseous exchange takes place.

In Chapter 4, the digestive tract is discussed, starting with the oral cavity, where adaptations of the mucosa to mastication and secretion are pointed out. In Chapter 5, we learn about the esophagus and stomach, and the difference between stratified squamous epithelium and the glandular lining which secretes acid and enzymes. Chapter 6 overviews the small and large intestines, which have villi, crypts and specialized cells that help in absorption, lubrication and host defense.

Chapter 7 reflects on the lobular structure of the liver, centering on hepatocytes, sinusoids and biliary networks. Chapter 8 explains the pancreas, the difference between exocrine acini and endocrine islets, which control glucose metabolism. Chapter 9 discusses the gallbladder, which stores and concentrates bile and releases it into the duodenum. In Chapter 10, the urinary system is introduced, including the glomerular filtration units of the kidney, through to the transitional epithelium that lines the bladder.

Chapter 11 is devoted to the male reproductive system, where seminiferous tubules, accessory glands, and ductal structures are described. In Chapter 12, the female reproductive system is looked at, where ovarian follicles, uterine lining cycles, and glandular components of the mammary tissue are discussed. Lastly, Chapter 13 provides an overview of the endocrine system, which combines histological aspects of the pituitary, thyroid, parathyroids, adrenal glands, and other organs that secrete hormones.

The book is compiled to meet the needs of medical and dental students, graduate students in biomedical and health sciences, who need a thorough knowledge of organ-system histology. It will also become a useful resource to practicing clinicians, trainee pathologists, and researchers requiring an in-depth atlas of human tissue organization. This book, with its systematic coverage and rich illustrations, serves equally well as a basis of learning and as a guide to advanced research and clinical practice, preparing its readers to read micrographs with understanding and to employ the principles of histology in research and clinical practice.

INTEGUMENTARY SYSTEM

1

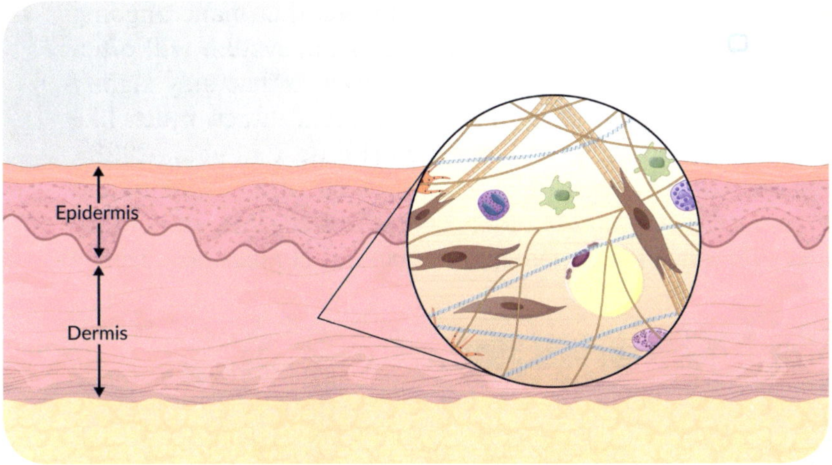

LEARNING OBJECTIVES

After studying this chapter, you will be able to:

1. Understand the structure of the skin
2. Describe the functions of the integumentary system
3. Describe the accessory structures of the skin
4. Learn about common integumentary disorders
5. Understand the role of the integumentary system in homeostasis
6. Discuss the advances in integumentary system research

Introduction

The integumentary system is the par excellence defense mechanism of the body, made up of skin, hair, nails, and associated glands. It is multi-functional, performing a critical function to sustain homeostasis, affording a shield for defense against external damage, temperature, and the sense of perception. The skin also has a number of layers, each being infused with certain functions that are geared towards making systems' overall performance effective. In addition to playing a barrier role against pathogens and chemicals, the integumentary system has a significant role in preventing dehydration and facilitating thermoregulation by controlling sweat production and blood flow. This barrier function is similar to those found in other biological systems, such that boundaries serve to preserve the integrity of the organism, as is the case with the oral mucosa's role in preserving against pathogens and allergens. These revelations provide insight into the integrative functions of other systems, particularly pointing to the role of the integumentary system in overall physiological health. Further inspection reveals the complexity of the integumentary system, i.e., its involvement in other biological functions. The role of the skin transcends protection, as it involves itself in metabolic functions such as vitamin D production, which has a key role in the metabolism of calcium and bone health. Furthermore, the integumentary system plays an important role in immunity by virtue of specialized cells with the ability to identify and respond to foreign substances. The ability of the system to feed back to other processes within the body is comparable to the networked systems identified in other crucial physiological barriers, such as the oral mucosa, the portal of entry to the body's immune system (Kordestani et al., 2023). Thus, a complete understanding of the integumentary system involves an awareness of its several functions and interaction with other body systems in concert to enhance well-being. The value of studying the integumentary system is emphasized by its applicability to disease and health. Disruptions in its integrity lead to many diseases and states, including infections, dermatitis, and skin cancers, that make ongoing research into prevention and therapy worthwhile. Further, the condition of the system will often signify overall health issues, as seen with changes in skin coloration or texture that may signify systemic illness. A dynamic management of keeping the integumentary system intact, much like the culture of health surveillance and management of other body systems (Kordestani et al., 2023), can greatly enhance the quality of life in individuals. This intersection of structure, function, and health impact highlights the need for an interdisciplinary understanding of the integumentary system, as it continues to be the focus of interest within medical science and clinical practice.

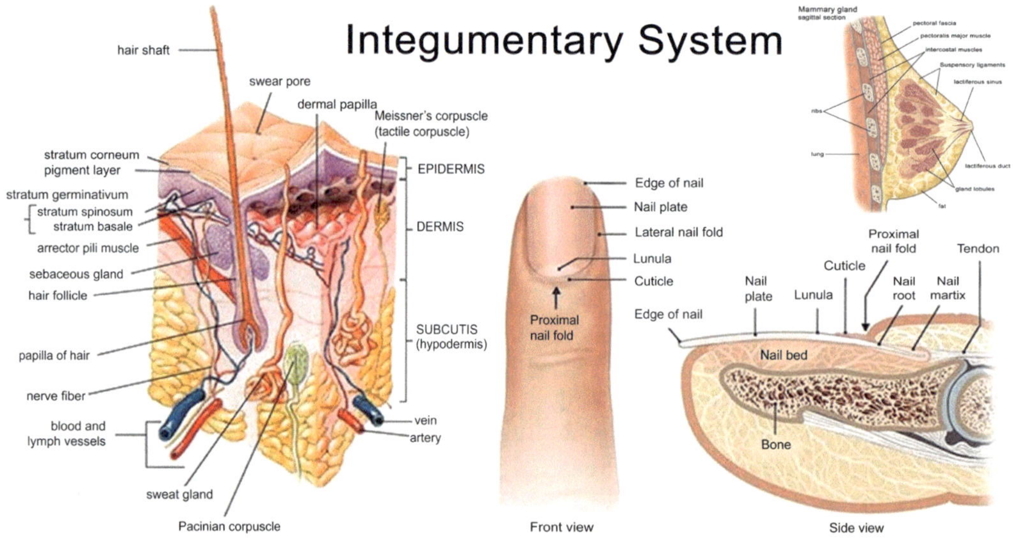

Figure 1.1. Integumentary system.

Source: https://microbenotes.com/wp-content/uploads/2020/06/Integumentary-System.jpg

Importance of the Integumentary System in Human Health

The integumentary system is the body's first line of defense against the environment, highlighting the necessity of overall health. The skin, hair, nails, and the glands accompanying them comprise the system that protects internal organs from pathogens, chemicals, and physical injury. The multi-layered state of the skin, particularly the epidermis, provides a strong barrier against infectious agents. Moreover, the system is also responsible for keeping the body temperature and hydrating the body through sweat and sebaceous glands. The effective functioning of these systems is essential not only to ward off disease but also to maintain homeostasis, underscoring their role in safeguarding health in everyday life. Moreover, the integumentary system is directly linked to immune health and overall health, as recent studies have identified how crucial the skin microbiome is. Dysbiosis of the skin microbiome can lead to various skin diseases, such as atopic dermatitis and psoriasis, showing just how crucial this ecosystem still is to the skin. Two-way communication between the skin microbiome and the systemic immune response highlights the importance of maintaining a balanced microbial community. The interface states that dysfunction of the integumentary system has the potential to potentiate not only local dermatological illnesses but also systemic illness, since the immune responses are highly interdependent. A healthy integumentary system is thus a key determinant in disease avoidance and wellness maintenance. Besides its defensive and immunological role, the integumentary system is a critical sensory interface for sensory perception that contributes to emotional and physical health. The skin is rich in sensory receptors that respond to touch, temperature, pain, and pressure, allowing an individual to interact constructively with his or her environment. The sensory input is vital for survival as it sensitizes the body to threats and influences behavioral activities. The psychological dimension of healthy skin is also significant; integumentary disease may lead to isolation and emotional upset. By an appreciation of these various aspects of the integumentary system, e.g., that it includes the microbiome and sense modalities, we are better able to appreciate its general role in the improvement of human health and well-being and the value of preventative treatment and consequent therapeutic interventions (Pessemier et al., 2021; Yang et al., 2021).

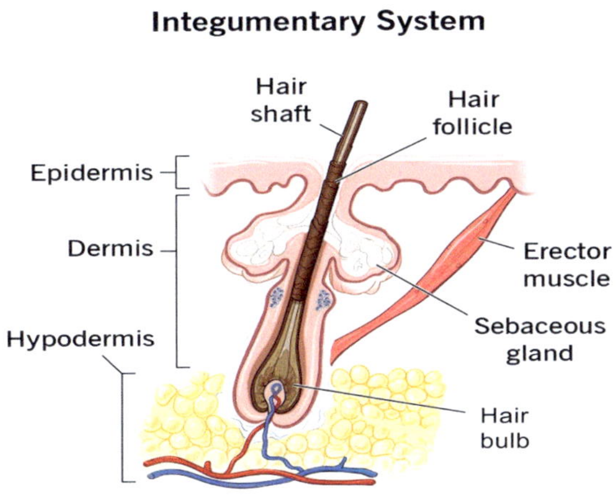

Figure 1.2. Your integumentary system consists of your hair, skin and nails. It's your body's outer layer and first line of defense against bacteria and injury.

Source: https://my.clevelandclinic.org/-/scassets/images/org/health/articles/22827-integumentary-system

1.1. Structure of the Skin

Learning Outcome

1. Describe the layers and functions of the epidermis
2. Understand the composition and role of the dermis
3. Understand the connection to the underlying structures of the hypodermis

The skin is an integumentary multicategory organ with a sophisticated organization that displays three principal layers: epidermis, dermis, and hypodermis. The epidermis, which is the outermost layer, is primarily composed of keratinized stratified squamous epithelium, which offers protection from external insults such as chemicals and pathogens. This layer also plays an important role in the regulation of water and is responsible for vitamin D production when exposed to ultraviolet radiation. Specialized epidermal cells like keratinocytes, melanocytes, and Merkel cells play many roles, ranging from pigmentation to the reception of sensory inputs. This unique ability of this layer to rapidly regenerate is indicative of the resiliency and compensability of the skin in response to injury and environmental stimulus, making it an essential element in homeostasis of the human organism. Below the epidermis lies the dermis, a fibrous layer of connective tissue that serves to provide structural support and elasticity. This layer, rich in elastin and collagen fibers, contains numerous blood vessels, nerves, and appendages such as sweat glands and hair follicles.

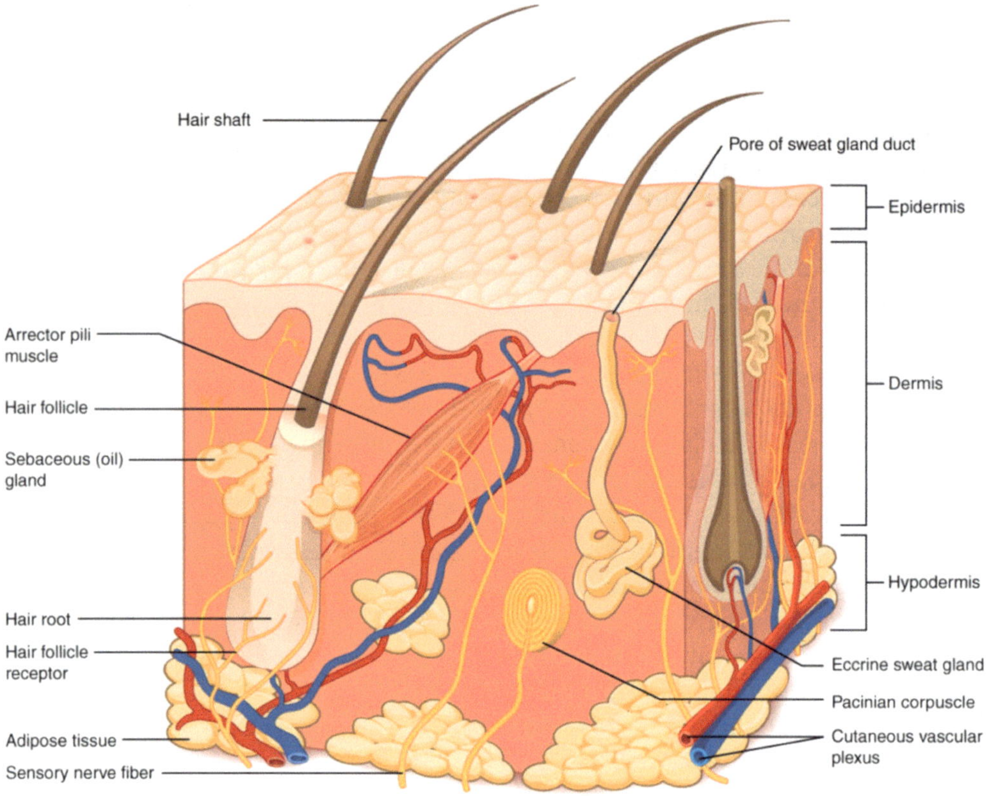

Figure 1.3. The skin is composed of two main layers: the epidermis, made of closely packed epithelial cells, and the dermis, made of dense, irregular connective tissue that houses blood vessels, hair follicles, sweat glands, and other structures. Beneath the dermis lies the hypodermis, which is composed mainly of loose connective and fatty tissues.

Source: https://s3-us-west-2.amazonaws.com/courses-images/wp-content/uploads/sites/1223/2017/02/08004822/501_Structure_of_the_skin-1024x803.jpg

The dermis can further be divided into two regions: papillary dermis and reticular dermis. The papillary layer, consisting of loose connective tissue, houses capillaries as well as sensory neurons, providing the skin its sense of touch. Conversely, the reticular layer, composed of dense, irregular connective tissue, gives the skin its strength and flexibility. Not only does the layered organization facilitate epidermis function, but also thermoregulation, nutrient delivery, and immunity. This kind of dermal complexity shows how interactive the various features of the skin are in establishing overall skin health and function. The hypodermis, or subcutaneous tissue, is a significant skin-deep structure interface comprised mostly of loose connective tissue and fat tissue. The hypodermis possesses rudimentary functions of insulation, energy storage, and cushioning above deeper structures such as muscles and bones. The function of the presence of fat tissue in the hypodermis is also to aid in thermoregulation by acting as a barrier to temperature changes. Interestingly, different species have different skin structures that reflect their adaptive and behavioral modifications in response to the environment. For instance, adaptive pigmentation and keratinization, as observed in reptilian species *Acanthodactylus boskianus* and *Ptyodactylus guttatus*, demonstrate how skin structure adjusts to ecological demands (Saber et al., 2018). These remarks underscore the evolutionary significance of the skin and suggest how its form is not anatomical in itself but essentially functional in the context of the organism's survival and interaction with the world.

1.1.1. Epidermis: Layers and Functions

The epidermis, which is the outermost layer of the integumentary system, has different layers that have different roles to play in the protection of the body. The major cells found in this structure are keratinocytes, and they undergo a differentiation process as they move up the structure's basal layer to the surface. There are four main layers of the epidermis, namely stratum basale, stratum spinosum, stratum granulosum, and stratum corneum. Cellular proliferation takes place in the stratum basale, resulting in an unending supply of new cells. As these cells rise, they pass through the other layers, in which they lose moisture and become gradually more keratinized. This process plays an important role in preserving the skin barrier that helps defend against environmental aggressors, pathogens, and mechanical damage, thus playing an important role in homeostasis. The specific structure of every epidermal layer also increases its protective properties. The spiny layer, also known as stratum spinosum, is where desmosomes are found, which are responsible for binding the keratinocytes together and giving it structural strength. The layer is also involved in the immune response since Langerhans cells that are vital in detection and presentation of antigens are found there. As they enter the stratum granulosum, keratinocyte cells start to dehydrate, and keratohyalin granules start to accumulate in the cell. These granules contain proteins essential to the process of keratinization and the water barrier property. Lastly, the stratum corneum is the most important barrier of the skin, which is made of dead keratinized cells that are constantly shed and renewed.

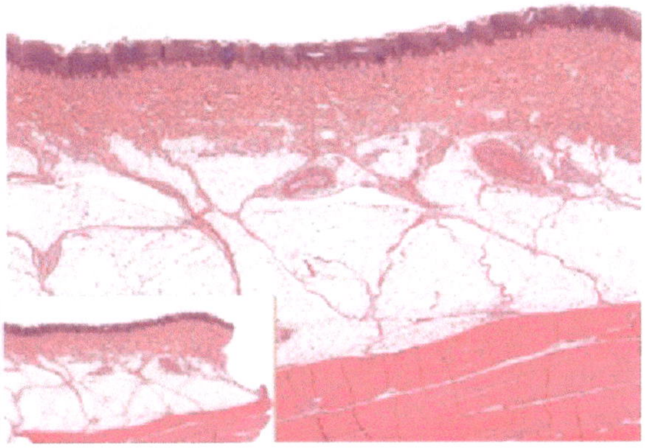

Figure 1.4. The epidermis is epithelium composed of multiple layers of cells. The basal layer consists of cuboidal cells, whereas the outer layers are squamous, keratinized cells, so the whole epithelium is often described as being keratinized stratified squamous epithelium.

Source: https://s3-us-west-2.amazonaws.com/courses-images/wp-content/uploads/sites/1223/2017/02/08005325/503_Epidermis.jpg

This careful stratification also helps in safeguarding the tissues beneath it, as well as is the basis of the capacity of the skin to hold moisture and control permeability, an essential aesthetic and physical phenomenon. Recent dermatological research has provided novel in vitro models, which improve our knowledge of the epidermis. For instance, the development of organotypic skin models has allowed researchers to accurately replicate the complex architecture of the epidermis, as well as its barrier functions (Li et al., 2023). Different environmental conditions can be modeled and provide insightful information on topical treatment efficacies and the penetration of drug substances. Research indicates that while human and reconstructed skin models demonstrate unique compositional characteristics, they provide reproducible data crucial for evaluating drug delivery systems (Kocsis et al., 2022). With such technological innovations, researchers will be in a better position to estimate skin absorption and irritation potential, which will eventually lead to the production of more effective and safer skincare products and treatment of dermatological diseases.

1.1.2. Dermis: Composition and Role

The dermis is a very important part of the integumentary system, a layer underneath the epidermis, and is composed mainly of dense connective tissue. A complex network of collagen and elastin fibers gives it structural integrity, resilience, and elasticity of the skin.

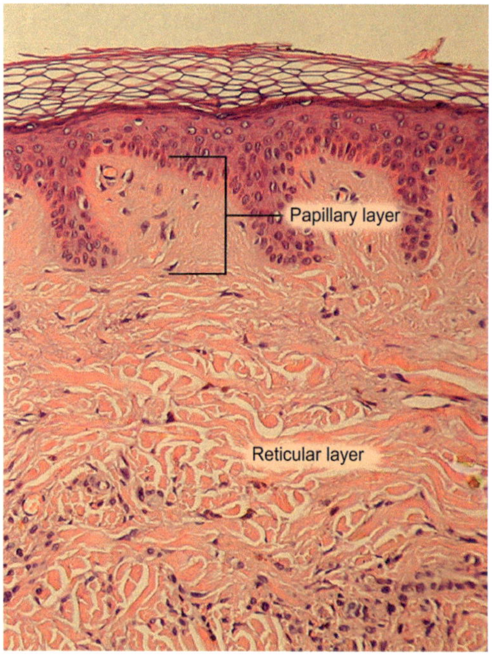

Figure 1.5. This stained slide shows the two components of the dermis—the papillary layer and the reticular layer. Both are made of connective tissue with fibers of collagen extending from one to the other, making the border between the two somewhat indistinct. The dermal papillae extending into the epidermis belong to the papillary layer, whereas the dense collagen fiber bundles below belong to the reticular layer.

Source: https://s3-us-west-2.amazonaws.com/courses-images/wp-content/uploads/sites/1223/2017/02/08005943/506_Layers_of_the_Dermis.jpg

This layer is characterized by the fact that it has an abundant extracellular matrix that not only provides support to the skin cells but also helps in the communication between the different cellular components. Moreover, the dermis has vital components including fibroblasts, mast cells, and immune cells which play a role in the defense mechanisms of the skin. The dermis plays a large part in the health of the skin in general by keeping it hydrated and elastic as well as playing a central role in the process of wound healing since scars form as the dermis heals over. The intricate structure of the dermis thus plays a pivotal role in both the mechanical and biological functions of the skin (Fina, 2024). Besides its structural purpose, the dermis is essential because it accommodates several appendages that play a role in the functionality of the skin. This layer has hair follicles, sebaceous glands, and sweat glands, which have different physiological functions. The hair follicles serve the sense and warmth, and the sebaceous glands produce oils that make the skin hydrated and prevent the invasion of microbes. Instead, sweat glands are vital in thermoregulation because they secrete perspiration, which helps in losing heat via evaporation. These appendage structures are part of the dermis, hence the multifunctional property of this skin layer. Beyond these roles, the dermis contains a network of blood vessels that supply nutrients and oxygen, reinforcing the skin's metabolic activities and enabling the efficient removal of waste products (van der Meer et al., 2022). In addition, the dermal layer plays an important role in the sensory activity of the skin, which hosts a number of mechanoreceptors, which enable the skin to sense touch, pressure, and temperature. Such sensory receptors include Meissner's corpuscles and Pacinian corpuscles which are highly complex in design to enable the body to react to the stimuli in the environment, enabling effective interaction of the body with the environment. Sensory feedback integration via the dermis provides the central nervous system with information, which influences reflexes and protective reactions. This ability highlights the dermis' role not only in the protection of the skin but also in homeostasis by means of sensory data. The intricate balance of the composition and functionality of the dermis illustrates its unmatched importance within the larger context of the integumentary system, highlighting how disruptions in this layer can lead to significant pathological conditions (Fina, 2024).

1.1.3. Hypodermis: Connection to Underlying Structures

The hypodermis, or subcutaneous tissue, is a vital interface between skin and underlying support structures, including muscles and bones. Composed primarily of loose connective tissue and adipose tissue, this layer provides essential insulation and energy storage in addition to acting as a shock absorber for the body. This protection of the body is also provided to inner organs, lessening what might result in injury from external impacts. In addition, the hypodermis is filled with an interconnected network of blood vessels and nerves to facilitate communication between the skin and internal structures for effective temperature management and sense perception. The intricacy of the function of the hypodermis reveals its importance not only in structural support but also in metabolic processes in the integumentary system, which offers a sophisticated relationship that requires more studies (Carvajal et al., 2024). Also, the hypodermis plays a crucial role in the vascularization of the skin because it has the larger vessels that supply oxygen and nutrients to the dermal layer. The vascular supply is important to the maintenance of health and functionality of the skin to enable repair processes in the event that the skin is injured. Also, the layered structure of the hypodermis allows it to have various levels of movement and pressure, thus making the strength and elasticity of the skin more efficient. These mechanical properties are achieved by the connective tissue fibers present in the hypodermis, including collagen and elastin, which allow the skin to interface with muscular and other systems beneath. Thus, hypodermic knowledge is significant in understanding many medical ailments and injuries of the skin and percutaneous structures, emphasizing its pivotal role in the integumentary system (Benner et al., 2024). Additionally, the hypodermis also has a role in thermoregulation and overall metabolic health of the body. The fat tissue of this layer not only provides energy but is also a thermal insulator, conserving body heat. This function is particularly important under diverse conditions of the environment, where the body must adapt in order to regulate homeostasis. Endocrine messaging from fat tissue also has the potential to influence systemic metabolism, and a complex relationship between the endocrine system and the integumentary system is observed. Through its provision of access to deeper structures, including the varied range of organs and systems, the hypodermis is then seen to be a powerful force in environmental adjustment and physiology. With advancing research, increased study of the hypodermis' multifaceted role can lead to new avenues for understanding health, illness, and the overall function of the integumentary system (Carvajal et al., 2024).

1.2. Functions of the Integumentary System

Learning Outcome

1. Protect the body against various environmental hazards
2. Understand the regulation of body temperature
3. Describe the sensory perception and communication

The integumentary system is responsible for a variety of crucial functions essential to the maintenance of homeostasis and protection of the body from external damage. It serves, in the first instance, as a barrier function, excluding pathogens, chemicals, and physical trauma from deep tissues. This is largely a consequence of the stratified layers of epidermis and associated lipids, which collaborate to waterproof the skin. The integumentary system also plays a critical role in thermoregulation. Through mechanisms such as sweating and the dilation or constriction of blood vessels, the skin regulates body temperature, a need for metabolic processes. This thermoregulatory process is particularly important in the ability to adapt to changing environmental conditions, thus signifying the importance of integumentary systems in attaining physiological stability and overall wellness. The integumentary system is also important for sense perception. The skin contains a wide range of nerve endings and sensory receptors that allow it to perceive stimuli, such as pressure, temperature, and pain. The sensing functions allow the organism to interact with the environment appropriately, providing the necessary information that affects behavior and reflexes. Sensory information that the skin gathers is deciphered by the nervous system, allowing it to determine body position and environmental hazards. Moreover, the system is also involved in vitamin D production, which is a critical component for calcium metabolism and bone health. This multiple functional role further increases the importance of the integumentary system, transcending its protective functions, to expose its involvement in overall physiological processes. Apart from protection and sensory roles, the integumentary system is also an important component in the body's immune defense. The epidermal skin is the first line of defense against microbial infection, with immune cells in its layers, i.e., Langerhans cells. These cells are the ones that detect and respond to pathogens and initiate an immune response that guards against infections. Further, the recent findings highlight the use of the integumentary system in drug delivery, particularly through developments like transdermal systems. These systems provide new pathways for drug administration, enhancing therapeutic outcomes without the constraints of standard delivery. As seen through advances in technologies like microneedle technology, the integumentary system has expanded its function, undoubtedly demonstrating its central role in modern pharmaceutical applications, thus merging biology and technology in a never-before-seen harmony (Ménard et al., 2021; Ramadon et al., 2021).

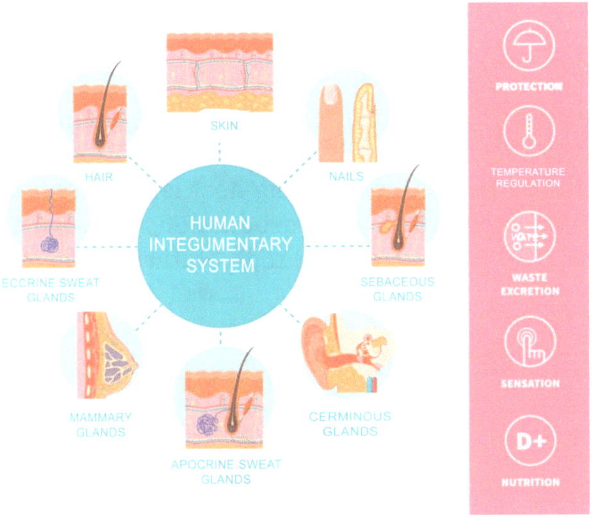

Figure 1.6. Functions of the Integumentary System.

Source: https://stgaccinwbsdevlrs01.blob.core.windows.net/newcorporatewbsite/blogs/october2023/Human-Integumentary-System.jpg

1.2.1. Protection Against Environmental Hazards

The integumentary system is of prime importance in defending the body against a number of environmental threats. The skin, as the primary component, serves as a physical barrier that safeguards internal structures from harmful agents such as pathogens, chemicals, and ultraviolet (UV) radiation. The epidermis, in its stratified architecture, offers toughness, and the dermis, in its turn, accommodates such important processes as thermoregulation and sensitivity. Another major cell type in the epidermis is keratinocytes that synthesize keratin that strengthens the skin's barrier to water loss and external irritants. Therefore, the anatomy of the skin is highly constructed in such a way that it not only ensures protection against immediate danger, but also ensures general homeostasis. In this connection, the knowledge of the protective mechanisms of the skin is crucial in the creation of effective interventions in people exposed to environmental aggressions, which would play an important role in the health of the population and the individual's safety in different situations. In addition, the integumentary system must deal with numerous environmental insults that may interfere with its protective roles. As an illustration, skin may be damaged due to exposure to pollution, extreme weather conditions, hazardous substances, etc., and become more vulnerable to infections. The risks are further aggravated by climate change, whereby increasing temperatures and changing precipitation patterns lead to a more unstable environment. The importance of efficient protection measures can be proven, especially because some groups of the population might be unable to access essential resources to take care of their skin and protect it. Efforts to create awareness about skin protection measures, such as the application of sunscreen and wearing protective clothes, are important in reducing the effects of these hazards. This knowledge is in line with other wider health agendas to treat not only the physical, but also the socio-economic factors that determine the health of the skin, which supports the relationship between the environment and skin health. Lastly, the other measure that is instrumental in protecting the environment-related hazards to the integumentary system is the protective legislation and policies. Legal instruments can facilitate the implementation of precautionary measures to provide safe working environments, control hazardous substances, and facilitate greener environments. As an example, the passing of laws, which have environmental protection and public health provisions, plays a critical role in alleviating the toxic exposures, that come with an industrial or urban environment. In some jurisdictions, including Indonesia, some special safeguards, including the ANTI-SLAPP laws, exist to protect environmental activists against any legal consequences, thus creating a strong environmental health advocacy. Further, there is a growing emphasis on urban resilience approaches to develop infrastructure that minimizes vulnerability to environment-related catastrophes, which is evident in such cities as New York and Lagos. Learning and applying these defense mechanisms in regard to the integumentary system is fundamental not only to personal health but also to the overall strength of communities exposed to environmental hazards, and eventually to the improved quality of life in general.

1.2.2. Regulation of Body Temperature

The regulation of body temperature is one of the main functions of the integumentary system and serves as the basis for homeostasis in the human body. Skin, which is made up of multiple layers, plays a most significant role in the process of thermoregulation by facilitating heat loss as well as conservation. Consequently, by the mechanisms of vasoconstriction and vasodilation, the dermal blood vessels react by elevating blood supply to the skin surface as body temperature increases or as a result of shivering and heat conservation in cold.

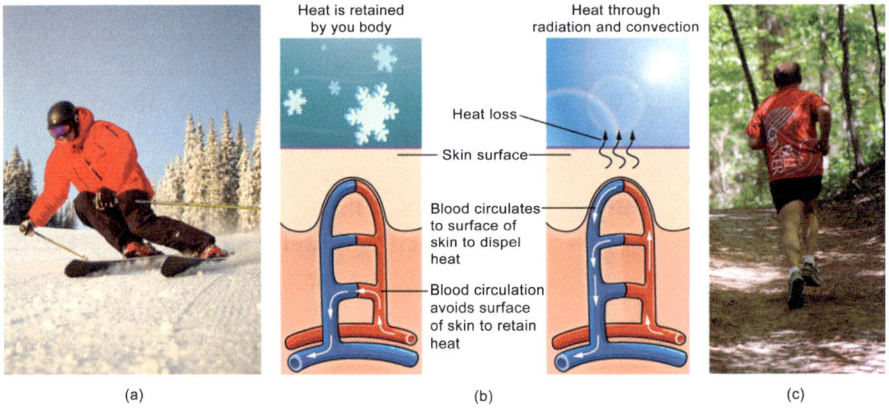

Figure 1.7. During strenuous physical activities, such as skiing (a) or running (c), the dermal blood vessels dilate and sweat secretion increases (b). These mechanisms prevent the body from overheating. In contrast, the dermal blood vessels constrict to minimize heat loss in response to low temperatures (b).

Source: https://s3-us-west-2.amazonaws.com/courses-images/wp-content/uploads/sites/1223/2017/02/08172355/515_Thermoregulation-1024x453.jpg

This active response makes apparent the skin's function not only as a barrier but as an active participant in the regulation of heat balance. Furthermore, sweat glands make their contributions by producing perspiration, which cools the body by evaporation. It is important to understand these processes in order to know how the integumentary system ensures overall physiological stability and reaction against changes in the environment. Apart from vascular compensations and sweating, circadian rhythms also play a role in maintaining body temperature. The internal clock of the body coordinates a number of physiological processes during the course of the day, including temperature fluctuations that have a characteristic pattern. At night, for example, the core body temperature typically drops, which correlates with the body's requirement for sleep and recuperation.

This periodic fluctuation is important not just for thermoregulation but also for efficient metabolic activity and nighttime activities. Studies using mathematical models, including the Duffing equation, have explained the intricate dynamics of such circadian rhythms, showing that parameter changes can have a profound effect on temperature control (Lin, 2024). An understanding of circadian rhythms enables a holistic view of how the integumentary system develops and responds to internal and external stimuli. Moreover, the intricate mechanisms of temperature control are not confined to the skin but involve neural circuits that integrate the sensory data to maintain thermal homeostasis. Thermosensitive TRP channels, particularly TRPV4, play a critical role in transducing temperature variations into electrical impulses, which ultimately decide the activity of neurons (Shibasaki, 2024). This integration of the integumentary system and the nervous system bears testimony to the intricate processes of thermoregulation. Abnormalities in these pathways have the potential to predispose individuals to a number of conditions, making their further investigation important. Because the integumentary system plays an active role in these regulatory processes, it is clear that the regulation of optimal body temperature is a multifaceted interplay of physiological processes and highlights the significance of this system in maintaining health and wellness.

1.2.3. Sensory Perception and Communication

The body's first line of defense, but also contributing largely to the sense of perception and communication, is the integumentary system, which comprises skin, hair, nails, and the glands associated with them. The buried sensory receptors in the skin can detect various stimuli such as pressure, temperature, and pain, and help individuals interact with their environment effectively. This sensory information is vital for survival as it conveys threat to the brain, aids in social interaction, and also promotes well-being. In addition, the sense functions of the integumentary system are directly related to communication, with non-verbal information being conveyed through touch and other forms of contact. Through such processes, not only does the integumentary system protect, but also protects interpersonal relationships, enhancing the quality of life. The relationship between sensory perception and communication within the integumentary system is of utmost significance in the context of Autism Spectrum Disorder (ASD). The majority of individuals with ASD exhibit atypical sensory processing, which also influences their social communication ability and interpretation of social signals. Emerging evidence has highlighted sensory alterations, particularly in auditory and visual modalities, which may exacerbate communication challenges of such individuals. For instance, hypo- or hyper-reactivity to sensory input can lead to heightened anxiety or indifference towards social relationships. An understanding of these sensory problems facilitates the development of more accommodating methods of communication that account for the unique sensory needs of individuals with ASD and promote social integration and enhanced quality of life. Such surmounting of sensory challenges bespeaks the pervasive impact of the integumentary system on social interactions and communications. In examining the sensory perception role of the integumentary system, it is essential to recognize the broader physiological and neurological systems that control these mechanisms. The visual cortex, for example, deciphers data from retinal inputs as well as non-visual inputs, including auditory inputs and motor outputs. This multiple integration demonstrates that sensory perceptions are not individual functions; rather, they are in an extended network with greater than one modality for intensive processing. Research has proven that this interaction might strengthen perception and interaction functions, showing the significant role of the integumentary system in informing sensory perceptions. By appreciating the intricacy of sensory integration, one can better appreciate how the integumentary system facilitates communication as well as supports interpersonal relations in an ever-changing environment through a focus on incorporating holistic approaches to sensory processing, given human behavior.

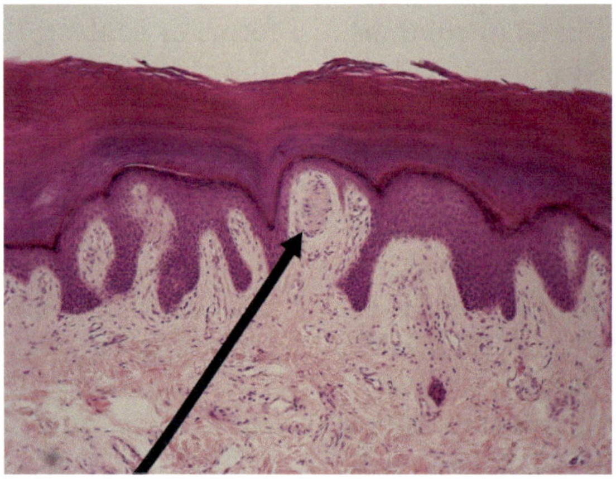

Figure 1.8. In this micrograph of a skin cross-section, you can see a Meissner corpuscle (arrow), a type of touch receptor located in a dermal papilla adjacent to the basement membrane and stratum basale of the overlying epidermis.

Source: https://s3-us-west-2.amazonaws.com/courses-images/wp-content/uploads/sites/1223/2017/02/08172240/514_Light_Micrograph_of_a_Meissner_Corpuscle.jpg

Test Your Knowledge

1. How to protect against an environmental hazard?
2. What is the regulation of body temperature?

1.3. Accessory Structures of the Skin

Learning Outcome

1. Describe the types and functions of hair
2. Understand the structure and significance of nails
3. Describe the sweat and sebaceous glands

The integumentary system consists of the skin, as well as numerous accessory structures, which are extremely important in terms of homeostasis and general health. Such structures are the hair, nails, sweat glands, and sebaceous glands, which add to the functional integrity of the skin. The hair follicles grow hair, which serves as a covering to the skin against environmental factors and the nails cover the tips of the fingers and toes. In addition to this, these accessory structures also provide sensory feedback, which improves the interaction with the environment. Sensory perception is enhanced by the existence of specialized nerve endings in the skin, which enable organisms to respond quickly to stimuli. Appreciation of the significance of these accessory structures provides clues as to their role not just in physical protection, but also in sensory and thermoregulatory processes, which are essential to well-being. Among other accessory structures of the skin, special mention should be made of sweat glands and sebaceous glands that are involved in thermoregulation and skin moisturizing, respectively. Sweat glands are profusely present all over the body and assist in controlling the body temperature by perspiration, which aids in losing the heat by evaporation. This process is needed when performing exercises or being in hot conditions. On the other hand, sebaceous glands produce sebum, which is an oily liquid that hydrates the hair and skin, and does not allow it to dry out, and serves as a protective layer against environmental pathogens. Such dual roles of moisture retention and thermoregulation show a high level of balance that the integumentary system performs, which explains the significance of the accessory structures in maintaining skin health and contributing to the overall comfort and functionality of the body. Tissue engineering and regenerative medicine are among the fields where the reconstruction of accessory structures is extremely difficult. The conventional skin grafts might not contain the skin appendages that are essential in the recovery of complete sensory functions and structural composition of the skin. New insights into the basic biology of these structures have been used to develop novel strategies to attempt to regenerate hair follicles, sweat glands, and sensory nerves. Effective replacement of these structures not only enhances the cosmesis result of skin regeneration, but also sensory activities and quality of life of the patients. Studies of seeding of particular cell types, scaffold materials and bioactive factor use have held promise in recapitulating these accessory structures. Addressing the restoration of sensory nerve function is also critical, as it directly impacts the patient's experience of pain, temperature, and touch (Weng et al., 2020).

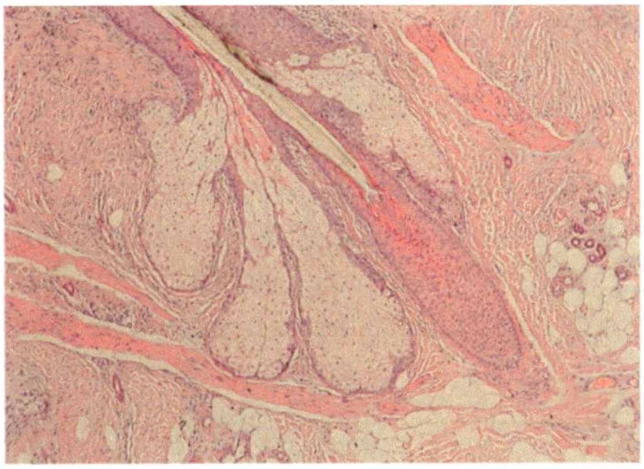

Figure 1.9. The slide shows a cross-section of a hair follicle. Basal cells of the hair matrix in the center differentiate into cells of the inner root sheath. Basal cells at the base of the hair root form the outer root sheath.

Source: https://s3-us-west-2.amazonaws.com/courses-images/wp-content/uploads/sites/1223/2017/02/08171036/511_Hair_Follicle.jpg

1.3.1. Hair: Types and Functions

In delving into the nature and purpose of hair in the integumentary system, it is important to demarcate the different forms that hair takes across species. Hair can be divided into three main categories: guard hair, underfur, and vibrissae. The guard hairs are longer and thicker, conferring initial protection against environmental conditions, whereas underfur offers insulation against cold and heat. Vibrissae or sensory hairs are typically associated with heightened sensitivity to touch, allowing the animal to navigate through its environment in a more sensitive manner. The exact configuration and character of such hairs are typically established by genes and the environment, which, to some extent, contribute to an organism's general adaptation to the environment, a finding attested by studies on the genetic underpinnings of such traits (Gong et al., 2022). The physiological function of hair goes beyond mere protection and insulation, having important contributions to thermoregulation and social communication. Hair traps air against the skin, thus creating an insulating layer that aids in maintaining the body's warmth. For instance, thick-pelage animals can tolerate more frigid environments, while those with less hair are likely to exhibit larger behavioral adaptations to prevent overheating. Apart from this, hair color and texture can influence species' social patterns in impacting patterns of mating as well as territoriality.

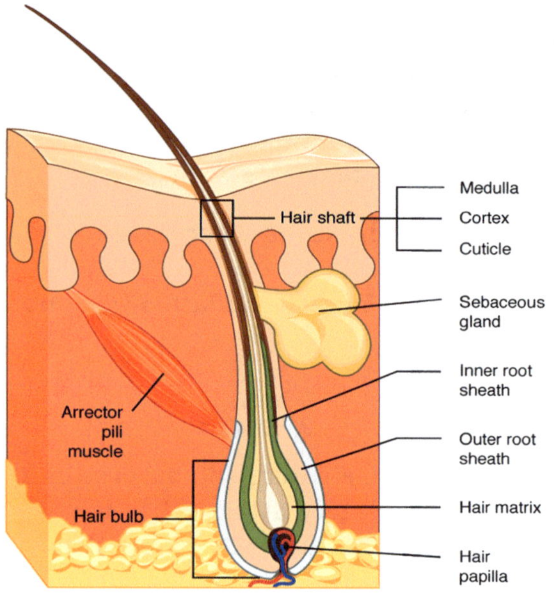

Figure 1.10. Hair follicles originate in the epidermis and have many different parts.

Source: https://s3-us-west-2.amazonaws.com/courses-images/wp-content/uploads/sites/1223/2017/03/28185157/506_Hair.jpg

The combination of such functions gives rise to the intricate relationship between the environmental pressures and hair characteristics, highlighting the evolutionary function of hair in the animal kingdom (Saber et al., 2018). In structural as well as molecular analysis of hair, it is observed that hair types not only fulfill functional requirements but also possess distinctive biochemical properties. For example, differences in the keratin architecture of thick guard hairs and more delicate underfur decide their elasticity and foaming ability, and genetic elements like those of Inner Mongolia cashmere goats account for the molecular basis of hair differentiation (Gong et al., 2022). Moreover, genes have been identified to be accountable for controlling these variations, providing doors for further research into livestock improvement and textile production. Knowledge of these biological activities can clarify the evolutionary activities that facilitate survival and reproduction in various ecological niches, validating the importance of hair as a complicated component of the integumentary system.

1.3.2. Nails: Structure and Significance

The anatomy of nails, which is part of the integumentary system, boasts a remarkable sophistication that serves numerous functional purposes. Composed primarily of keratin, a fibrous protein, nails grow out of the nail matrix, an area below the cuticle. This matrix makes the nails grow, producing new cells that force the older cells forward to form the hard nail plate seen at the tip of the fingers and toes. Beneath the nail plate lies the nail bed formed by a rich supply of blood vessels and nerves, contributing to the nails' sensitivity and health. The unique structure of cells within the nail matrix and bed ensures nails remain robust and, upon injury, allows repair mechanisms to function effectively. Considering their composition and structure, nails not only offer physical protection to the distal phalanges but also facilitate tactile functions that are vital for grip and manipulation of objects. Nails also possess physiological and social importance in addition to their structural role. Their inherent biological function is to be protective, covering the delicate ends of fingers and toes against harm and from external threats. However, their beauty aspect also plays a critical function in self-presentation since most individuals perform nail care and decoration as ways of expressing personal style. On this day, nails can even be psychosocial, with an influence on perceptions of beauty and professionalism. It has been hypothesized by researchers that the health of the nail can be a marker of overall health, with changes in color, texture, or growth rate being a potential indication of systemic disease. Thus, nails are not only physical barriers but also windows into the patient's overall health status and are functionally important in the integumentary system. Further, the treatment implications related to nail health have begun to draw interest in dermatology and psychology as well. For instance, improved nail health due to proper care can enhance a person's social life and self-esteem and influence mental health. Little-known to many, nails can also be of significant value in the diagnosis of certain medical conditions; irregularities in these may reveal nutritional deficiencies or skin conditions, where early detection may result in timely interventions. Recent studies highlight the significance of valuing nail structure from a biological perspective, yet also in clinical practice, with clinicians needing to consider the integumentary system's approach to patient inspection. Ultimately, the structure and function of nails encapsulate an intersection of biology, health, and social dynamics, which underscores their significance in the context of human physiology and interaction.

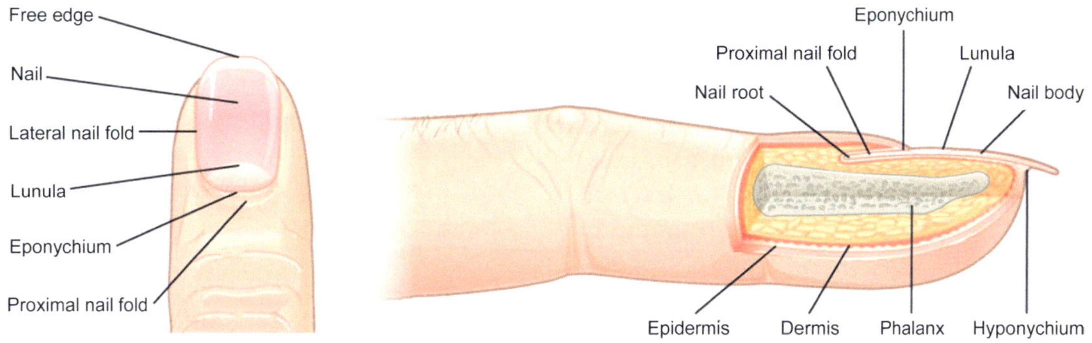

Figure 1.11. The nail is an accessory structure of the integumentary system.

Source: https://s3-us-west-2.amazonaws.com/courses-images/wp-content/uploads/sites/1223/2017/02/08171245/507_Nails-1024x309.jpg

1.3.3. Glands: Sweat and Sebaceous Glands

The integumentary system plays a crucial role in homeostasis through a number of special structures, primarily sweat and sebaceous glands. The sweat glands are predominantly eccrine and apocrine, which are involved in thermoregulation and excretion. The ubiquitous presence of eccrine glands across the body secretes a fluid that is largely water and electrolytes in nature. Its secretion plays a significant role in the control of body temperature by evaporative cooling. In comparison, apocrine glands located in areas such as the axillae and groin produce a thicker, milky substance that emerges at puberty. Not only does this secretion cause body odor, but it is also functioning in concert with the skin's microbiome, illustrating the complex interdependence between skin glands and microbial activity beneath the surface. Knowledge of these functions is integral to the understanding of how the body reacts to environmental stress and maintains its internal environment at homeostasis. Sebaceous glands, which are distinct from sweat glands, secrete largely an oily substance called sebum. Its secretion plays a significant role in lubricating the hair and the skin, hence forming a protective covering from environmental injury. The sebum, being lipid-rich, contributes to the natural barrier function of the skin, preventing loss of moisture and inhibiting the growth of pathogenic microorganisms. In addition, the interaction of sebum with the skin's microbiome is critical; for example, dysregulation of sebum production may lead to diseases such as acne, which is characterized by follicular blockage and inflammation. Both microbial systems and sebum excretions are related to various skin illnesses, therefore emphasizing homeostatic equilibrium within the integumentary system. With further studies, the interaction among sebaceous gland activity, microbiome, and general skin well-being becomes increasingly significant in framing effective treatment strategies for skin illness. Recent studies have established that an altered microbiome in the healthy skin context can play a significant role in sweat and sebaceous gland functionality. Dysbiosis, or imbalance of microbe composition, has been linked with various skin conditions such as acne, atopic dermatitis, and psoriasis, suggesting that a dysfunctional skin barrier might be a downstream effect of glandular dysfunction. The sweat and sebum glands do not act independently; their functioning can influence, and be influenced by, the skin microbiome. For instance, the lipid composition of sebum can provide a source of nutrients for microbial communities, and the water produced by sweat reduces the pH value of the skin, which directly influences the growth of microbes. This intricate interplay points to the necessity of taking into consideration the microbiome while examining glandular function and its relevance to skin pathology and well-being, as emphasized by recent study recommendations towards microbiome-centered therapeutic interventions (Lee and Kim, 2022; Pessemier et al., 2021).

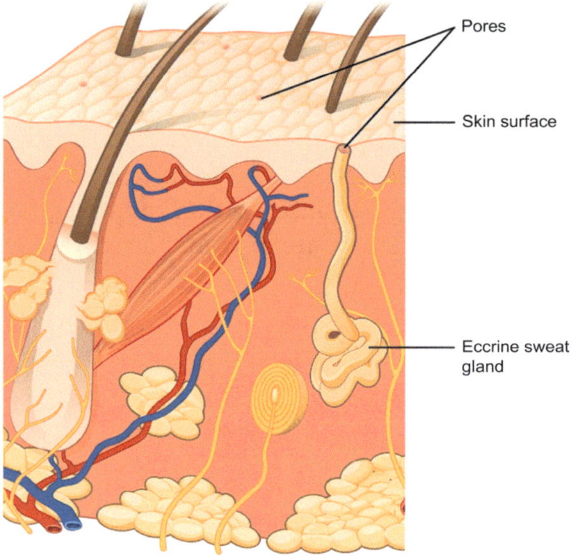

Figure 1.12. Eccrine glands are coiled glands in the dermis that release sweat that is mostly water.

Source: https://s3-us-west-2.amazonaws.com/courses-images/wp-content/uploads/sites/1223/2017/02/08171347/508_Eccrine_gland.jpg

Test Your Knowledge

1. What are the types of hair?
2. What is the significance of nails?

1.4. Common Integumentary Disorders

Learning Outcome

1. Learn about causes and treatments of acne
2. Describe the symptoms and management of eczema
3. Describe the types and prevention of skin cancer

Common integumentary disorders have a major bearing on people's health, mainly expressed as different types of skin problems. One of the most common disorders is psoriasis, involving rapid growth of skin cells to form red, scaly patches on the skin. This autoimmune disorder typically occurs chronically and recurrently, mostly on the elbows, knees, and scalp. Social stigmatization and decreased quality of life may result from the psychological effects of visible lesions. Educating patients regarding psoriasis and why it is caused, such as by stress and specific medications, can empower patients to better manage their own symptoms. Treating the psychosocial components of psoriasis is also crucial, since studies have determined that this condition can lead to increased instances of anxiety and depression, making integrative management strategies involving both physical and mental health imperative. Another common integumentary disorder is eczema, also known as atopic dermatitis, seen in millions of individuals all over the globe. It is defined by red, pruritic lesions of the skin, which are frequently stimulated by environmental stresses such as allergens, irritants, and climatic changes. In children, eczema can result in long-lasting effects on self-esteem due to visible skin lesions and accompanying stigma. Treatment for eczema typically involves a combination of topical treatments, skin care practices, and lifestyle modifications to reduce exposure to precipitating factors. Furthermore, awareness of the patient's psychosocial status is important since patients with eczema become increasingly socially isolated and emotionally distressed. Research indicates that intensive care, like counseling and support groups, significantly increases coping mechanisms for those suffering from eczema, enhancing their quality of life. Acne is among the most prevalent integumentary diseases, primarily affecting teenagers but sometimes persisting into adulthood. Caused by overproduction of sebum and plugging of hair follicles, acne manifests itself in pimples, blackheads, and cysts, causing bodily discomfort and psychological distress.

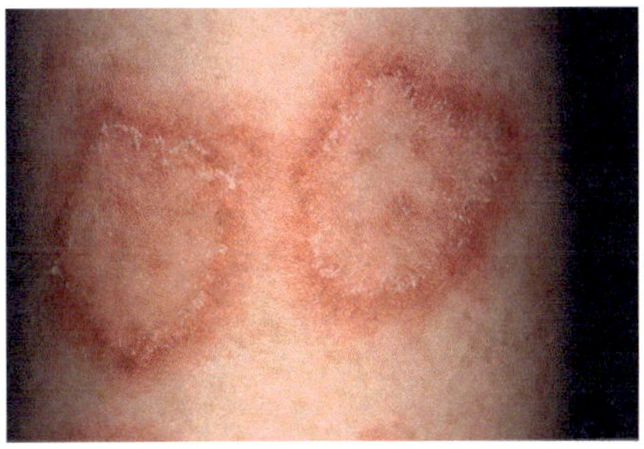

Source: https://www.health.com/thmb/XQgfO15UvHX5V84ph4VB952p_r8=/1500x0/filters:no_upscale():max_bytes(150000):strip_icc()/GettyImages-128548623-2000-ac49621a51ad4fdabfe3045cf3e56676.jpg

The psychosocial impact of the conditions is significant because chronic acne can lead to low self-esteem, anxiety, and even depression in the affected individuals. There are numerous treatment options, from topical retinoids to systemic medications, and the treatment can be tailored according to the severity of the condition. Further, recent evidence suggests that the psychological aspect of acne treatment needs to be addressed because the patient's emotional condition can have a direct impact on his/her compliance and outcome of treatment. Both physical and psychological aspects of acne need to be treated to offer an integrated approach towards its management and healing and finally to ensure enhanced patient outcomes and satisfaction.

1.4.1. Acne: Causes and Treatments

The pathophysiology of acne is mainly linked to excessive production of sebum, abnormal shedding of skin cells, and overgrowth of Propionibacterium acnes, which is a skin bacterium. These elements play a role in clogging the hair follicles, thereby resulting in comedones, cysts, and inflamed lesions. Moreover, acne is highly likely to be experienced during hormonal changes, mostly in puberty, because it stimulates the production of oil. The connection between the psychological aspect and acne cannot be underestimated; the disease can seriously affect self-esteem and social life, especially in teenagers who are more susceptible to emotional disorders. The psychological complexities inherent in treating acne necessitate a multifaceted approach that addresses not only the physical symptoms but also the emotional well-being of patients, as highlighted in contemporary dermatological discussions (Kibitska, 2024).

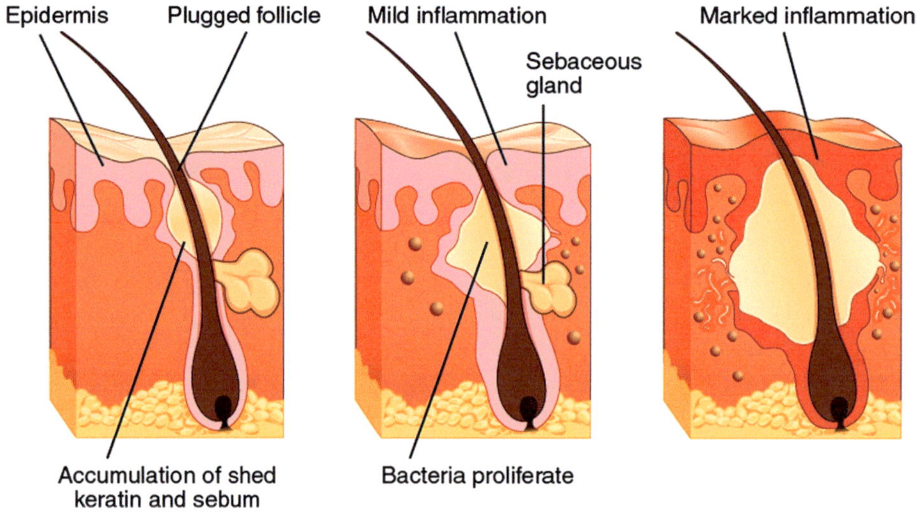

Figure 1.13. Acne is a result of over-productive sebaceous glands, which leads to formation of blackheads and inflammation of the skin.

Source: https://s3-us-west-2.amazonaws.com/courses-images/wp-content/uploads/sites/1223/2017/02/08175301/515_Acne_formation.jpg

There is no single effective treatment of acne, and any treatment should be selected individually depending on the severity of the disease, the type of skin, and the psychological requirements of the person. Topical retinoids, benzoyl peroxide, and antibiotics are commonly used treatments, all targeted at decreasing inflammation and bacterial colonization. In moderate to severe cases, oral drugs such as isotretinoin can be used, although the possible side effects are taken into consideration. Besides, acne treatment requires an interdisciplinary effort on the part of healthcare specialists, including dermatologists, cosmetologists, and psychologists. This interdisciplinary strategy ensures that the treatment plan is holistic, addressing both the physical manifestations of acne and the psychological impact it can impose on patients, particularly adolescents who may experience heightened emotional distress (Dhaheri et al., 2024). Early and effective treatment is important because it may help to avoid long-term effects, which include scarring and hyperpigmentation that can worsen the psychosocial problem. A stepwise implementation of therapies, as supported by clinical guidelines, can provide improved patient outcomes, especially when early psychological support and cosmetic intervention are involved. Such a gradual process not only prevents the negative effects but also makes the patient more motivated and positive about the treatment process. Such comprehensive management strategies are effective tools in the fight against acne because they stabilize the psychological state, as well as the general quality of life. It is essential for future research to continue exploring integrative methodologies that bridge dermatological and psychological disciplines, ultimately optimizing care for those suffering from this prevalent condition (Kibitska, 2024).

1.4.2. Eczema: Symptoms and Management

Atopic dermatitis, also known as eczema, has a wide range of symptoms that really affect the way of life of many individuals. Dryness, itchiness, and inflammation are the primary symptoms and it exists in various forms ranging from mild to severe. There often are periods of intense itching, and it will hurt the skin through scratching and cause secondary infections. Other symptoms of presentation may be redness, scaly lesions, and weeping lesions, depending on the stage of the disease. The chronic course of eczema can also lead to psychological consequences, such as anxiety and low self-esteem, particularly among children. A proper understanding of the clinical presentation of eczema is essential for successful management and intervention programs aimed at minimizing symptoms and improving patient outcomes. Eczema control typically must be multi-factorial and tailored to the individual's unique symptoms and provoking factors. Therapy typically involves the use of topical corticosteroids to reduce inflammation and moisturizing preparations to maintain hydration of the skin. Emollients are especially valuable in barrier repair, reducing flare and discomfort. In severe disease, systemic treatment, e.g., immunomodulators or phototherapy, can be utilized to control extensive disease. Additionally, it is also important to identify and rule out known precipitating factors, such as allergens and irritants, which can further aggravate the condition. Alternative newer therapies, such as homeopathy and Ayurveda, are also being investigated for their effectiveness in the treatment of eczema. These modalities provide different avenues for adding to conventional therapies with emphasis on the importance of customized treatment (Patil, 2024; Kapatkar et al., 2024).

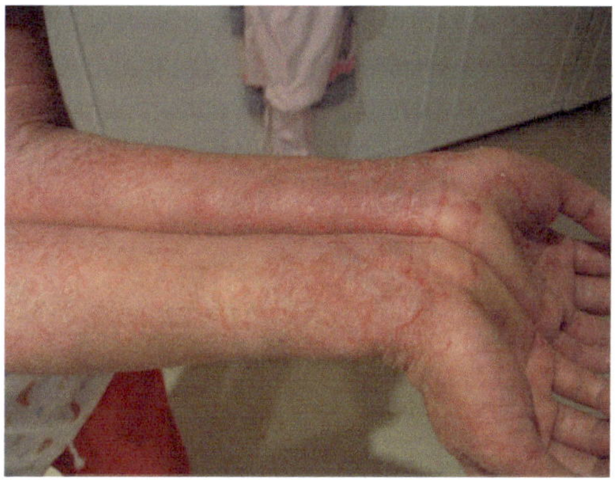

Figure 1.14. Eczema is a common skin disorder that presents as a red, flaky rash.

Source: https://s3-us-west-2.amazonaws.com/courses-images/wp-content/uploads/sites/1223/2017/02/08175217/520_Eczema.jpg

These new paradigms have only just been tested for effectiveness in the treatment of eczema. For instance, Ayurvedic and homeopathic therapies, as applied to Vicharchika, have demonstrated the ability to reduce symptom intensity as well as enhance patient satisfaction. Elements of tailored treatment, such as the identification of unique exacerbating factors and fine-tuning intervention protocols to the individual patient, are emphasized within these paradigms. Although the alternative treatments' evidence base is generally unclear, some studies have shown substantial improvement in the quality of life and overall well-being of patients. The inclusion of both conventional and alternative care strategies within an integrated model of care may, therefore, bring broad benefit to those suffering from eczema. This calls for constant communication between the healthcare professionals on the safety and effectiveness of the available therapies (Patil, 2024; Kapatkar et al., 2024).

1.4.3. Skin Cancer: Types and Prevention

Skin cancer is one of the most prevalent forms of cancer that arises from the components of the skin, and it can primarily be divided into three main forms: basal cell carcinoma (BCC), squamous cell carcinoma (SCC), and melanoma. BCC is the most common one, and it typically happens on areas of the skin with maximum sunlight exposure and seldom metastasizes, although it has a tendency to cause severe tissue destruction. On the other hand, SCC is more aggressive and metastasizes to other parts of the body if left untreated. Melanoma, though less common, has the worst outcomes because metastatic spread occurs at a high frequency. Understanding these distinctions is highly critical in preventing and treating skin cancer because early detection is commonly thought to significantly enhance patient outcomes and enable more intervention strategies. Prevention of skin cancer is most crucial as it involves lifestyle modification and defensive measures against harmful ultraviolet (UV) radiation.

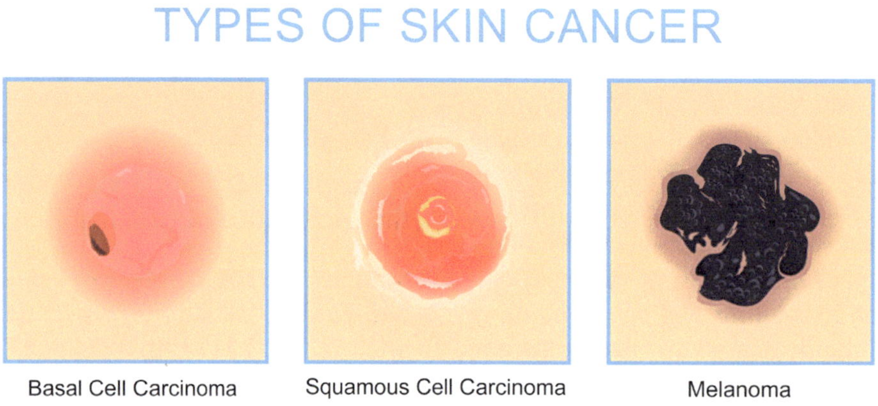

Figure 1.15. Types of skin cancer.

Source: https://news.christianacare.org/wp-content/uploads/2024/05/GettyImages-1404462398.jpg

Adherence to using sunscreens, wearing protective clothing, and seeking shade during sunlight hours are some of the essential ways of limiting UV radiation exposure. Additionally, periodic checks of the skin—either self-screening or by a physician—constitute an essential way of early discovery (Rahman et al., 2024). The importance of early diagnosis cannot be overstated; it directly influences treatment and survival rates. Notably, better medical technology has made possible automated machines based on machine learning, such as Deep Convolutional Neural Networks (DCNN), to enhance the detection rate of skin cancer through dermoscopic image analysis. These technological advancements have great potential to enable people even more in the fight against skin cancer as well as offer assistance for ongoing preventive action. One should not downplay the influence of public education campaigns in sensitizing people to skin cancer. By circulating facts about the different types of skin cancer and the implicated risks, the campaigns encourage preventive practices among risk groups. Teen and young adult educational programs are particularly necessary, since increased sun exposure at these age ranges can raise the probability of melanoma occurrence in the future considerably

(Aishasiddhika and Jenovajosephine, 2024). In addition, health system intervention to establish routine screening and patient education about self-examination is a critical step in lowering incidence rates. It also enhances screening and preventive care access by involvement in community resources such as dermatology clinics and outreach programs, hence contributing to proactive skin health preservation as part of the culture required to counteract the daunting threat of skin cancer.

Test Your Knowledge

1. What treatment for acne?
2. What are the types of skin cancers?

1.5. The Role of the Integumentary System in Homeostasis

Learning Outcome

1. Maintain the hydration and barrier function
2. Understand the immune response and skin health
3. Describe the vitamin D synthesis and its importance

The skin, hair, nails, and associated glands form the integumentary system that plays a central role in the human body's homeostasis. Temperature regulation is one of its most important functions, and this is maintained by a highly-regulated mechanism of vasodilation and vasoconstriction. When body temperature increases, blood vessels in the skin are dilated, so that heat can be lost through the surface, usually accompanied by the opening of the sweat glands. On the other hand, when temperatures are low, vasoconstriction reduces the amount of blood flowing to the skin and conserves core body temperature. This adjustable control is necessary in order to avoid hyperthermia or hypothermia, which can drastically affect the physiological processes and even create life-threatening conditions. Skin serves as a border between the body and the environment, and, therefore, its contribution to the thermoregulation process is critical to the overall condition and internal stability. Moreover, the integumentary system plays a role in defense against pathogens and environmental threats, which is part of homeostatic processes. The outer layer of skin, which is known as the epidermis, has cells that are packed tightly together, and thus they offer a formidable barrier against the entry of harmful microorganisms and chemicals. There are also other types of immune cells that play a role in this detection and response to a potential threat, e.g., Langerhans cells in the skin. Failure of this barrier may cause infections, inflammations, and serious health problems, and hence disturbs homeostasis. In addition to this, the fact that the skin can produce vitamin D when exposed to sunlight only serves to highlight the significance of the skin in terms of the achievement of a homeostatic balance, since vitamin D is vital in the absorption of calcium and the health of our bones. The integumentary system, therefore, plays a very vital role not only in providing physical protection, but also in providing a means through which required physiological activities can occur. Last but not least, the integumentary system is also crucial in sensory perception, which also leads to homeostasis. The skin is well equipped with a number of receptors which help in the detection of stimuli like temperature, pressure, and pain, enabling individuals to react to their surroundings. This sense feedback plays an important role in causing behaviors that enhance homeostasis, like moving into shade on a hot day or moving out of noxious stimuli. Also, the sense of touch and pressure is relevant to social life and well-being, which demonstrates the mutual influence of sensory inputs and emotional well-being. The coordination of the sensory information with the physiological actions, such as the change of posture or the adjustment of the activity level, helps the body to overcome environmental challenges. Therefore, the diversified roles of the integumentary system demonstrate the critical importance of this system in the process of balancing the wider scope of human health and life.

1.5.1. Maintaining Hydration and Barrier Function

The integumentary system, which consists of the skin, hair, nails, and accessory glands, plays a significant role in the supply of hydration and barrier protection. The system is an outer protective covering against environmental attackers, excluding the entry of pathogenic microorganisms and toxic substances. The stratum corneum is the external covering of the skin, and it plays a key role in this protection. It consists of dense keratinocytes that are rich in lipids, a tight barrier to the evaporation of moisture and external toxins. Furthermore, hydration of this layer is essential for the maintenance of its integrity.

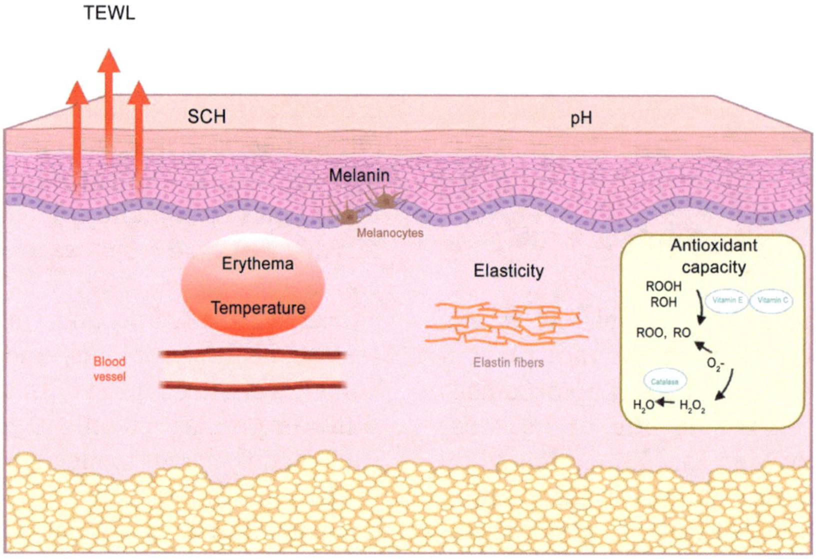

Figure 1.16. Skin barrier function parameters that can be evaluated non-invasively at the skin surface.

Source: https://www.mdpi.com/ijerph/ijerph-19-16678/article_deploy/html/images/ijerph-19-16678-g001.png

A compromised barrier can lead to TEWL, not only distorting the appearance of the skin but also leading to various dermal disorders and hence emphasizing the need for optimal methods of hydration to preserve skin wellness. Hydration in the integumentary system is inherently connected with its barrier function. The skin's retention of moisture relies upon a system of natural moisturizing factors (NMFs) that absorb and adhere water molecules in order to keep the stratum corneum soft and flexible. Interactions between these factors and the intercellular lipids also protect against dehydration and strengthen the epidermal barrier. There has also been growing evidence regarding the gut microbiome's function in skin hydration and the integrity of the barrier as a whole. As implications, the gut microbiome plays a conclusive part in metabolite production to enhance skin health, implying a complex relationship between the gastrointestinal tract and integumentary system. The consequences of such a connection illustrate that proper hydration is not simply an outcome of external interventions but a holistic approach to skin care. Moreover, the role of micronutrients and essential fatty acids cannot be left out, as far as hydration and barrier function are involved. Vitamins A, E, and C all contribute significantly to skin repair and maintenance, while omega fatty acids strengthen the lipid barrier, thus sustaining retention of hydration. Well-balanced nutrition, in addition to adequate water intake, plays a critical role in supporting the biochemical processes that help maintain the health and integrity of the skin. New evidence also indicates that modulation of the microbiota – gut – brain axis holds an appealing therapeutic approach to enhancing the barrier function of the skin. Appreciation of the interrelationship between skin hydration, nutrition, and microbial health is the foundation upon which an integrative approach to skin care is based, justifying the importance of maintaining integrative body function in order to attain optimal integumentary function (Nakamura and Matsumoto, 2025; Zhuang et al., 2024).

1.5.2. Immune Response and Skin Health

The integumentary system functions as the first barrier against all forms of external threats, including pathogens, toxins, and physical injury. Skin immunity plays a significant role in maintaining skin integrity and systemic immunity. Breakdown of the skin barrier enhances the risk of infections, including bacterial and fungal skin infections. This is particularly evident in conditions like atopic dermatitis, in which inflammatory responses lead to skin irritations and increased susceptibility to infectious agents. Understanding of the immune mechanisms engaged is significant because it is a highly developed interaction between innate immunity and adaptive immunity. Determinants such as cytokines and immune cells regulate local response and systemic cues to monitor infection, thereby maintaining the skin as an impenetrable cover over attacking pathogens. The immune response in skin health is both proactive and reactive. Cells of the skin, such as keratinocytes and resident immune cells, such as Langerhans cells, have sentinel roles, identifying possible threats prior to their reaching deeper tissues. The activation of these cells triggers the release of various cytokines alongside chemokines that cause inflammation and also result in the recruitment of additional immune cells to the site of injury or infection. This interactive mechanism lends itself to the need for a suitably regulated immune response in order to prevent chronic skin diseases. Additionally, external stimuli such as UV radiation may result in oxidative stress, which can complicate the immune response with the progression of premature aging, along with other dermatological diseases. Protection of the skin by antioxidants, such as tocotrienols and squalene, has taken center stage for their role in lowering oxidative damage as well as supporting the skin's immune function (Silva et al., 2025). Further, the influence of systemic immune responses on skin health cannot be overemphasized. Leishmaniasis is but one disease that highlights the connection between cutaneous immunity and wellness, and how systemic immune adaptations may enhance skin pathologies. The interaction of Leishmania RNA virus (LRV) with the influence on immune modulation underscores the complexity of immune-related interactions in skin tissues. As further research on the immune mechanisms involved in skin health proceeds, the understanding of how the pathways influence susceptibility to disease and therapeutic response becomes increasingly more important. This emerging body of knowledge suggests potential ways to enhance skin immunity and better control skin disease. Overall, establishing a healthy immune climate within the integumentary system is key to enhancing skin condition and managing dermatologic disease (Silva et al., 2025).

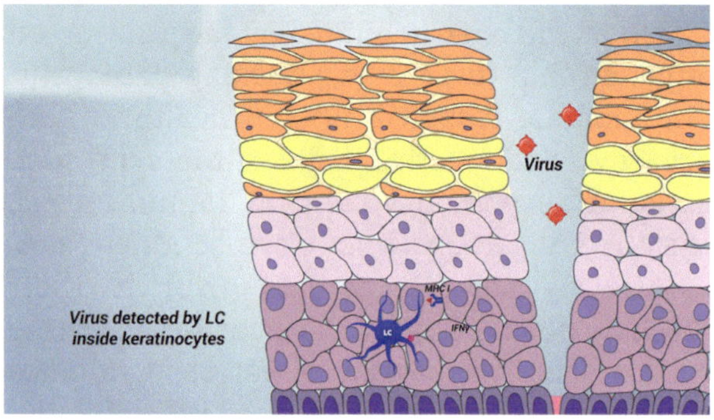

Figure 1.17. Immune response in the skin.

Source: https://i.ytimg.com/vi/SXLGgVcN3-E/maxresdefault.jpg

1.5.3. Vitamin D Synthesis and Its Importance

Vitamin D production is one such process that occurs in the skin upon exposure to ultraviolet B (UVB) light of the sun. Such a unique function of the integumentary system also highlights its important role as not just a barrier, but also an active participant in metabolic processes. When UVB rays penetrate the skin, they turn 7-dehydrocholesterol into pre-vitamin D3, which is subsequently altered into active vitamin D after a cascade of biochemical transformations in the liver and the kidneys. The transformation is crucial because vitamin D helps in calcium absorption and bone growth and strengthens the skeleton. Insufficient sunlight exposure can cause deficiencies, raising the prevalence of osteoporosis and rickets among vulnerable populations. Thus, the capacity of skin to synthesize vitamin D emphasizes the reciprocal relationship between integumentary functioning and bodily physiological functioning. The biological functions of vitamin D have implications wider than the maintenance of bone because it influences various body functions and processes. Vitamin D affects the immune system greatly, which governs the body's defense against infection and inflammation. Research has shown that optimal levels of vitamin D are likely to lower the risk of autoimmune disorders and respiratory tract infections.

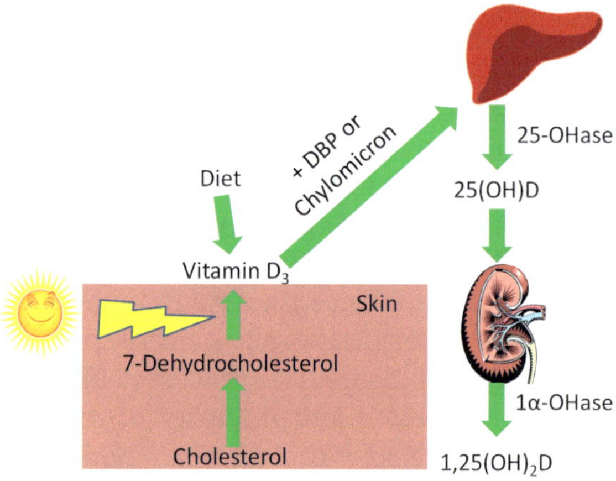

Figure 1.18. Vitamin D synthesis and activation.

Source: https://s3-us-west-2.amazonaws.com/courses-images/wp-content/uploads/sites/2569/2017/10/26165247/100000000000047300000359430FD8BF.png

In addition, growing evidence points towards a possible involvement of vitamin D in mood, brain function, and thus mental health. With its diverse biological functions, the importance of upholding optimal levels of vitamin D ensues. These are geographical position, skin color, and living conditions, which have a substantial influence on the ability of individuals to synthesize vitamin D, thus emphasizing the necessity of public health training on proper sunlight exposure and dietary intake of vitamin D to prevent deficiency. In the endeavor to develop medical science, new strategies are being planned for the improvement of vitamin D supply and metabolism. New research has been conducted into biotechnological approaches to vitamin D synthesis and delivery that may enhance its bioavailability and efficacy in the body. This is at a time when liver or renal failure can compromise endogenous biosynthesis of vitamin D, leading to deficiencies requiring therapeutic intervention. Research on altered vitamin D metabolism attempts to resolve these problems, potentially constraining the hypercalcemic action of supplementation while ensuring adequate physiological effects. As researchers investigate microbial bioconversions and enzymatic conversions further, vitamin D delivery becomes a very promising field in the future, targeting various subjects with varied health profiles and diet restrictions. This convergence of scientific progress maintains the importance of vitamin D as a bioactive molecule within the realm of human health and integumentary physiology, providing avenues for enhanced clinical practice (Mía-Domínguez et al., 2024;Neharkar et al., 2024).

Test Your Knowledge

1. How does the immune system affect the skin?
2. Why is vitamin D synthesis important?

1.6. Advances in Integumentary System Research

Learning Outcome

1. Describe the innovations in skin care and treatment
2. Understand regenerative medicine and skin grafts
3. Know the impact of technology on dermatology

Recent studies on the integumentary system have highlighted the importance of the skin microbiome in homeostasis and the consequences of its disruption in a number of dermatological diseases. Skin microbiome is a community of various microorganisms that participate in protective and immune activities and creates a multilayered defense against exogenous pathogens. Dysbiosis of this microbiome may lead to the induction of inflammatory processes that play a key role in the pathogenesis of chronic diseases such as psoriasis, in which case the immune system starts attacking harmless skin flora. This pathological reaction explains the complexity of the links between microbial composition and skin health, stating the need for further research to disentangle the details of such interactions. By understanding these mechanisms, researchers can identify novel therapeutic targets and potentially mitigate the onset of inflammatory skin diseases, paving the way for innovative treatments that leverage the natural defenses of the skin microbiome (Celoria et al., 2023). The development of biomaterials has dramatically changed the concepts of wound healing in the integumentary system, which should focus on their biocompatibility and biodegradability. These materials play a central role in the natural healing processes, which entail intricate interactions among cytokines, macrophages, and fibroblasts. Recent research has been aimed at the synthesis of biopolymer-based matrices which can be customized to promote cellular responses important in wound repair. The different methods used in the creation of advanced wound dressings have created products with differentiated features, where each product has its own strengths and weaknesses. The future studies have to focus on the investigation of cost-effective and eco-friendly methodologies and improving the efficiency of these materials. The potential of biomaterials could revolutionize wound care, ultimately leading to improved patient outcomes in the management of integumentary injuries (Prete et al., 2023). In addition, the incorporation of nanotechnology in the manufacture of wound care products heralds a new breakthrough in integumentary research. This is a novel technology whereby nanoparticles and nanoscale materials can be developed to improve the delivery of bioactive molecules to the target sites in the skin. With nanotechnology, the researchers see the possibility of having a wound dressing that does not simply cover the wound, but takes an active part in the healing process by stimulating cellular functions and limiting the possibilities of infections. The intersection between nanomaterials and more natural healing approaches is an optimistic horizon, as it will allow the creation of customizable treatments that can be much more aligned with the needs of particular patients. With ongoing advancements in this field, it is essential to evaluate the efficacy and safety of these novel approaches to ensure that they effectively contribute to the broader goals of integumentary system health and disease management (Prete et al., 2023).

1.6.1. Innovations in Skin Care and Treatment

The field of treatment and skincare has witnessed significant advancements that reflect growing appreciation for the complexity of integumentary systems and the need for novel therapies. Novel advancements in biomaterials have been shown to be highly significant in terms of constructing more efficient wound healing processes. These biodegradable, biocompatible compounds can be precisely used to develop innovative wound dressings that actively support the body's intrinsic healing capabilities. Through the combination of various biopolymers with therapeutic properties, researchers have begun producing matrices that not only provide a physical barrier but also trigger cellular reactions essential in the healing of wounds properly. Such innovations signal a shift from conventional therapies to more biologically relevant interventions that recognize the interconnected processes involved in skin repair, thereby enhancing recovery rates among patients with cutaneous injuries and pathologies (Prete et al., 2023). Besides biomaterials, advancements in traditional systems of medicine are now being integrated into modern skincare routines. The utilization of Traditional Chinese Medicine (TCM) and its food medicines has also become more accepted, especially when dealing with post-COVID syndromes, which affect skin health. The theory of Medicine and Food Homology in TCM suggests that certain foods are able to elicit therapeutic effects, offering a less artificial means of long-term skin treatment. These medicinal foods have also been found to cure various skin conditions by promoting overall wellness and speeding up the body's natural healing processes. With holistic health growing in significance, exploring the incorporation of TCM practices promises promising territories for effective skincare treatments harnessing the interconnectivity of dietary habits and dermatology (Ng et al., 2023). Furthermore, novel technologies such as drug-delivery systems and nanotechnology are revolutionizing skincare treatments. Topical application of nanoparticles makes it possible to have selective drug delivery, improve the bioavailability of active ingredients, and increase the efficacy on the skin. Such advances not only allow one to attain targeted treatment of diseases like acne, psoriasis, and eczema but also minimize side effects generally associated with conventional therapy. As researchers continue to investigate other means of synthesizing and utilizing such technologies in skin treatment regimens, the potential for more effective and specific skincare solutions draws nearer. Through a synthesis of scientific advances and increased understanding of holistic well-being, the future of skin treatment appears destined for sweeping transformation, ultimately to the advantage of many who suffer from skin conditions (Prete et al., 2023).

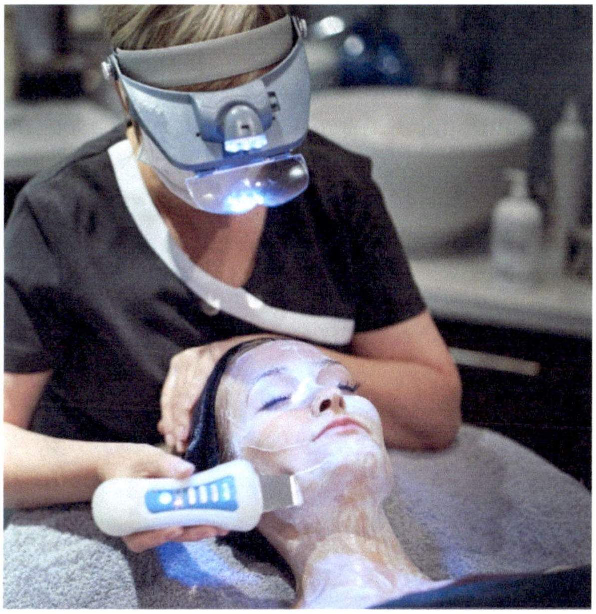

Figure 1.19. Latest innovations in skincare treatments.

Source: https://www.cortiva.edu/wp-content/uploads/sites/2/2025/01/Cortiva.Blog_.Latest-Innovations-in-Skincare-Treatments-What-Estheticians-Need-to-Know.FINAL_-scaled.jpg

1.6.2. Regenerative Medicine and Skin Grafts

The evolution of regenerative medicine revolutionized the process of wound repair and skin injury treatment, particularly in the use of skin grafts. Skin grafting refers to the transplantation of tissue to repair or replace damaged skin, which is primarily utilized for burn patients, trauma wounds, or surgical wounds. The integration of regenerative medicine protocols enhances the functions of conventional grafting procedures through the adoption of advanced cellular therapies, such as the utilization of epidermal stem cells. The cells share the proliferative and self-renewal ability, allowing for rapid and efficient healing processes. By leveraging these cellular attributes, physicians can minimize the size of donor sites and the risks of immune rejection, allowing for a patient-specific remedy for skin repair. Evolution of regenerative techniques in skin grafting remaps the treatment standards of the integumentary system in a way that not only is healing efficient but also sustainable. Moreover, research into extracellular vesicles (EVs) of stem cells presents a new addition to the uses of regenerative medicine. With preconditioning of such stem cells, researchers have observed an enhancement of the functional performance of EVs as a potential therapeutic agent for tissue repair. In skin transplantation, EVs have the potential to dominate wound healing by promoting angiogenesis, which is critical for the establishment of a stable blood supply to the graft tissue. This capability is essential in ensuring that the skin transplanted can survive and be incorporated into the recipient's body. Through this, application of stem cell-derived EVs not only complements existing skin graft methods but also opens new avenues for personalized medicine approaches with a bright future awaiting the treatment of integumentary system diseases (Yoo et al., 2025). Skin graft efficacy is further improved by an understanding of the skin's extracellular matrix (ECM) component, which is also a critical structural and biochemical supporter of cells involved in the cellular interactions of wound healing. ECM comprises various components that influence cellular proliferation, differentiation, and migration. By incorporating ECM elements into skin grafting, clinicians can achieve a healing-conducive environment while simultaneously minimizing complications associated with grafting techniques. Various sources of cultured skin cells, such as autologous keratinocytes, have been more solidified, offering a substitute for traditional skin grafts. These techniques ensure that the transplant is tailored to the specific patient's requirements, echoing the general goals of regenerative medicine. The novel applications of ECM and its components in skin grafting reflect a revolutionary era in regenerative therapy to enhance recovery and patient outcomes within the integumentary system (Fina, 2024).

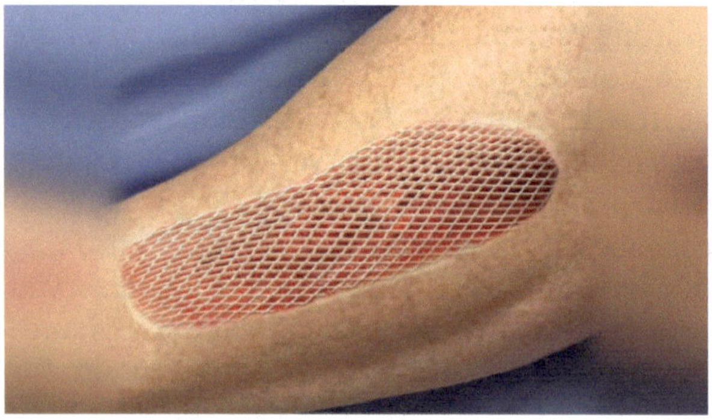

Figure 1.20. Skin grafting.

Source: https://d2yjegym0lbr1w.cloudfront.net/thumbs/skingraft_1280.jpg?v=201404114

1.6.3. The Impact of Technology on Dermatology

Technological progress has significantly transformed dermatology practice, both diagnostic and treatment strategies. One of the most significant advances is the implementation of teledermatology, which allows patients access to specialist advice without necessarily attending clinics. This has improved access to dermatological care, particularly among patients residing in rural or underserved communities. Teledermatology not only streamlines the diagnostic process but also enhances chronic skin disease monitoring by enabling frequent imaging and patient contact via internet-based platforms. Thus, patients are able to achieve better outcomes due to early interventions as well as enhanced knowledge about their disease. Also, artificial intelligence-driven integration in dermatological diagnosis holds much promise since algorithms can classify images of skin lesions with high accuracy, enabling early disease detection for diseases such as melanoma. In addition to diagnostic enhancement, the treatment areas of dermatology have also changed with technology. Emerging technologies, such as 3D printing, are revolutionizing the production of custom-made implants and prosthetics for dermatology. Furthermore, the coming of age of personalized medicine based on genomic technology promises the possibility of patient-specific treatment regimens based on patient-specific genetic signatures.

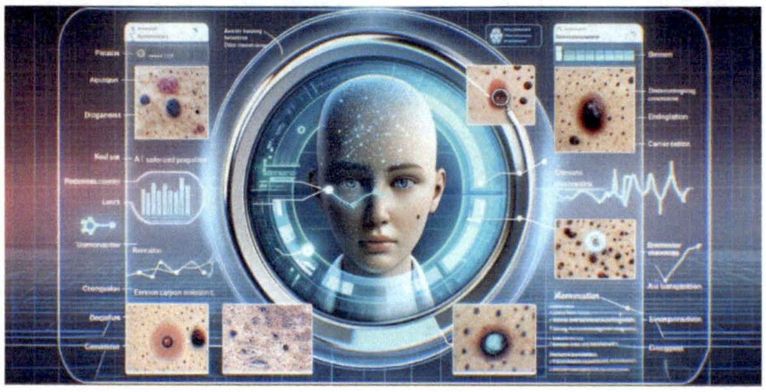

Figure 1.21. AI-based support system for skin cancer diagnostics.

Source: https://img.chemie.de/Portal/News/65a8fd37044ee_oxRiYp0_n.png?tr=w-1792,h-896,cm-extract,x-0,y-32:n-news_teaser

The result of such interventions can yield more efficiency and less toxicity, particularly for diseases such as psoriasis, where elucidation of the gene-microbiome interactions is key to guiding therapeutic strategies. Increased research into the skin microbiome demonstrates its role in inflammatory skin diseases, with the diverse community of microorganisms that exist on the skin playing an important aspect of immune function, as well as the origination of skin disease, highlighting the potential for new therapeutic and management strategies (Celoria et al., 2023). Another mind-boggling technological advancement in dermatology lies in the development of new drug delivery systems, e.g., hydrogels derived from Aloe vera, which have been identified to promote accelerated mechanisms of wound healing. Not only do such hydrogels provide a biocompatible platform for healing, but they also deliver therapeutic agents in a targeted manner to combat inflammation and infection at the site of injury. Moreover, their antimicrobial activity makes them extremely useful for wound healing and skin infection treatment. Incorporating various bioactive agents in hydrogel forms offers greater regenerative effects, emphasizing the significance of technology for higher efficacy in therapy. As with continuous research into the multi-purposive applications of Aloe vera-based hydrogels, the hope for new therapies is created that is destined to transform treatments for a myriad of dermatological conditions (Chelu et al., 2023).

Test Your Knowledge

1. What is skincare innovation?
2. How does technology affect dermatology?

SUMMARY

The integumentary system, which incorporates the skin, hair, nails, and associated glands, is a critical interface between the human being and the external world. Due to its varied functions, such as protection, regulation, and sensation, the integumentary system forms an integral part of homeostasis. With increasing research, it is increasingly important to appreciate the impact of external factors, such as pollution and synthetic materials, on this critical system. Notably, the detection of microplastics in human tissues by recent studies clearly indicates the long-term health implications environmental toxins may have, such as potential skin function and inflammatory alterations. This finding emphasizes the necessity for ongoing research and public education to guard against compromising the integrity of the integumentary system in an increasingly polluted environment, and it implies a pressing need for preventive measures and regulatory control of environmental exposures (Roslan et al., 2024).

Aside from this, the presence of microplastics and nanoplastics in cosmetics also highlights a hitherto less-focused area of dermatology, raising concerns about long-term skin health. The ability of such particles to break the cutaneous surface barrier is not just a threat to dermatological homeostasis but also raises the demand for thorough research into their effects. Long-term exposure is depicted by evidence to trigger inflammatory responses and affect physiological processes, thereby contributing significantly to the integumentary system's health (Aristizabal et al., 2024). These findings reaffirm the importance of challenging cosmetic formulations and environmental policies, encouraging an outlook that prioritizes both individual and environmental well-being. Even though these consequences are recognized, the academic community has to campaign for stricter policies and consumer education in order to minimize the threat from microplastics and nanoplastics. In a nutshell, the integumentary system is faced with new challenges posed by environmental and man-made contaminants, necessitating research with a science-backed approach, along with public discourse. The interface of microplastics in human tissues and their potential implications on skin health underscores the critical need for a comprehensive understanding of their impact on the integumentary system. Coordinated efforts among researchers, physicians, and regulatory agencies are needed in order to produce strategies that effectively counteract these changing threats. Through enhanced collaboration and enhanced public awareness about these factors, we are able to more effectively maintain the integrity of the integumentary system and, therefore, individual and community health. Ongoing research into the interfaces of dermatology and environmental science will guide future practice and guidelines in the field and ultimately lead the discussion toward a healthier future (Roslan et al., 2024; Aristizabal et al., 2024).

The integumentary system, made up of the skin, hair, nails, and associated glands, serves several important functions that are central to homeostasis and health maintenance. The function of the skin is mainly protective, covering up the underlying tissues from mechanical trauma, disease-producing organisms, and harmful chemicals. This protective function is essential in preventing infection and disease, underscoring the integumentary system's role in immunity. In addition, the skin also regulates temperature by secreting sweat and dilating or narrowing blood vessels, a process that becomes increasingly significant in altering environmental conditions. Overall, this intricate role emphasizes the underlying significance of integumentary systems in physical protection and physiological regulation. In the same manner, the integumentary system is also significant in sensory perception, which allows organisms to react to their surroundings. Skin is also equipped with multiple receptors that detect variations in pain, pressure, and temperature, facilitating a quick response necessary for survival. For instance, the detection of a pointed object or an abrupt change in temperature may enable people to avoid being hurt and promote adaptive behavior. Data gained through sensory inputs also enhances the richness of one's perception of the environment to permit more interaction with the world. This sensory function is particularly pertinent in the context of social interaction because it facilitates communication through nonverbal cues, once again emphasizing the pivotal role of the skin in human experience and relation. Moreover, the integumentary system's excretory and production functions for essential compounds, such as vitamin D, also demonstrate its higher pertinence beyond protection. Skin plays a role in the excretion of metabolic waste products, such as salts and urea, thus contributing to the regulation of internal health and equilibrium. In addition, vitamin D formation on exposure to ultraviolet light contributes to calcium absorption and has direct implications for immune competence and bone health. The recognition of these multifaceted functions emphasizes the integumentary system's critical contribution to homeostasis, affirming its pivotal position in disease prevention and promotion of health. Being the initial defense of the body, the roles of the integumentary system reveal its importance in sustaining life and at the same time enabling interaction with the environment (Shelton et al., 2024; Apaydin et al., 2024).

KEY TERMS FROM THIS CHAPTER

- Adipose tissue
- Dermatitis
- Environmental hazards
- Hypodermis
- Integumentary system
- Pathogens
- Skin cancer
- Thermoregulation
- Allergens
- Dermis
- Epidermis
- Infections
- Loose connective
- Sebaceous glands
- Sweat glands

CRITICAL THINKING QUESTIONS

1. **The integumentary system primarily includes:**
   a. Skin, hair, nails, sweat glands, and sebaceous glands
   b. Bones, muscles, and cartilage
   c. Blood vessels, lymph nodes, and heart
   d. Eyes, ears, and nose
2. **The largest organ of the human body is:**
   a. Liver
   b. Skin
   c. Heart
   d. Brain
3. **The primary function of the integumentary system is:**
   a. Blood circulation
   b. Gas exchange
   c. Protection against environmental hazards
   d. Hormone production
4. **The three main layers of the skin are:**
   a. Dermis, hypodermis, and epidermis
   b. Epidermis, dermis, and subcutaneous tissue
   c. Stratum basale, stratum corneum, and dermis
   d. Epidermis, dermis, and cartilage
5. **The outermost layer of the skin is the:**
   a. Dermis
   b. Epidermis
   c. Hypodermis
   d. Stratum basale

Short Answer Questions

1. What is the integumentary system?
2. How is the integumentary system important to the human health?
3. What is the structure of the skin?
4. What are the functions of the integumentary system?
5. What is the role of the integumentary system in homeostasis?

Answer to Critical Thinking Questions

1. (a) 2. (b) 3. (c) 4. (b) 5. (b)

REFERENCES

1. Aishasiddhika, N., & Jenovajosephine, P. (2024). Skin cancer detection using image processing. *International Research Journal of Modernization in Engineering Technology and Science*. https://www.semanticscholar.org/paper/08eeaa22c7704bb2f9d447098f061c7bc059c287 (accessed on 15th June 2025).
2. Al Dhaheri, A., Ameen, A., Reda, A. M., Alnaeem, A., Al Nuaimi, K., Marzooqi, F. A., Albreiki, F., et al. (2024). United Arab Emirates consensus recommendations for management of acne vulgaris. *Journal of Drugs in Dermatology: JDD, 23*(8), 653–660. https://www.semanticscholar.org/paper/d5bb6e8fda41ed7af6e1c2967ca3dad5656bfb1f (accessed on 15th June 2025).
3. Anders, P., Bissantz, N., Boysen, L., Grijs, R., Astrophysik, U. F. I. F. I., Goettingen, U., Sterrenkundig Instituut, et al. (2007). The young star cluster system in the Antennae: Evidence for a turnover in the luminosity function. *Monthly Notices of the Royal Astronomical Society, 377*, 91–106. https://www.semanticscholar.org/paper/7e3cab02075990a639bb7a6ec00d55902631fd58 (accessed on 15th June 2025).
4. Apaydin, N., Crosthwait, R., & Pire-Smerkanich, N. (2024). 539 Identifying best practices: Content analysis of Plain Language Summary (PLS) resources for disseminating study results to participants. *Journal of Clinical and Translational Science, 8*, 160–161. https://www.semanticscholar.org/paper/aadbe9a182d5acbdec10e1928fa36d556a265c00 (accessed on 15th June 2025).
5. Aristizabal, M., Jiménez-Orrego, K. V., Caicedo-León, M. D., Páez-Cárdenas, L. S., Castellanos-García, I., Villalba-Moreno, D. L., Ramírez-Zuluaga, L. V., et al. (2024). Microplastics in dermatology: Potential effects on skin homeostasis. *Journal of Cosmetic Dermatology, 23*, 766–772. https://doi.org/10.1111/jocd.16167 (accessed on 15th June 2025).
6. Benner, P., Goyal, P., & Pontes Duff, I. (2024). Identification of dominant subspaces for model reduction of structured parametric systems. *International Journal for Numerical Methods in Engineering, 125*. https://www.semanticscholar.org/paper/64b68b0b112bb1af9f9e18d3eeeb39e98c9b207c (accessed on 15th June 2025).
7. Carvajal, M. A., Oates, W., & Pahari, B. (2024). Multifractal analysis of heat transport in DLA structures. *12947*, 1294707–1294707-12. https://www.semanticscholar.org/paper/551cd138ace0978714583a82d1a8e5acc5c9288c (accessed on 15th June 2025).
8. Celoria, V., Rosset, F., Pala, V., Dapavo, P., Ribero, S., Quaglino, P., & Mastorino, L. (2023). The skin microbiome and its role in psoriasis: A review. *Psoriasis: Targets and Therapy, 13*, 71–78. https://doi.org/10.2147/ptt.s328439 (accessed on 15th June 2025).
9. Chelu, M., Musuc, A. M., Popa, M., & Calderon Moreno, J. (2023). *Aloe vera*-based hydrogels for wound healing: Properties and therapeutic effects. *Gels, 9*, 539. https://doi.org/10.3390/gels9070539 (accessed on 15th June 2025).
10. da Silva, A. A., de Castro, M. C. A. B., de Freitas e Silva, R., de Oliveira, B. C., Werkhauser, R. P., Brito, M. D., Gil, L. H. V. G., et al. (2025). A strategic conflict between two sides: Host immune cells vs. viral symbiont of *Leishmania* spp. in cutaneous leishmaniasis. *Brazilian Journal of Health Review*. https://www.semanticscholar.org/paper/eeb62b01187d7f8e4ad9a8faba5b663732ec35f7 (accessed on 15th June 2025).

11. De Pessemier, B., Grine, L., Debaere, M., Maes, A., Paetzold, B., & Callewaert, C. (2021). Gut–skin axis: Current knowledge of the interrelationship between microbial dysbiosis and skin conditions. *Microorganisms, 9*, 353. https://doi.org/10.3390/microorganisms9020353 (accessed on 15th June 2025).

12. Fina, S. T. (2024). Exploring the potential of skin cell culture and the vital role of skin grafts in regenerative medicine and biology. *Journal of Clinical and Medical Research*. https://www.semanticscholar.org/paper/78aa1278c5235e21896a3b4508c80ab506f977dc (accessed on 15th June 2025).

13. Finnerty, C., Jeschke, M., Herndon, D., Gamelli, R., Gibran, N., Klein, M., Silver, G., et al. (2008). Temporal cytokine profiles in severely burned patients: A comparison of adults and children. *Molecular Medicine, 14*, 553–560. https://www.semanticscholar.org/paper/1a53932f22ce24c7607376a6083d538573ce084c (accessed on 15th June 2025).

14. García-Domínguez, M., Gutiérrez-del-Río, I., Villar, C. J., Pérez-Gómez, A., Sancho-Martinez, I., & Lombó, F. (2024). Structural diversification of vitamin D using microbial biotransformation's. *Applied Microbiology and Biotechnology, 108*. https://www.semanticscholar.org/paper/fcdc74590575e2c3949587b203c221aa34dbc8fe (accessed on 15th June 2025).

15. Gong, G., Fan, Y., Li, W., Yan, X., Yan, X., Zhang, L., Wang, N., et al. (2022). Identification of the key genes associated with different hair types in the Inner Mongolia cashmere goat. *Animals: An Open Access Journal from MDPI, 12*. https://www.semanticscholar.org/paper/799e356deb58ceba24eb0ce8cf1f385a533be33c (accessed on 15th June 2025).

16. Hartvigsson, T., Sandman, L., Bergström, G., & Brämberg, E. (2024). Cooperation in return-to-work interventions for common mental disorders: An ideal theory analysis of actors, goals, and ethical obstacles. *Health Care Analysis, 33*, 173–191. https://www.semanticscholar.org/paper/a26593480ffec1e56245e01fcf9c55700f8c88a6 (accessed on 15th June 2025).

17. Kapatkar, S., Deshmukh, S., Thakre, T., & Rathi, R. (2024). Management of Vicharchika (eczema) by multi-model Ayurveda intervention: A case report. *Journal of Clinical and Diagnostic Research*. https://www.semanticscholar.org/paper/7342db74f8481929003872f0c24a935032504394 (accessed on 15th June 2025).

18. Kibitska, H. (2024). Acne in adolescents: How emotional support improves treatment outcomes. *Journal of Medical–Clinical Research & Reviews*. https://www.semanticscholar.org/paper/2c69821b1d41eccb37216b866f5b4ac30fcaf381 (accessed on 15th June 2025).

19. Kocsis, D., Kichou, H., Döme, K., Varga-Medveczky, Z., Révész, Z., Antal, I., & Erdő, F. (2022). Structural and functional analysis of excised skins and human reconstructed epidermis with confocal Raman spectroscopy and in microfluidic diffusion chambers. *Pharmaceutics, 14*. https://www.semanticscholar.org/paper/e9b04b6a8509e75cb42fff830ded65e1302b09b7 (accessed on 15th June 2025).

20. Kordestani, M., Orchard, M., Khorasani, K., & Saif, M. (2023). An overview of the state of the art in aircraft prognostic and health management strategies. *IEEE Transactions on Instrumentation and Measurement, 72*, 1–15. https://www.semanticscholar.org/paper/8b773301b1b4606905117baf507f94baa28c25bd (accessed on 15th June 2025).

21. Kritsilis, M., Vanherle, L., Rosenholm, M., In 't Zandt, R., Yao, Y., Swanberg, K. M., Weikop, P., et al. (2024). Loss of glymphatic homeostasis in heart failure. *Brain, 148*, 985–1000. https://

www.semanticscholar.org/paper/b109b614fccffc928172022b75785b4f50fa9e49 (accessed on 15th June 2025).

22. Lee, H. J., & Kim, M. (2022). Skin barrier function and the microbiome. *International Journal of Molecular Sciences, 23*, 13071. https://doi.org/10.3390/ijms232113071 (accessed on 15th June 2025).

23. Li, Q., Wang, C., Li, X., Zhang, J., Zhang, Z., Yang, K., Ouyang, J., et al. (2023). Epidermis-on-a-chip system to develop skin barrier and melanin mimicking model. *Journal of Tissue Engineering, 14*. https://www.semanticscholar.org/paper/4dd9d1bacb5daab91367b19e24df9ee7ebd3539c (accessed on 15th June 2025).

24. Lin, F. (2024). Obscured complexity: How external cycles simplify the dynamics of the endogenous circadian oscillator–Take the time series of body temperature records as an example. *bioRxiv*. https://www.semanticscholar.org/paper/ee9ec21806369509b186633657b7fe992fbe340f (accessed on 15th June 2025).

25. Ma, W., Zhan, Y., Zhang, Y., Mao, C., Xie, X., & Lin, Y. (2021). The biological applications of DNA nanomaterials: Current challenges and future directions. *Signal Transduction and Targeted Therapy, 6*. https://doi.org/10.1038/s41392-021-00727-9 (accessed on 15th June 2025).

26. Ménard, G., Rouillon, A., Cattoir, V., & Donnio, P. Y. (2021). *Galleria mellonella* as a suitable model of bacterial infection: Past, present and future. *Frontiers in Cellular and Infection Microbiology, 11*. https://doi.org/10.3389/fcimb.2021.782733 (accessed on 15th June 2025).

27. Morgan, N. R., Magalingam, K. B., Radhakrishnan, A., Arumugam, M., Jamil, A., & Bhuvanendran, S. (2024). Explicating the multifunctional roles of tocotrienol and squalene in promoting skin health. *Skin Health and Disease, 4*. https://www.semanticscholar.org/paper/6dbe5a8c74de5e16d00994b305bbbdde37f793fc (accessed on 15th June 2025).

28. Nakamura, A., & Matsumoto, M. (2025). Role of polyamines in intestinal mucosal barrier function. *Seminars in Immunopathology, 47*. https://www.semanticscholar.org/paper/9cb614bbb7da442b36834fc34df2553c1c78b887 (accessed on 15th June 2025).

29. Neharkar, N., Dalvi, S. Y., Chaudhari, M. A., Chaudhari, G. D., & Chaudhary, J. (2024). Exploring the vital role of vitamins in disease prevention and health maintenance. *International Journal of Advanced Research in Science, Communication and Technology*. https://www.semanticscholar.org/paper/2b5eda3fcd22c9064ca62ce1709221b63cf89705 (accessed on 15th June 2025).

30. Ng, C. Y., Bun, H., Zhao, Y., & Zhong, L. L. D. (2023). TCM "medicine and food homology" in the management of post-COVID disorders. *Frontiers in Immunology, 14*. https://doi.org/10.3389/fimmu.2023.1234307 (accessed on 15th June 2025).

31. Nikolenko, V. N., Borminskaya, I. D., Nikitina, A. T., Golyshkina, M. S., Rizaeva, N., & Oganesyan, M. (2024). Locus coeruleus-norepinephrine system: Spheres of influence and contribution to the development of neurodegenerative diseases. *Frontiers in Bioscience, 29*(3), 118. https://www.semanticscholar.org/paper/b1b7ee6287b1f3117feb2e9edb7b1b99aea2fb51 (accessed on 15th June 2025).

32. Patil, P. C. (2024). Evaluating the efficacy of homeopathic treatments in the management of eczema: A comprehensive review. *International Journal for Multidisciplinary Research*. https://www.semanticscholar.org/paper/8f4a01354c3c9b0214441ee81210e205bde587e1 (accessed on 15th June 2025).

33. Pennartz, C., oude Lohuis, M. N., & Olcese, U. (2023). How 'visual' is the visual cortex? The interactions between the visual cortex and other sensory, motivational and motor systems as enabling factors for visual perception. *Philosophical Transactions of the Royal Society B: Biological Sciences, 378*. https://www.semanticscholar.org/paper/a3b03010617e8988c363f0cb6768aad5ee71f0c4 (accessed on 15th June 2025).

34. Prete, S., Dattilo, M., Patitucci, F., Pezzi, G., Parisi, O. I., & Puoci, F. (2023). Natural and synthetic polymeric biomaterials for application in wound management. *Journal of Functional Biomaterials, 14*, 455. https://doi.org/10.3390/jfb14090455 (accessed on 15th June 2025).

35. Rahman, M. A., Bazgir, E., Hossain, S. M. S., & Maniruzzaman, M. (2024). Skin cancer classification using NASNet. *International Journal of Science and Research Archive*. https://www.semanticscholar.org/paper/f0ce9212189220965fa2edaa681936dbf6d29d7e (accessed on 15th June 2025).

36. Ramadon, D., McCrudden, M., Courtenay, A. J., & Donnelly, R. F. (2021). Enhancement strategies for transdermal drug delivery systems: Current trends and applications. *Drug Delivery and Translational Research, 12*, 758–791. https://doi.org/10.1007/s13346-021-00909-6 (accessed on 15th June 2025).

37. Roslan, N. S., Lee, Y. Y., Ibrahim, Y. S., Anuar, S. T., Ku Yusof, K. M. K., Lai, L. A., & Brentnall, T. A. (2024). Detection of microplastics in human tissues and organs: A scoping review. *Journal of Global Health, 14*. https://doi.org/10.7189/jogh.14.04179 (accessed on 15th June 2025).

38. Saber, S. A., ElSalkh, B. A., Gadel-Rab, A. G., Mahmoud, F. A., El-Dahshan, A. A., & Gewily, D. I. (2018). Comparative and functional study of integumentary system of two different reptiles: Adaptation to their different modes of life. *The Egyptian Journal of Hospital Medicine, 73*, 6802–6811. https://doi.org/10.21608/ejhm.2018.16723 (accessed on 15th June 2025).

39. Salari, N., Heidarian, P., Jalili, F., Babajani, F., Shohaimi, S., Nasirian, M., & Mohammadi, M. (2024). The sexual dysfunction in women with thyroid disorders: A meta-analysis. *BMC Endocrine Disorders, 24*. https://www.semanticscholar.org/paper/fbe1f48edc63e505f47af949c0aa6f9a7728b37d (accessed on 15th June 2025).

40. Schmidt, T., Dahlberg, A., Berthold, E., Król, P., Arve-Butler, S., Rydén, E., Najibi, S. M., et al. (2023). Synovial monocytes contribute to chronic inflammation in childhood-onset arthritis via IL-6/STAT signaling and cell-cell interactions. *Frontiers in Immunology, 14*. https://www.semanticscholar.org/paper/e78e04562e7cabe6dacaaeaa0fecf74d66517a1f (accessed on 15th June 2025).

41. Shelton, S. R., Nelson, C. D., Sullivan, M., Wroblewski, K., Mueller, E., & Wolford, T. (2024). Strengthening the US public health lab system: Summary of Coronavirus Disease (COVID-19) After Action Review Workshop. *Journal of Public Health Management and Practice, 30*, 710–717. https://www.semanticscholar.org/paper/e7610aceaf05d3360c5f280ba1b084a4500ecc78 (accessed on 15th June 2025).

42. Shibasaki, K. (2024). TRPV4 activation by core body temperature has multimodal functions in the central nervous system. *The Journal of Physiological Sciences: JPS, 74*. https://www.semanticscholar.org/paper/0266090bd5284ecdcec5bddf5fb995cb3fbc00a7 (accessed on 15th June 2025).

43. Taylor, A. B., Holmes, M. A., Laird, M. F., & Terhune, C. E. (2025). Jaw-muscle structure and function in primates: Insights into muscle performance and feeding-system behaviors.

Evolutionary Anthropology, 34. https://www.semanticscholar.org/paper/35597e49a3d26f727f2fdacdef388f11cd167d55 (accessed on 15th June 2025).

44. van der Meer, D., Gurholt, T., Sønderby, I., Shadrin, A., Hindley, G., Rahman, Z., de Lange, A. D., et al. (2022). The role of liver fat in cardiometabolic diseases is highlighted by genome-wide association study of MRI-derived measures of body composition. *bioRxiv*. https://www.semanticscholar.org/paper/b677fe30546502f8b643e27a8098636af01909c3 (accessed on 15th June 2025).

45. Vestby, L. K., Grønseth, T., Simm, R., & Nesse, L. L. (2020). Bacterial biofilm and its role in the pathogenesis of disease. *Antibiotics, 9*, 59. https://doi.org/10.3390/antibiotics9020059 (accessed on 15th June 2025).

46. Weng, T., Wu, P., Zhang, W., Zheng, Y., Li, Q., Jin, R., Chen, H., et al. (2020). Regeneration of skin appendages and nerves: Current status and further challenges. *Journal of Translational Medicine, 18.* https://doi.org/10.1186/s12967-020-02248-5 (accessed on 15th June 2025).

47. Yang, D., Zhou, Q., Labroska, V., Qin, S., Darbalaei, S., Wu, Y., Yuliantie, E., et al. (2021). G protein-coupled receptors: Structure- and function-based drug discovery. *Signal Transduction and Targeted Therapy, 6.* https://doi.org/10.1038/s41392-020-00435-w (accessed on 15th June 2025).

48. Yoo, D., Jung, S. Y., Go, D., Park, J. Y., You, D., Jung, W. K., Li, Y., et al. (2025). Functionalized extracellular vesicles of mesenchymal stem cells for regenerative medicine. *Journal of Nanobiotechnology, 23.* https://www.semanticscholar.org/paper/fed7a2dba34389b7f4651df184dd173aa1e02a0b (accessed on 15th June 2025).

49. Zhuang, M., Zhang, X., & Cai, J. (2024). Microbiota–gut–brain axis: Interplay between microbiota, barrier function and lymphatic system. *Gut Microbes, 16.* https://www.semanticscholar.org/paper/ca10eadc0b458111ff74b401cd9a77638aa237df (accessed on 15th June 2025).

CIRCULATORY SYSTEM

2

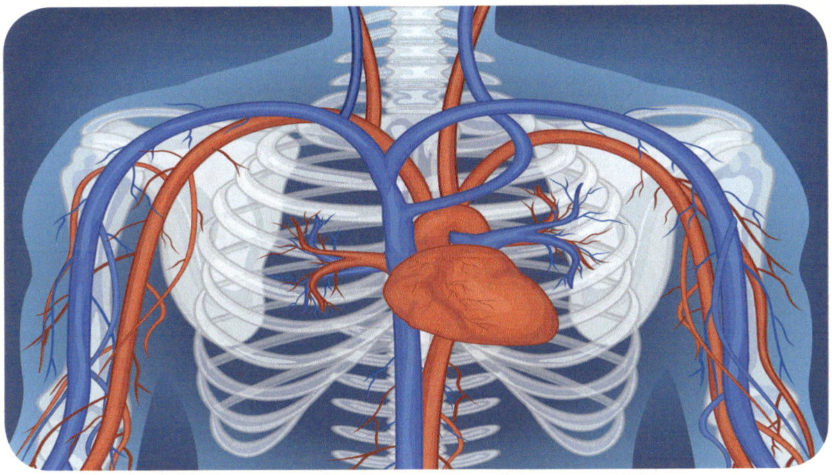

LEARNING OBJECTIVES

After studying this chapter, you will be able to:

1. Understand the anatomy of the circulatory system
2. Understand the blood composition
3. Describe the circulatory pathways
4. Explain the regulation of blood flow
5. Describe the common circulatory system disorders
6. Discuss the advances in circulatory system research

Introduction

The circulatory system is a complex network that is vital for maintaining life, conducting the delivery of nutrients, gases, hormones, and waste products throughout the body. The system consists of the heart, blood vessels, and blood and plays vital functions that contribute to overall well-being and homeostasis. At its center lies the heart itself, a muscular organ that acts as a pump, forcing blood through an extensive network of arteries, veins, and capillaries. The study of the structure and dynamics of the circulatory system teaches us about how this complex system is capable of maintaining the body in equilibrium and responding to varying physiological demands. In particular, studies on fluid dynamics nonholonomic constraints, as in Borisov et al. (2013), may explain the interaction between blood flow and vascular resistance and how these forces regulate circulatory efficiency. In additional studies, the circulatory system's relevance is not only transportation but also interdependent with other body systems, e.g., the immune system. For instance, the immune system is tasked with keeping an organism healthy by conferring immunity against pathogens and allowing for cellular waste to be removed through the bloodstream. As noted in Conrad and Gillen (2014), the immune system's structure allows it to have a harmonious interaction with various body functions, which symbolizes interdependence between physiological processes. Such a collaboration highlights the importance that circulatory system disruptions, such as hypertension or atherosclerosis, can exert on a cascade of effects on immune reactions and health.

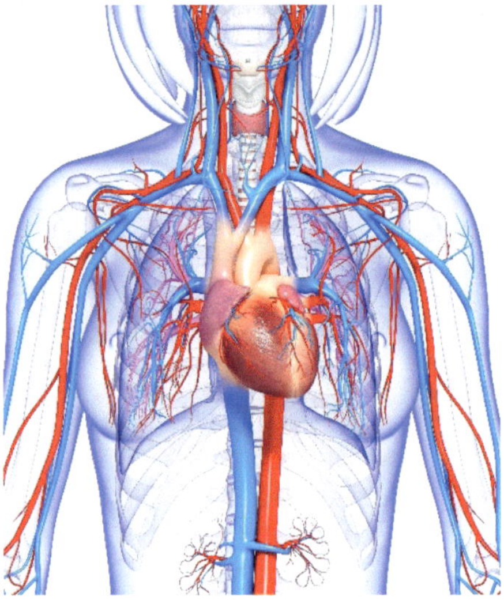

Figure 2.1. Illustration showing the circulatory system.

Source: https://media.healthdirect.org.au/images/inline/original/d65krw-(1)_d9750aa7-7903-4ed0-936e-70d01b22e08f-5ff882.png

An understanding of this interrelation is thus imperative to biomedical studies and therapeutic innovations aimed at improving cardiovascular and immune function. The multifaceted relationships within the circulatory system serve as a reminder of human physiology's complexity. With the ongoing growth of our understanding of circulatory dynamics and its cross-talk with other systems, it is evident that possessing an optimally efficient circulatory system is imperative to maintain health and prevent disease. The application of fluid mechanics in circulatory system studies is particularly promising; for example, the developments in blood flow dynamics that have implications for the management of cardiovascular diseases. Investigation of these dimensions, in combination with technological developments like imaging and computational modeling, permits a broader perspective of the circulatory system's contribution to health and disease control. Therefore, the study of the circulatory system paves the way for further investigation into the circulatory system's complex functions and how environmental and genetic influences impact its efficiency and health.

Importance of the Circulatory System in Human Physiology

The circulation system is basically intrinsic to the human body in the sense that it is a well-evolved network which ensures the continuous transport of vital material throughout the body. It consists of the heart, blood vessels, and blood, each functioning together to supply oxygen and nutrients and to exchange metabolic waste products. Tissue and organ oxygenation are critical to cellular respiration, a process necessary for energy generation. Through its role of transporting hormones and enzymes, the circulatory system also maintains homeostasis, regulates body temperature, and reacts to infection and trauma. It also maintains the immune system by transporting white blood cells and antibodies, and thus shields the body from infections. The health of an individual is dependent upon the proper operation of this system as any interference will lead to extreme physiological consequences. The circulatory system's dynamic behavior can be understood through mathematical modeling, enhancing our comprehension of its physiological processes. Recent advances in the field place emphasis on adopting a reduced-order model with the basis on Pulsed Flow Equations (PFE). These models include blood flow movement within various arterial networks and take into consideration fluctuations in velocity and pressure throughout the cardiac cycle. The proposed mathematical model introduces a new approach to modeling physiological fluid flow in one-dimensional networks, enabling researchers to explore the dynamics of the cardiovascular system with greater specificity. By incorporating such models into the context of human physiology, researchers can explore diseases such as hypertension or atherosclerosis, in which blood flow dynamics are compromised. This synergy of biology and mathematics reveals how mathematical models can lead to useful insight into vitality and the control of disease (San et al., 2012).

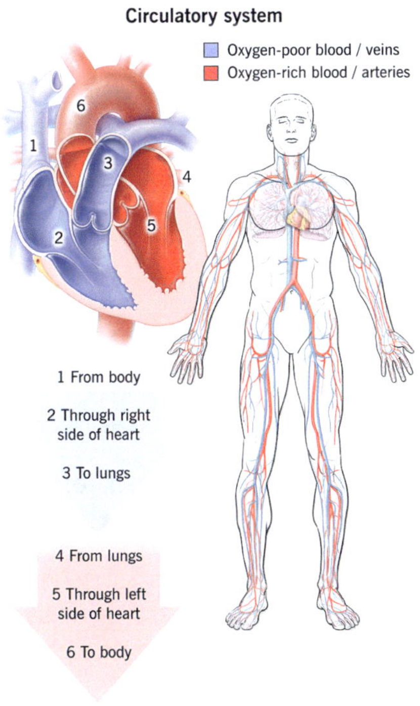

Figure 2.2. Your circulatory system (heart and blood vessels) works to move blood and oxygen through your entire body.

Source: https://my.clevelandclinic.org/-/scassets/images/org/health/articles/circulatory-system

A general overview of the circulatory system's function in human physiology also underscores its applicability across extensive medical science. A functional-based global classification system can facilitate easier organization of knowledge regarding cardiovascular health. An integrated model is able to include both the physiological processes and the objects that are in charge of their realization. This type of model will help to enhance diagnostics and therapeutic interventions, thus helping all life sciences. Since circulatory health usually indicates overall well-being, medical experts have to understand the system's complexities in order to effectively identify potential health threats. Therefore, ongoing research into the ability of the circulatory system, both biologically and mathematically, is a testament to its utility to humanity and in terms of disease avoidance (Smith et al., 2005).

2.1. Anatomy of the Circulatory System

Learning Outcome

1. Describe the major components of the circulatory system
2. Understand the structure and function of the heart
3. Describe the types of blood vessels

The circulatory system has a complicated anatomy that is designed in such a way that it allows the efficient delivery of blood, nutrients, and oxygen to the body. The heart is a muscular organ at the center of which there are four chambers: the right and left atria, and the right and left ventricles. This compartmentalization enables an orderly circulation of blood: blood with low oxygen levels flows into the right atrium via the body and is pumped into the right ventricle, which channels it to the lungs to be oxygenated. Once oxygenated, the blood flows back into the left atrium, into the left ventricle, and is then pushed with force into the aorta to be carried throughout the body via the systemic circulation. Appreciation of this compartmentalization illustrates the importance of the heart in creating a highly regulated circulatory environment essential to life and adaptations to body needs. The vascular network that makes the circulatory system complete includes veins and arteries, each type of vessel having specific but complementary roles. Arteries are thick-walled (muscular) vessels that transport oxygenated blood out of the heart, and they adjust to the different blood pressures produced in the cardiac cycles. Conversely, thinner-walled and valved veins carry deoxygenated blood back toward the heart, usually against gravity. This two-way interaction is fundamental not just to daily operability but also to the bigger physiological functions that manage the body. Moreover, there are also specific adaptations like the introduction of valves into veins that allow the blood to flow only in one direction. This is particularly important when we are talking about extremities, where blood has to flow long distances against gravity. Thus, the anatomy of the vessels is an important aspect that should be considered in detail to understand the way the circulatory system maintains adequate blood flow. Further, the circulatory system can be said to have a further level of complexity in terms of its anatomy, the study of blood itself, its make-up and its job. Blood is a connective tissue that is fluid in nature and consists of red blood cells, white blood cells, platelets, and plasma. All of the components have their own role in homeostasis and responding to physiological needs. As an example, red blood cells have hemoglobin, which is crucial in the transportation of oxygen, whereas the white blood cells play a significant role in the immune response. Furthermore, the Turkic and Mongolian peoples of Inner Asia offered a unique perspective on blood, viewing it not only as a biological fluid but also as a vital essence that intertwines with societal beliefs and health interpretations, illustrating the cultural significance and mythological dimensions associated with human anatomy (Sodnompilova and Nanzatov, 2020). Thus, the study of the anatomy of the circulatory systems does not only dwell on the physiological structures but rather on the wider cultural and social concepts of blood and health.

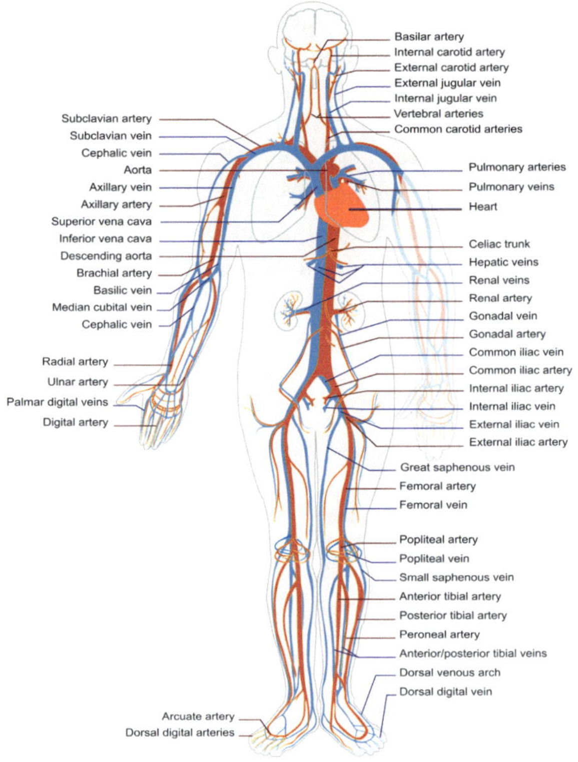

Figure 2.3. Simplified diagram of the human circulatory system in anterior view.

Source: https://bio.libretexts.org/@api/deki/files/12171/Circulatory_System_en.svg?revision=1&size=bestfit&width=711&height=988

2.1.1. Major Components: Heart, Blood Vessels, and Blood

The heart is the central organ of the circulatory system and is a muscular pump that circulates blood throughout the entire body. Having four chambers, namely two atria and two ventricles, it is held accountable for maintaining efficient blood circulation. The right heart gets the body's oxygen-poor blood and directs it to the lungs to be oxygenated, while the left gets oxygenated blood from the lungs and distributes it to the other tissues. The rhythmic beating of the heart is regulated through electrical impulses to drive the circulation of blood efficiently. Furthermore, acquiring knowledge about how the heart functions is of relevance since abnormalities lead to cardiovascular diseases (CVDs), which are a primary source of morbidity and mortality globally. Consequently, ongoing research into heart functionality, in addition to new monitoring techniques, remains critical towards enhancing cardiovascular disease prevention and improved cardiovascular health. Blood vessels form the intricate network that transports blood around the body, connecting the heart to every cell. The network consists of arteries, veins, and capillaries, each serving a distinct function. Arteries receive oxygenated blood from the heart, and deoxygenated blood is returned to the heart through veins. The smallest vessels, capillaries, exchange nutrients and gases at the cellular level. The regulation of blood flow through these arteries is based on various factors, including blood pressure as a measure of cardiovascular status. In line with studies involving the employment of new algorithms in determining blood pressure, for example, from the application of photoplethysmogram and electrocardiogram signals, growing awareness of the imperative for accurate measurement and monitoring of blood vessel function has been achieved (Géraud Bossavi et al., 2023). It is imperative for the development of effective treatments for vascular dysfunction-related ailments. The blood itself is a specialized tissue with a connective type that is crucial for transporting oxygen, nutrients, hormones, and waste products around the body. Comprised of red blood cells, white blood cells, platelets, and plasma, the blood works relentlessly to maintain life by managing homeostasis and facilitating immune function. The physiology and function of blood play a central role in the understanding of different health disorders, with any variations indicative of possible disorders. New research has highlighted the unification of circulatory and respiratory processes in newborns, with significant priority to studies of blood dynamics alongside other physiological aspects (Skazkina et al., 2020). Such a cross-disciplinary strategy not only enriches our knowledge of blood's function in the circulatory system but also facilitates the creation of early diagnostic tools for disorders that can interfere with normal autonomic control. Ultimately, it is the appreciation of the interdependence of the heart, blood vessels, and blood that is at the heart of enhancing cardiovascular healthcare.

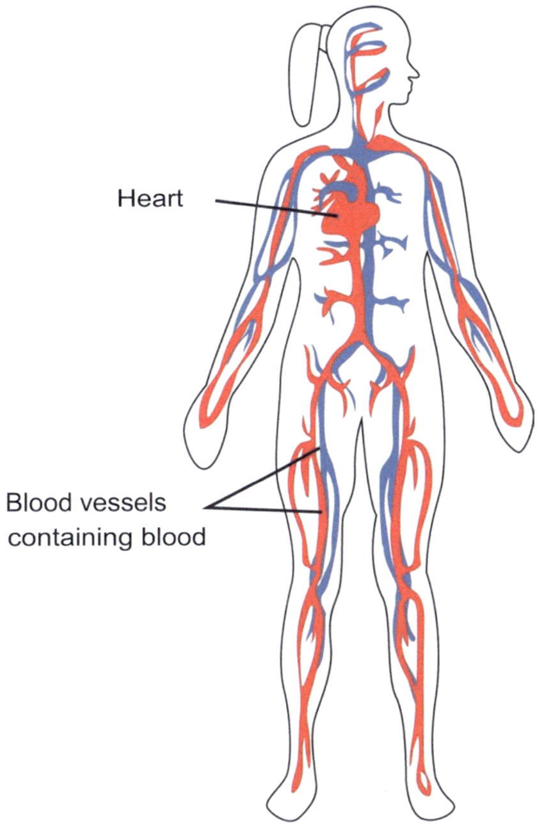

Figure 2.4. Major components of the circulatory system.

Source: https://cms-media.bartleby.com/wp-content/uploads/sites/2/2021/09/24104517/Circulatory-System-1-687x1024.jpg

2.1.2. Structure and Function of the Heart

The heart is the integrating organ of the circulatory system and has an incredibly efficient structure to facilitate perpetual circulation of blood throughout the body. Made up of four chambers—two atria and two ventricles—the structure allows for the separation of oxygenated and deoxygenated blood, which is a major part of its function. The right-hand side of the heart receives deoxygenated blood from the body and pumps it to the lungs to be oxygenated, whereas the left-hand side receives oxygenated blood from the lungs and pumps it to the rest of the body. This system of two pumps is required to provide the flow and pressure necessary to meet the metabolic demands of organs and tissues, and in the end the life of cells by providing nutrients and removing waste (Smith et al., 2005). The physical structure of the heart is augmented by its intricate valvular system, which maintains blood flow and backflow prevention during the cardiac cycle. The atrioventricular valves, which lie between atria and ventricles, ensure one-way atrial flow into ventricles, whereas semilunar valves prevent return flow into the heart after ventricular ejection. During each heartbeat, muscular contraction is exactly synchronized by the hearts electrical conduction system with the sinoatrial node acting as the intrinsic pacemaker initiating the rhythm of contraction. This remarkable synergy of structural and functional elements ensures smooth flow and adequate perfusion to all body tissues in support of the hearts position as the central piece of the circulatory system (Smith et al., 2005). In addition to its anatomical structure, the heart function has varied across millions of years to accommodate various physiological needs and demands. The evolutionary change from more rudimentary heart configurations in older vertebrates to the advanced mammalian four-chambered heart demonstrates significant adaptations enhancing general circulatory efficiency. Each improvement accounted for the hearts ability to handle increasing rates of metabolism and environmental pressures, as exemplified by the development of the conduction system facilitating rapid electrical conduction. This evolutionary perspective underscores the functionality and resilience of the heart; any failure or collapse in any section of its structure can lead to poor health, underscoring the balance of the cardiovascular system needed for the maintenance of life (Ustroi et al., 2024).

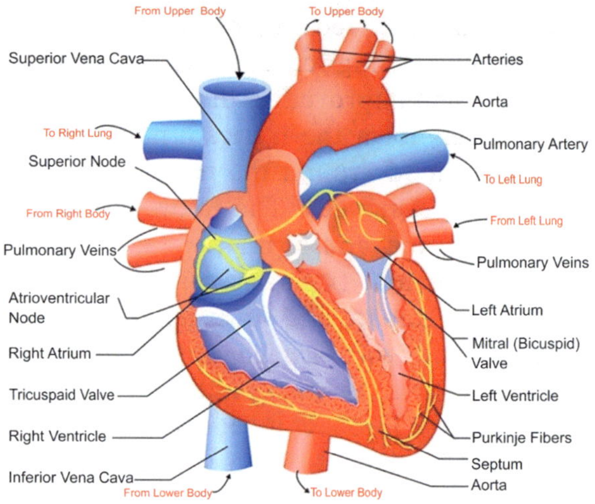

Figure 2.5. Structure and Function of the Heart.

Source: https://d2jx2rerrg6sh3.cloudfront.net/image-handler/picture/2018/7/shutterstock_139537109.jpg

2.1.3. Types of Blood Vessels: Arteries, Veins, and Capillaries

The circulatory system can be described as a complicated system of blood transmission involving the use of distinct varieties of blood vessels, i.e., arteries, veins, and capillaries. Arteries are the vessels that have thick and elastic walls and whose duty is to transport oxygenated blood out of the heart to different body tissues. The anatomical modifications of arteries enable them to resist and control high-pressure blood flow, which is produced by the contraction of the heart. Moreover, arteries are divided into smaller and smaller arterioles and finally end in capillaries, where nutrient and gas exchanges occur. The fact that the walls of the arteries can stretch and recoil is very important in the smooth flow of blood and the delivery of oxygen and nutrients to the tissues involved in metabolic processes. Unlike the arteries, the veins are developed in a manner that allows the oxygen-depleted blood to flow back to the heart. The walls of veins are less muscular and thinner than those of the arteries, indicating the low pressure at which blood flows in these vessels. Veins have a set of one-way valves that allow free flow, but no back flow to ensure effective blood returning, particularly in limbs where gravity is a major factor. Also, veins have a greater luminal diameter, which enables them to act as blood reservoirs to compensate for changes in blood volume. The importance of the veins in the circulatory system is not just limited to the transportation process, but it is also important in the overall balance of hemodynamics that is critical to the homeostasis of the body, especially during situations of exercise or inactivity. The smallest and most numerous blood vessels are the capillaries which form the point of interaction between the circulatory system and the tissues of the body. These small vessels have walls just a single cell thick, and allow the ready transfer of gases, nutrients, and waste products by diffusion. The microcirculation network maximizes the exchange surface area and enhances the delivery of oxygen and the elimination of carbon dioxide in tissues. Additionally, the morphological characteristics of capillaries, including the presence of endothelial cells and glycocalyx, significantly influence their functional capabilities (Tsapaeva and Tsapaev, 2024). Recent studies also highlight the role of capillaries in regulating blood flow through myogenic and metabolic mechanisms, contributing to the nuanced interplay between vascular health and systemic function (Elmira et al., 2024). This extensive knowledge on the types of blood vessels is essential in dealing with cardiovascular health and establishing specific medical interventions.

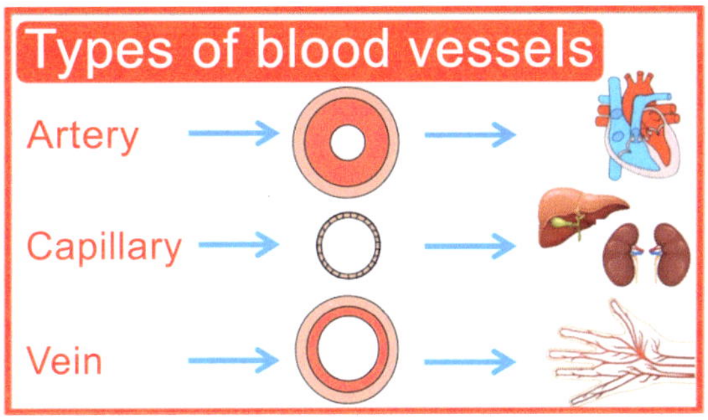

Figure 2.6. Types of blood vessels.

Source: https://i.ytimg.com/vi/Oq3SbxO8RB0/maxresdefault.jpg

Test Your Knowledge

1. What are the main components of the circulatory system?
2. What are the three main types of blood vessels?

2.2. Blood Composition

Learning Outcome

1. Describe the components of blood
2. Understand the role of plasma in the circulatory system
3. Understand the importance of hemoglobin and oxygen transport

Blood composition is a component of the circulatory system that plays various physiological functions required for homeostatic maintenance. Blood is composed of a liquid phase, plasma, and cellular elements, including red blood cells, white blood cells, and platelets. Plasma accounts for approximately 55% of blood, and it is largely composed of water, electrolytes, proteins, hormones, and waste products. The plasma proteins include albumin, which makes a contribution to oncotic pressure, and globulins, with roles in immune responses. This intricate blend allows blood to function well as a transporting medium, carrying nutrients, gases, and waste materials to and from cellular environments, thereby being a significant component of general body function. Red blood cells, or erythrocytes, are the most common component of blood and are oxygen-transport specialized cells. They possess hemoglobin, a specialized protein that grabs oxygen in the lungs and delivers oxygen to tissues throughout the body. Quantity and quality of RBCs are needed for the delivery of adequate oxygen supply; thus, any change in their constitution may lead to severe diseases such as anemia or polycythemia. Their production, or erythropoiesis, is regulated by advanced physiological mechanisms that reflect the intricate interactions among blood constituents. Mathematical models and simulations facilitate understanding of these processes, giving insight into the circulatory dynamics as outlined in the extensive treatise on blood physiology models (Leonard et al., 2025a). Models allow for an accurate analysis of blood flow and composition, a factor of the utmost importance when solving many health problems. The role of white blood cells (WBCs) is also significant, as they are central to the immune system. WBCs have the job of detecting and responding to pathogens, thus being an integral component of the body's protective system. There are numerous WBCs, each with diverse functions, including neutrophils, lymphocytes, and monocytes, which collectively provide a sophisticated response to infections and foreign objects. Second, platelets or thrombocytes have a significant function in hemostasis, the process that prevents excessive bleeding following vascular injury. Coordination among these cellular components and their distinct function means complex physiological systems, which lends itself to the argument that blood composition should be viewed as a whole and not as its elements (Barnaby R Hutchins et al., 2015). From this perspective, one better understands the holistic relationship between blood composition and its relevance to overall health and circulatory system efficiency.

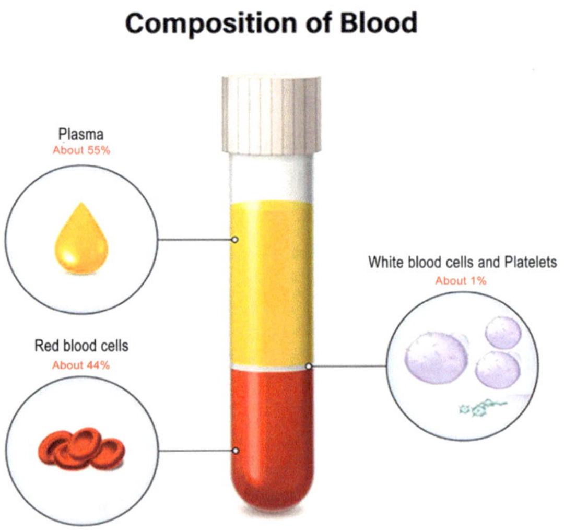

Figure 2.7. The composition of blood.

Source: https://www.hematology.org/-/media/hematology/images/patients/blood-composition.png?la=en&h=501&w=872&hash=04A91A7CB1617CEB0595141AA9C10955

2.2.1. Components of Blood: Red Blood Cells, White Blood Cells, and Platelets

The circulatory system is a fundamental process that distributes vital substances in the body through its primary elements: red blood cells (RBCs), white blood cells (WBCs), and platelets. Red blood cells, or erythrocytes, constitute the biggest population of cells in blood, taking up approximately 40-45% of the total volume. Their primary function is to transport oxygen from the lungs to the tissues and collect carbon dioxide and transport it back to the lungs for exhalation. Hemoglobin, an iron-containing protein in RBCs, facilitates this gas exchange by binding oxygen efficiently. Red blood cell health and function are essential to maintain overall oxygenation of the body, and pathology can lead to various conditions, i.e., anemia or polycythemia (Fahed et al., 2022).

On the other hand, white blood cells are part of the immune system, providing immunity against infections and foreign invaders. While red blood cells are lower in number, WBCs are important for the body's immune response. They can be classified into several types, i.e., lymphocytes, neutrophils, monocytes, eosinophils, and basophils, each having a unique function of surveillance, identification, and killing of harmful pathogens. Lymphocytes, particularly T cells and B cells, are vital in adaptive immunity, establishing a memory against specific pathogens. The roles of these immune cells are closely related to the circulatory system, with the latter acting as a conduit for their migration towards injury or infection sites (Emma J Schuster et al., 2021).

Platelets, or thrombocytes, are the smallest of blood components and play a very important role in hemostasis—the process that prevents hemorrhage when the blood vessels are damaged. When they are damaged, platelets adhere to the injured tissue and become activated, forming an initial temporary plug that stops bleeding. They secrete growth factors and cytokines, which stimulate healing and tissue repair. The platelet mechanism is crucial to the integrity of the circulatory system, as deficiency or dysfunction leads to abnormal bleeding or to thrombosis. An understanding of the interactions among platelets, WBCs, and RBCs is necessary to understand how the circulatory system can achieve homeostasis and assist the body's response to physiological stress (Fahed et al., 2022; Emma J Schuster et al., 2021).

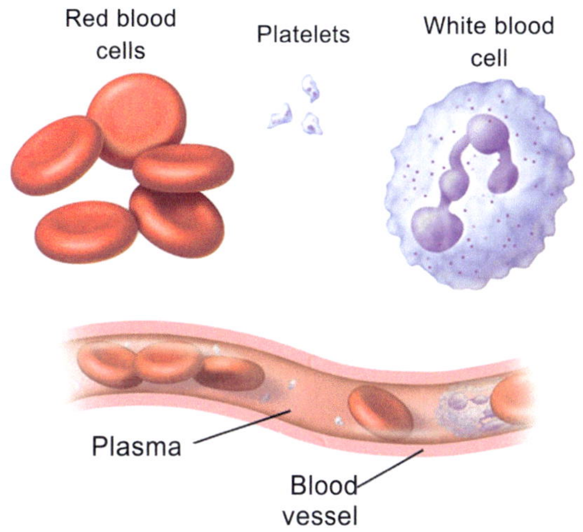

Figure 2.8. Components of blood.

Source: https://api.kramesstaywell.com/Content/6066ca30-310a-4170-b001-a4ab013d61fd/ucr-images-v1/Images/image-176940

2.2.2. Role of Plasma in the Circulatory System

In the intricate structure of the circulatory system, plasma is a very important component as the fluid part that sustains and supports cellular and metabolic processes in the body. Since roughly 55% of all the blood content, plasma contains mostly water with additional required proteins, nutrients, hormones, and waste. This yellowish fluid not only serves to transport red and white blood cells but also to supply the proper amount of nutrients and hormones to organs and tissues. One of the major functions of plasmas is a result of its capability to maintain osmotic pressure, a process which equalizes fluid flow between the tissue surrounding the blood vessels and the blood vessels themselves. This osmotic balance is vital to blood pressure and circulation maintenance, illustrating plasma's intrinsic connection to body homeostasis. Plasma proteins are also significant in many bodily processes, such as immune protection, coagulation, and colloidal osmotic pressure control. Proteins like albumin regulate fluid distribution and blood volume by drawing water into circulation. Additionally, globulins are essential in immune defense, while clotting factors are essential in hemostasis following injury. The interactive dynamic between these proteins enables the plasma to respond favorably to physiological stresses, like hemorrhage or infection, to enhance the circulatory system's resilience. The presence of these proteins in the plasma reflects the sophistication and diversity of the circulatory system and its emphasis on the function of plasma as a transport medium but also as a participant in the body's defense mechanisms—a fact reinforced by recent findings on cardiovascular health and disease regulation (Scott W Biggins et al., 2021). Above all, plasma is also involved in the removal of metabolic waste products and, therefore, is critical to homeostatic control. As cells digest nutrients to supply energy, they produce waste products, such as carbon dioxide and urea, which must be removed from the body to prevent toxic accumulation. Plasma transports these waste products to organs of elimination, primarily the kidneys and lungs, where they are excreted. The economy of the transport process operates to highlight plasma's inherent contribution to the circulatory system's total function. Also, plasma's fluid-like nature guarantees that it is able to flow freely through the intricate network of blood vessels, allowing for the unhindered distribution of nutrients as well as the elimination of wastes. This critical function of plasma in the sustenance of metabolic balance is highlighted in the ongoing research into finding out how plasma composition varies with various states of pathology, for example, systemic inflammatory responses (Ponikowski et al., 2016).

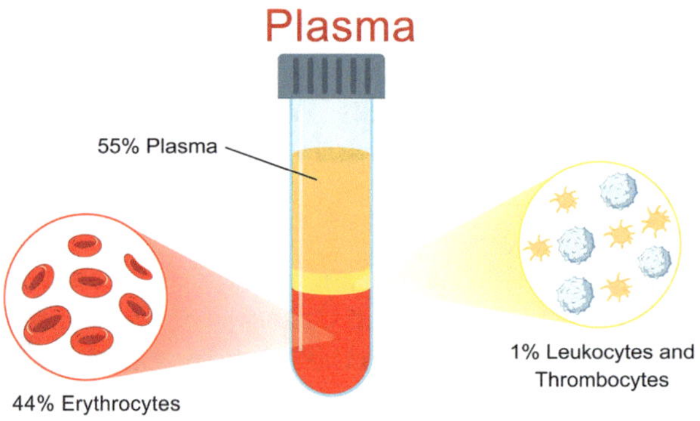

Figure 2.9. Plasma.

Source: https://assets.lybrate.com/imgs/tic/enadp/image-of-the-plasma.jpg

2.2.3. Importance of Hemoglobin and Oxygen Transport

The process of circulation is fundamentally reliant on hemoglobin's role in oxygen delivery, a critical function that underlies cellular respiration and general metabolic homeostasis. Hemoglobin, a protein complex molecule within erythrocytes, possesses a unique property to bind oxygen in oxygen-rich environments such as lungs and release it in low-oxygen tissue environments. This process is essential because oxygen is needed for the formation of adenosine triphosphate (ATP), the energy currency of the cell. Abnormalities in hemoglobin function, particularly due to alterations in erythrocyte morphology or membrane composition, can adversely impact oxygen delivery and thereby tissue function and health. Research indicates that patients with cardiovascular diseases (CVD) are prone to show impressive changes in erythrocyte properties that prevent efficient delivery of oxygen, indicating the need for treatments that restore hemoglobin's capacity for efficient oxygen delivery (Gromova et al., 2016). Additionally, research on synthesizing new treatments to enhance oxygen transport is becoming increasingly prominent as an agenda in healthcare settings, particularly under conditions of anemia and other blood-related disorders. Traditional methods of increasing oxygen transport have involved erythrocyte transfusions, but the generally limited effectiveness of hemoglobin-based products has led to reconsideration of methods to increase oxygen-carrying capacity (OCC). Current research into hemoglobin-based oxygen therapeutics seeks to enhance these products with higher oxygen affinity and focused delivery to oxygen-deficient regions in the body. But the problem is in dealing with the resulting adverse functional effects of these therapeutic approaches, pointing to the challenge of achieving enhanced oxygen delivery without exacerbating vascular issues (Acharya et al., 2014). In addition to developing hemoglobin-based treatments, other methods also aim to increase the overall oxygen delivery capacity (ODC) through increased blood flow and the normalization of microvascular function. One of the most hopeful strategies is the use of hyperviscous plasma expanders, which increase ODC via enhanced perfusion and oxygenation of tissues. These drugs, like polyethylene glycol conjugate albumin (PEG-Alb), improve blood shear properties to enable greater blood flow and thereby increase oxygen delivery to organs and tissues. This multi-dimensional approach not only minimizes the risks of anemia but also enhances the clearance of metabolic waste products in tissues that are deficient in oxygen. Therefore, integrative approaches that target optimizing hemoglobin function as well as perfusion are among the vanguard approaches to treatment alternatives in clinical circulatory disease management (Acharya et al., 2014).

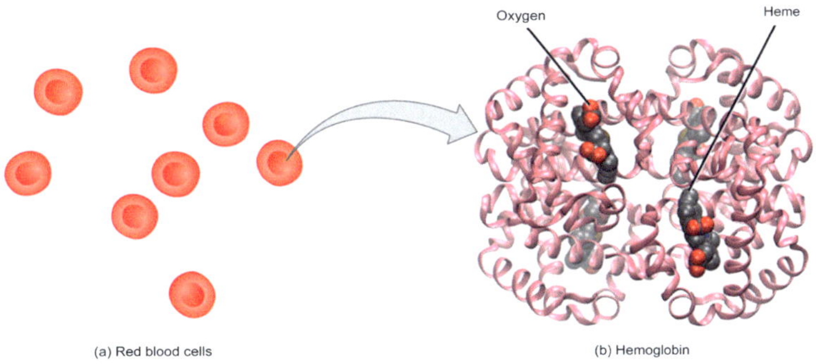

Figure 2.10. The protein inside (a) red blood cells that carries oxygen to cells and carbon dioxide to the lungs is (b) hemoglobin. Hemoglobin is made up of four symmetrical subunits, each containing a heme group. Iron in heme binds oxygen. It is the iron in hemoglobin that gives blood its red color.

Source: https://s3-us-west-2.amazonaws.com/courses-images/wp-content/uploads/sites/1223/2017/02/08195831/Figure_39_04_01-1024x432.jpg

Test Your Knowledge

1. What are the 3 components of blood?
2. What is the role of plasma in the circulatory system?

2.3. Circulatory Pathways

Learning Outcome

1. Understand the function and significance of systemic circulation
2. Describe the process and importance of pulmonary circulation
3. Describe the coronary circulation

Circulatory pathways are vital in the function as the necessary pathways for the distribution of blood, nutrients, and other essentials to the rest of the body. This intricate system includes the cardiovascular system, which includes the heart, blood vessels, and blood. It begins with oxygen-laden blood pushed out of the left ventricle into the aorta, then travels through progressively smaller arteries, arterioles, and to the capillaries. These micro-capillaries are used in exchanging gases, nutrients, and waste products between the tissues and the blood. On the way back, the blood that is deoxygenated moves from the capillaries through the venules and veins and ends up entering the heart through the superior and inferior vena cava. Such a lifelong cycle, pivotal to homeostasis, exemplifies the dynamic nature of circulatory pathways, which are fundamental to maintaining life. Spleen, as a significant component of circulatory pathways in the body, unites immunologic response with its primary role of filtration of blood. As the largest lymphoid secondary organ, the spleen accommodates various immune cells to engage with blood-borne infections and abnormal red blood cells. The unique structure of the spleen enhances filtration of blood, which promotes low-probability encounters between antigen-presenting cells (APCs) and lymphocytes. These contacts are crucial for the activation of the adaptive immune response to infections of the system. The spleen anatomy allows it to provide a specialized setting where T and B cells can be activated and differentiated in response to antigenic targets within the blood. The normal operation of the spleen demonstrates the connection between circulatory pathways and immune system activation, emphasizing the importance of the organ in a person's health (Steven M Lewis et al., 2019). Angiogenesis, or new blood vessel formation, is a key function of circulatory systems that is important for maintaining the health and functioning of tissues.

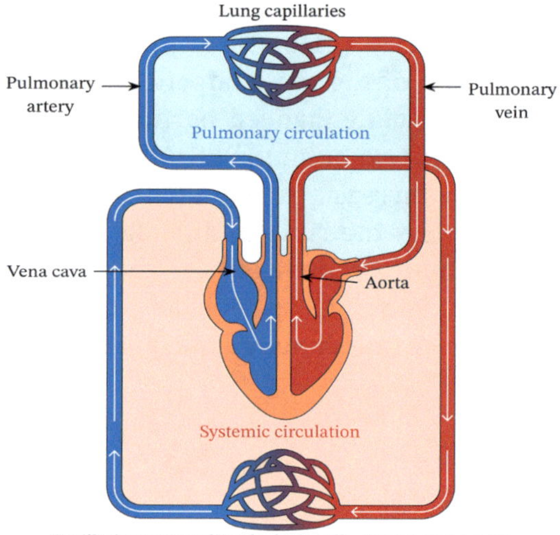

Figure 2.11. A diagram representing the two pathways involved in the double circulatory system—pulmonary circulation and systemic circulation.

Source: https://images.nagwa.com/figures/explainers/912123271719/5.svg

This is a process not only critical in development but also of very critical significance in wound healing and response to hypoxia. Angiogenesis is the growth and migration of endothelial cells to form new capillaries. Understanding angiogenesis is critical because it addresses disease conditions such as cancer, where tumor growth relies on the formation of new blood vessels for the supply of nutrients and oxygen. Bioassays of angiogenesis have now become a focus point in biomedical studies, revealing its mechanism and therapeutic targets. Through its investigation, scientists are increasingly unraveling how circulatory pathways adapt during disease and health, ultimately leading to advances in medical treatment (Nowak P-Sliwinska et al., 2018).

2.3.1. Systemic Circulation: Function and Significance

Systemic circulation is the primary pathway through which oxygenated blood is delivered to the entire body and gives vital organs and tissues adequate nourishment. Oxygenated blood from the left ventricle of the heart flows into the aorta, then divides into various arteries, arterioles, and finally capillaries. The capillaries facilitate the oxygen, nutrient, and waste exchange at a cellular level. Besides transferring required materials, systemic circulation is needed for the maintenance of homeostasis, regulation of blood pressure, and coordination of physiological reactions. The relationship between cardiac output and peripheral vascular resistance regulates the efficiency of this circulatory route, highlighting its significance for maintaining life. As the central oxygen source for the body and the primary means of nutrient supply, systemic circulation is not simply a biomechanical phenomenon; it is fundamental to overall health and well-being. Systemic circulation may be more satisfactorily explained by mathematical modeling, which models the dynamics of blood flow and pressure control. A good example is the closed-loop mathematical model of the cardiovascular system that explains mechanisms for generating signals such as the ballistocardiogram (BCG). The model describes how arterial pressure waveforms are influenced by many factors, including the contractility of the heart and vascular stiffness. This modeling not only predicts the characteristic BCG peaks but also detects variations in these signals that agree with pathological states. Therefore, the use of this model extends far beyond theoretical application; it has direct practical application in clinical settings, as it can be utilized to maximize BCG sensing devices for enhanced diagnosis. Thus, mathematical modeling of systemic circulation adds a quantitative procedure to the assessment of circulatory health, revealing the intricate nuances underlying the mundane processes of physiology (Despins et al., 2019). Furthermore, the overall explanation of systemic circulation typically gains from well-established paradigms, like the Guyton model, which is especially robust in modeling human cardiovascular responses under varied conditions.

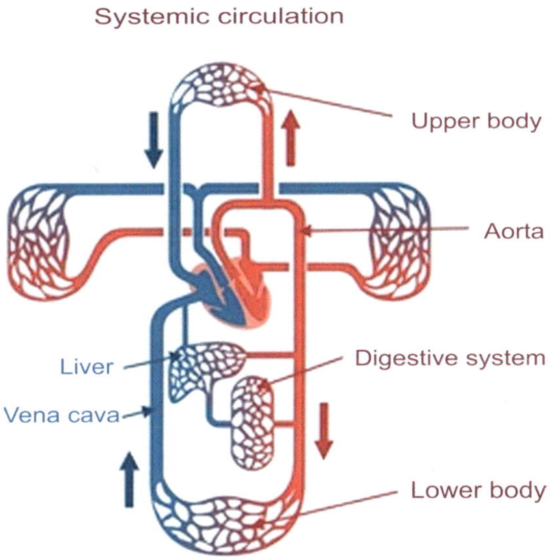

Figure 2.12. Systemic circulation.

Source: https://www.shutterstock.com/image-vector/circulatory-system-260nw-366326216.jpg

This model nicely portrays how the fluid dynamic phases, the balance of electrolytes, and circulatory regulation interact, particularly under stressors like weightlessness. Research on such interactions may enable scientists to gain insight into the test imposed by such conditions on circulatory efficiency and regulation. Guyton's model not only clarifies the physiological significance of systemic circulation but also highlights its importance in diverse conditions, including space-flight studies that require alterations in cardiovascular control.

For the most part, systemic circulation importance is irrevocably linked to health consequences as well as the comprehension of complex biological systems and is thus a crucial subject in human physiology discussion (Leonard et al., 2025a,b).

2.3.2. Pulmonary Circulation: Process and Importance

Pulmonary circulation represents an essential part of the entire circulatory system, as it performs the key role in the gas exchange, making sure that oxygen is delivered to the tissues and carbon dioxide is eliminated. The process starts as the deoxygenated blood flows back to the heart through the systemic circulation and gets into the right atrium and then the right ventricle. This blood is then pumped by the right ventricle into the pulmonary arteries that carry it to the lungs. Blood is circulated through complex networks of capillaries in the lungs, around the alveoli, where it takes up oxygen and gives out carbon dioxide. The effective operation of this system stresses the significance of the pulmonary circulation in the provision of homeostasis and satisfaction of the metabolic needs of the body.

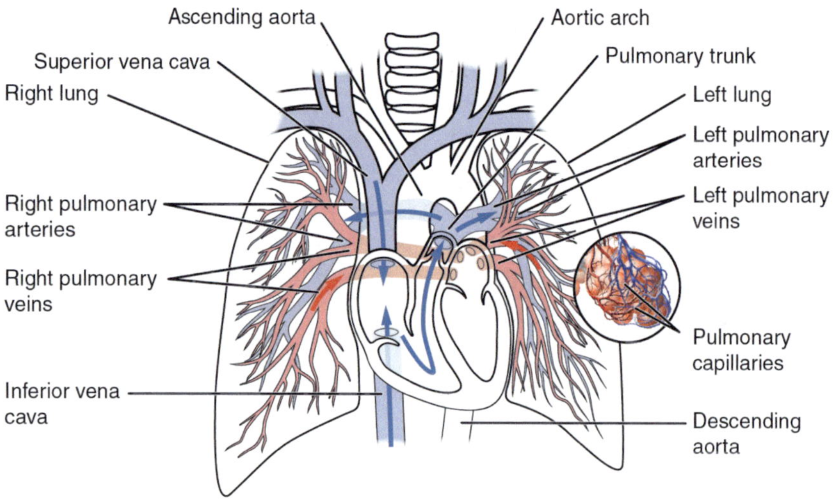

Figure 2.13. Pulmonary circulation.

Source: https://upload.wikimedia.org/wikipedia/commons/3/36/2119_Pulmonary_Circuit.jpg

After being oxygenated, the blood is drained out of the lungs via the pulmonary veins back into the heart, into the left atrium. This circulation stage is critical, since it leads to the distribution of freshly oxygenated blood to the systemic circulation, which nourishes vital organs and tissues. Any compromise of this circulation can carry important implications for health. For instance, conditions such as pulmonary hypertension or chronic obstructive pulmonary disease (COPD) can disrupt normal pulmonary circulation, leading to insufficient oxygen supply to the body. The significance of the strong pulmonary circulation in the physiology of the body and the wider perspective of cardiopulmonary wellbeing can be explained by the knowledge of these relations. Moreover, unlike the systemic circulation, the pulmonary circulation dynamics are affected by numerous external forces, among which are gravitational and inertial forces, that may change the hemodynamics in various conditions, e.g., in weightlessness in space. Physiological investigations have provided evidence that the consequences of these forces can have important implications on cardiovascular and respiratory interactions, and this underlines the sophisticated interactions of the circulatory system. The importance of these nuances is that they will allow finding effective solutions in the treatment of pulmonary disorders and the normal operation of the circulatory system as a whole. As the Guyton model and related studies illustrate, the mathematical models of circulatory and fluid regulation provide essential frameworks for analyzing these processes, particularly in scenarios that challenge the body's physiological norms, such as in space (Leonard, 2025c; Wood et al.).

2.3.3. Coronary Circulation: Blood Supply to the Heart Muscle

The coronary circulation is the critical system that ensures the myocardium, a requirement for preserving the integrity of the heart's function and of the circulatory system as well, is kept healthy. Comprising the two coronary arteries and their subsequent branches, this blood vessel network allows for oxygen- and nutrient-enriched blood to be supplied to the heart muscle. The left and right coronary arteries are aortic branches that serve the respective sides of the heart. Worth noting is that the left coronary artery also further divides into the circumflex artery and anterior interventricular artery, which serve important regions such as the left atrium and ventricle. Disruptions in coronary flow can lead to ischemia, a condition that underscores the interdependence of coronary flow and cardiac health, illustrating its significance within the grand framework of circulatory function.

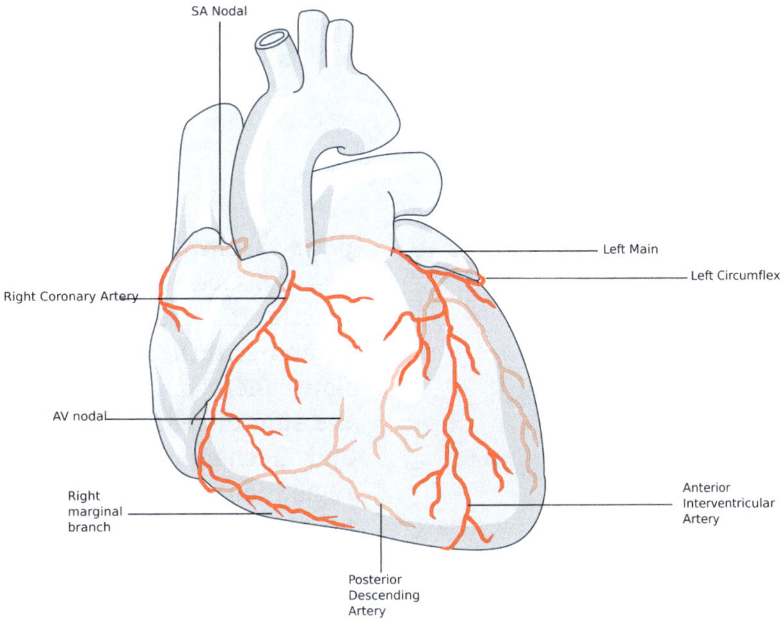

Figure 2.14. Coronary circulation.

Source: https://partone.litfl.com/resources/coronary.svg

In explaining the function and potential pathology of coronary flow, one must comprehend the intricacy of this system. Coronary arteries not only provide oxygenated blood but also help remove waste products of metabolism from cardiac tissue. Importantly, the dense capillary network in the myocardium permits maximum exchange of nutrients. Various factors, like coronary artery disease (CAD), may interfere with blood flow, leading to severe end effects such as myocardial infarction. The necessity to maintain a coronary circulation free of any unhealthy situation cannot be exaggerated, as seen in numerous clinical guidelines. The health practitioners are advised to observe established guidelines to know that complexities concerning coronary arteries and blood supply should be their benchmark for preventive and therapeutic treatment of patients as they work on individual cases (Members ATF et al., 2014) (Windecker et al., 2014). An understanding of the physiology of coronary circulation is reinforced with an appreciation of the interface between this system and broader metabolic activities. The heart, more often than not a muscle of muscles, requires a massive blood supply to maintain its relentless rhythmic contractions. During physical exercise, the myocardial requirement for oxygen rises and demands moment-to-moment control of coronary blood flow. Endothelial cells lining coronary arteries secrete vasodilators such as nitric oxide in response to an increased workload of the heart, demonstrating the perfect versatility of this vascular bed. Paradoxically, whereas physical exercise is performed, coronary flow increases, whereas to avoid potential ischemic events, the underlying tissues must be healthy. Therefore, the intricate relationship between coronary perfusion, cardiac function, and metabolic need remains the focus of research and clinical activity, with important implications for cardiovascular health in the circulatory system.

Test Your Knowledge

1. What is the significance of systemic circulation?
2. What is the importance of pulmonary circulation?

2.4. Regulation of Blood Flow

Learning Outcome

1. Know the mechanisms of blood pressure regulation
2. Understand the role of the autonomic nervous system
3. Describe the hormonal influences on circulation

The circulatory system plays a critical role in regulating circulation to supply tissues with oxygen and nutrients and effectively remove products of metabolism. Regulation is mostly concerned with the integration of local, hormonal, and neural mechanisms to regulate the diameter and distribution of blood vessels. For instance, during exercise, the autonomic nervous system plays a central role. The sympathetic nervous system is activated, which causes vasodilation of muscles that are exercising and vasoconstriction of non-critical areas, hence optimizing blood flow where it is needed the most. Moreover, the sum of reactions of many chemoreceptors and mechanoreceptors allows for continuous regulation of blood pressure and blood flow, essentially responding in real time to both internal and external needs. The fine balance maintained by these mechanisms is an indication of the intricacies of circulatory blood flow regulation. A key aspect of blood flow control is the operation of reflexive control mechanisms. Central command, baroreflex, and chemoreflex are essential neural pathways that provide cardiovascular regulation during exercise and at rest. Central command causes alterations in blood pressure and heart rate in anticipation of exercise, essentially preparing the cardiovascular system for increased demand. The baroreflex is aware of changes in arterial blood pressure and takes action to re-establish homeostasis, such as modifying heart rate and vessel diameter. These are especially important during dynamic exercise when metabolic demand by the muscle increases significantly, as outlined in Crisafulli et al. (2014). Understanding these neural reflexes enhances our knowledge of the ways that the body maintains balance in various circumstances and helps to develop effective interventions for cardiovascular illnesses. Additionally, mathematical modeling has provided insightful information regarding the regulation of blood flow, particularly in harsh conditions such as space travel. The Guyton model is a groundbreaking theory for understanding the circulatory system and its control mechanisms, as presented in Leonard et al. (2025c) This model gives a complete description of fluid dynamics, cardiovascular regulation, and electrolyte balance that allows researchers to model the physiological response to stressors like microgravity. Researchers can predict how blood flow adapts in new environments through the application of such models and thus enlarge our knowledge of human physiology beyond Earth's limits. Lastly, the integration of empirical evidence and mathematical modeling enhances our understanding of blood flow control within the cardiovascular system, with its importance for maintaining global health as well as adapting to environmental stresses.

2.4.1. Mechanisms of Blood Pressure Regulation

Regulation of blood pressure is a complex process involving multiple mechanisms that are regulated based on physiological needs and maintain homeostasis within the circulatory system. Regulation mechanisms are mostly divided into neural, hormonal, and intrinsic. Neural regulation is primarily achieved by the autonomic nervous system, which regulates vascular tone via sympathetic and parasympathetic systems. The sympathetic stimulation results in vasoconstriction by releasing norepinephrine, thereby increasing the blood pressure. Hormonal regulation, such as that by the renin-angiotensin-aldosterone system, helps maintain blood pressure by regulating fluid balance and vascular resistance. Such intricate relationships illustrate the maintenance of proper blood pressure in the body under various conditions of stress and activity, culminating in perfusion of tissues to maintain optimal function. Body-mechanism-based mechanisms, particularly those that involve microvascular regulation, are significant regulators of blood pressure homeostasis. The microcirculation provides exchange of blood-borne nutrients and waste products with tissues at a level necessary for cellular health and integrity. Central regulatory mechanisms in microcirculation are neurohumoral, myogenic, and metabolic regulation that control arteriolar blood flow according to local tissue requirements. The endothelium is an active tissue-blood interface that controls vascular responses by releasing signaling molecules. Strikingly, glycocalyx on endothelial cells regulates fluid flow and vascular permeability, emphasizing its vital function in sustaining hydrostatic and osmotic pressure equilibrium of the circulatory system. Clarification of these microscopic processes illuminates how local conditions affect overall blood pressure regulation and overall health (Tsapaeva and Tsapaev, 2024). Developmental alterations also have an effect on blood pressure control, demonstrating the importance of considering life stages in the investigation of vascular function. In the neonatal period, structural and functional characteristics of the cardiovascular system are greatly altered compared to adults, and lower values of blood pressure follow as a consequence of them. In growth, mechanisms controlling contraction of vascular smooth muscle, such as alterations in ion channel activity and calcium sensitivity, become mature. These changes are vital for synchronizing the regulation of blood pressure with the growing demands of the developing organism. Moreover, they reflect the complexity of blood pressure control throughout life, and how the combination of vascular smooth muscle cell differentiation and maturation illustrates this. The developmental approach underscores the importance of accounting for age-related factors in the investigation of the pathophysiological mechanisms of hypertension and cardiovascular disease (Gaynullina et al., 2024).

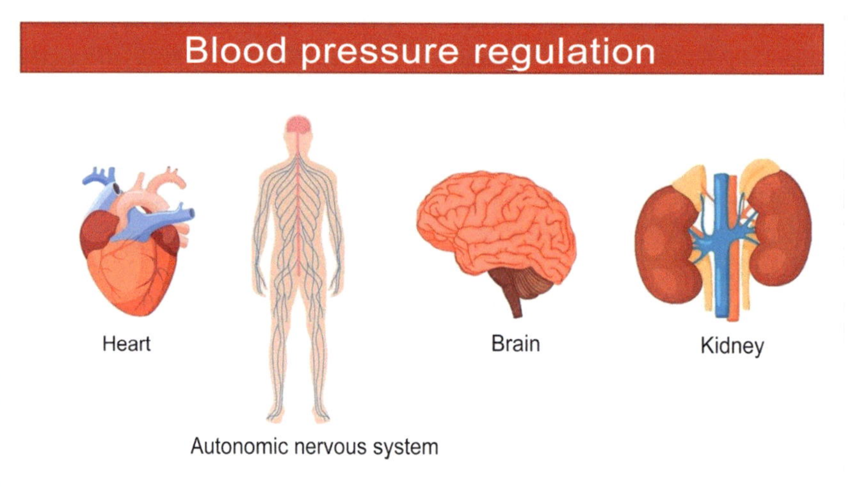

Figure 2.15. Blood pressure regulation.

Source: https://i.ytimg.com/vi/6n2aKipt4U0/maxresdefault.jpg?sqp=-oaymwEmCIAKENAF8quKqQMa8AEB-AH-CYAC0AWKAgwIABABGH8gFSgTMA8=&rs=AOn4CLAYYUu1Ys-PHH9EWUrJzSKDw9_uqQ

2.4.2. Role of the Autonomic Nervous System

The autonomic nervous system (ANS) plays a pivotal role in regulating the functions of the circulatory system, influencing both heart rate and vascular tone. It has two major branches that include the sympathetic and parasympathetic nervous systems that act in an antagonistic manner to ensure homeostasis. The sympathetic nervous system stimulates the fight or flight response, which results in tachycardia, contractility, and vasoconstriction of some vascular beds. On the other hand, the parasympathetic nervous system generates the rest and digest condition that decreases the heart rate and induces vasodilation. This is a fine balance between sympathetic stimulation and parasympathetic inhibition, which is important to maintain adequate blood flow and pressure changes in response to various physical and emotional stressors, and to ensure that tissues receive just the right amount of oxygen and nutrients as required. More recent research has employed mathematical modeling (e.g., Guyton model) to highlight the significance of the ANS in the analysis of the cardiovascular system. Simulation and analysis can allow the researcher to investigate the effect of changes in autonomic tone on hemodynamic parameters during different stresses. For instance, during weightlessness, the mathematical models adapt to analyze how cardiovascular fluid and electrolyte regulation is maintained, shedding light on the intricate connections between the ANS and circulatory responses to environmental changes (Leonard et al., 2025a,b,c). This modelling strategy has enabled a better comprehension of the cardiovascular systems adaptations during duress, which has indicated the need for the autonomic nervous system in facilitating favorable physiological adjustments when external circumstances change. To enlarge on the role of the ANS, empirical research has proved the great impact of the ANS on the individual cardiovascular performance through the measurement of dominant autonomic patterns. In a study of medical students under examination stress, the students with sympathetic predominant activity had divergent hemodynamic parameters from those who had vagotonic regulation. The findings were that people with high sympathetic tone exhibited high stroke volumes and cardiac outputs, but presented with low diastolic blood pressure. These findings elucidate the relevance of neurohumoral mechanisms in cardiovascular regulation and adaptation, emphasizing that variations in autonomic influence substantially affect circulatory efficiency (Spitsin et al., 2023). This highlights the significance of the autonomic nervous system not only in the maintenance of cardiovascular function but also in providing optimal flexibility to stressors, which is imperative for general health and performance.

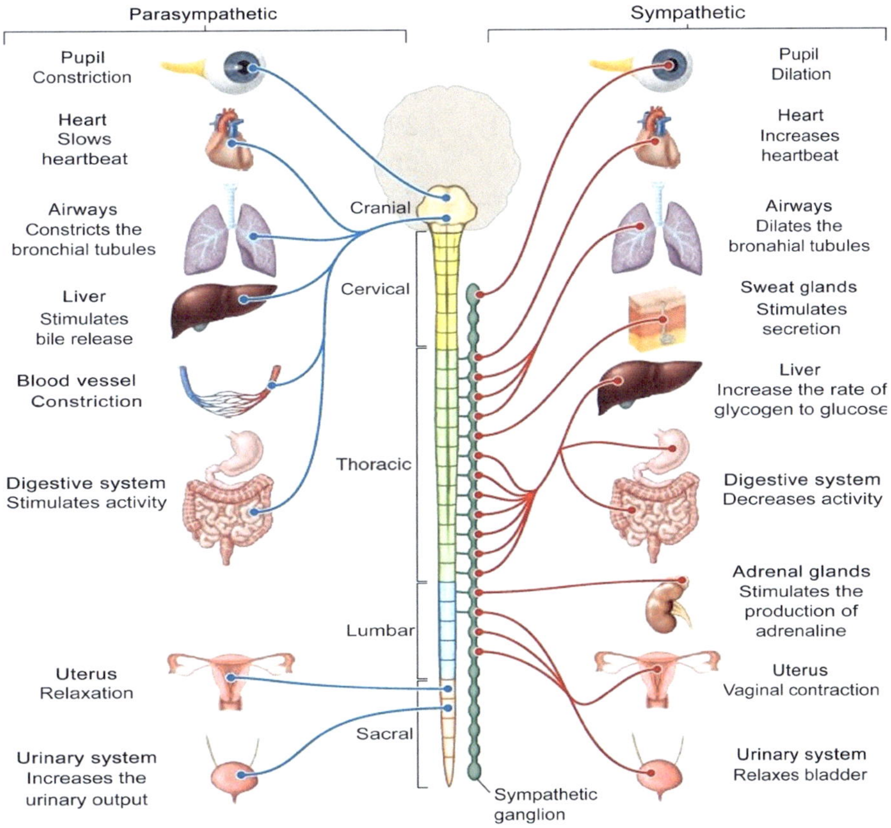

Figure 2.16. Autonomic nervous system.

Source: https://www.shutterstock.com/image-illustration/parasympathetic-sympathetic-nervous-systems-various-600nw-2464371745.jpg

2.4.3. Hormonal Influences on Circulation

The action of hormones with circulation is a built-in characteristic of the circulatory system's function. Adrenaline, norepinephrine, and angiotensin II are hormones that have significant effects on regulating blood flow and vascular resistance. For instance, under stress or exercise, adrenaline secreted by the adrenal glands increases heart rate and contractility, thus increasing cardiac output. This regulation is required to provide tissues with an adequate amount of oxygen and nutrients within a proper time. The RAAS also delicately maintains blood pressure by controlling blood volume and vascular tone. The complex action of these hormones allows the body to promptly respond to various physiological demands, proving the need for hormonal regulation in achieving circulatory homeostasis. Fluid and electrolyte balance is also closely linked to hormonal action, particularly under physiological stress. Aldosterone and antidiuretic hormone (ADH) are some of the hormones that have a key function in regulating the activity of the kidneys in the conservation of water and electrolytes, thus affecting blood volume and tension. For instance, aldosterone promotes sodium reabsorption and potassium secretion in the renal system, leading to expanded blood volume and, consequently, blood pressure. Similarly, ADH enhances the reabsorption of water from the kidney collecting ducts to maintain fluid in dehydrated conditions. All of them work together, as implied by simulations accounting for their regulatory networks under various scenarios. These endocrine responses can have a significant impact on circulation, particularly during space travel, where fluid distribution is influenced by microgravity, underscoring the key role of these hormones in systemic circulation (Leonard et al., 2025b). In addition, the interaction of multiple hormonal inputs imparts a significant impact on cardiovascular dynamics. The synergy of multiple hormones has the potential to alter circulatory variables in ways that enhance total physiological performance. For example, the complex mathematical models that examine fluid and electrolyte balance in space flight physiology illustrate how the pulsatile cardiovascular model may be affected by the interaction between hormones like ADH and renin-angiotensin (Leonard et al., 2025b). The models become essential to the understanding of systemic circulation changes, particularly in extreme environments where conventional physiological condition-based responses may be compromised. By utilizing advanced simulation techniques, researchers can investigate the function of hormonal regulation to maintain blood pressure and flow and, in doing so, increase our understanding of circulatory adaptations. Such knowledge is vital to the implementation of countermeasures against coping with physiological challenges under harsh conditions, validating the extreme influence of hormones on the circulatory system.

Test Your Knowledge

1. What are the mechanisms that regulate blood pressure?
2. What is the role of the autonomic nervous system?

2.5. Common Circulatory System Disorders

Learning Outcome

1. Know the causes and effects of hypertension
2. Describe the development and consequences of atherosclerosis
3. Describe the risk factors associated with heart attacks and strokes

The circulatory system is predisposed to a variety of disorders that can lead to serious disability in its function and result in serious complications. Some of the most common circulatory system disorders include heart failure, coronary heart disease, and high blood pressure or hypertension. Hypertension, which has been referred to as the silent killer, is a highly dangerous state because it is non-symptomatic in nature, leading to long-term heart and blood vessel damage when not corrected. Similarly, coronary artery disease is caused by the deposition of plaque in the coronary vessels, reducing the supply of blood to the heart muscle and leading to angina and myocardial infarction. Such conditions bear testimony to the fact that early detection and treatment are necessary to offset the consequences of chronic circulatory diseases, which eventually take the form of severe cardiovascular events. The second important disorder of the circulatory system is cardiomyopathy, in which the heart muscle wears out, ultimately compromising its pumping ability. The disorder can have various causes, from genetic to viral infections to long-term exposure to toxic agents. Studies have shown that neuregulin-1 (NRG 1), secreted by endothelial cells, is involved in cardiomyocyte health and repair, particularly in cardiomyopathy (Sh W. Al – Sh Z. Al – Zuhairi et al., 2024). Identification of molecular pathways, such as the NRG 1/ErbB pathway, is crucial to fashion therapeutic interventions that can potentially reverse or alleviate the severity of cardiomyopathy and recover cardiac function. Inflammatory pathways also contribute to circulatory system disease, and an excellent example is atherosclerosis. Atherosclerosis is defined as the formation of plaques on arterial walls, leading to narrowed arteries and reduced blood flow. Atherosclerosis is typically linked with metabolic disorders and inflammatory bowel disease (IBD), indicative of a sophisticated interaction of body systems. Recent research suggests the Western lifestyle and diet are perpetuators of metabolic inflammation responsible for causing or exacerbating atherosclerosis (Adolph et al., 2024). Thus, controlling these underlying lifestyle problems is vital not only for circulatory but also for general metabolic health, implying the utility of holistic approaches in treatment as well as prevention.

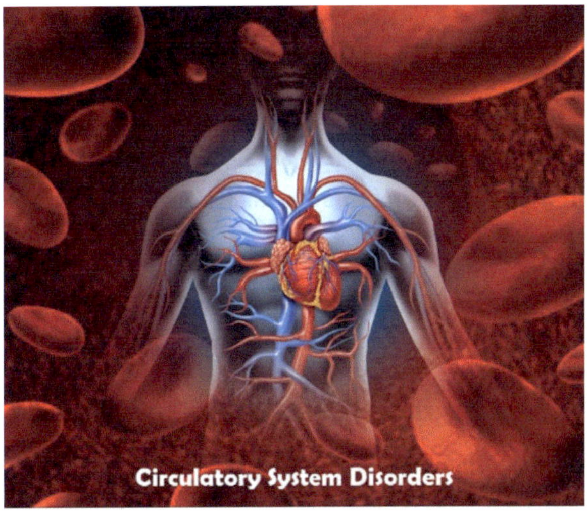

Figure 2.17. Circulatory System Disorders.

Source: https://d1qumhq2zx0vxs.cloudfront.net/ArticleImages/CirculatorySystemDis_19-08-2016_01-56-50-PM.jpg

2.5.1. Hypertension: Causes and Effects

High blood pressure, also known as hypertension, is a multifactorial health condition, and its etiological factors are varied, contributing to the development of this health condition. Among them, lifestyle habits, including high salt consumption, inactivity, and obesity, have leading roles. Additionally, these environmental factors can be further enhanced by genetic orientations, resulting in greater tendencies to develop hypertension. Psychosocial factors such as stress and socioeconomic status also play an important role in the regulation of blood pressure. This kind of complex interaction of factors requires extensive measures of public health that are oriented to prevention. Both modifiable and non-modifiable risk factors should be addressed by effective management strategies that are aimed at decreasing the occurrence of hypertension and its complications, which means that more attention should be drawn to awareness and health education programs in different populations. Consequences of hypertension go well beyond short-term unpleasant sensations and severely affect the state of cardiovascular health and well-being in general. When hypertension becomes persistent, it exerts long-term pressure on the heart and may cause some conditions like left ventricular hypertrophy and heart failure, among others. The connection between hypertension and the emergence of coronary artery disease is especially problematic, since high blood pressure is a decisive factor in atherosclerosis. The subsequent stiffening and constriction of arteries may lead to dire developments like a heart attack or a stroke. Notably, epidemiological studies indicate that high blood pressure-related cardiovascular diseases are a leading cause of morbidity and mortality globally (Parveen and Devika 2022). The health consequences are immense, and thus, further research and specific treatment strategies are needed to alleviate these risks. The existing sources stress that there is a strong correlation between hypertension and a range of cardiovascular conditions, which creates the need to address this issue with specific medical tools as soon as possible. Studies have shown that hypertensive patients may experience structural and functional alterations in the heart, as illustrated in the context of the Chornobyl disaster survivors (N/A, 2021). Such changes usually appear in the form of augmented left ventricular hypertrophy and impaired heart functioning, which aggravate the dangers of hypertension. Therefore, it is necessary to identify people with comorbid conditions to maximize treatment plans. The most important to enhancing the outcomes in patients with hypertension and preventing the development of cardiovascular diseases is interdisciplinary treatment that combines lifestyle changes with medication therapies. These complex dynamics are important to understand in the continuing strategy of public health with regard to hypertension as a major modifiable risk factor in the bigger picture of the health of the circulatory system.

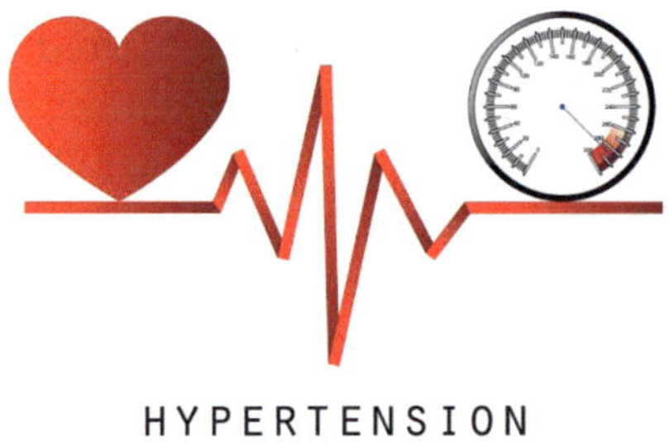

Figure 2.18. Hypertension.

Source: https://ijcscardiol.org/wp-content/uploads/2021/02/shutterstock_411862570-1024x737.x61798.jpg

2.5.2. Atherosclerosis: Development and Consequences

Atherosclerosis development is a complex process that involves several biochemical and physiological changes in the arterial wall. The disease is largely characterized by the accumulation of lipids, inflammatory cells, and fibrous materials, and atherosclerosis often begins with endothelial injury resulting from conditions such as hypertension, smoking, and hypercholesterolemia. These factors result in endothelial dysfunction, which allows low-density lipoprotein (LDL) cholesterol to penetrate into the arterial wall. Over time, these lipids are oxidized and activate inflammatory responses, attracting macrophages that phagocytose the oxidized lipids and subsequently become foam cells. This foam cell buildup, together with smooth muscle cell growth, forms atheromatous plaque, destabilizes, and leads to significant cardiovascular events, highlighting the complex pathogenesis of atherosclerosis (Sh W. Al – Sh Z. Al – Zuhairi et al., 2024).

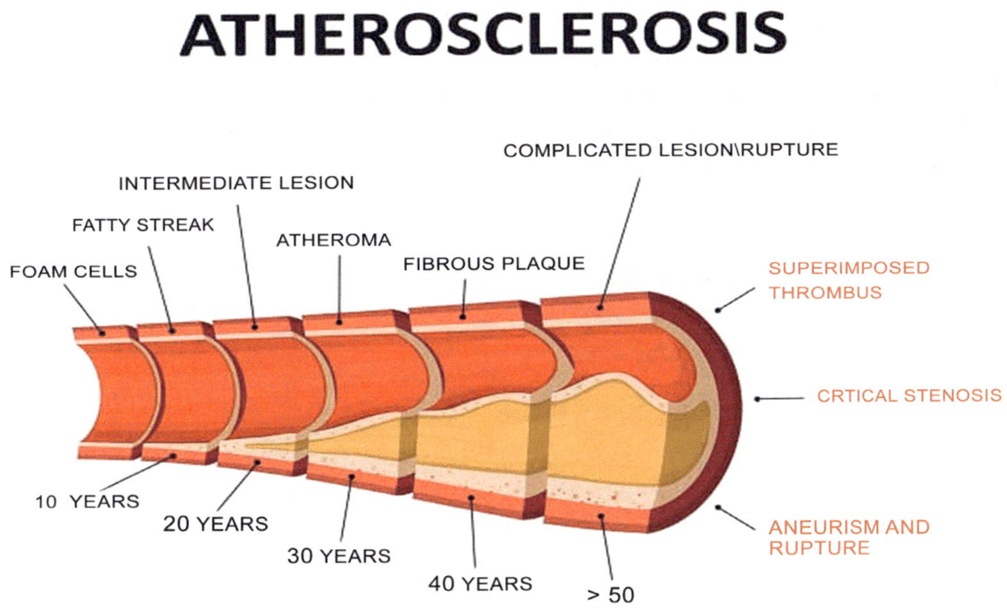

Figure 2.19. The Progression of Atherosclerosis.

Source: https://biologydictionary.net/wp-content/uploads/2017/03/The-Progression-of-Atherosclerosis.jpg

The manifestations of atherosclerosis extend beyond the mere accumulation of plaques within the arteries; they have profound consequences for overall cardiovascular health as well as systemic physiology. As atherosclerotic plaques become larger, stenosis, or narrowing of the arteries, can result, thereby compromising blood flow to vital organs. This reduction in perfusion can cause ischemic conditions, such as angina pectoris or myocardial infarction, and considerably increase the morbidity and mortality risk of cardiovascular disease. Moreover, the rupture of the plaque can cause thrombosis, possibly resulting in a complete obstruction of blood flow, further increasing the risk of heart attacks and strokes. The dynamic understanding of the causes of atherosclerosis, such as the functional aspect of Neuregulin-1 (NRG 1) in cardiac performance, highlights the importance of integrated prevention and treatment of atherosclerotic disease (Sh W. Al – Sh Z. Al – Zuhairi et al., 2024). An interfactorial understanding is essential to comprehending atherosclerosis and creating effective public health and therapeutic interventions. It has been established through research that dyslipidemia remains a key cause of the disease, though other conditions, genetic predisposition, and lifestyle also play crucial roles. Lifestyle modification is now advocated, such as the use of a heart-healthy diet, exercise, and stress reduction, which cumulatively contribute to lowering lipid levels and overall cardiovascular well-being. Also, recent studies on the molecular mechanisms of atherosclerosis reveal the need for new pharmacological agents that target the underlying processes rather than symptomatic relief alone. Targeting both the conventional and emerging risk factors, the management and treatment of atherosclerosis can be altered and improved, leading to improved prevention and management outcomes against cardiovascular disease (Askerov et al., 2024).

2.5.3. Heart Attacks and Strokes: Risk Factors and Prevention

The risk factors of heart attacks and strokes are complex, and more than one may overlap and combine in physical health issues that have a great influence on the circulatory system. Risk factors commonly seen are high blood pressure or hypertension, elevated cholesterol levels, smoking, diabetes, and obesity. High blood pressure creates greater stress on the heart and arteries, potentially causing heart attacks or strokes when the arteries become weakened. Similarly, high cholesterol results in atherosclerosis, i.e., the deposition of fatty plaques in arteries, with resulting arterial narrowing.

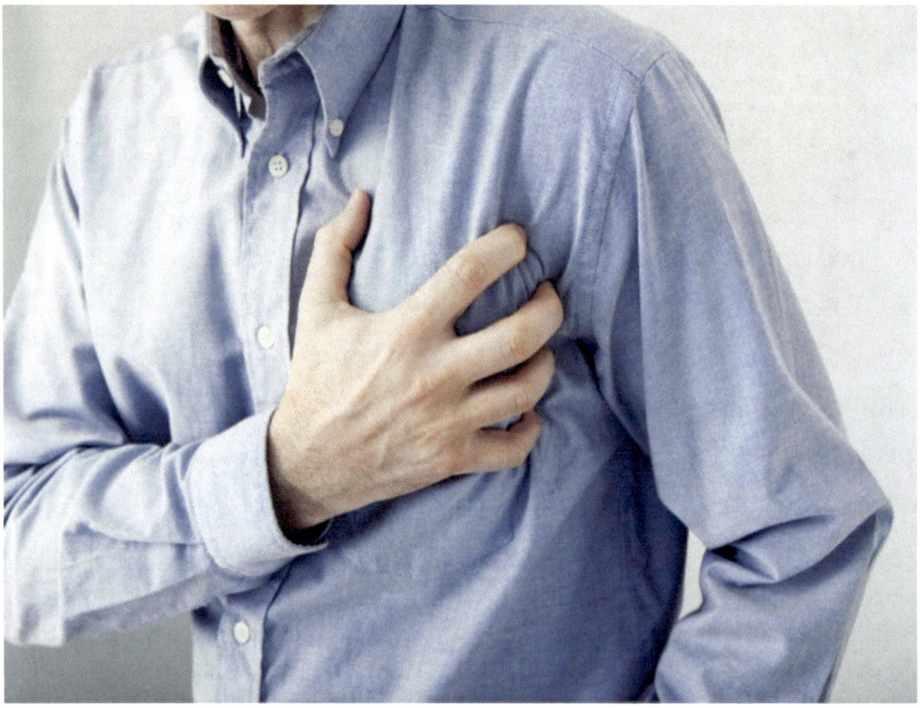

Source: https://www.tricitymed.org/wp-content/uploads/2018/06/shutterstock_174191435.jpg

These are further augmented by lifestyle factors such as physical inactivity and a diet high in saturated fats, and a multimodal approach to prevention must involve lifestyle modification as well as pharmacologic interventions, as appropriate, particularly among risk groups such as the elderly and the chronically ill. Prevention strategies play an important part in reducing the occurrence of heart attacks and strokes, particularly through the alteration of key risk factors. Consumption of a balanced diet of fruits, vegetables, whole grains, and healthy fats can significantly minimize cardiovascular risks. Regular physical activity is also necessary, as it serves to control weight not only but also overall cardiovascular wellbeing through circulation improvement and blood pressure reduction. Moreover, medical therapy progress also contributes to prevention. Studies have shown that appropriate medical therapy, such as beta-blockers, aspirin, and ACE inhibitors, can effectively reduce the risk of future cardiovascular events (David M Cutler et al.). These medications improve prognosis in patients and expand quality-adjusted survival, which highlights the worth of therapy targeted to individuals at greatest risk. The connection between migraine and stroke also deserves mention in the discussion of cardiovascular disease, as it has implications for prevention. Fresh studies show that migraine may be a standalone risk factor for ischemic stroke, particularly in some groups of patients (Balzo et al., 2016). Clinicians must keep this association in mind when assessing the risk of stroke, especially in patients with established migraines. Monitoring and treating comorbid conditions, such as patent foramen ovale (PFO), can better clarify the link between strokes and migraines, providing potential intervention strategies. In-depth comprehension of the intricacies can lead to more effective prevention measures and improved health outcomes for populations at risk, with ultimate effect towards the reduction of morbidity and mortality associated with cardiovascular diseases in the United States and globally.

Test Your Knowledge

1. What are the main causes of hypertension?
2. What is the development of atherosclerosis?

2.6. Advances in Circulatory System Research

Learning Outcome

1. Know the innovations in cardiovascular treatments
2. Understand the role of technology in monitoring heart health
3. Describe the future directions in circulatory system research

The study of developments in circulatory system research has provided significant information on molecular mechanisms underlying heterogeneous vascular diseases, of especial interest being deep vein thrombosis (DVT). Researchers have come to understand somewhat the dynamics of how thrombi might form and, depending on conditions, become dislodged and cause life threatening diseases such as pulmonary embolism. At the forefront of these findings is the delineation of the role of vascular endothelial cells (VECs) in hemostasis. These cells not only form the barrier of the vascular wall but also release regulatory factors, which maintain a balance of coagulation-anticoagulation. Furthermore, recent developments in molecular biology have placed emphasis on the pathogenesis of DVT by microRNAs (miRNAs). miRNAs are found to control VEC activity, which has great potential for understanding the pathogenesis of thrombotic disease and the development of new therapies that could better treat patients with circulatory disease (Fang et al., 2024). In addition to understanding thrombotic conditions, circulatory system research has also involved technological innovations that enhance vascular health. For instance, magnetorheological polishing technology is a new frontier in ultra-precision machining with a possible area of application in the manufacture of medical devices used for circulatory system interventions. The new development involves the employment of magnetorheological fluids that adjust their viscosity when a magnetic field is applied, resulting in improved processing accuracy and efficiency of vascular devices. By concentrating on finishing processes that accommodate the curvature of different vascular implants, scientists are capable of providing high-quality surfaces lowering the chances of thrombus formation upon implantation of these devices in the human body. This progress is a direction towards higher biocompatibility and performance of circulatory system implants, ultimately upgrading patient care quality (Lu M-M et al., 2024). The intersection of molecular science and technological innovation yields a comprehensive study of nascent and future opportunities for research in circulatory systems. An understanding of what molecules like miRNAs do enables scientists to potentially uncover new biomarkers for vascular disease and even set direct therapeutic targets. In parallel to this, the use of new manufacturing techniques also ensures that the devices intended for interfacing with the circulatory system are not only effective but safe for patients to use. As the studies continue, the collaboration of molecular biology and engineering disciplines will likely lead to increasingly sophisticated interventions for circulatory disease, holding a bright future for therapeutic opportunities. By bridging the gap between basic research and clinical practice, such breakthroughs can dramatically improve diagnostics and treatment procedures, eventually transforming patient outcomes in victims of vascular disease.

2.6.1. Innovations in Cardiovascular Treatments

The cardiovascular treatment field has seen revolutionary developments that aim to maximize patient outcomes and the efficacy of existing treatments. Of these advances, the progression of minimally invasive therapies has transformed the traditional method of managing cardiovascular illnesses. Catheter-based interventions like procedures have minimized recovery times, decreased complications, and provided patients with less traumatic avenues for compensation instead of open-heart surgeries. In addition, these innovations have also led to better precision of targeting compromised areas, thereby improving the overall safety profile of interventions. With patient-centered care being given priority, these technological advancements are a part of broader trends in healthcare aimed at more personalized treatment strategies that allow for unique patient requirements to achieve an improved cardiovascular health profile. The second significant area of innovation in cardiac therapy includes the management of acute illnesses like pulmonary embolism (PE). Severe pulmonary embolism, with the potential for creating severe complications in the form of right ventricular dysfunction, poses a significant challenge for practitioners. Traditional thrombolysis remains a common intervention; nevertheless, recent developments highlight the importance of surgical therapy as an effective option, particularly in scenarios where thrombolytic treatment is contraindicated or unsuccessful. Studies have indicated that effective risk stratification and multidisciplinary team use are able to reduce PE-related mortality from 1% in small cases to 65% for massive ones (Bellis et al., 2018). It emphasizes the need for constant enhancement of the diagnostic and management techniques, hence improving cardiovascular interventions to be safer and more efficient. Furthermore, treatment of traumatic hemorrhagic injury has emerged as an imperative area of research in cardiovascular innovation. Current treatment technologies are often inefficient, particularly in the treatment of high-pressure arterial bleeding. In addressing this challenge, researchers are producing low-cost models that are similar to the human circulatory system to allow researchers to test new treatments for bleeding in a secure environment. Such models not only reduce the barriers of entry to innovation but also enable smaller players to contribute towards developments in the treatment options at the cost of affordable, non-prohibitive simulators. Emphasized by recent studies, one of the innovative methodologies included a tripartite model used to establish the efficiency of various solutions, thus establishing effective interventions that safely translated into clinical practice (Choy et al., 2016). This spiral cycle of testing and innovation is important to the progression of the science of cardiovascular treatment, and especially in emergency and trauma environments.

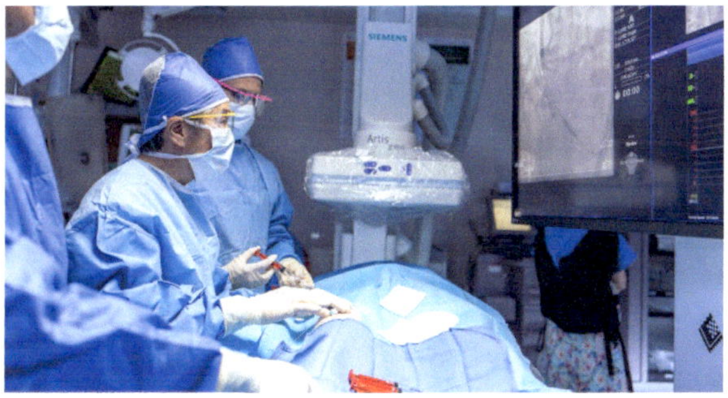

Figure 2.20. Innovations in cardiology.

Source: https://www.elcaminohealth.org/sites/default/files/2023-02/cardiology-1200x630.jpg

2.6.2. Role of Technology in Monitoring Heart Health

Technology development has greatly changed the game in the field of heart health monitoring, offering new ways of constant patient observation to both patients and medical professionals. One of the most notable developments is the introduction of Internet of Things (IoT)-enabled heart monitoring systems, which utilize pulse sensors to track heart rates in real-time. These systems enable distant monitoring, and healthcare professionals are able to detect irregularities in good time, thus enhancing patient outcomes. These sensors send the collected data that is processed and relayed to cloud platforms or mobile apps, where vital signs can be visualized and analyzed by both the patient and doctor. This non-invasive approach not only enhances patient care but also supports proactive interventions, making it a pivotal tool in managing cardiovascular health, particularly in an era where instant access to medical information is increasingly paramount (Bujunuru et al., 2025). Wearable devices, including smartwatches and fitness trackers, have also been important in keeping track of heart health. These devices are equipped with sensors that can track heart rate, rhythm, and even offer electrocardiogram (ECG) capabilities, allowing users to measure their cardiovascular metrics conveniently throughout the day. The integration of artificial intelligence (AI) algorithms further enhances the functionality of these devices, enabling them to analyze collected data and provide users with personalized feedback on their heart health. The innovation promotes individual engagement in personal wellness by empowering them with knowledge about making appropriate choices on physical exercise and lifestyle. More importantly, the immediate feedback mechanism helps in identifying potential health concerns before they escalate, showcasing how technology can empower users to maintain their heart health effectively (Bujunuru et al., 2025). The importance of technology in heart health monitoring is not limited to its personal use as it also affects the population health approach and the entire healthcare system. Using big data collected by wearable devices and IoT systems, researchers have an excellent opportunity to discover useful information about the health status of the population and the risks of developing cardiovascular diseases. Such data-driven solutions will help to create specific interventions and preventive strategies and eventually decrease the load of heart disease on the health systems. Moreover, the expandability of these monitoring solutions is in line with the increasing popularity of telehealth services, especially in rural or underserved regions. The implementation of such health monitoring technologies in daily life not only promotes improved patient outcomes but also leads to the creation of a more proactive public health system that is committed to fighting heart-related diseases.

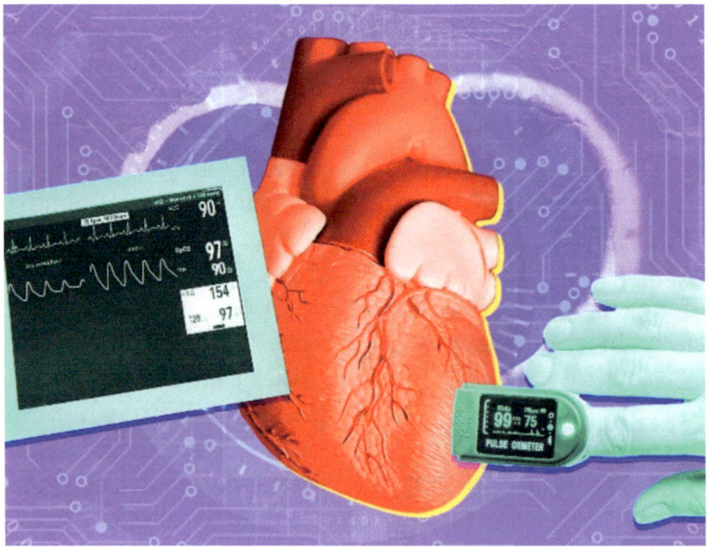

Figure 2.21. IoT monitoring devices and early detection of heart diseases.

Source: https://cdn.ai-forall.com/ifa_dev_media/How_Io_T_monitoring_devices_are_used_in_real_time_for_early_detec_787d199b2e.jpg

2.6.3. Future Directions in Circulatory System Research

With growth in circulatory system research, various advancements in mechanical circulatory support (MCS) devices are emerging as vital for cardiovascular disease control. As cardiovascular disease remains a leading cause of mortality in the United States, technological advancements in MCS are essential to care for the increasing population of patients, predicted to reach over 8 million heart failure patients by the year 2030. Evidence has indicated that heart rate variability (HRV), an objective diagnostic criterion recorded by MCS devices, can provide useful information on patient prognostics. This emergent technology, combined with machine learning software, holds the potential to make HRV into an adaptive biomarker that could optimize device responsiveness and improve patient outcomes. Validating HRV indices' predictive validity would be paramount in subsequent studies that could potentially redefine the clinician's method of monitoring and treating MCS-therapied patients (Aras et al., 2020). Another promising area of research in circulatory systems is the fusion of engineering developments with biological systems. For instance, the study of artificial organs like artificial blood and lungs points to the union of regenerative medicine and biomedical engineering. Developments in 3D bioprinting and the use of sophisticated biomaterials aim to enhance biocompatibility, coupled with the minimization of immune rejection in artificial implantable devices. These advances are particularly relevant in the context of the chronic shortage of suitable donor organs. Methods such as donor organ decellularization followed by autologous cell repopulation offer a solution that is sustainable, with the possibility of providing patients with tailored therapy with reduced immunosuppression. Multidisciplinary teams of researchers will be instrumental in surmounting the complex problem of creating functional artificial organs (Gutiérrez et al., 2025). Finally, the circulatory system's complexity necessitates ongoing exploration of system-wide responses to varied interventions and pathologies. Investigation of endothelial function in the context of vascular health is most critical, especially in aging and chronic disease. Additional research investigating the mechanistic pathways involving endothelial response can potentially provide novel therapeutic targets for cardiovascular diseases, including heart failure and peripheral artery disease. By studying the interactions between endothelial cells and the remainder of the vascular system, strategies can be formulated to optimize vascular resilience. By further research into patient-specific factors influencing vascular responses, personalized medicine strategies can be formulated to optimize treatment for individual conditions, thereby improving circulatory system therapies across a broad patient population.

Test Your Knowledge

1. What is the new technology for heart treatment?
2. What is the role of technology in monitoring heart health?

SUMMARY

In looking at the intricacies of the circulatory system, one can see that its multifaceted nature is essential to the maintenance of life. The interaction between the heart, blood vessels, and blood highlights the need to know how these elements interact both in healthy and diseased states. Since the circulatory system is essential for transporting oxygen and nutrients and eliminating waste products, any interruption can be detrimental to health. The study of conditions such as cardiac arrhythmias and valvular stenosis underscores the demand for novel methods in medical technology. Such diseases, though common, have in the past lacked adequate documentation, and hence there is a need to drive research models to better mimic such conditions. The creation of mock circulatory systems presents a viable option for testing devices that can assist and augment cardiovascular function, and this underscores the importance of ongoing study in this area. As the discussion surrounding the circulatory system is ongoing, the examination of diagnostic and therapeutic developments is increasingly important. The integration of hybrid mock circulation loops that mimic pathological conditions, as seen in recent studies, foretells a new era in the approach to cardiovascular well-being. These models, in addition to providing accurate simulation of cardiac events, also facilitate validation and verification of circulatory assist technologies like ventricular assist devices (VADs). By ensuring that the technologies are tested rigorously under conditions very similar to real life scenarios, researchers have a chance of being more adequately prepared to face the complexities that are prevalent in clinical practice. This commitment to developing credible, evidence-based solutions will ultimately improve patient outcomes, pointing to the value of aligning technological advancement with clinical realities. Taken collectively, the advances in understanding and modeling the circulatory system provide the foundation for the future of cardiovascular treatment and research. Next-generation medical devices depend increasingly on advancing technologies that credibly reflect cardiac conditions. This merger of advanced engineering and medicine not only enhances the reliability of equipment performance but also enhances the scientific knowledge of heart disease. As highlighted by many studies, cardiac disease recording and the development of successful interventions are of critical importance for optimizing the treatment of patients. Through continuous research and practice development in these disciplines, the potential for maximizing critical thinking and clinical outcomes, as in education models, also exists. Lastly, the interconnectedness of these disciplines necessitates a sustained emphasis on interdisciplinary education, innovation, and patient-centered care in the treatment of circulatory systems (Ethan S Rapp et al., 2022; Rahmatika et al., 2020).

The circulatory system is the essential system in the human body that transports blood, oxygen, and nutrients to tissues and facilitates the removal of waste products. Its efficiency relies on an efficient cooperation of components, including the heart, blood vessels, and blood itself. The muscular pump of the heart generates the force that enables the circulation of blood in the body and creates a system of arteries, veins, and capillaries for timely delivery to all cells. During heart contraction, oxygen-rich blood is supplied to various organs, where it performs vital functions, thereby highlighting cardiovascular health and fitness as essential aspects for general health. Not only does this system provide essential nutrients, but it also controls body pH and temperature and therefore affects homeostasis. Beyond its overall task of delivering nutrients and oxygen, the circulatory system is very closely linked to other systems of the body, particularly for physical fitness and intelligence. Current research, for example, on physical education's contribution to the school environment, recognizes that higher physical fitness is positively linked with good academic performance. It has been established that formal physical education can enhance physical fitness, which can in turn enhance cognitive performance. Children who were involved in daily fitness programs recorded improvements in their overall academic performance, particularly in subjects like math and reading, according to studies that combined physical education with the curricular subject matter (Lynch et al., 1980). The link underscores the necessity for implementing good physical fitness programs in schools in attempts to capitalize on the benefits that physical fitness both enables towards health and academic performance. Secondly, the modifications to the general circulation model (GCM) used in atmospheric research are an example of circulatory principles outside the human body, namely the identification of systemic flow and patterns. In Martian science, the GCM has been adapted to examine dynamic interactions of flows within different atmospheres, which is a method of understanding circulatory phenomena in other contexts. The main conclusions of these models describe cycles of circulation intensification, just like those in Earth systems, and suggest that there is a better understanding of circulation processes that can yield meaningful information on planetary environments (Mischna et al., 2016). This new approach not only consolidates our knowledge of circulatory systems but also highlights the potential interlinkage of circulatory structures across domains, ultimately serving to highlight the importance of cross-disciplinary study in advancing the boundaries of knowledge of our understanding of circulatory mechanics.

KEY TERMS FROM THIS CHAPTER

- Arteries
- Blood
- Blood vessels
- Capillaries
- Cardiovascular diseases
- Circulatory system
- Electrocardiogram
- Erythrocytes
- Fluid dynamics
- Gases
- Hormones
- Nutrients
- Photoplethysmogram
- Plasma
- Veins

CRITICAL THINKING QUESTIONS

1. **The main components of the circulatory system are:**
   a. Heart, lungs, and brain
   b. Heart, blood vessels, and blood
   c. Kidneys, liver, and blood vessels
   d. Brain, spinal cord, and heart
2. **The circulatory system is responsible for:**
   a. Transporting oxygen, nutrients, and waste products
   b. Digesting food and absorbing nutrients
   c. Regulating body temperature only
   d. Producing hormones
3. **The two main types of circulatory systems are:**
   a. Open and closed
   b. Arterial and venous
   c. Pulmonary and systemic
   d. Single and double
4. **Arteries carry blood:**
   a. Away from the heart
   b. Toward the heart
   c. Between the lungs and the heart
   d. Only to the lungs
5. **Which blood vessels have valves to prevent backflow?**
   a. Arteries
   b. Capillaries
   c. Veins
   d. Arterioles

Short Answer Questions

1. What is the circulatory system?
2. Why is circulatory system important in the human body?
3. What is the circulatory pathway?
4. What are the regulations of blood flow?
5. Describe the common disorders that affect the circulatory system.

Answer to Critical Thinking Questions

1. (b) 2. (a) 3. (a) 4. (a) 5. (c)

REFERENCES

1. Acharya, S. A., Cabrales, P., Intaglietta, M., Kistler, et al. (2014). Replacing the transfusion of 1–2 units of blood with plasma expanders that increase oxygen delivery capacity: Evidence from experimental studies. https://core.ac.uk/download/323065176.pdf (accessed on 15th June 2025).
2. Adolph, T., Meyer, M., Jukic, A., & Tilg, H. (2024). Heavy arch: From inflammatory bowel diseases to metabolic disorders. *Gut, 73*, 1376–1387. https://www.semanticscholar.org/paper/291b0f43a2f660a5140078683b50fe9e3eaa2adb (accessed on 15th June 2025).
3. Al-Zuhairi, W. Sh., Sadeghi, L., & Hassan, E. A. (2024). Neuregulin-1, or NRG 1, is a powerful cardiomyocyte proliferator that impacts the circulatory system. *Academic Science Journal*. https://www.semanticscholar.org/paper/9b2c6c4b42591c5859d006a277f2cfd7aca08a53 (accessed on 15th June 2025).
4. Aras, S., Khalpey, Z., & Lin, T. (2020). Heart rate variability: A possible machine learning biomarker for mechanical circulatory device complications and heart recovery. https://core.ac.uk/download/287891095.pdf (accessed on 15th June 2025).
5. Askerov, E. M., Utkina, V. A., Filich, A. S., & Fisyuk, Ye. A. (2024). Modern ideas about the development of atherosclerosis. *Meditsinskaya Sestra*. https://www.semanticscholar.org/paper/f29b1ceb10b3173640ebae8e8080860ca195433e (accessed on 15th June 2025).
6. Biggins, S. W., Angeli, P., García-Tsao, G., Ginés, P., Ling, S. C., Nadim, M. K., Wong, F., et al. (2021). Diagnosis, evaluation, and management of ascites, spontaneous bacterial peritonitis and hepatorenal syndrome: 2021 practice guidance by the American Association for the Study of Liver Diseases. *Hepatology, 74*, 1014–1048. https://doi.org/10.1002/hep.31884 (accessed on 15th June 2025).
7. Borisov, A. V., Borisov, A. V., Shashikanth, B. N., Shashikanth, B. N., Zenkov, D. V., Kanso, E., Fassò, F., et al. (2013). The motion of the 2D hydrodynamic Chaplin sleigh in the presence of circulation. https://core.ac.uk/download/41772804.pdf (accessed on 15th June 2025).
8. Bossavi, G., Yan, R., & Irfan, M. (2023). A novel convolutional neural network deep learning implementation for cuffless heart rate and blood pressure estimation. *Applied Sciences*. https://www.semanticscholar.org/paper/6e3b981779167bc55f2e13ec9e25392c6861ff90 (accessed on 15th June 2025).
9. Bujunuru, A., Challa, A. R., Arepally, S., & Arrabojju, S. (2025). Smart heart monitoring system using IoT and pulse sensor technology. *International Journal on Science and Technology*. https://www.semanticscholar.org/paper/406f5151a3faeb82fb57253ec2d46fba431711fa (accessed on 15th June 2025).
10. Choy, J. A. I., Domek, N., & Tavelli, J. P. (2016). Innovations in traumatic hemorrhage. https://core.ac.uk/download/72852887.pdf (accessed on 15th June 2025).
11. Conrad, J., & Gillen, A. L. (2014). Our impressive immune system: More than a defense. https://core.ac.uk/download/220159125.pdf (accessed on 15th June 2025).
12. Crisafulli, A., Marongiu, E., Nobrega, A. C. L., et al. (2014). Neural regulation of cardiovascular response to exercise: Role of central command and peripheral afferents. https://core.ac.uk/download/pdf/54599119.pdf (accessed on 15th June 2025).

13. Cutler, D. M., Stewart, K. A., & Landrum, M. B. (2025). Intensive medical care and cardiovascular disease disability reductions. https://core.ac.uk/download/pdf/6819629.pdf (accessed on 15th June 2025).

14. De Bellis, A., D'Abramo, M., Frati, G., et al. (2018). Surgical embolectomy for acute massive pulmonary embolism: State of the art. https://core.ac.uk/download/188822613.pdf (accessed on 15th June 2025).

15. Del Balzo, F., Duse, M., Nicita, F., et al. (2016). Stroke and migraine: Is there a possible comorbidity? https://core.ac.uk/download/154947765.pdf (accessed on 15th June 2025).

16. Despins, L., Enayati, M., Guidoboni, G., et al. (2019). Cardiovascular function and ballistocardiogram: A relationship interpreted via mathematical modeling. https://core.ac.uk/download/228101928.pdf (accessed on 15th June 2025).

17. Fahed, G., Aoun, L., Bou Zerdan, M., Allam, S., Bou Zerdan, M., Bouferraa, Y., & Assi, H. (2022). Metabolic syndrome: Updates on pathophysiology and management in 2021. *International Journal of Molecular Sciences, 23*, 786. https://doi.org/10.3390/ijms23020786 (accessed on 15th June 2025).

18. Fang, C., Huang, F., Yao, M., Wang, Z., Ma, J., Wu, D., Guo, T., et al. (2024). Advances in microRNA regulation of deep vein thrombosis through venous vascular endothelial cells (Review). *Molecular Medicine Reports, 29*(6). https://www.semanticscholar.org/paper/e25014d9b6e9e5c15a1c540854a7a89788c758c9 (accessed on 15th June 2025).

19. Gaynullina, D., Tarasova, O. S., & Shvetsova, A. (2024). Regulation of vascular smooth muscle cell contraction during early postnatal ontogenesis. *Vestnik Moskovskogo Universiteta. Seria 16. Biologia*. https://www.semanticscholar.org/paper/bc76ab52bdfd8b09400297e37b8b2417672aa663 (accessed on 15th June 2025).

20. Gromova, N. V., Imarova, O. G., Martynova, M. I., et al. (2016). Role of membrane lipids in the regulation of erythrocytic oxygen-transport function in cardiovascular diseases. https://core.ac.uk/download/228177833.pdf (accessed on 15th June 2025).

21. Gutiérrez, Y., Lugo, C., & Rondón, J. (2025). Artificial lung: A biomedical engineering approach. https://core.ac.uk/download/652359337.pdf (accessed on 15th June 2025).

22. Hutchins, B. R., Brown, D., Buchwald, D., Clarke, D., et al. (2015). Descartes, corpuscles and reductionism: Mechanism and systems in Descartes' physiology. https://core.ac.uk/download/147061302.pdf (accessed on 15th June 2025).

23. Leonard, J. I. (2025). An integrated analysis of the physiological effects of space flight: Executive summary. https://core.ac.uk/download/pdf/42844718.pdf (accessed on 15th June 2025).

24. Leonard, J. I. (2025). Description, validation, and modification of the Guyton model for space-flight applications. Part A. Guyton model of circulatory, fluid and electrolyte control. Part B. Modification of the Guyton model for circulatory, fluid and electrolyte control. https://core.ac.uk/download/pdf/42845535.pdf (accessed on 15th June 2025).

25. Leonard, J. I. (2025). The behavior of renal-regulating hormones during hypogamic stress. https://core.ac.uk/download/pdf/42845534.pdf (accessed on 15th June 2025).

26. Lewis, S. M., Williams, A., & Eisenbarth, S. C. (2019). Structure and function of the immune system in the spleen. *Science Immunology, 4*. https://doi.org/10.1126/sciimmunol.aau6085 (accessed on 15th June 2025).

27. Lu, M. M., Yang, Y. K., Lin, J., Du, Y. S., & Zhou, X. Q. (2024). Research progress of magnetorheological polishing technology: A review. *Advances in Manufacturing*. https://www.semanticscholar.org/paper/cfee1493a287a67958dcdfd37fa808bd9f4fb33f (accessed on 15th June 2025).

28. Lynch, C. J. (1980). Measures of the efficacy of a daily fifteen-minute fitness programmed for intermediate school children: A thesis presented in partial fulfilment of the requirements for the degree of Masterate in Education at Massey University. https://core.ac.uk/download/157568860.pdf (accessed on 15th June 2025).

29. Mischna, M. A., & Shirley, J. H. (2016). Numerical modeling of orbit-spin coupling accelerations in a Mars general circulation model: Implications for global dust storm activity. http://arxiv.org/abs/1602.09137 (accessed on 15th June 2025).

30. Nowak-Sliwinska, P., Alitalo, K., Allen, E., Anisimov, A., Aplin, A. C., Auerbach, R., Augustin, H. G., et al. (2018). Consensus guidelines for the use and interpretation of angiogenesis assays. *Angiogenesis, 21*, 425–532. https://doi.org/10.1007/s10456-018-9613-x (accessed on 15th June 2025).

31. Parveen, A., & Devika, R. (2022). Fibrinolytic enzyme–An overview. *Current Pharmaceutical Biotechnology*. https://www.semanticscholar.org/paper/319739b1b809fb6036d3d97548978c2374ae86ed (accessed on 15th June 2025).

32. Peak, P., Tedesco, V., Kiang, S., Smith, P. A., Nissim, L., Fraser, K., Frazier, O., et al. (2022). Physiological control algorithm for a pulsatile-flow 3D printed circulatory model to simulate human cardiovascular system. *2022 44th Annual International Conference of the IEEE Engineering in Medicine & Biology Society (EMBC)*. https://www.semanticscholar.org/paper/28e70fa00dfeaaf7c9656dc017fe86c8f6179581 (accessed on 15th June 2025).

33. Ponikowski, P., Voors, A. A., Anker, S. D., Bueno, H., Cleland, J. G. F., Coats, A. J. S., Falk, V., et al. (2016). 2016 ESC guidelines for the diagnosis and treatment of acute and chronic heart failure. *European Heart Journal, 37*, 2129–2200. https://doi.org/10.1093/eurheartj/ehw128 (accessed on 15th June 2025).

34. Rahmatika, H., Lestari, S., & Sari, M. (2020). A PBL-based circulatory system e-module based on research results to improve students' critical thinking skills and cognitive learning outcome. *9*, 565. https://www.semanticscholar.org/paper/db169174ca647ffe05fcc5f9f0d577e2528c49f5 (accessed on 15th June 2025).

35. Rapp, E. S., Pawar, S. R., & Longoria, R. (2022). Hybrid mock circulatory loop simulation of extreme cardiac events. *IEEE Transactions on Biomedical Engineering, PP*, 1. https://www.semanticscholar.org/paper/8f9813aa1672fa9c22a17e897bf439b4ddb109f2 (accessed on 15th June 2025).

36. San, O., & Staples, A. E. (2012). An improved model for reduced-order physiological fluid flows. http://arxiv.org/abs/1212.0188 (accessed on 15th June 2025).

37. Schuster, E. J., Taftaf, R., Reduzzi, C., Albert, M. K., Romero-Calvo, I., & Liu, H. (2021). Better together: Circulating tumor cell clustering in metastatic cancer. *Trends in Cancer, 7*, 1020–1032. https://doi.org/10.1016/j.trecan.2021.07.001 (accessed on 15th June 2025).

38. Simion, M. (2018). Epistemic trouble for engineering 'woman.' https://core.ac.uk/download/161770716.pdf (accessed on 15th June 2025).

39. Skazkina, V., Mureeva, E. N., Karavaev, A., Kiselev, A., Panina, O., Gridnev, V., Galushko, T. A., et al. (2020). Development of features of the autonomic circulatory regulation in late premature and full-term infants. *2020 4th Scientific School on Dynamics of Complex Networks and their Application in Intellectual Robotics (DCNAIR).* https://www.semanticscholar.org/paper/840afac0b6c14ed7defd5c105e80f09c02b13204 (accessed on 15th June 2025).

40. Smith, B., Siebert, D., Ernst, D., Johansson, I., Munn, K., Elsner, K., & Tsikolia, N. (2005). Functional anatomy: A taxonomic proposal. https://core.ac.uk/download/131215354.pdf (accessed on 15th June 2025).

41. Sodnompilova, M., & Nanzatov, B. (2020). Human body in traditional views of Turkic and Mongolian peoples: Blood and circulatory system. *Bulletin of the Irkutsk State University. Geoarchaeology, Ethnology, and Anthropology Series.* https://www.semanticscholar.org/paper/09e6d0f65fdee556c71b39c61897a4b574c0f6fb (accessed on 15th June 2025).

42. Spitsin, A. P., Knyazhev, I. S., Karaulova, L. V., & Reztsov, O. V. (2023). Econometric predictive model for assessing the functional state of students during the examination period: A cross-sectional exploratory pilot study. https://core.ac.uk/download/591233166.pdf (accessed on 15th June 2025).

43. Tambe, S., Sawant, S., Sonawane, S., Ghodake, S., & Kawade, S. B. (2025). Animal health monitoring system using IoT technology. *International Journal of Advanced Research in Science, Communication and Technology*. https://www.semanticscholar.org/paper/970f6ed21bd11e5444e2fc1aa326f3a2a5c3d026 (accessed on 15th June 2025).

44. Task Force Members, Erbel, R., Aboyans, V., Boileau, C., Bossone, E., Di Bartolomeo, R., Eggebrecht, H., et al. (2014). 2014 ESC guidelines on the diagnosis and treatment of aortic diseases. *European Heart Journal, 35*, 2873–2926. https://doi.org/10.1093/eurheartj/ehu281 (accessed on 15th June 2025).

45. Tsapaeva, N. L., & Tsapaev, V. G. (2024). Microcirculation (Part 1–Main players and their role in the circulatory system). *Emergency Cardiology and Cardiovascular Risks.* https://www.semanticscholar.org/paper/c9c052a189b505a2897d485bf1ad6b9379104814 (accessed on 15th June 2025).

46. Ustroi, L. (2024). The histological miracle of the circulatory system. https://core.ac.uk/download/642804958.pdf (accessed on 15th June 2025).

47. Windecker, S., Kolh, P., Alfonso, F., Collet, J.-P., Cremer, J., Falk, V., Filippatos, G., et al. (2014). 2014 ESC/EACTS guidelines on myocardial revascularization. *European Heart Journal, 35*, 2541–2619. https://doi.org/10.1093/eurheartj/ehu278 (accessed on 15th June 2025).

48. Wood, E. H. (2025). Studies of the effects of gravitational and inertial forces on cardiovascular and respiratory dynamics: Semiannual status report. https://core.ac.uk/download/pdf/85246868.pdf (accessed on 15th June 2025).

RESPIRATORY SYSTEM

3

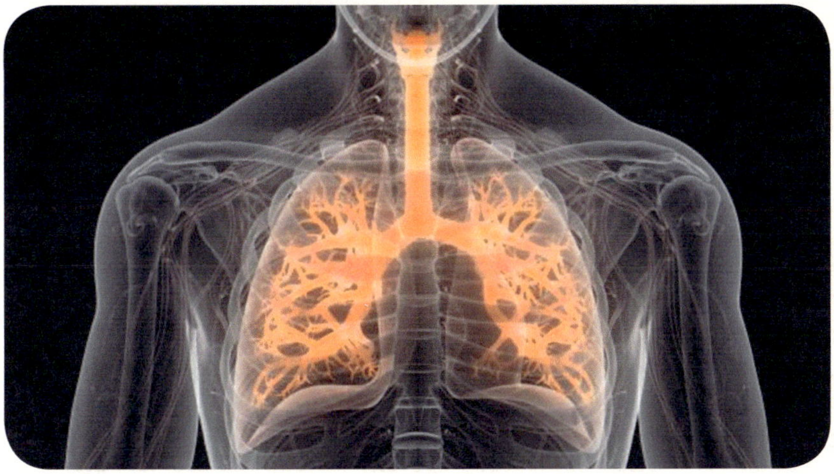

LEARNING OBJECTIVES

After studying this chapter, you will be able to:

1. Understand the anatomy of the respiratory system
2. Describe the function of the respiratory system
3. Describe the respiratory pathways
4. Learn about respiratory health and diseases
5. Understand the role of the respiratory system in homeostasis
6. Discuss the advances in respiratory medicine

Introduction

In the investigation of the human respiratory system, it is critical to acknowledge its complexity and the critical role it plays in sustaining general well-being. The respiratory system is not merely charged with the uptake of oxygen and the excretion of carbon dioxide, but plays a considerable role in the maintenance of homeostasis, blood pH, and multiple metabolic processes. The elaborate anatomy that exists to service this system, such as structures such as the lungs, bronchi, and alveoli, is a sophisticated network specifically designed to optimize gas exchange. This delicate interaction between anatomy and function serves to highlight the significance of valuing respiratory health, particularly in the context of environmental stressors and novel pathogens. Understanding the mechanisms underlying the respiratory tract's interactions with internal and external agents opens the door to a more detailed investigation of its role in human physiology and medicine. Further, the interface between microbiology and respiratory health is another critical region of investigation.

The human respiratory system is more than a series of anatomical structures; it also hosts a sophisticated microbiome, particularly in the nose, which plays a critical role in immune system regulation and protection against pathogens. Colonization of the upper respiratory tract in early life with beneficial microbes may influence immune responses, offering early protection against potentially lethal infections, while preserving mucosal integrity (Gillen, 2017). Understanding, therefore, the dynamics of the nasal microbiome and its resident bacterial population provides critical information pertaining to the prevention and treatment of respiratory disease. Additionally, the development of research into microbiota and its effect on respiratory function may have the potential to lead to revolutionary therapeutic strategies, revolutionizing our attempts to counteract respiratory disease and enhance patient outcomes. Understanding of the anatomical organization of the respiratory system forms a fundamental foundation to comprehend how disease can threaten its operation.

Familiarity with the anatomical parts is required to investigate their response to disease states and the consequent effect on therapeutic intervention (Mejino et al., 2007). Advances in anatomical studies have reaffirmed the value in pursuing a holistic and systematic method of describing respiratory anatomy, of the utmost importance for clinical practice. Tools like the Foundational Model of Anatomy (FMA) seek to develop a systematic method of better comprehending anatomical and physiological correlation, and therefore clinical diagnosis and treatment. By integrating such anatomical understanding and further research into respiratory health, improved comprehension of respiratory function and disease, and ultimately, a more informed strategy to health care and policy development can be achieved based on human respiratory health.

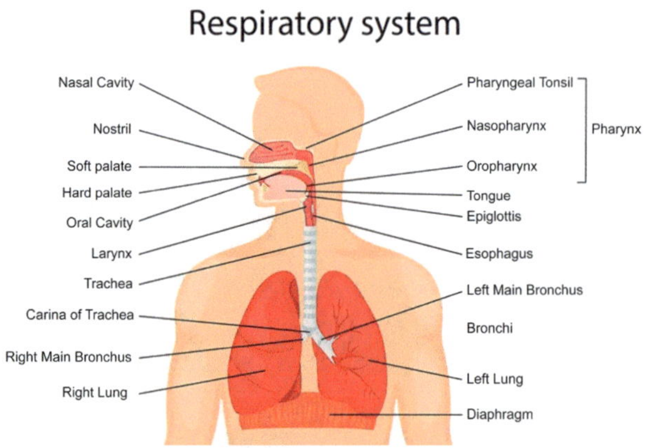

Figure 3.1. Respiratory System.

Source: https://img.lb.wbmdstatic.com/vim/live/webmd/consumer_assets/site_images/article_thumbnails/BigBead/respiratory_system_bigbead/1800x1200_respiratory_system_bigbead.jpg?resize=750px:*&output-quality=75

Importance of the Respiratory System in Human Physiology

The respiratory system is responsible for the provision of homeostasis in the human body through the facilitation of gas exchange, which is of pre-eminent importance in cellular respiration. This system is responsible for ensuring oxygen in the air is delivered to the bloodstream and the efficient removal of carbon dioxide, a by-product of metabolism. The complex structures of the respiratory system, such as the lungs, bronchi, and alveoli, function coordinately to ensure the maximum surface area for gas exchange. The respiratory system also dynamically modulates to changing physiological requirements, especially with exercise. With increasing workload, rates of ventilation are regulated via an advanced control system, ensuring proper oxygenation and carbon dioxide removal. Dynamic regulation is the key to preserving acid-base balance in the body and justifies the respiratory system's prevalence in human physiology. Respiratory control complexity is also increased with exercise. It has been demonstrated that the human body utilizes an open-loop control system for ventilation with heavy exercise, which substantially contrasts with the negative feedback system used at rest (Murray-Smith et al., 2009). This open-loop system enables quick modulation of respiratory rate and depth and thereby satisfies the growing metabolic requirements of contracting tissues. Moreover, interconnection of respiration with other physiological systems is essential; for example, during breathing, heart rhythms and changes in blood pressure are seen, and this is indicative of the coordination required to maximize oxygen delivery and resource allocation within the body.

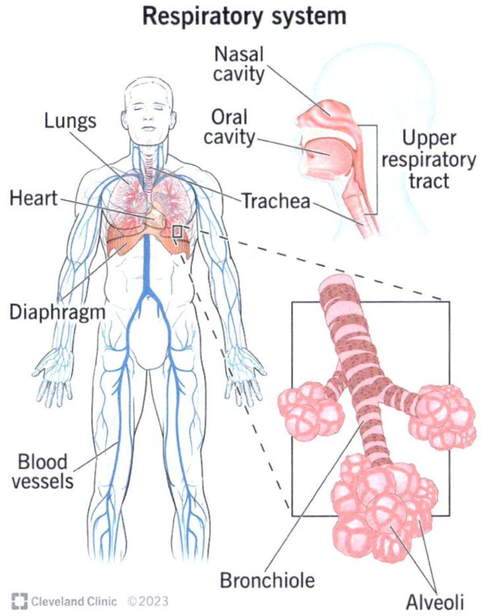

Figure 3.2. Your respiratory system — lungs, airways, pharynx, larynx, nose, and mouth — brings in oxygen and gets rid of carbon dioxide.

Source: https://my.clevelandclinic.org/-/scassets/images/org/health/articles/respiratory-system

Elucidation of these interactions not only serves to underscore the pre-eminent position of the respiratory system but also to guide disease management and optimization of athletic performance. In exploring the extended influence of respiratory health, it is evident that changes in respiratory function have significant implications for overall health. Respiratory disease, such as asthma or COPD, is characterized by abnormal gas exchange, with increased risk of systemic sequelae. Physiological control of heart rate and blood pressure with respiration underscores the importance of maintaining respiratory health in safeguarding optimal cardiac function (Barnes et al., 2014). Moreover, data derived from examining intracellular ionic changes in breathing mechanisms may provide new therapeutic interventions for a wide range of diseases. With more exploration of the intricacy of the respiratory system, researchers can further determine its function as a regulator of varied body functions and improve health outcomes in a wide range of medical conditions.

3.1. Anatomy of the Respiratory System

Learning Outcome

1. Describe the major components of the respiratory system
2. Describe the role of the diaphragm and intercostal muscles
3. Understand the structure of the alveoli and gas exchange

The human respiratory system is a delicate network of structures coordinated for respiration and homeostasis. The lungs, the core of the system, are the main location of oxygen-carbon dioxide exchange. The anatomy of the lungs is made up of a series of lobes, bronchi, and alveoli, each of which is specialized to perform a specific function. The alveoli, small air sacs at the terminal end of the bronchioles, are extremely important because of the enormous surface area they contain, making the process of gas exchange extremely efficient. Furthermore, the coordination of the respiratory and cardiovascular systems, where oxygen-rich blood is circulated to tissues, is an extension of the complexity of the system. As the lungs expand and contract during respiration, they not only make breathing easier but are also involved in essential biochemical reactions, which reflect the importance of this system in maintaining life. Anatomical structures like the diaphragm and intercostal muscles are significant in the process of respiration, as this makes the respiratory system functionally effective. The diaphragm—a dome-shaped muscle below the lungs—contracts during inhalation, increasing thoracic volume and sucking air into the lungs. Exhalation happens when the diaphragm relaxes, reducing thoracic volume and forcing air out. These repeated contractions and relaxations are essential for effective ventilation. The coordination of the movement of these muscles reflects the relationship between anatomy and physiology in the respiratory process. Furthermore, the protective structures, like the rib cage and pleural membranes, ensure physical protection to the lungs and prevent lung collapse, reflecting the reliance of most anatomical structures in the respiratory system. These features unveil an extremely efficient system that has developed to maximize respiratory effectiveness in humans. The evolutionary aspect of the anatomy of the respiratory system uncovers impressive adaptations to maximize its function. As studied in recent research, the dimensions and shape of the thoracic cavity and nasal passages have developed to enable bipedal walking and high metabolism (Bastir et al., 2022). These anatomical structures not only facilitate airflow but also enable effective temperature and humidity control of inspired air. The respiratory system also dynamically interacts with other organ systems, such as the cardiovascular and nervous systems, to maximize respiratory homeostasis. Through the study of fossil evidence and present-day anatomy, scientists have identified diverse configurations of the respiratory system in hominins, offering avenues for future research into human evolution (Awoyomi, 2020). This integrative approach indicates the need for further research into the respiratory system to explain its intricate integration into human biology and evolution.

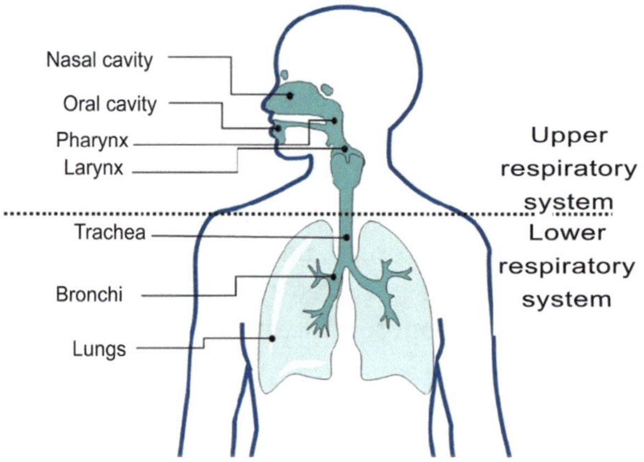

Figure 3.3. Anatomy of respiratory system.

Source: https://www.researchgate.net/profile/Jesus-Lujan-Montelongo/publication/357470377/figure/fig1/AS:1121095860142082@1644301490964/Anatomy-of-respiratory-system.png

3.1.1. Major Components: Lungs, Trachea, Bronchi

The respiratory system is primarily structured around three mandatory elements: the lungs, trachea, and bronchi, each of which is essential to enabling gas exchange. The windpipe or trachea is the primary airway descending from the larynx down to the bronchi. Composed of C-shaped rings of cartilage, the trachea is kept rigid and open for inhalation and exhalation. A mucous covering of cilia and mucus cells lines the trachea and captures and expels foreign particles and pathogens from inhaled air. This protective system illustrates the body's capability to filter danger from the environment prior to reaching the sensitive spaces of the lungs. An understanding of how the trachea is structured and functions is important to understanding how it maximizes respiratory health and reduces risk of associated diseases (Miller et al., 2017). The bronchi, which branch off from the distal end of the trachea, further subdivide into smaller tubes called bronchioles, which ultimately bring air to the alveoli—small air sacs where gas exchange is facilitated. The main bronchi are protected by the same mucous lining as the trachea, extending protection of filtering and humidification of inspired air. As the bronchi subdivide into bronchioles, their diameter narrows, which facilitates a vast surface area for gas exchange. This complex network of bronchi and bronchioles is important to ensuring effective delivery of oxygen to pulmonary alveoli as well as carbon dioxide removal from the blood, a function important to the maintenance of homeostasis. The structural design of the bronchi and the components of smooth muscle enable dynamic regulation of airflow, complementing the effectiveness of the respiratory system (Ackermann et al., 2001). Finally, the lungs hold the majority of the respiratory tract's gas exchange activity. Composed of millions of alveoli, they offer a massive surface area for the diffusion of carbon dioxide and oxygen. The pulmonary structure, consisting of a right and left lung each with various lobes, emphasizes the adjustment of the organ to respiratory demand. In addition to basic ventilation, the lungs are involved in other activities, such as the maintenance of blood pH concentration and as a pulmonary pathogen barrier. From research, it has been determined that compromised lung function results in severe health complications, as evidenced by the prevalence of chronic lower respiratory diseases, which are leading causes of morbidity and mortality globally (Miller et al., 2017). Thus, understanding the intricate anatomy and physiology of the lungs and connectivity to the trachea and bronchi is of paramount concern in respiratory complication management and the prevention of disease.

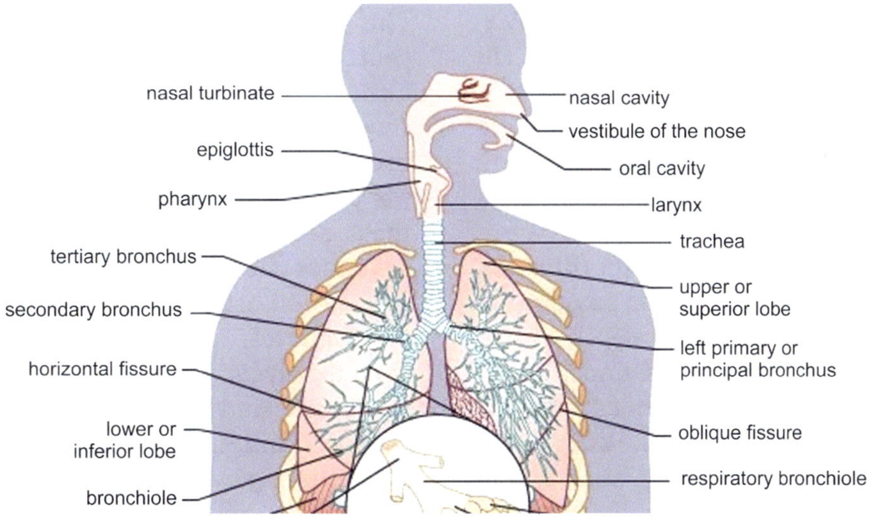

Figure 3.4. Components of the human respiratory system.

Source: https://cdn.britannica.com/17/72217-035-1C2827DB/air-nasal-cavity-nostrils-mucous-membranes-nasal-turbinates-pharynx.jpg?w=740&h=416&c=crop

3.1.2. Role of the Diaphragm and Intercostal Muscles

The diaphragm and intercostal muscles are the major players in the respiratory mechanics, coordinating the delicate process of ventilation. The diaphragm, a muscular dome-shaped organ at the bottom of the thoracic cavity, is the chief respiratory muscle. When it contracts, it flattens and descends, pulling the thoracic cavity with it. This lowers intrathoracic pressure, and air enters the lungs, a process known as inhalation. But when exhaling, the diaphragm relaxes, while the elasticity of the lungs assists in expelling air. The intercostal muscles, between the ribs, synergize with the action of the diaphragm. The external intercostals assist during inhalation by raising the ribs, which causes the thoracic cavity to expand further, while the internal intercostals are used in forceful exhalation, maximizing flow. These muscles, collectively, enable effective respiratory function, essential for optimal gas exchange in the human body. New research suggests that non-invasive techniques might be effective alternatives for inspiratory muscle function testing, particularly in the case of the intercostal and diaphragm muscles. New techniques like mechanomyography (MMG) and electromyography (EMG) usher in new possibilities in assessing such muscle activity without involving invasive techniques. The research has shown significant correlations between these non-invasive techniques vs. traditional measurements of transdiaphragmatic pressure (Pdi) and crural diaphragm EMG. These findings underscore the significance of diaphragm and intercostal muscle coordination, not only for breathing but also for posture and movement, marking their critical role in full muscular dynamics during rest and activity, particularly as people perform various voluntary movements (Jané Campos et al., 2018). The intricate interaction provided by such testing reveals the muscle's role beyond breathing, expanding our understanding of their complex roles within human physiology. The role of the diaphragms also extends beyond simple respiratory functions, playing a significant role in maintaining postural stability through movement. As examined within research into voluntary movement of the body, diaphragmatic function is regulated through the central nervous system's control strategies, showing an integration of respiratory and non-respiratory function. This interaction is best observed during the transition from rest to movement in humans, where diaphragmatic activation is complemented by trunk muscle activation to support upright posture and initiate movement. Asymmetrical diaphragm activity within dynamic movements such as rotation also illustrates this complexity, with changes in muscle usage enabling effective body mechanics (Masatoshi et al., 2010). It is within this comprehension that we can observe the viewpoint of how respiratory muscles adapt in a way that assists in maintaining functional integrity throughout the range of physical demands made upon the body, thereby cementing the diaphragm and intercostal muscles' significant role within the overall context of human respiratory physiology.

3.1.3. Structure of the Alveoli and Gas Exchange

The alveoli are the microscopic units at the center of the respiratory system, enabling the all-important process of gas exchange. The tiny, balloon-shaped sacs at the end of the bronchioles double the exchange surface area for oxygen and carbon dioxide. The walls of these sacs consist of a thin layer of epithelial cells that allows for efficient diffusion of gases. The alveoli are also surrounded by a network of capillaries, such that the oxygen transferred from the alveoli can be efficiently channeled into the blood, and carbon dioxide released from the blood into the alveoli to be eliminated. This spatial configuration highlights how the alveolar structure is optimized for maximal facilitation of gas exchange, reflecting its all-important role in ensuring optimal respiratory function. Gas exchange in alveoli is made possible by the process of diffusion, fueled by partial pressure gradients between the alveolar air within and the capillary blood. Oxygen, more dense in alveolar air than in deoxygenated blood, diffuses into the blood, while carbon dioxide, more dense in the blood as a cellular waste product of cells, diffuses in the opposite direction. The immeasurable importance of accurate gas exchange cannot be overstated, such that any deviation from this process can have disastrous physiological consequences. For instance, conditions that compromise the integrity of the alveolar and capillary membranes can disrupt this process, resulting in compromised oxygen delivery to tissues and potential respiratory distress. An understanding of this mechanism highlights the imperative of healthy alveolar structures to enable effective gas exchange. Alveolar complexity is further made apparent with reference to parameters of respiratory efficiency under the control of varied physiological states and airway gas exchange. Research has shown, for instance, that respiratory patterns can significantly influence the concentration of gases exchanged in the alveoli. Composition and exhaled breath concentrations of metabolites, such as acetone, have been shown to vary across metabolic states and exercise protocols. Methods such as measurements of nitric oxide have also been automated to aid clinical diagnostics, demonstrating the dynamic coexistence of gas exchange and metabolic activity. Such a multidisciplinary approach to the alveolar function necessitates the need for thorough study over superficial structural anatomy due to the interdependence of structure and function to enable effective respiration (Amann et al., 2010; Brown et al., 1990).

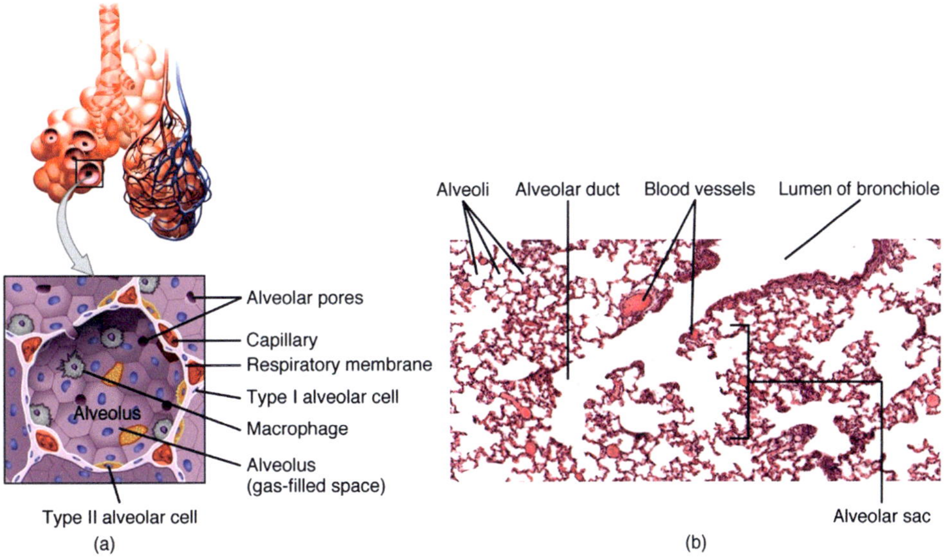

Figure 3.5. (a) The alveolus is responsible for gas exchange. (b) A micrograph shows the alveolar structures within lung tissue.

Source: https://s3-us-west-2.amazonaws.com/courses-images-archive-read-only/wp-content/uploads/sites/403/2015/04/21031640/2310_Structures_of_the_Respiratory_Zone.jpg

Test Your Knowledge

1. What are the major components of the respiratory system?
2. What is the role of the diaphragm and intercostal muscles?

3.2. Function of the Respiratory System

Learning Outcome

1. Know the process of inhalation and exhalation
2. Describe the mechanism of gas exchange in the alveoli
3. Understand the regulation of blood pH through respiration

At the very center of human survival, the respiratory system is the body's primary machinery of gas exchange that enables oxygenation and carbon dioxide elimination. The system functions through complex coordination among many anatomical structures in the form of the lungs, trachea, bronchi, and alveoli. Inhaling brings air into the alveoli, in which oxygen diffuses through their membranes into the blood. On the other hand, carbon dioxide, a by-product of cellular metabolism, diffuses from the blood into the alveoli to be eliminated. Such gas exchange performance is essential to maintaining cellular respiration and the body's acid-base balance, ultimately to maintain overall metabolic processes for life continuation. In addition to the vital function of gas exchange, the respiratory system also regulates blood pH and defends against environmental pathogens. Accumulation of carbon dioxide in the blood triggers changes in blood pH, for which the respiratory system forms a rapid response to achieve homeostasis. Moreover, the system contains defense mechanisms in the form of mucous membranes, cilia, and immune cells that filter out pathogens and particulates from inspired air. Such defense mechanisms not only defend the respiratory system against infections but also stimulate overall immunity, which is particularly important in the age of viral pandemics, such as the interactions of the immune response and respiratory viruses, such as coronaviruses. This is a testament to the multi-role importance of the respiratory system in maintaining respiratory as well as systemic health (Amodio et al., 2021). Furthermore, its impact on respiratory health transcends functional roles, influencing entire physiological systems such as circulatory and muscular functions. Disease states such as spinal cord injury can severely compromise respiratory function, with complications in other organ systems. Autonomic dysfunction, potentially from such trauma, can interfere with respiratory control and thereby affect cardiovascular well-being. Interdependence of such systems is a testament to the significance of respiratory integrity. Respiratory dysfunction can lead to metabolic complications, such as the impairment of effective gas exchange, which can trigger a cascade of health complications. It is therefore essential to comprehend the enormity of the functions of the respiratory system to develop intervention models for disease states that violate respiratory integrity and overall health (N/A, 2023).

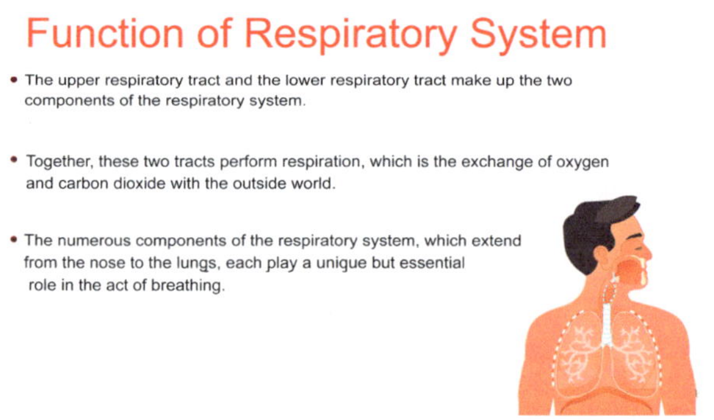

Figure 3.6. Function of the Respiratory System.

Source: https://assets.lybrate.com/imgs/tic/enadp/function-of-respiratory-system.webp

3.2.1. Process of Inhalation and Exhalation

The process of inhalation initiates the beginning of the respiratory cycle, where air enters the lungs, making room for gas exchange that is required for cellular respiration. Inhalation is facilitated when the diaphragm, a dome-shaped muscle at the bottom of the thoracic cavity, contracts and moves downwards. This decreases the pressure inside the thoracic cavity, creating a vacuum that draws the atmospheric air into the airways. The intercostal muscles, located between the ribs, also aid the process by opening the ribcage, hence increasing the volume of the lungs. The effect of the contraction of these muscles is to increase the volume in the thoracic cavity, hence causing air to enter the alveoli, small air sacs where oxygen is taken in and carbon dioxide is expelled. This critical process not only starts the respiratory process but also provides homeostasis by keeping the level of oxygen adequate for the body's metabolic requirements. Exhalation, however, is a process where carbon dioxide, the body's metabolic waste, is expelled from the body. This is an involuntary process in which the diaphragm relaxes and moves upwards, accompanied by the relaxation of the intercostal muscles, hence making the thoracic cavity smaller. Due to the higher pressure in the lungs, the air is forced out through the trachea and out of the body. The process is also aided by the contraction of stomach and abdominal muscles in forceful exhalation, further decreasing the thoracic cavity and accelerating the expulsion of the air. Smooth coordination of the inhalation and exhalation process is needed in order to have effective gas exchange, and the body's tissues are oxygenated with sufficient oxygen while the carbon dioxide is efficiently expelled. An imbalance in this relationship can result in respiratory distress and a host of health complications. New monitoring technology has made a greater understanding of inhalation and exhalation mechanisms possible to provide useful information about respiratory health. Real-time monitoring equipment that tracks airflow rates and respiratory cycles allows clinicians to track lung function and diagnose respiratory illness with greater accuracy. Advanced measurement equipment involves one-way valves and flowmeters to measure the movement of inhalation and exhalation with great accuracy. For instance, using a mass spectrometer, the content of exhaled gases can be determined, providing a greater understanding of gas exchange in the lungs (Liu, 1973). Additionally, the anatomy of the nasal cavity, which warms and humidifies air, illustrates the anatomical and functional differences that influence the efficiency of air intake (Brenner et al., 2017). The interdisciplinary study of the respiratory process illustrates its importance in maintaining health and treating disease.

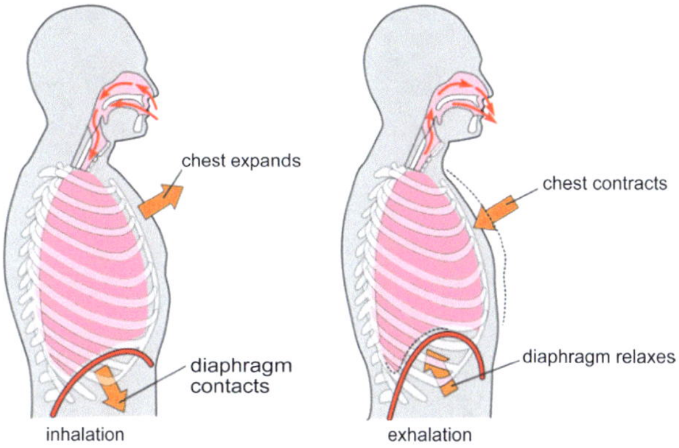

Figure 3.7. Process of inhalation and exhalation.

Source: https://infinitylearn.com/surge/wp-content/uploads/2023/09/Breathing.png.webp

3.2.2. Mechanism of Gas Exchange in the Alveoli

The mechanism of gas exchange in alveoli is a critical component of the human respiratory system, enabling oxygen and carbon dioxide exchange between the air and blood. This takes place in the alveolar sacs, where they are surrounded by a dense network of capillaries. Inspired air oxygen diffuses across thin alveolar membranes into capillary blood through a partial pressure gradient, while carbon dioxide diffuses in the opposite direction, from blood to alveoli to be expelled. Efficiency in gas exchange is governed by surface area, membrane thickness, and respiratory gas partial pressures, emphasizing the role of the alveoli in homeostasis through the regulation of blood gas levels and stability of pH. Furthermore, the structural integrity of the alveoli and the surrounding tissues is an important determinant of the efficiency of gas exchange. Alveoli walls are formed of a single layer of diffusional epithelial cells, while surfactant, an alveolar cell secretion, reduces surface tension to avoid collapse of these microscopic structures during exhalation. Interestingly, changes in respiratory status, e.g., progression of chronic obstructive pulmonary disease (COPD) or aging, can have extreme consequences on this mechanism of gas exchange.

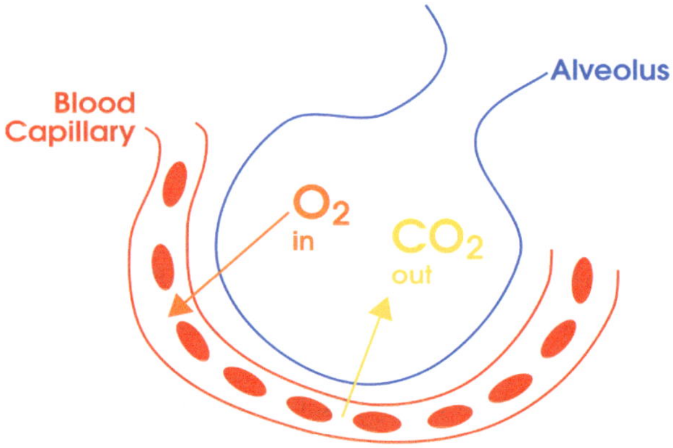

Figure 3.8. Gas exchange in humans. Oxygen and carbon dioxide switch places between a capillary (part of the bloodstream) and an alveolus (an air sac in the lungs).

Source: https://upload.wikimedia.org/wikipedia/commons/thumb/c/c4/Gas_exchange_in_the_aveolus_simple_%28en%29.svg/1280px-Gas_exchange_in_the_aveolus_simple_%28en%29.svg.png

As discussed, aging of the lung involves structural and physiological changes that diminish pulmonary reserve and modify efficiency of gas exchange, making it difficult to evaluate respiratory function in elderly patients, who can present in a myriad of ways with symptoms of gas exchange dysfunction (Ebejer and Lesauskaite, 1999). Current work has recognized the significance of airway gas exchange and its role in generating the variability of exhaled gases, such as acetone, that indicates the body's ongoing metabolic activity. The variability implies that changes in breathing behaviors can alter the gas amounts in the exhaled breath, and hence it is important to have a sensitive perspective of the dynamics between the alveoli and systemic levels of metabolites. The Farhi equation, the conventional gas exchange model, may not be able to capture the dynamics, a compartmental model may be able to yield more realistic models (Amann et al., 2010). As research into the complexities of alveolar gas exchange continues, the correlation between airway function and the gases in exhaled breath will become increasingly relevant to applications in respiratory diagnostics and disease.

3.2.3. Regulation of Blood pH Through Respiration

Blood pH control is an important physiological process that has a direct influence on the metabolic processes of the human body. The respiratory system plays a central role in this control by regulating the blood concentration of carbon dioxide (CO_2). With rising levels of CO_2, it combines with water to form carbonic acid that reduces pH levels. The respiratory system thus enhances ventilation to remove more CO_2 and normalize pH. The intricate relationship between respiration and pH control illustrates the respiratory system's immediate feedback control mechanisms responding to metabolic needs. An illustration is that during exercise, when the body's oxygen demand rises, the rise in breathing rates assists in the efficient removal of CO_2, thereby stabilizing blood pH levels within the tightly regulated range required for normal cell function. During exercise, blood pH regulation is also complexly coordinated by the simultaneous interactions of multiple physiological systems. The autonomic nervous system regulates cardiovascular support through sympathetic stimulation and parasympathetic withdrawal, providing the required blood flow to essential organs while responding to changes in blood pressure. The central command, as well as reflexes such as the baroreflex and chemoreflex, coordinates these adjustments, illustrating how synergistic body responses work together to regulate metabolic by-products. The adaptive capability of these systems illustrates the importance of maintaining homeostasis in physical stress conditions in which the respiratory system's contribution to blood pH control becomes intrinsically coupled with exercise performance and recovery, illustrating the importance of efficient carbon dioxide removal and oxygen delivery to exercising tissues (Crisafulli et al., 2014). Modeling of the respiratory control system also accounts for the dynamics of blood pH regulation at levels of activity, i.e., above lactate threshold. A simulation of respiratory response to ramp exercise has demonstrated that with varied control strategies, the body adapts when transitioning from rest to exercise. The findings provide that at rest, ventilation is controlled by negative feedback control reacting to blood acid and CO_2 changes in an appropriate way. During physical exercise, the body uses an open-loop control strategy, where ventilation is predominantly controlled by the added metabolic needs, compared to necessarily tracking feedback signals. The dual regulation indicates that, in addition to CO_2 production, blood acid also independently controls respiratory rates, expanding our understanding of how the human body maintains pH homeostasis in the presence of stressors like exercise (Murray-Smith et al., 2009).

Test Your Knowledge

1. Describe the process of inhalation and exhalation.
2. What is the mechanism of gas exchange in the alveoli?

3.3. Respiratory Pathways

Learning Outcome

1. Understand the upper respiratory tract
2. Understand the lower respiratory tract
3. Describe the role of mucous membranes and cilia in protection

The human respiratory pathways are essential to global respiratory system function, ensuring the continuation of gas exchange and homeostasis within the body. Air is filtered, warmed, and humidified through the nasal cavity and into the trachea, branching into the bronchi. The pathways become smaller and smaller into smaller bronchioles, eventually into the alveoli, where gas exchange is the essential process. The complex structure of the pathways, for example, ciliated epithelial cells and mucus secretion, is intended to trap pathogens and particulate material. This feature becomes increasingly important in the modern environment, with pollutants and engineered nanoparticles able to interfere with normal respiratory function. As documented in the literature, exposure to nanoparticles/nanotubes of carbon can cause gross respiratory toxicity, further highlighting the necessity for understanding how the pathways can be adaptive as well as susceptible to external influences (Kafoury et al., 2016). As well as air filtration, the respiratory pathways also constitute a complex interface to the entry of a variety of pathogens, including viruses. The coronavirus disease (COVID-19) provides a graphic example of a critical dynamic within the pathways, where the virus exploits natural entry routes. Evidence indicates the virus leads to dysfunction of the respiratory system, giving rise to critical health complications. The expression of bitter taste receptors, for example, TAS2Rs, in airway smooth muscle has been found to be an interesting area of study, suggesting these receptors may be protective against viral infection. TAS2R activation has been documented to stimulate host-defense pathways, thus enhancing immune responses and reducing the inflammatory cascades associated with diseases such as COVID-19. This is in accordance with the importance of respiratory pathways not only for gas exchange, but as front-line defense mechanisms against infectious disease (Bansal and Sharma, 2020). Secondly, interdependence between respiratory pathways and external agents implies the intricacy of respiratory health. The implication of engineered nanoparticles on breathing pathways implies the possible impact of industrial development on human health. Descriptions of the pathways by which particles impact biological tissues are crucial, as they can cause chronic respiratory disease. Observations of studies exploring the implications of carbon nanofibers on the respiratory system imply that rigorous safety measures are in place in the production and application of such materials. While health practitioners demand heightened sensitization and regulation of environmental pollutants, advocating for a holistic conceptualization of respiratory pathways is crucial. Further investigation in this direction will not only enhance our knowledge of respiratory pathology but also come up with innovative therapeutic approaches that put respiratory health at the center of contemporary challenges (Kafoury et al., 2016).

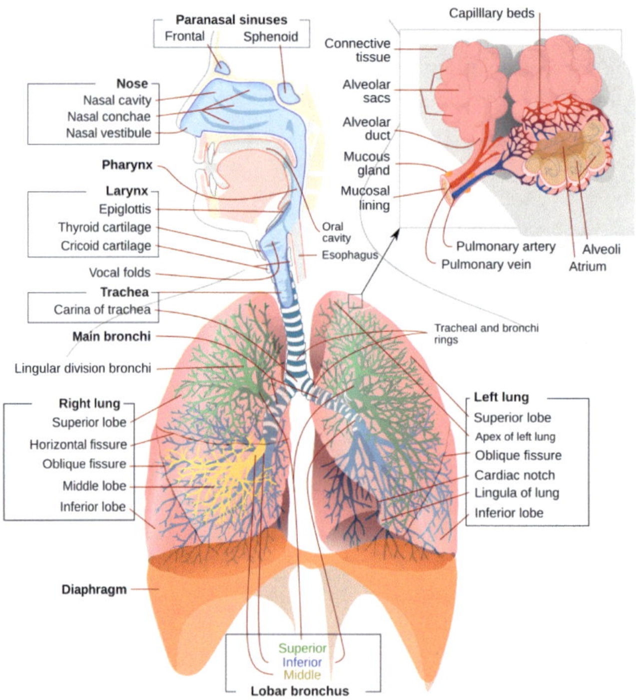

Figure 3.9. The respiratory system consists of the airways, the lungs, and the respiratory muscles that mediate the movement of air into and out of the body.

Source: https://upload.wikimedia.org/wikipedia/commons/5/5e/Respiratory_system_complete_en.svg

3.3.1. Upper Respiratory Tract: Nose, Nasal Cavity, Pharynx

The upper respiratory system, consisting of the nose, nasal cavity, and pharynx, is crucial to the general functioning of the respiratory system. The nose is the point of entry of air, where the nasal structure is such that the air entering is filtered, warmed, and humidified. The nasal passages consist of mucous membranes and cilia that filter out particulates and pathogens. This is crucial for maintaining respiratory health, as it helps protect against the risk of infection and other dangers when unfiltered air enters the lower respiratory system. During inhalation, airflow passes through the nasal cavity, which not only influences the quality of air but also plays a role in olfaction, which enhances the sense of smell through the assistance of special receptors in the nasal passages. The intricacy of the nasal cavity extends beyond the mere passage of airflow; it is also a significant place for airflow dynamics modulation. Computational models, such as those that have been created in current research, demonstrate the way airflow interacts with the different anatomical structures of the nasal cavity, influencing particle deposition in the event of inhalation. For instance, research has utilized computational fluid dynamics (CFD) to investigate the patterns of airflow, which demonstrate that local deposition efficiencies are highly responsive to particle size and flow rate, as demonstrated in (3rd Micro and Conference NF (MNF2011) et al., 2011). This is significant in fully understanding the implications of health in the event of particles inhaled into the system, bringing to the forefront the importance of the upper respiratory system in protecting the body from harmful particles in the environment. Finally, the pharynx further reinforces the position of the upper respiratory system in protecting the body from pollutants in the air. Being a conduit from the nasal cavity to the esophagus and larynx, the pharynx facilitates not only respiratory but also digestive and voice function. The function of air quality in the pharyngeal space is vital—poor air quality has been linked to increased rates of respiratory disease (e.g., asthma and COPD). Literature has indicated a correlation with airborne pollutants and increased morbidity and emphasized the significance of effective filtration and humidification mechanisms initiated within the upper respiratory tract in minimizing this threat to health, emphasizing the importance of these structures within public health interventions against air pollution, as detailed by Filipović et al. (2022).

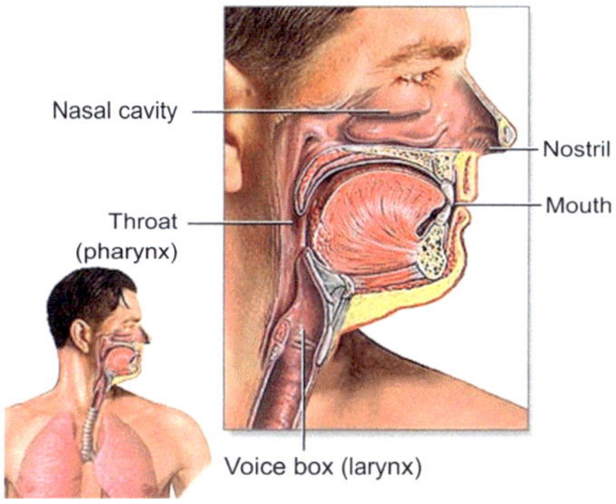

Figure 3.10. Upper Respiratory Tract.

Source: https://medlineplus.gov/ency/images/ency/fullsize/19378.jpg

3.3.2. Lower Respiratory Tract: Larynx, Trachea, Bronchi

The lower respiratory tract, consisting of the larynx, trachea, and bronchi, is an intrinsic part of the overall respiratory system functioning. The larynx, or voice box, is an important passageway between the trachea and pharynx, providing for airflow while protecting the airway from aspiration during swallowing. This complex structure of cartilage and muscle, contributing to phonation as well as containing the vocal cords, ensures the generation of sound with the vibration of the vocal cords with exhalation, used for communication. The larynx's function in controlling airflow and preventing aspiration implies its dual role as a respiratory and a phonatory organ, indicating the complex interplay of the respiratory system. The trachea, taking over from the larynx, is a rigid tube supported by C-shaped cartilaginous rings. This anatomical arrangement ensures the airway remains in an open state for the success of air passage. The trachea runs from the larynx to the bronchi, where it bifurcates into two large bronchi, leading to the left and right lungs. It is lined with mucous membrane and cilia, and the trachea also acts as a trap to eliminate foreign bodies and pathogens, hence acting as one of the body's defense mechanisms.

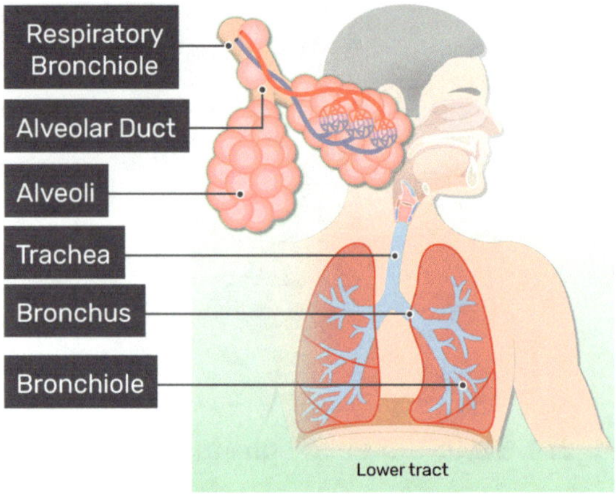

Figure 3.11. Lower respiratory tract.

Source: https://www.getbodysmart.com/wp-content/uploads/2017/09/Respiratory-lower-tract-1024x732.png

The anatomy and physiology of the trachea are of special interest, as congenital tracheal malformations can lead to serious complications. For instance, studies show that complete tracheal ring deformity (CTRD) is a cause for concern and warrant investigation into its etiology, especially in neonates and children, who are more commonly affected (Fockens et al., 2024). The bronchi further branch into smaller bronchioles, leading to the alveolar sacs, where gas exchange occurs. This branching system optimizes surface area and allows for efficient air flow through the lungs. Both bronchi have the same ciliated epithelium and smooth muscle, allowing for control of air flow into the alveoli. During respiratory distress, abnormalities such as tracheobronchomalacia can occur, leading to collapse and blockage of the airways. Such abnormalities highlight the need for structural integrity in the lower respiratory system. They often require advanced medical interventions, such as surgical interventions to remove obstructions resulting from abnormalities such as severe tracheobronchomalacia (Fockens et al., 2024). Increased knowledge of these abnormalities and treatment enhances clinical outcomes for affected children, illustrating the complex interplay between structure and function in the lower respiratory system.

3.3.3. Role of Mucous Membranes and Cilia in Protection

The respiratory system also depends on mucous membranes and cilia to offer a protective barrier against environmental irritants and pathogens. Mucous membranes line the nasal passages, trachea, and bronchi, secreting mucus which traps foreign particles, such as dust, allergens, and microbes. Not only does sticky mucus prevent harmful agents from sneaking into the deeper areas of the lungs, but it also plays an important function in keeping the airways moist, a critical parameter in successful gas exchange. Furthermore, these membranes are not inert; they are colonized by a dense microbiome that plays an important function in immune modulation and respiratory health. The presence of microbes, such as helpful *Staphylococci*, functions to stimulate the immune system, demonstrating the symbiotic relationships between the microbial and our body's defense, and the important function of the nasal microbiome in the health of human beings (Gillen, 2017). In conjunction with mucous membranes, cilia play an important function in the respiratory tract's protective function. These microscopic hair-like appendages project from the airway epithelial cells and are highly coordinated in their motion. Cilia beat in a rhythmic coordination, moving the mucus and trapped particles and pathogens up toward the throat, where they may be swallowed or expelled. This function is critical in maintaining a cleared and unobstructed airway, minimizing the occurrence of respiratory infections and other complications. Furthermore, the function of cilia can be compromised by numerous factors, including environmental toxins and smoking, which may lead to ineffective mucociliary clearance.

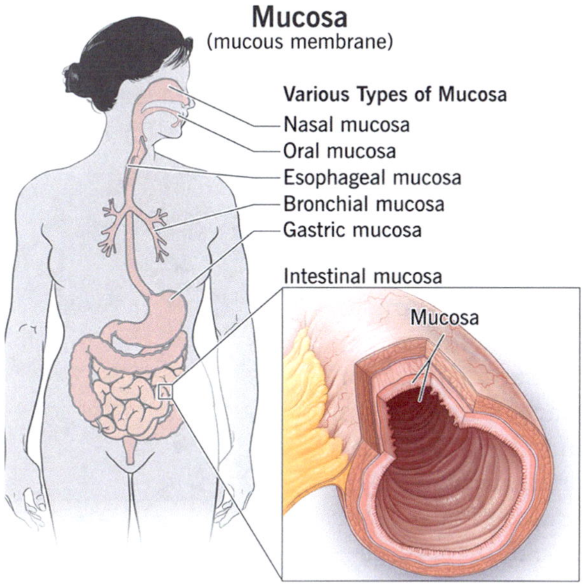

Figure 3.12. Mucosa is a mucus-secreting membrane that lines your body cavities and organs.

Source: https://my.clevelandclinic.org/-/scassets/images/org/health/articles/23930-mucosa

This highlights the importance of healthy ciliary function, as dysfunctional cilia can lead to illness such as chronic bronchitis or pneumonia, and emphasizes the importance they have in defending human respiratory health (Gokcimen, 2019). This relationship of mucous membrane, cilia, and microbiome demonstrates an intricate defense mechanism in the respiratory system. Effective mucociliary clearance plays a crucial role in maintaining lung health by directly determining the susceptibility of the body to infection. For instance, an intact barrier of mucosa functions synergistically with the cilia's protective function and beneficial microorganisms, leading to a condition that reduces the effect of pathogenic microbes. Furthermore, the fine balance of this system emphasizes the importance of normal respiratory function, particularly in instances where mucosal integrity is potentially at stake. Through an appreciation of these interactions, we are better able to appreciate how these protection mechanisms contribute to overall health and emphasize the importance of the means by which respiratory function can be maintained and enhanced against environmental harm (Gillen, 2017).

Test Your Knowledge

1. What is the upper respiratory tract?
2. What is the lower respiratory tract?

3.4. Respiratory Health and Diseases

Learning Outcome

1. Describe the common respiratory diseases
2. Know the impact of smoking and air pollution on respiratory health
3. Describe the preventive measures and treatments for respiratory conditions

The respiratory system is pivotal to human health as the primary system of gas exchange, critical to survival. It includes a highly specialized group of organs, such as the lungs, bronchi, and trachea, which together facilitate the intake of oxygen and the elimination of carbon dioxide. This is imperative not only to attain physiological homeostasis but also to facilitate the multifaceted metabolic processes conducted in the body. Significantly, the susceptibility of the respiratory system to environmental exposures—like air pollutants, allergens, and pathogens—dramatizes its susceptibility to disease, which is a persistent public health concern. Statistics testifying to this fact reveal that chronic lower respiratory diseases are the third most common cause of death in the United States. From the crossroads created by environmental exposure and disease manifestation, the need for ongoing studies continues to elucidate the pathogenesis of respiratory disease and develop effective interventions (Miller et al., 2017).

In the last decade, biomedical research breakthroughs have considerably enhanced our understanding of respiratory disease pathogenesis. Of specific mention, biologic research with nonhuman primate models has become invaluable, since such animals have lung anatomy and immune potential closely similar to that of humans. Such models provide important insights into how airborne microbes and pollutants induce respiratory disease. For example, research on the interaction of respiratory tract toxins identifies potential molecular targets for therapeutic interventions. Such findings open doors to novel treatment strategies that can impede the acceleration of diseases like asthma, COPD, and lung cancer. Secondly, application of vaccine trials in such models also serves to verify safety and efficacy against other infectious diseases and thereby translate basic research to improved clinical practices for human health (Miller et al., 2017).

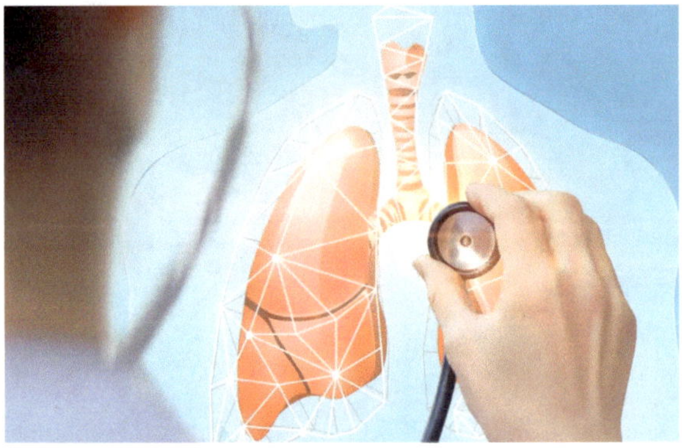

Source: https://www.visbymedical.com/wp-content/uploads/elementor/thumbs/doctor-checking-lungs-qohojwol3vm3qwv9v0wmu6ba0kq3jrui43754nvv4o.webp

The experience of viral respiratory disease, particularly by the coronaviruses, has highlighted other challenges for respiratory health. Such viruses' ability to mutate and cross species boundaries makes the public health response complex and necessitates a multidisciplinary approach to disease management. Research has sought to implement therapeutic protocols to address the viral life cycle, with the aim of inhibiting viral adhesion and replication and modulating the host's immune system. Such an One Health approach serves to highlight the interlinkage of human and animal health, necessitating the exploration of viral pathogenesis in both these areas to protect public health. Understanding the implications of such pathogens and the related therapeutic strategy is essential to optimizing respiratory health outcomes. Lastly, collaborative research and intervention strategies targeting environmental and viral aspects are key to combating respiratory disease and for maximizing overall human health.

3.4.1. Common Respiratory Diseases: Asthma, COPD, Pneumonia

The respiratory system is a critical mediator of oxygen exchange, and common diseases can disrupt this vital process. Asthma, a hyperreactive and inflammatory airway disorder, is a common disease in millions of sufferers worldwide. Asthma is a chronic disease most commonly resulting from the interaction of genetic susceptibility and environmental stimuli like allergens and irritants. Asthma leads to frequent wheezing, coughing, and shortness of breath secondary to bronchial constriction. The aggravation of asthma's conditions may severely compromise one's activity level and may lead to severe health consequences if left under treatment. Asthma's pathophysiologic process is a critical determinant of effective treatment programs and, hence, the significance of ongoing education and research to further optimize patient management and outcome. COPD is a common respiratory illness that is predominantly characterized by high morbidity and mortality, predominantly due to chronic exposure to hazardous particulate matter or gases. Tobacco smoking is the most common etiology of COPD, but air pollution, occupational dust, and passive smoke exposure non-smokers as well, rendering them susceptible.

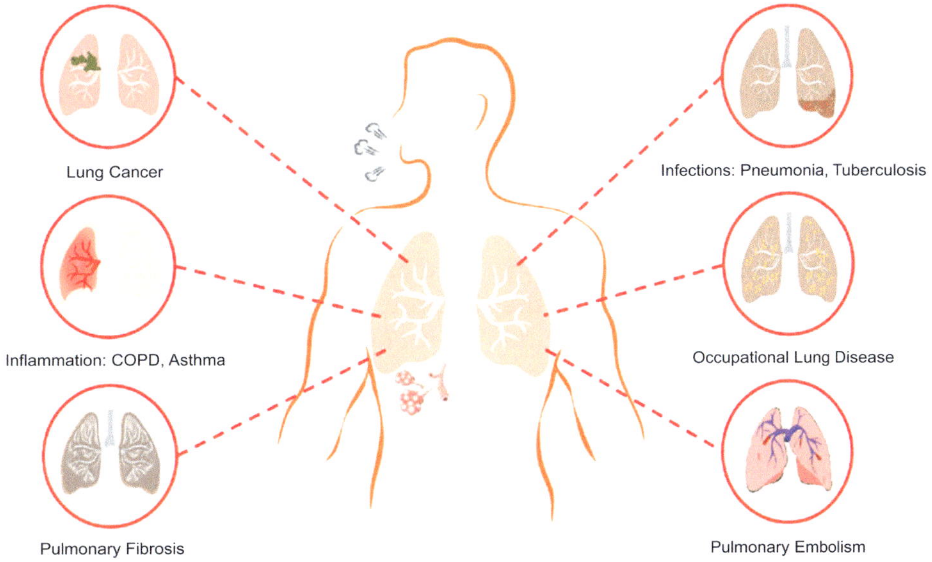

Figure 3.13. Common respiratory diseases: respiratory diseases are among the leading causes of death worldwide. Chronic respiratory conditions, including COPD and asthma, affect most people. All respiratory diseases have symptoms varying from mild to severe and can also be life-threatening.

Source: https://www.researchgate.net/profile/Jesus-Shrestha/publication/338429576/figure/fig1/AS:847043081797634@1578962216226/Common-respiratory-diseases-respiratory-diseases-are-among-the-leading-cause-of-deaths.png

The chronic, progressive illness is characterized by airflow limitation and a chronic inflammatory response, resulting in symptoms of chronic cough, sputum production, and dyspnea. With progressive age, COPD may result in severe impairment of lung function, compromising quality of life and placing a tremendous burden on health expenditure. COPD is treated with a multi-faceted approach, including smoking cessation, pharmacotherapy, and pulmonary rehabilitation to control symptoms and slow disease progression, with an emphasis on prevention and early intervention in respiratory disease. Pneumonia, a parenchymal infection of the lung, is a pandemic global public health issue, and several etiologic pathogens, including viruses, bacteria, and fungi, are responsible for its etiology. The disease can present acutely with fever, chills, cough, and shortness of breath, and, in most cases, patients present early in the illness. In vulnerable populations, such as the elderly and those with underlying diseases, pneumonia can cause dire complications and high morbidity and mortality. The respiratory tract-microbiota interaction is important in health and disease because dysbiosis can predispose a patient to respiratory infections, including pneumonia (Hou et al., 2022). Finally, the transmission of respiratory viruses, such as SARS-CoV-2, has fueled the pandemic public health issue of pneumonia, frightening healthcare systems across the globe (Gao et al., 2020). The understanding of pneumonia's pathophysiology and prevention is, therefore, critical in the development of public health programs and enhancing patient care in respiratory disease.

3.4.2. Impact of Smoking and Air Pollution on Respiratory Health

The respiratory health of individuals is negatively affected by both air pollution and smoking, which are major public health concerns. Smoking is a central cause of respiratory diseases, including COPD and lung cancer. The inhalation of tobacco toxicants results in extreme physiological changes within the lung, leading to inflammation and impaired gas exchange. Such damage is exacerbated in vulnerable populations, including children, with developing respiratory organs. The link between air pollution and respiratory health is evidenced through research, which indicates that high levels of particulate matter are linked to increased incidence of respiratory disease. Specifically, studies have established that children living in polluted areas have high rates of restricted activity days (RAD) for respiratory disease, indicating the need to address environmental reasons for declining respiratory health (Amalia et al., 2013). As one moves to more urban settings with higher levels of automotive and industrial emissions, the impact of air quality on respiratory health becomes more pronounced. The multipollutant mixture of pollutants in the air, including PM10 and PM2.5, has the potential to produce a range of health effects, of particular concern in vulnerable populations like children and the elderly. Children with high exposure levels to these particulates tend to develop asthma or experience worsening of underlying respiratory disease. Further, evidence shows children are most vulnerable as their respiratory organs are more susceptible to the damaging effects of air pollution. In comparative studies of rates of pollution in urban areas, high PM10 levels have been directly linked to the prevalence of respiratory disease, and regulatory measures for improving air quality have been emphasized as a protective factor to public health (Amalia et al., 2013). Alternative smoking products have raised concerns regarding their comparative safety compared to traditional cigarettes. Although e-cigarettes and other non-combustion products release lower amounts of harmful particles, they are not completely risk-free. Studies have found that even in non-combustion products, particulate emissions released can lead to respiratory distress, particularly in infants. Dosimetry studies demonstrate that infants receive much higher doses of particles in cigar and traditional cigarette exposure, and small particles can crosslocate to the brain through the olfactory pathway. This demonstrates that even if e-cigarettes emit lower particle levels, exposure to any form of aerosol is dangerous to respiratory health. The comparative analysis of risk exposure between alternative smoking methods emphasizes the importance of identifying the total effects of smoking and air pollution with respect to respiratory health.

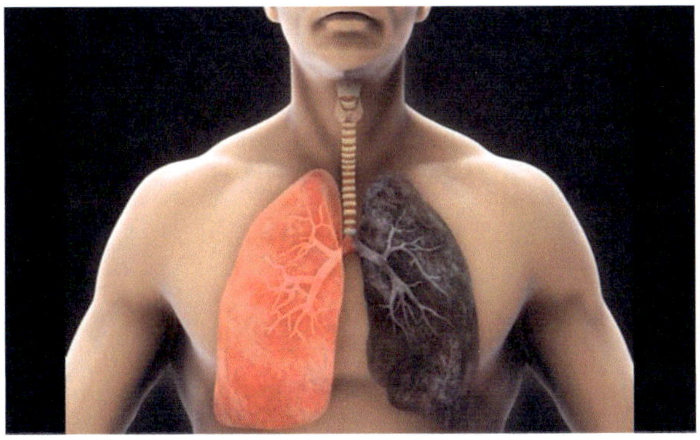

Source: https://articles-1mg.gumlet.io/articles/wp-content/uploads/2019/05/smoking-lung.jpg?compress=true&quality=80&w=640&dpr=2.6

3.4.3. Preventive Measures and Treatments For Respiratory Conditions

Preventive interventions form a crucial part of the management of respiratory conditions, both individual and public health interventions. Immunization against causal agents such as influenza and pneumococcus decreases the incidence of respiratory infection in high-risk groups. Public health interventions aim at mobilizing the population in terms of the importance of stopping smoking, purifying the air, and maintaining hygiene to reduce exposure to respiratory irritants and pathogens. Evidence has been established to show that communities with lower pollutant concentrations result in lower respiratory morbidity, highlighting the role of ambient air quality, particularly in respiratory conditions. Early detection and control of chronic diseases such as asthma and COPD through follow-up and individualized health plans also decreases rates of acute exacerbation and hospitalization, with greater long-term health benefit to the patient. Treatment-wise, it adopts an approach of multi-disciplinary intervention in handling respiratory conditions optimally. Pharmacologic interventions such as bronchodilators and corticosteroids form a crucial part of the management of conditions such as asthma and COPD, as these alleviate symptoms and improve lung function. Further, newer therapies such as monoclonal antibodies that block unique inflammatory pathways have been promising in managing severe asthma. Non-pharmacologic interventions such as pulmonary rehabilitation include exercise training, nutrition counseling, and education in disease management, with positive effects on physical function and quality of life.

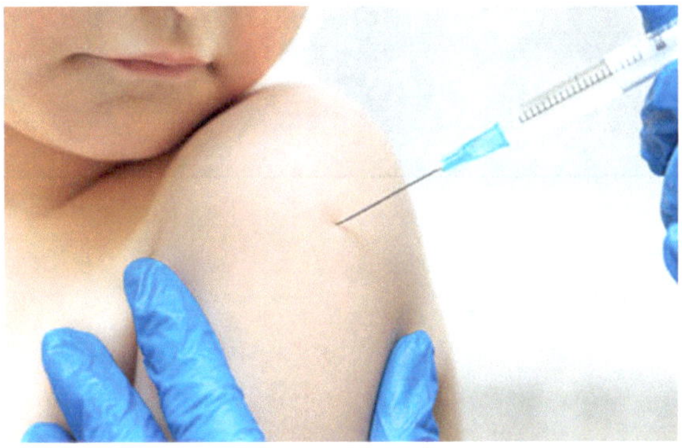

Figure 3.14. Vaccination and prevention of respiratory diseases.

Source: https://www.kauveryhospital.com/wp-content/uploads/2023/12/88-3.jpg

Research evidence indicates that treatment programs incorporating medication adherence and lifestyle modification can lead to better control of respiratory symptoms and overall patient well-being (Lundborg, 2004). Lastly, careful monitoring practices form an integral part of the management of respiratory conditions, as this results in timely intervention and judicious utilization of therapies. The use of antibiotic surveillance systems facilitates the role of antibiotic stewardship in preventing increased resistance, particularly for respiratory infections. Interventions like the Defined Daily Doses (nDDDvet) provide information on treatment frequency and facilitate the enhanced understanding of trends in the use of antibiotics (Merle and Meyer-Kühling, 2019). By implementing antimicrobial stewardship practices, healthcare professionals can enhance public health by reducing the burden of resistant pathogens and maintaining the sustainability of effective therapy. Hence, an integrated system involving preventive interventions, new therapies, and cautious monitoring practices can enhance the outcome of respiratory disease patients and community health.

Test Your Knowledge

1. What are the common respiratory diseases?
2. What is the impact of smoking and air pollution on respiratory health?

3.5. The Role of the Respiratory System in Homeostasis

Learning Outcome

1. Understand the interaction between the respiratory and circulatory systems
2. Understand the regulation of body temperature through respiration
3. Describe the role of respiratory system in maintaining acid-base balance

The respiratory system has a central role in the homeostatic control of the human body in regulating the concentrations of oxygen (O2) and carbon dioxide (CO_2) in the blood. There must be dynamic control of these concentrations so that cells have a continuous supply of oxygen for aerobic metabolism, and carbon dioxide, a by-product of metabolism, could induce acidosis if not adequately removed. The lungs facilitate gas exchange through intricate networks of alveoli, maximizing surface area and facilitating more efficient diffusion of O2 and CO_2. Also, the nervous system closely controls blood concentrations of gases, transmitting signals for compensation in respiratory rates where necessary, to maintain homeostatic equilibrium during a variety of physiological situations, e.g., rest or maximal exercise. The newer literature indicates a more intricate interaction between the respiratory system and other body systems, e.g., the cardiovascular system. For instance, the von Hippel–Lindau tumor suppressor protein–hypoxia-inducible factor (VHL–HIF) pathway has been identified as a key mediator of human systemic physiology, bridging oxygen sensing and vascular tone regulation. Chuvash polycythemia patients exhibit abnormal respiratory and pulmonary vascular control, indicating the respiratory system's integrative role in responding to systemic hypoxia. This implies that the respiratory system does not operate independently but is instead an essential interface by which various physiological systems communicate with each other to maintain overall homeostasis. Through modulation of ventilatory and vascular responses to a change in oxygen availability, the body is able to adapt to prevent harmful metabolic disturbances. Also, the microbiota-gut-brainstem axis introduces an additional dimension of complexity into the respiratory system's contribution to homeostasis. New findings from chronic intermittent hypoxia (CIH) studies reveal that gut microbiota dysregulation is able to impact respiratory function and, as a consequence, autonomic heart rate and blood pressure regulation. These findings refer to the function of the gut microbiome in respiratory and general homeostatic regulation. In this context, enhanced carotid body signaling emerges as a probable mechanism for regulating respiratory and autonomic homeostasis. These findings demonstrate that the respiratory apparatus is not an inert gas-exchange pipe but a central organ that integrates information from multiple organ systems to perform complex homeostatic processes required for survival and adaptation in various environmental niches.

3.5.1. Interaction With the Circulatory System

The interaction of the circulatory and respiratory systems is an intrinsic process of human physiology that enables the important exchange of gases for life's maintenance. The primary role of the respiratory system is focused on oxygen consumption and carbon dioxide expulsion via ventilation, diffusion, and perfusion. This gas exchange primarily occurs in the lung's alveoli, where oxygen is transferred into the blood and carbon dioxide is removed. The efficacy of this interaction largely relies on the circulatory system, where oxygen-rich blood is transported from the lungs to tissues while concurrently bringing carbon dioxide-rich blood back to the lungs. Through this dynamic interaction, the tissues of the body are assured of adequacy in oxygen for cellular metabolism and effectively remove metabolic waste. At the center of this interaction is how the brain regulates the two systems through an exquisite neural control system. The respiratory control system is ready to respond within an instant to the body's metabolic needs, where rates of ventilation are appropriately modified. For instance, during exercise, the brain increases respiratory rate to enhance oxygen consumption and reduce carbon dioxide accumulation. Such adaptations are the interdependence of the circulatory and respiratory systems, wherein respiratory function can directly influence arterial as well as compartmental gas tensions. As demonstrated. The respiratory control system, as an independent system, must cope with variations of the exercise subroutine, demonstrating our body's capacity to fine-tune these interdependent processes to respond to physiological needs (Gallagher, 2025). In addition, the effectiveness of gas exchange relies on the integrity of the two systems functioning in harmony. The circulatory system is also significant in the sense that it regulates blood supply to the organs based on their oxygen needs. The dynamic process of this regulation is one where, when body stress or activity is on the rise, blood supply goes to the muscles, which in turn demands more respiratory effort to ensure sufficient oxygen. Any malfunction in any of the parts in this system leads to tissue insufficiency of oxygen, whose health implications are dire. From extensive amounts of research and reports, one can learn that these systems are interdependent and extremely important to health, making their interaction of the utmost importance to ensure proper oxygenation of the whole human body (N/A).

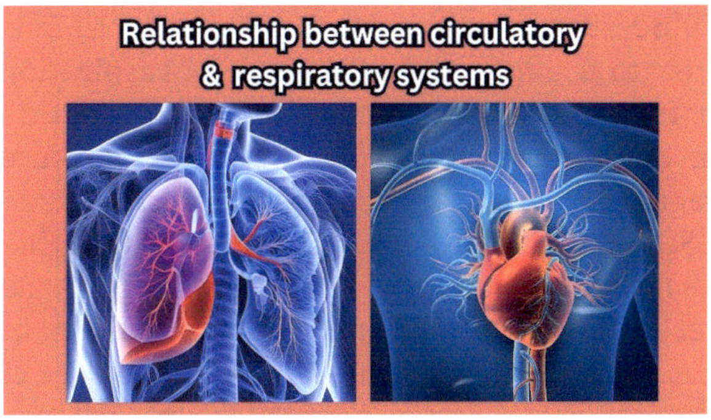

Figure 3.15. Understanding the relationship between respiratory and circulatory systems.

Source: https://i.ytimg.com/vi/nRrosNll6CQ/hq720.jpg?sqp=-oaymwEhCK4FEIIDSFryq4qpAxMIARUAAAAAGAElAADIQj0AgKJD&rs=AOn4CLCFHw6p_xxue3GH8zBHGAi1Ol4l0A

3.5.2. Regulation of Body Temperature Through Respiration

Body temperature control is an integral physiological process that requires coordination of a number of systems, including the respiratory system. In the process of air inhalation, the lungs not only facilitate gas exchange but also play a vital role in body temperature control. In situations where the body is exposed to high temperatures, the respiration rate increases, leading to greater heat loss. This is facilitated by removing warmer air and introducing cooler air into the lungs, creating a gradient through which the loss of excess body heat is facilitated. The water content in the air that is being exhaled is also responsible for evaporative cooling, a vital mechanism in body temperature control. Recognition of the mechanisms involved demonstrates the role of the respiratory system in temperature control, affirming its bifunctional role in respiration and thermoregulation. Research on the intricacies of heat transfer in medicine also establishes the role of respiration in body temperature regulation. Computational Fluid Dynamics (CFD) has also been used in simulating heat and mass transfer, with afocus on neonatal medicine, where the infant is highly vulnerable to temperature instability. CFD is easy to use in exploring the role of respiration patterns on thermal dynamics in incubators or oxygen hoods, which are vital temperature regulation devices. Research conducted using CFD has established the role of varying airflow and humidity levels in changing the respiratory function and thermal stability of patients. This demonstrates the versatility of the respiratory system's regulatory capacities in the clinical setting and establishes its imperative in the maintenance of thermal homeostasis in vulnerable populations (Fic et al., 2010). Furthermore, the application of sophisticated model-based methods to clinical care further elucidates the respiratory contribution to thermoregulation. The Infant Heat Balance Module, which was developed from CFD software, is a prime example of this paradigm shift in the inclusion of several thermal transfer processes inherent to efficient neonatal care. Simulating respiratory patterns and their effects on thermal management enables clinicians to provide concrete data to guide the design of medical devices such as incubators and radiant warmers. The predictability of thermal responses as a function of respiratory factors allows caregivers to provide optimal environmental conditions for infants and, consequently, avoid hypothermia and its complications. This integration of respiratory science and state-of-the-art technology not only underscores the multidimensional function of respiration in thermoregulation but also lays the groundwork for future advancements in medical equipment design and patient care (Ginalski et al., 2008).

3.5.3. Role in Maintaining Acid-Base Balance

The respiratory system is responsible for maintaining acid-base balance in the human body, an essential component of metabolic homeostasis. During the gas exchange process, the respiratory system controls carbon dioxide (CO_2) in the blood. During cellular metabolic processes, when carbon dioxide is produced, it combines with water to form carbonic acid, which tends to decrease blood pH. By removing carbon dioxide during exhalation, the respiratory system effectively neutralizes such acidifying processes and maintains a stable range of pH levels necessary for normal physiological processes. The efficiency of the process is crucial, especially when the body is under metabolic derangement or increased physical activity, when oxygen demand is increased, and CO_2 production is also increased. In acid-base balance, when the respiratory system is considered, it acts in combination with the renal system to correct any variation from normal pH levels. While the lungs ensure an immediate response to variations in CO_2 levels through adjustments in ventilation, the kidneys ensure regulation in the long term by reabsorbing bicarbonate ions and secreting protons. Such dual coordination ensures that any imbalance in acid-base status is corrected immediately, thereby preventing extreme physiological outcomes. Certain respirocytic changes in respiratory rates can correct acidosis or alkalosis rapidly, showing how the respiratory system can adapt to restore homeostatic balance. Such mechanisms form the basis of the significance of respiratory function not only in the uptake of oxygen but also in the regulation of pH balance in the body, which signifies its central role in human physiology. Recent research has emphasized the complexity of these interactions and the overall significance they have for health, especially in respiratory diseases. Diseases that affect lung function, for example, COPD or pulmonary fibrosis, can severely affect acid-base balance by restricting the elimination of carbon dioxide. Abnormal respiratory function can cause respiratory acidosis or defective compensation of metabolic derangement, with hazardous systemic consequences. As explored in studies intent on examining the interaction between respiratory function and acid-base homeostasis, the understanding of these mechanisms may result in novel treatment strategies. For example, newer medications aimed at reducing inflammation and respiratory efficiency have been shown to restore acid-base balance and enhance patient outcomes in conditions that test the respiratory system's capacity to maintain optimal pH levels (Ding et al., 2025; Gantsova et al., 2024).

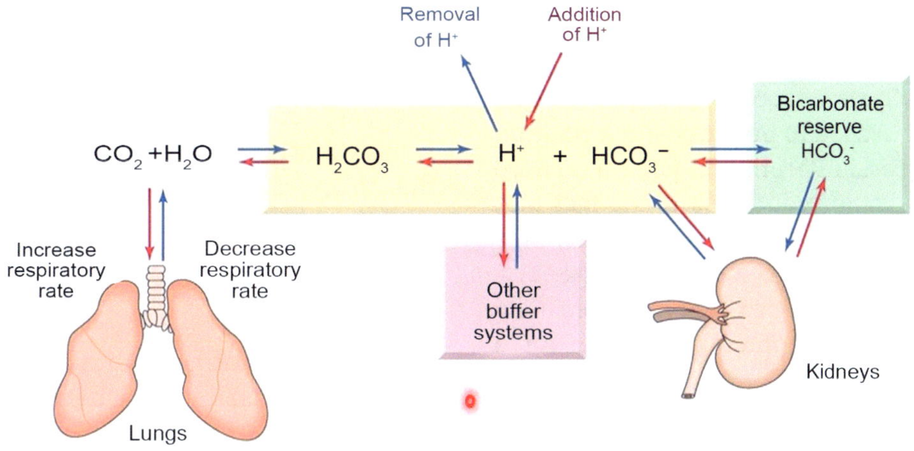

Figure 3.16. Acid Base Balance.

Source: https://i.ytimg.com/vi/GKFxuHKVh10/maxresdefault.jpg

Test Your Knowledge

1. Describe the regulation of body temperature through respiration.
2. What is the role of respiratory system in maintaining acid-base balance?

3.6. Advances in Respiratory Medicine

Learning Outcome

1. Understand the innovations in diagnostic tools
2. Know the development of treatments for respiratory ailments
3. Describe the research on lung transplantation and regenerative medicine

Excellent advances in respiratory medicine in the past half-century have transformed understanding and management of most respiratory diseases, most notably acute respiratory distress syndrome (ARDS). Significant effort in the past five decades has gone into defining ARDS risk factors and pathogenic processes and has led to better characterization of protein expression profiles in patients. There has been an advancement despite the fact that successful pharmacologic therapy remains limited, primarily due to ARDS heterogeneity and variability of patient drug response. The heterogeneity has prompted the search for a precision medicine strategy, where therapy tailored to the patient's biomarker profile would optimize therapy. With biomolecular measurements of increased complexity, scientists in the present era are more likely to discover new targets for therapy, which could facilitate personalized therapy to revolutionize ARDS therapy and improve patient outcomes (Calfee and Meyer, 2017). Another innovative front in respiratory medicine innovation is innovation in non-invasive monitoring devices that improve respiratory function monitoring. One of the new technologies is the use of electrocardiogram (ECG)-derived respiration (EDR) methods, where respiratory data can be derived from flexible electrodes on standard ECG locations. More recent literature has described novel techniques with miniaturized sensors with decreased inter-electrode distance, such that more precise monitoring can be done in a broad range of environmental conditions, from standard physiological monitoring to sleep studies. The new technique has special promise when implemented in smart clothing, where standard respiratory monitoring methods would be impractical. By providing real-time and precise respiratory data, such technology improves clinical monitoring as well as enables individuals to gain more control over their respiratory status (Daříček et al., 2018). Interfacing such cutting-edge methodologies and precision medicine strategy depicts a paradigm seismic shift in the direction of an integrative model of respiratory health. As research continues to deconstruct the complexity of respiratory disease, cross-disciplinary cooperation will be important to translating such scientific advances into beneficial clinical applications. Progress of respiratory medicine requires a multidisciplinary approach, not merely to the biological determinants of heterogeneous disease but also to the psychological and environmental determinants of respiratory health. As this specialty continues to progress, the potential to improve patient outcomes grows, necessitating healthcare professionals to keep abreast of such developments. With the application of innovation and a patient-centered model, respiratory medicine is set to revolutionize care and improve the quality of life for patients with respiratory disease.

3.6.1. Innovations in Diagnostic Tools: Spirometry, Imaging

The specialty of respiratory diagnostics has seen historic advances, primarily through technological advancements in spirometry, which measures lung function and air flow patterns. Traditional spirometry is limited in that it is patient-dependent and effort-dependent, leading to variable findings. Recent technological advances, including the availability of portable spirometers with mobile phone software, have made accessibility and ease of use simpler. In addition to being able to measure respiratory function in real-time, the devices also allow for patient-to-clinician transmission of data. Computerized algorithms of spirometric interpretation have also improved the accuracy of diagnosis, particularly in challenging conditions such as asthma and COPD. The advances underscore the importance of integrating more advanced spirometric technology into routine clinical practice, thereby allowing for earlier diagnosis and better management of respiratory disease. Imaging modalities of respiratory diagnostics have also seen significant advances to allow for better comprehension of pulmonary disease. HRCT and MRI have been effective diagnostic tools, allowing clinicians to visualize complex lung structures and surrounding tissues with high sensitivity. The advances not only improve lesion or abnormality detection but also allow for assessment of disease progression, such as in interstitial lung disease and thoracic endometriosis. As noted in recent research, imaging has the potential to allow for therapeutic intervention and improvement in patient outcomes through the detection of specific morphological changes characteristic in various respiratory diseases. Integrated approaches that integrate imaging findings with appropriate biomarkers are likely to increase diagnostic accuracy, allowing for individualized treatment regimens that account for the structural as well as biological characteristics of respiratory disease (Ba Jłoniak et al., 2025). The application of machine learning algorithms to respiratory diagnosis represents a paradigm shift to more efficient and accurate assessment processes. For instance, research on spirometry data for silicosis has demonstrated the potential of machine learning for enhancing the interpretability and accuracy of oscillometric parameters. Through the processing of large data sets, algorithms like Explainable Boosting Machines (EBM) and HyperTab can predict respiratory changes accurately, contributing to improved diagnostic accuracy for associated conditions that are frequently impacted by environmental exposure. These advancements not only enable the streamlined diagnostic process but also assist clinicians in making informed decisions based on detailed data analysis. With advances in machine learning, its application to respiratory diagnosis will increase further, harnessing emerging data interpretation methods into clinical practice, hence improving the management of complicated conditions (Lu Jís Machado do Amaral et al., 2025).

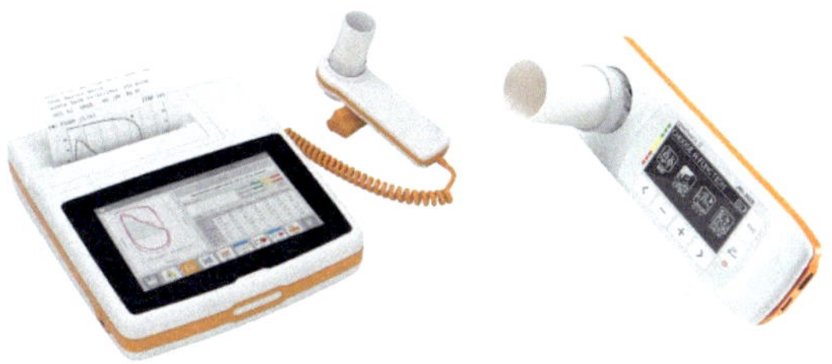

Figure 3.17. Spirometry.

Source: https://respiratory-therapy.com/wp-content/uploads/2024/07/SpiroPFT__MIR__Spirolab-Spirobank2-1280x640.jpg

3.6.2. Development of Treatments: Inhalers, Oxygen Therapy

The history of inhalers is a giant step forward in the development of treatments for respiratory disease, primarily asthma and COPD. Early attempts at inhalation therapy were primitive and often ineffective, but the introduction of metered-dose inhalers (MDIs) lent a new level of sophistication to the delivery of bronchodilators, including beta$_2$-agonists. Research shows that these inhalers, when used with a holding chamber or spacer, are as effective as nebulizers in acute situations without the logistical hassle of nebulizer therapy, such as power supply and maintenance needs (Ba et al., 2013). In addition, the convenience of MDIs allows patients to self-administer medication and, in doing so, enhance compliance while optimizing acute and chronic care outcomes in patients suffering from respiratory disease. In addition to inhalers, oxygen therapy is an integral part of the management of severe respiratory disease. This therapy involves the delivery of supplemental oxygen to hypoxemic patients, a condition common in diseases such as pneumonia, acute respiratory distress syndrome, and COPD. The therapeutic administration of oxygen not only calms symptoms but also maximizes patient survival by enhancing oxygenation to vital organs. Recent studies affirm the efficacy of oxygen therapy when administered with inhaled medication as a holistic approach to treatment.

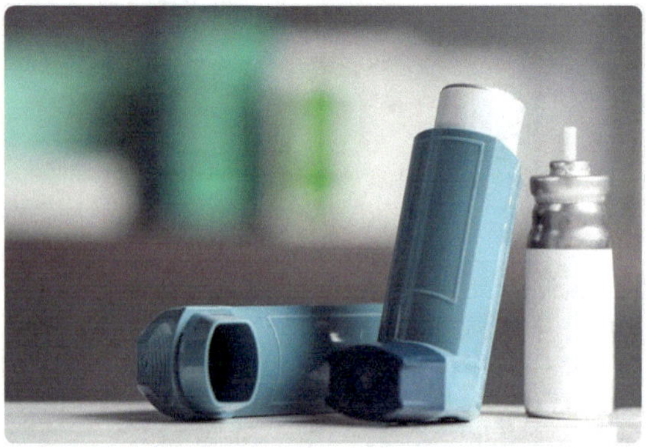

Figure 3.18. Inhalers.

Source: https://d2jx2rerrg6sh3.cloudfront.net/image-handler/picture/2021/1/shutterstock_1258402990.jpg

The inclusion of pulse oximetry technology has further optimized oxygen therapy, enabling clinicians to continuously monitor patients' oxygen saturation and adjust treatments accordingly (Ba et al., 2006). This dynamic management is central to preventing exacerbations and optimizing pulmonary function. Treatment for patients suffering from respiratory disease continues to evolve, most notably through the synergy of inhalers and oxygen therapy. Technological advancements in inhalation devices, such as dry powder inhalers and soft mist inhalers, are designed to provide optimal drug delivery efficiency and the least side effects, to adapt to variable patient needs. At the same time, new evidence regarding high-flow oxygen therapy has demonstrated promising benefits in acute respiratory failure, which reflects ongoing interest in the improvement of treatment modalities. With new emerging technologies and treatments, there is potential to improve personalized care strategies individually aimed at individual patient profiles and thereby improve overall treatment efficacy for respiratory disease. These developments underscore the pivotal role of research and innovation in shaping the future of respiratory care, thereby improving the quality of life for millions of patients worldwide.

3.6.3. Research on Lung Transplantation and Regenerative Medicine

Lung transplant and regenerative medicine are on the increase, with chronic respiratory disease and organ demand continuing to influence patient outcomes worldwide. The imperative demand for successful alternative lung transplantation has pushed innovation in the development of artificial lungs, where techniques like extracorporeal membrane oxygenation (ECMO) are temporary measures for desperately ill patients. Revolutionary progress has been achieved, overcoming the constraints of biocompatibility and the risk of immune rejection. For instance, the use of advanced biomaterials and technologies like 3D bioprinting has shown promise for the development of implantable artificial lungs that can mimic critical respiratory function autonomously. This multi-disciplinary area of study brings together engineering, technology, and biomedical sciences, potentially revolutionizing the treatment of respiratory patients with chronic lung disease or at risk of respiratory failure (Gutiérrez et al., 2025). Another promising breakthrough within the regenerative medicine field is the generation of organoids—miniaturized, self-assembling tissues that replicate the three-dimensional anatomy of human organs. Organoids have revolutionized the investigation of lung development and lung disease, giving scientists one platform to observe the development of disease and reaction to potential therapeutic compounds. As organoids are grown from stem cells or tissue, they can maintain the properties of their parent tissue, and thus they are very useful in research into a number of respiratory diseases as well as in drug screening. Organoid technology also serves the search for functional transplant mechanisms by offering insight into how lung tissue can be engineered or regenerated, thus setting the stage for alternatives to decrease dependence on donor organs (Freilich et al., 2020).

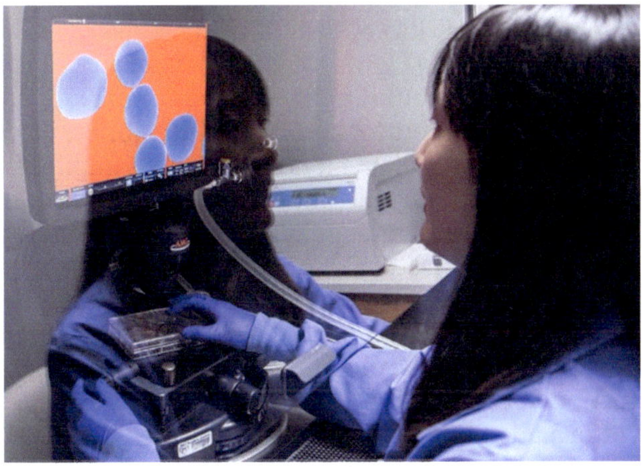

Figure 3.19. Regenerative medicine in lung diseases.

Source: https://www.mayoclinic.org/-/media/kcms/gbs/medical-professionals/images/2020/03/31/18/10/stem-cell-lab-767px.jpg

In addition, the advancement of lung transplantation research to the field of regenerative medicine is also an indication of the potential of an integrated approach to the treatment of respiratory disease. The challenge of organ availability can be addressed by techniques such as decellularization of donor lungs, where cellular material is removed, and patient-specific cells repopulate the lung scaffold. Not only does this increase the likelihood of transplant success by lowering rejection, but it also enables sustainability in organ transplantation. Current research in these regenerative techniques, coupled with synergistic artificial lung and organoid development, is a vital frontier in the development of treatments for chronic lung disease and the way forward for personalized medicine (Gutiérrez et al., 2025; Freilich et al., 2020).

Test Your Knowledge

1. What are the advances in diagnostic tools?
2. What are the development of treatments for respiratory ailments?

SUMMARY

In summarizing an analysis of the human respiratory system, it becomes apparent that this intricate system is at the heart of maintaining individual health and the overall dynamics of community health. The respiratory system performs gas exchange—infusing oxygen and expelling carbon dioxide—and thus immediately influences metabolic processes and overall homeostasis. Further, the intricate interplay between respiratory function and the immune response underscores the importance of respiratory health as protection against disease. As demonstrated in research, the role of specialized cells derived from bone marrow assists the immune system in the deployment of effective immunological attacks against pathogens, testifying to a direct relationship between respiratory mechanisms and immunological function, as demonstrated in granulopoiesis research (Burvenich et al., 2002). Such observation underscores the importance of understanding the complexity of the respiratory system to develop medical interventions and treatment for public health. More importantly, understanding the respiratory system is not anatomy and physiology; it is all about the implications of external influences, including environmental forces and pathogenic threats. Research into the spread of respiratory infection, such as grippe and acute respiratory tract infection, underscores the importance of understanding how and in what ways respiratory infection may affect large segments of the population and social structures. The use of statistical models in describing processes of epidemics underscores the importance of the relationship between respiratory health and societal resilience. This, in turn, underscores the respiratory system's central role in public health outcomes (Demin et al., 2004). The dynamics of respiratory infection in the community environment underscore the importance of active interventions in health and informed public policy in the prevention of infection. Finally, the complexity of the respiratory system necessitates an integrated response in its functioning and operation. Not just an important aspect of individual health and metabolism, but community health dynamics as well, the respiratory system is worthy of priority attention in research and focus. The association of respiratory physiology and the immune system, and regulation by external regulators, points to the necessity of ongoing research and attention to respiratory health. Refining our knowledge in this system and in the appropriate utilization of public health interventions is crucial in the prevention of respiratory disease and general health in society. An integrated response to respiratory health is therefore necessary to build resilience against possible health crises through respiratory infection and disease.

The respiratory system is essential to the gas exchange that forms the foundation of the body's homeostasis. The complex system consists of a chain of anatomical structures, the alveoli, bronchi, trachea, and lungs, functioning in series to facilitate efficient air passage in and out of the body. As one inhales air, air full of oxygen is swallowed into the lungs where it is channeled into thin-walled alveoli, facilitating diffusion into the blood. At the same time, carbon dioxide, a product of cellular metabolism, is expelled from the blood into the alveoli and exhaled. Process efficiency is of utmost importance, as human cells require a continuous supply of oxygen to facilitate energy production, and the function of the respiratory system in maintaining life and metabolic activities. In addition to gas exchange, the respiratory system also plays an essential role in the modulation of other physiological activities. It facilitates olfactory perception, or the sense of smell, through the inhalation of odor molecules in the air. This association of respiration and perception of odors is suggestive of a more profound physiological interconnection, with experiments showing changes in respiratory parameters with odors and olfactory imagery. Such respiratory responses might modulate sensory perception, demonstrating the way in which the respiratory system facilitates not only mere survival but also the human experience of the world. Perception of how such interactions play a part in the understanding of the function of the respiratory system to overall health and well-being further underscores its multifunctional nature beyond mere gas exchange

(Kleemann, 2010). The respiratory system is also of critical significance in the immune defense against pathogens, particularly in diseases such as influenza infection. Vaccination strategies, such as those that induce both mucosal and systemic immunity, highlight the respiratory system's ability to communicate with the immune system. The emphasis on cellular immunity in the induction of long-term protection against respiratory viruses in recent studies highlights that the respiratory system is more than just a conduit for air, but also a protective covering against infectious etiologies. Therefore, the progress achieved in vaccine development, such as the design of recombinant T cell-inducing vaccines, highlights the continued endeavor to optimize our immune defenses by understanding more about the respiratory system's inherent functions (Glezen et al., 2016). This interface highlights the respiratory system's important functions in oxygenation and immunity, and its relevance to human longevity and quality of life.

KEY TERMS FROM THIS CHAPTER

Alveoli
Bacteria
Bronchi
Electromyography
Lungs
Nervous systems
Respiratory system
Trachea
Asthma
Breathing disorders
Diaphragm
Heart rhythm
Mechanomyography
Respiratory diseases
Thoracic cavity

CRITICAL THINKING QUESTIONS

1. The primary function of the respiratory system is:

a. Digestion of food
b. Exchange of oxygen and carbon dioxide
c. Circulation of blood
d. Production of energy

2. The process of breathing is called:

a. Respiration
b. Ventilation
c. Inhalation
d. Diffusion

3. The respiratory system consists of:

a. Heart, lungs, and diaphragm
b. Nasal cavity, lungs, and diaphragm
c. Kidneys, lungs, and esophagus
d. Brain, spinal cord, and lungs

4. The upper respiratory tract includes:

a. Lungs and trachea
b. Nose, nasal cavity, and pharynx
c. Bronchi and alveoli
d. Lungs and diaphragm

5. The trachea is commonly known as:

a. Windpipe
b. Food pipe
c. Voice box
d. Nasal passage

Short Answer Questions

1. What is the respiratory system?
2. Why is respiratory system important in the human body?
3. What is the function of respiratory system?
4. What are the pathways of respiratory?
5. What is the role of the respiratory system in homeostasis?

Answer to Critical Thinking Questions

1. (b) 2. (b) 3. (b) 4. (b) 5. (a)

REFERENCES

1. Ackermann, M. (2001). *Respiratory Tract*. https://core.ac.uk/download/128980233.pdf (accessed on 15th June 2025).

2. Adami, C., Casoni, D., Giovannini, A. E. J., et al. (2016). A possible case of neurogenic pulmonary edema in a sheep following intracranial surgery. https://core.ac.uk/download/157769133.pdf (accessed on 15th June 2025).

3. Amalia, M., Bennet, J., Resosudarmo, P. (2013). The consequences of urban air pollution for child health: What does self-reporting data in the Jakarta metropolitan area reveal? https://media.neliti.com/media/publications/151254-EN-the-consequences-of-urban-air-pollution.pdf (accessed on 15th June 2025).

4. Amann, A., Lumb, A. B., Schrikker, A. C., Mörk, A. K., Amann, A., et al. (2010). A mathematical model for breath gas analysis of volatile organic compounds with special emphasis on acetone. http://arxiv.org/abs/1003.4475 (accessed on 15th June 2025).

5. Amaral, J. L. M. do, Sousa, C. M. de S., Ribeiro, C. de O., Sá, P. M. de, Lopes, A. J., & Lopes de Melo, P. (2025). A diagnostic support system based on interpretable machine learning and oscillometer for accurate diagnosis of respiratory dysfunction in silicosis. *bioRxiv*. https://www.semanticscholar.org/paper/5540cadd9dba985d23bec661675e9998c776bccb (accessed on 15th June 2025).

6. Amodio, F., Brancaccio, M., Caiazza, M., Calabro, P., Cesaro, A., D'Alicandro, G., Di Micco, P., et al. (2021). Exercise, immune system, nutrition, respiratory and cardiovascular diseases during COVID-19: A complex combination. https://core.ac.uk/download/541666585.pdf (accessed on 15th June 2025).

7. Avino, P., Manigrasso, M., Protano, C., et al. (2017). Second-hand smoke generated by combustion and electronic smoking devices used in real scenarios: Ultrafine particle pollution and age-related dose assessment. https://core.ac.uk/download/98348903.pdf (accessed on 15th June 2025).

8. Awoyomi, T. (2020). An anatomy of the international financial system vis-à-vis the human body system. *Comparative Political Economy: Regulation eJournal*. https://www.semanticscholar.org/paper/56914b66431595eb5e325a7380616bdff3b2524a (accessed on 15th June 2025).

9. Bałoniak, J., Szymańska, Z., Leszyńska, A., Bałoniak, Z., Jonkisz, A., Skurzyńska, G., Stremel, A., et al. (2025). Diagnostic challenges and innovations in thoracic endometriosis (TE). *Quality in Sport*. https://www.semanticscholar.org/paper/01ba55451652b5914c1b6bbc9fe454278cfd7661 (accessed on 15th June 2025).

10. Bansal, A., & Sharma, D. (2020). The bitter the taste, the better is the medicine: Is caffeine the answer to COVID-19? https://core.ac.uk/download/334499981.pdf (accessed on 15th June 2025).

11. Barnes, V. A., Crawford, M. W., Harden, K., et al. (2014). Widespread depolarization during expiration: A source of respiratory drive? https://core.ac.uk/download/131210052.pdf (accessed on 15th June 2025).

12. Bastir, M., Sanz-Prieto, D., López-Rey, J. M., Palancar, C. A., Gómez-Recio, M., López-Cano, M., González-Ruiz, J. M., et al. (2022). The evolution, form and function of the human respiratory system. *Journal of Anthropological Sciences = Rivista di Anthropology: JASS, 100*, 141–172.

https://www.semanticscholar.org/paper/49509f495d36e3d7230268c641389226ee5e4537 (accessed on 15th June 2025).

13. Brenner, M. P., Lieberman, D. E., Ostilla-Mónico, R., et al. (2017). Physical and geometric constraints explain the labyrinth-like shape of the nasal cavity. http://arxiv.org/abs/1708.08966 (accessed on 15th June 2025).
14. Brown, N. J. (1990). *Health Hazard Manual for Firefighters*. https://core.ac.uk/download/5122113.pdf (accessed on 15th June 2025).
15. Burvenich, C., Meyer, E., & Van Merris, V. (2002). Functional maturation during bovine granulopoiesis. https://core.ac.uk/download/55786961.pdf (accessed on 15th June 2025).
16. Calfee, C. S., & Meyer, N. J. (2017). Novel translational approaches to the search for precision therapies for acute respiratory distress syndrome. https://core.ac.uk/download/323074546.pdf (accessed on 15th June 2025).
17. Campos, J., Jolley, J., Lozano, M., et al. (2018). Surface mechanomyography and electromyography provide non-invasive indices of inspiratory muscle force and activation in healthy subjects. https://core.ac.uk/download/187265990.pdf (accessed on 15th June 2025).
18. Cates, C. J., Welsh, E. J., & Rowe, B. H. (2013). Holding chambers (spacers) versus nebulizers for beta-agonist treatment of acute asthma. *Cochrane Database of Systematic Reviews, 2013*(9), CD000052. https://doi.org/10.1002/14651858.CD000052.pub3 (accessed on 15th June 2025).
19. Crisafulli, A., Marongiu, E., Nobrega, A. C. L., et al. (2014). Neural regulation of cardiovascular response to exercise: Role of central command and peripheral afferents. https://core.ac.uk/download/pdf/54599119.pdf (accessed on 15th June 2025).
20. Dařiček, M., Donoval, M., Kopáni, M., et al. (2018). Optimization of the position of single-lead wireless sensor with low electrodes separation distance for ECG-derived respiration. https://core.ac.uk/download/189852067.pdf (accessed on 15th June 2025).
21. Demin, S., Emelyanova, N., Gafarov, F., et al. (2004). Non-Markov stochastic dynamics of real epidemic process of respiratory infections. http://arxiv.org/abs/nlin/0402010 (accessed on 15th June 2025).
22. Ding, Z., Deng, Y., Luo, H., Liu, C., Yang, M., Xue, H., & Chen, Z. (2025). Progress of tanshinone IIA against respiratory diseases: Therapeutic targets and potential mechanisms. *Frontiers in Pharmacology, 16*. https://www.semanticscholar.org/paper/ddfc79950cd29024b7386b8187a521321bf54884 (accessed on 15th June 2025).
23. Ebejer, M. J., & Lesauskaite, V. (1999). Age-related changes in the respiratory system. https://core.ac.uk/download/46601782.pdf (accessed on 15th June 2025).
24. Fic, A. M., Ginalski, M. K., Ingham, D. B., et al. (2010). An overview of recent applications of computational modelling in neonatology. https://core.ac.uk/download/336770.pdf (accessed on 15th June 2025).
25. Filipović, N., Jaćimovski, S., Lamovec, J., et al. (2022). Transient numerical simulation of airflow characteristics in the mouth-throat 3D model. https://core.ac.uk/download/541412415.pdf (accessed on 15th June 2025).
26. Fockens, M. M. (2024). Anomalies of the larynx and trachea: Developmental aspects and treatment considerations. https://core.ac.uk/download/604736713.pdf (accessed on 15th June 2025).

27. Freilich, M. (2020). What is the future of organoids? https://core.ac.uk/download/428373201.pdf (accessed on 15th June 2025).

28. Gallagher, R. R. (2025). Evaluation of exercise-respiratory system modifications and preliminary respiratory-circulatory system integration scheme. https://core.ac.uk/download/pdf/42869640.pdf (accessed on 15th June 2025).

29. Gantsova, E., Serova, O. V., Vishnyakova, P., Deyev, I., Elchaninov, A. V., & Fatkhudinov, T. (2024). Mechanisms and physiological relevance of acid-base exchange in functional units of the kidney. *PeerJ, 12*. https://www.semanticscholar.org/paper/fb1d19562f283ed07b9ff426d1278f98e549af92 (accessed on 15th June 2025).

30. Gao, Y., Ding, M., Dong, X., Zhang, J., Azkur, A. K., Azkur, D., Gan, H., et al. (2020). Risk factors for severe and critically ill COVID-19 patients: A review. *Allergy, 76*, 428–455. https://doi.org/10.1111/all.14657 (accessed on 15th June 2025).

31. Gavazza, A., Rossi, G., Galosi, L., Cerquetella, M., & Mangiaterra, S. (2021). Therapeutic approaches to coronavirus infection according to "One Health" concept. https://core.ac.uk/download/541169295.pdf (accessed on 15th June 2025).

32. Gillen, A. L. (2017). Staph bacteria from first breath: The interweaving of the nasal microbiome with the intricate and complex nose. https://core.ac.uk/download/220159120.pdf (accessed on 15th June 2025).

33. Ginalski, M. K., Nowak, A. J., & Wrobel, L. C. (2008). Modelling of heat and mass transfer processes in neonatology. https://core.ac.uk/download/335471.pdf (accessed on 15th June 2025).

34. Gokcimen, A. (2019). Morphology of salivary and lacrimal glands. https://core.ac.uk/download/322442316.pdf (accessed on 15th June 2025).

35. Gutiérrez, Y., Lugo, C., & Rondón, J. (2025). Artificial lung: A biomedical engineering approach. https://core.ac.uk/download/652359337.pdf (accessed on 15th June 2025).

36. Hou, K., Wu, Z. X., Chen, X. Y., Wang, J. Q., Zhang, D., Xiao, C., Zhu, D., et al. (2022). Microbiota in health and diseases. *Signal Transduction and Targeted Therapy, 7*. https://doi.org/10.1038/s41392-022-00974-4 (accessed on 15th June 2025).

37. Kafoury, R., Lowe, K. L., Pacurari, M., et al. (2016). A review on the respiratory system toxicity of carbon nanoparticles. https://core.ac.uk/download/539653798.pdf (accessed on 15th June 2025).

38. Kleemann, A. M. (2010). Orientation in space using the sense of smell. https://core.ac.uk/download/11031812.pdf (accessed on 15th June 2025).

39. Liu, F. F. (1973). Respiratory analysis system and method. https://core.ac.uk/download/pdf/10304244.pdf (accessed on 15th June 2025).

40. Lucking, E. F., O'Connor, K. M., Strain, C. R., Fouhy, F., Bastiaanssen, T. F. S., Burns, D. P., Golubeva, A. V., Stanton, C., Clarke, G., Cryan, J. F., & O'Halloran, K. D. (2018). Chronic intermittent hypoxia disrupts cardiorespiratory homeostasis and gut microbiota composition in adult male guinea-pigs. *EBioMedicine, 38*, 191–205. https://doi.org/10.1016/j.ebiom.2018.11.010 (accessed on 15th June 2025).

41. Lundborg, K. (2004). Housing, management and health in Swedish dairy calves. https://core.ac.uk/download/11694701.pdf (accessed on 15th June 2025).

42. Mejino, J. L. V., & Rosse, C. (2007). The Foundational Model of Anatomy Ontology. https://core.ac.uk/download/pdf/9412334.pdf (accessed on 15th June 2025).

43. Merle, R., & Meyer-Kühling, B. (2019). Concepts, examples and discussion of influencing factors. https://core.ac.uk/download/288845806.pdf (accessed on 15th June 2025).

44. Miller, L., Pinkerton, K., Royer, C., et al. (2017). Nonhuman primate models of respiratory disease: Past, present, and future. https://core.ac.uk/download/323069778.pdf (accessed on 15th June 2025).

45. Murray-Smith, D. J., & Thamrin, H. (2009). A mathematical model of the human respiratory system during exercise. https://core.ac.uk/download/9399576.pdf (accessed on 15th June 2025).

46. N/A. (2023). Pathophysiology of spinal cord injury (SCI). https://core.ac.uk/download/553656710.pdf (accessed on 15th June 2025).

47. N/A. (2025). *Aerospace Medicine and Biology: A Continuing Bibliography with Indexes, Supplement 197, September 1979*. https://core.ac.uk/download/pdf/42868228.pdf (accessed on 15th June 2025).

48. Niwa, M., Ochiai, N., Sasaki, S. I., Uga, M. (2010). Activity patterns of the diaphragm during voluntary movements in awake cats. https://core.ac.uk/download/56644610.pdf (accessed on 15th June 2025).

49. Smith, T. G., Brooks, J. T., Balanos, G. M., Lappin, T. R., Layton, D. M., Leedham, D. L., Liu, C., Maxwell, P. H., McMullin, M. F., McNamara, C. J., Percy, M. J., Pugh, C. W., Ratcliffe, P. J., Talbot, N. P., Treacy, M., & Robbins, P. A. (2006). Mutation of von Hippel–Lindau tumor suppressor and human cardiopulmonary physiology. *PLoS Medicine, 3*(7), e290. https://doi.org/10.1371/journal.pmed.0030290 (accessed on 15th June 2025).

50. Spitaels, J., Roose, K., & Saelens, X. (2016). Influenza and memory T cells: How to awake the force. *Vaccines (Basel), 4*(4), 33. https://doi.org/10.3390/vaccines4040033 (accessed on 15th June 2025).

DIGESTIVE SYSTEM (ORAL CAVITY)

4

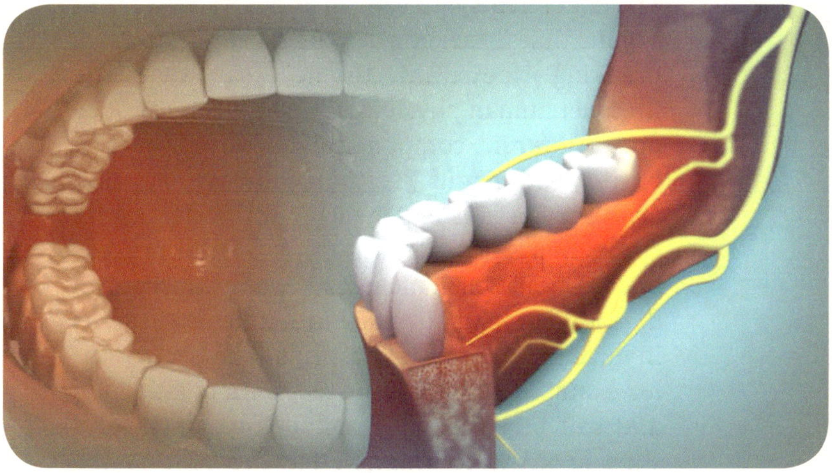

Introduction

The digestive system is a fundamental component of human physiology with the intrinsic role of breaking down food into available nutrients for the body. It is a complex system comprising a number of different organs, each with a specific function in the overall process of digestion. The oral cavity, or mouth, is where digestion first begins and is a fundamental component of the process. Not only is it responsible for initial mechanical breakdown of food by mastication, but it is also where enzymes and saliva enter the process to start chemical digestion. An understanding of the multifaceted role of the oral cavity in the process of digestion is the cornerstone of the study of how various pathological states can affect this critical system. In addition to mechanical and chemical roles, the oral cavity has an important role in the overall health and maintenance of the digestive system. The mouth is more than a gateway for food; it contains a mixed oral microbiota. This microbiota has a role in digestion, immune function, and systemic health through interaction with other systemic

LEARNING OBJECTIVES

After studying this chapter, you will be able to:

1. Describe the anatomy of the oral cavity
2. Learn about functions of the oral cavity
3. Know the salivary glands
4. Understand the process of digestion in the oral cavity
5. Describe the common disorders of the oral cavity
6. Describe the role of the oral cavity in overall health

components. Recent studies shed light on the oral and gut health complexities and show that dysregulation of oral health can have systemic implications on conditions, such as those arising from dysbiosis of the gut microbiome. As such, an understanding of the oral cavity's role is more than simple digestion and involves a more holistic understanding of health and disease. Additionally, implications of oral health continue to expand with responses to discussion in public health, including antimicrobial resistance (AMR) and diet influences on health outcomes.

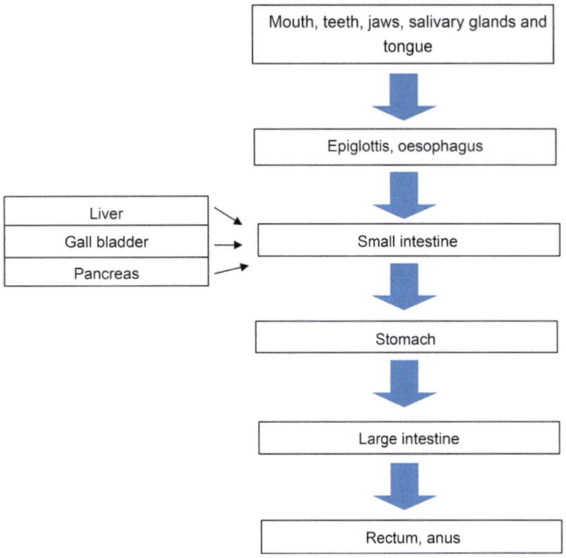

Figure 4.1. Flow chart of the digestive system.

Source: https://www.dental-nursing.co.uk/article-images/image-library/161/image_1_cea4740f.jpg

The oral cavity is a reservoir for many pathogens and thus carries a risk of infection that may complicate an underlying condition or initiate new health conditions. Studies reveal that the interaction among diet, oral health, and microbial interaction has a significant role in influencing digestive and systemic health outcomes. For example, consumption of high-sugar foods contributes to an elevated rate of dental caries, which, in turn, may trigger inflammatory reactions detrimental to overall health. A proper survey of the oral cavity and its significant role in digestion is thus essential to the development of more precise and effective health interventions, particularly in the context of adversity brought by diseases such as AMR (Christopher J L Murray at al., 2022) and new evidence-based understanding of the gut-brain axis (Silva YP at al., 2020).

Definition of the Digestive System

The digestive system is an intricate system of organs that is tasked with the digestion of food, breaking it down into the necessary nutrients that fuel human physiology. The system includes many different components, including the oral cavity, esophagus, stomach, intestines, and accessory organs like the liver and pancreas. All components are integral to the overall process of digestion, which includes not only mechanical digestion of food but also biochemical processes involved in nutrient absorption. The oral cavity, for example, starts the process with mastication and saliva release that includes enzymes, and thus lays the foundation for the rest of the digestive processes. The intricate interaction between these organs shows the importance of a highly coordinated system to allow for the efficient digestion and nutrient absorption, all of which is necessary for homeostasis as well as overall well-being. Beyond its physiological role, the digestive system contains a high concentration of microbes, also known as the gut microbiome. The microbiome is integral to digestion, with roles influencing metabolic processes and the operation of the immune system. Recent findings have indicated that the balance between the populations of the microbes may have a profound effect on the destiny of health, with alterations corresponding to a range of diseases, including obesity and inflammatory bowel disease. As an example, the balance of beneficial microbes and potentially disease-causing microbes, such as Candida species, demonstrates the importance of homeostasis of the microbes. Host-microbiome interaction diversity is a reflection of the dynamic nature of the digestive system in which every microbial component is an intrinsic part of the overall process of digestion and assimilation of nutrients (Dynowska et al., 2013). Growing research in host-microbiome interaction (HMI) continues to push forward knowledge about gastrointestinal disease and health. The advancement in molecular technologies and computational biology has allowed us to harvest and interpret large amounts of information on HMI. Standardization of data representation of HMI is required to further push forward knowledge on the effect of microbial communities on host physiology and susceptibility to disease. An example is the Ontology of Host-Microbiome Interactions (OHMI), which is essential progress toward formalization of knowledge on the interaction of host anatomy and gastrointestinal microbes during states of disease. These developments are indicative of the complexity and importance of the understanding of the digestive system, which is not anatomical structures per se but also complex biological interactions that determine the fate of health ultimately (Alekseyenko et al., 2019).

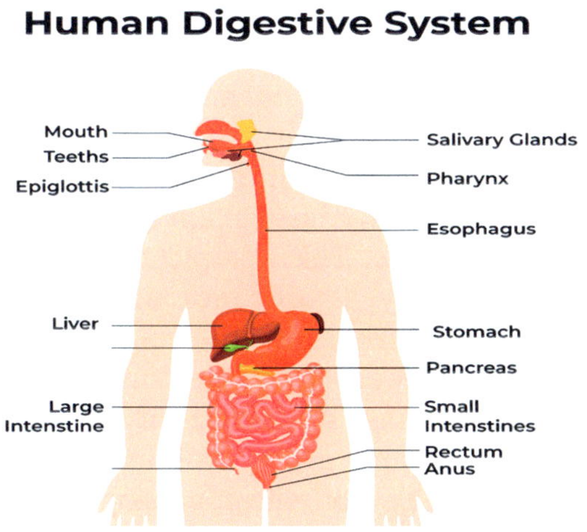

Figure 4.2. Diagram of the digestive system.

Source: https://media.geeksforgeeks.org/wp-content/uploads/20231113145954/Human-Digestive-System.png

Importance of the Oral Cavity in Digestion

The oral cavity serves as the initial site of the digestive process, where mechanical and chemical breakdown of food begins. Chewing, or mastication, is the mechanical phase that increases the surface area of food, allowing enzymes to act more effectively during digestion. Saliva, produced by the salivary glands, contains enzymes such as amylase, which initiates the breakdown of carbohydrates. As food is chewed, it is mixed with saliva, resulting in the formation of a bolus that is easier to swallow. This mechanical action is critical because it not only facilitates swallowing but also sets the stage for digestion, emphasizing the oral cavity's dual role as both a mechanical and chemical processor of food. The process of digestion begins in the mouth, underscoring its crucial role in the overall efficiency of nutrient absorption in subsequent digestive stages. Moreover, the oral cavity is essential for flavor perception, which plays a significant role in the digestive process. Taste buds located on the tongue help to identify the flavors of different foods, influencing our appetite and food choices. Flavor perception is directly linked to saliva production, as the act of tasting stimulates salivary glands to enhance secretion. This increase in saliva not only assists in the swallowing process but also promotes the enzymatic breakdown of food components, thereby optimizing nutrient availability. Furthermore, the presence of diverse bacteria in the oral cavity contributes to a balanced microbiome, which may have implications for digestion and overall health. An imbalance in microbial populations can lead to digestive issues, underscoring how crucial the oral cavity is not just mechanically, but also in fostering a healthy environment conducive to digestion. In addition to these mechanical and chemical functions, the oral cavity plays a significant role in swallowing and the transit of food into the digestive tract. The act of swallowing involves a complex interplay of muscle movements that transport the bolus from the mouth to the esophagus, initiating the involuntary swallowing reflex. The efficacy of this process is essential; any disruption can lead to aspiration or choking, highlighting the importance of coordinated oral and throat musculature. The design of the oral cavity, including the positioning of the tongue and the hard and soft palates, facilitates the proper routing of food during this transition. As food progresses further into the digestive system, the work that began in the oral cavity continues to influence digestion, demonstrating that the initial stages of the digestive process are foundational for overall digestive health and efficiency (Dallas et al., 2012; Bekish and Zorina, 2017).

4.1. Anatomy of the Oral Cavity

Learning Outcome

1. Describe the components of the oral cavity
2. Understand the role of the tongue
3. Describe the structure of the teeth

The anatomy of the oral cavity comprises several critical structures that facilitate its primary function in the digestive system: the ingestion and initial processing of food. The cavity is bounded anteriorly by the lips and posteriorly by the oropharynx, with the cheeks forming its lateral walls. The roof of the oral cavity consists of the hard palate, supported by bone, and the soft palate towards the back, which is muscular and plays a vital role in swallowing. The floor of the cavity houses the tongue, a complex muscular organ essential for the manipulation and sensory perception of food. This arrangement enables the oral cavity to blend mechanical and chemical digestion, emphasizing the need for proper nasal and oral coordination during the swallowing process, which prepares food for passage into the esophagus, thus illustrating the initial stage of the digestive journey. Within the oral cavity, numerous anatomical components contribute significantly to digestion, among which the teeth and salivary glands are paramount. Humans possess two sets of teeth throughout their lifetime—deciduous and permanent—each serving to break down food into smaller, more digestible pieces. The diverse types of teeth, including incisors, canines, premolars, and molars, are specifically adapted to perform these functions. Salivary glands, located around the oral cavity, produce saliva, which serves multiple purposes, including the enzymatic breakdown of starches, lubrication for easier swallowing, and antimicrobial action to protect oral tissues. Furthermore, ongoing research indicates that individual genetic factors affect taste perception, impacting food preferences and, consequently, dietary habits. Variants of the TAS2R38 bitter receptor, for example, demonstrate how taste sensitivity can influence a person's dietary choices, thereby affecting overall nutrition (Banni et al., 2014). In addition to its mechanical and chemical functions, the oral cavity plays a critical role in taste perception, which is integral to the digestive process. Taste buds, primarily located on the tongue, are responsible for detecting the five basic taste modalities—sweet, sour, salty, bitter, and umami. The interaction between taste stimuli and the gustatory system significantly influences food intake and dietary preferences, shaping the human eating experience. This complexity highlights the evolutionary significance of taste as a mechanism for promoting the consumption of nutrient-dense foods while deterring the intake of potential toxins. The oral cavity's interplay between anatomy and physiology extends beyond basic digestion, encompassing aspects of metabolism and homeostasis. Understanding the intricate relationships between its anatomical components emphasizes their collective role in maintaining human health and nutrition (Bochsler et al., 2007).

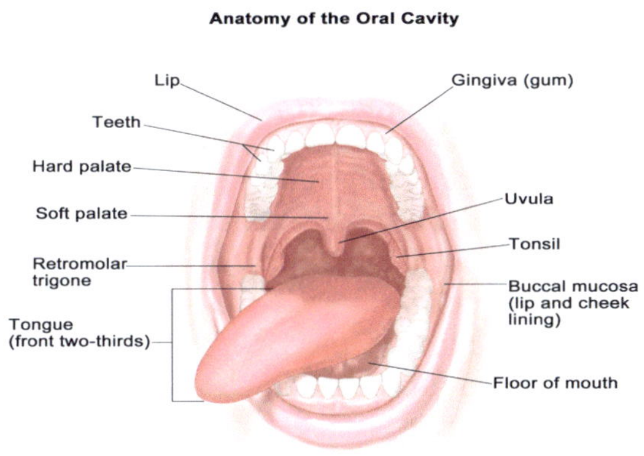

Figure 4.3. Anatomy of the Oral Cavity.

Source: https://nci-media.cancer.gov/pdq/media/images/716338.jpg

4.1.1. Components of the Oral Cavity

The oral cavity is an important port of entry in the gastrointestinal tract, and it is made up of integral structures that allow for the initial processes of food digestion. At the center of the space are the teeth, which play a central role in mechanically breaking down the food into tiny pieces, a process known as mastication. The varying types of teeth, incisors, canines, premolars, and molars all have varied shapes and functions tailored to specific dietary demands. The tongue is also an important contributor, not only in food manipulation for chewing and swallowing, but also in the sense of taste, which is vital in the determination of the palatability and safety of edible items. By undertaking these interrelated functions, the structures of the oral cavity act in harmony to transform food into an enhanced form that is more digestible, laying the groundwork for subsequent digestive processes along the gastrointestinal tract. Saliva from salivary glands in the oral cavity is another important structure that aids the digestive process. Saliva is a thick fluid that contains enzymes like amylase, which begins the breakdown of carbohydrates, and lipase, which begins the digestion of fat, although on a minimal scale in the mouth. The existence of saliva also moistens the food, facilitating its swallowing and aiding in the composition of the bolus—a dense mass of food ready for swallowing. Saliva is also antimicrobial, helping keep the oral cavity sanitary by neutralizing the acid produced by bacteria and breaking down food particles. The harmony of the mechanical process of the teeth and tongue, and the chemical process from the saliva, guarantees the significance of the oral cavity in allowing for the digestive process as well as the prevention of oral disorders. Oral cavity health has a significant impact on the well-being of the world since it not only serves a digestive purpose but also a systemic one. Conditions such as oropharyngeal candidiasis can be detrimental to normal functioning and thus, by extension, to greater digestive issues as well as immunosuppression. Studies have indicated a link between oral diseases and other body system disorders, such as thyroid disease, and it has been suggested that the oral cavity has an association with overall physiological health. The consumption of substances such as areca nut, while having some traditional medicinal benefits, is also known to have serious adverse effects in the form of inducing disorders such as Oral Submucous Fibrosis, illustrating how some aspects of the oral cavity can have a significant impact on health outcomes (Chatra et al., 2014). Awareness of these dynamics reiterates the importance of maintaining oral hygiene and the elimination of dental issues early on to promote overall health (Kushnirenko, 2016).

4.1.2. Function of the Tongue

The tongue is a vital part of the digestive process, specifically that of the oral cavity, being a multi-purpose organ that facilitates the ingestion of food and initial processing. Its surface, which is covered with papillae and taste buds, facilitates the perception and sensation of flavors, important for the modulation of food preference and choice. The presence of five principal taste modalities—sweet, salty, sour, bitter, and umami—plays an important role in the identification of nutrient foods and the avoidance of potentially toxic compounds. Recent research even suggests the tongue's involvement in the perception of fat as a sixth basic taste, challenging traditional notions of taste perception. This role affects not only individual food behavior but also its broader context with respect to health, obesity, and regulation of energy intake, emphasizing the fundamental role of the tongue in nutritional status and health (Costanzo and Keast, 2015). Moreover, the muscularity of the tongue provides essential mechanical functions that enhance food manipulation during mastication. Their coordinated movements play a key role in mixing food with saliva for the initiation of digestion by enzymic action, specifically involving amylase for the digestion of carbohydrates. The tongue also plays a vital role in the formation of a bolus—a cohesive bolus of masticated food easily translatable to the pharynx and thence to the esophagus. This activity not only allows for swallowing but is of vital importance for the prevention of choking and preparation of food for introduction into the stomach for further digestion. Such mechanical processing, combined with sensory feedback from taste buds, enhances the importance of wise food choice, as the tongue facilitates the assessment of palatability and safety of potential ingesta, emphasizing its key role in human digestion (Baptista et al., 2012). In addition, the function of the tongues in the perception of taste extends beyond the mere recognition of flavor. It is intricately associated with physiological mechanisms that affect satiation and the regulation of appetite. Recognition of fats by some receptors on the taste bud, for instance, initiates a physiological cascade that affects hunger and food intake behavior. Studies indicate oral stimulation with fatty acids results in blood triglyceride elevations, which shows that the sensory role of the tongue can significantly impact metabolic function. Finally, understanding the function of the tongues in the perception of taste is critical in addressing public health problems like obesity because individuals who are insensitive to some tastes may be more prone to overconsumption of calorically dense food. Finally, the tongue's multiple functions in the perception of taste, processing food, and metabolic signaling position the tongue in an important role in the functioning of the digestive system overall (Costanzo and Keast, 2015).

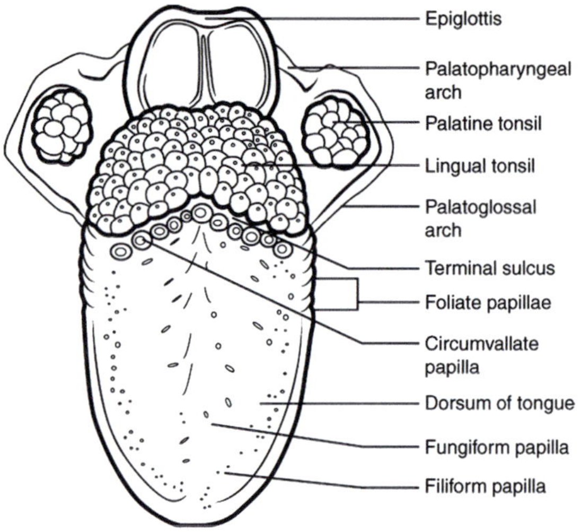

Figure 4.4. This superior view of the tongue shows the locations and types of lingual papillae.

Source: https://s3-us-west-2.amazonaws.com/courses-images-archive-read-only/wp-content/uploads/sites/403/2015/04/21031710/2407_Tongue.jpg

4.1.3. Structure of the Teeth

The dental anatomy of human teeth is highly specialized to complement their primary function in the digestive system—mechanical breakdown of food. There are various layers of each tooth, including enamel, dentin, and pulp. The outer layer, enamel, is the hardest substance of the body, protecting against physical and chemical destruction. Underlying the protective layer is the dentin, a calcified tissue that makes up most of the tooth and offers additional support and sensitivity. The pulp, in the inner layer, has blood vessels and nerves that are in charge of supplying the tooth with nourishment and sensing stimuli. This layered nature not only provides durability but also enables the teeth to withstand the great forces involved in mastication, indicating the evolutionary adaptability of human dental anatomy (Bekish and Zorina, 2017). The four general groups of teeth are specialized for specific tasks in the digestive process. Incisors, usually flat and tapering, are specialized in cutting food to enable precise bites of fruits and vegetables. Canines, tapering and hard, are efficient in tearing food, particularly meat, which indicates humans' omnivorous nature. Premolars and molars, with a broader, flatter surface area, are the major contributors to grinding and crushing food into small sizes, hence increasing the surface area available for digestive enzyme activity. The arrangement of these teeth in the oral cavity enables easy transition from tearing to grinding, complementing effective digestion. This shape and function diversity again indicates the accommodability of human teeth to diverse dietary demands over time (Bekish and Zorina, 2014). Besides, biological mechanisms of tooth formation and maintenance ensure their relevance to the human digestive system. Teeth undergo a complex process known as odontogenesis, in which enamel and dentin are produced through tightly regulated development during childhood. Oral health can also affect overall health directly, with poor oral health resulting in cavities and periodontal disease, ultimately inhibiting the chewing and digestion of food. Moreover, the morphology of the teeth also reflects eating behavior and nutritional status during a person's lifetime. Thus, the shape of teeth not only permits primary digestion but is a critical part of human nutrition and health, reflecting more general principles of biological organization and physiological adaptation (Bekish and Zorina, 2014, 2017).

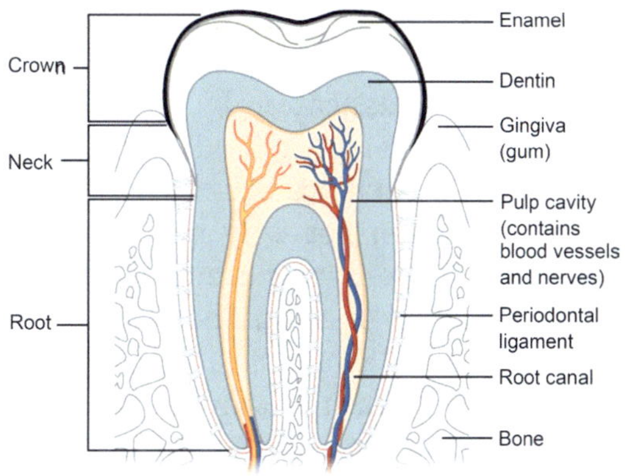

Figure 4.5. This longitudinal section through a molar in its alveolar socket shows the relationships between enamel, dentin, and pulp.

Source: https://s3-us-west-2.amazonaws.com/courses-images-archive-read-only/wp-content/uploads/sites/403/2015/04/21031715/2409_Tooth.jpg

Test Your Knowledge

1. What are the components of the oral cavity?
2. What is the role of the tongue?

4.2. Functions of the Oral Cavity

Learning Outcome

1. Describe the mechanical digestion through mastication
2. Understand the chemical digestion with saliva
3. Describe the role of the oral cavity in taste perception

The oral cavity is the start of the digestive tract and also an essential site for mechanochemical food processing. Within the oral cavity, food is chewed or masticated by the teeth by fracturing such complex food particles into smaller particles that are easy to handle. Such physical disruption not only maximizes food surface area for enzymatic activity but also facilitates mixing of solid food with saliva. Saliva, produced by a number of salivary glands, contains enzymes such as amylase that trigger the chemical digestion of carbohydrates when food is mixed and softened for easy swallowing. The complex coordination of oral cavity muscles also facilitates smooth food transport, leading to the pharynx for further digestion, hence showing the complexity of oral cavity functions in the digestive process. Apart from mechanical and enzymatic functions, the oral cavity is also crucial in sensory evaluation and initiation of swallowing. Taste buds on the tongue allow the individual to experience different tastes, which may contribute to food selection and eating behavior. Sensory input from such food tasting is an essential function in initiating salivary gland secretion and stimulating gastric secretions for further digestion. Such a sensory function shows the interdependency of the oral cavity and the entire digestive process. In addition, after food is chewed well and mixed with saliva, the tongue assists in shaping the food mass into a bolus, triggering the swallowing reflex. Upon swallowing, a highly intricate interaction between muscle contractions guarantees safe passage of the bolus into the esophagus, showing the oral cavity's role in smooth digestion. Apart from that, the oral cavity is the defense mechanism of the digestive system, supporting the immune system in several ways. Saliva not only houses digestive enzymes but also antimicrobial agents like lysozyme and immunoglobulin A (IgA) that inhibit bacterial growth and pathogens that come into the body with food. The protective role highlights the importance of oral health, with an imbalance or disruption in this defense mechanism resulting in increased susceptibility to infection and gastrointestinal disease. Apart from that, the composition of the oral microbiome is also an important factor that guarantees oral and overall well-being. The oral cavity, thus, not only carries out basic digestive functions but also plays a critical role in guarding the individual from harm, hence showing its importance in the overall picture of the digestive system, as evident from studies of dietary patterns and immune response in infants where protein digestion and salivary composition are critical (Dallas et al., 2012), (Patwardhan, 2008).

4.2.1. Mechanical Digestion Through Mastication

The initial step of digestion, mechanical digestion, begins with mastication within the mouth. This is significant because it physically breaks down food into small particles, making it more favorable for subsequent enzymatic action. Mastication is characterized by the coordinated jaw, tongue, and teeth movement, which, in concert, grind and tear food. Physical breakdown not only facilitates easier food mixing with saliva but also aids in the formation of a cohesive bolus that can be swallowed. Further, the mechanical action of mastication increases the surface area of food particles, which is significant for the release of nutrients. Disregarding the significance of this initial step could compromise understanding of the total process of digestion, nutrient bioavailability, and the related physiological processes of the digestive system (Adlercreutz et al., 2014). The mastication process also plays a part in other aspects of the food once initial chewing occurs, such as its bioavailability and release of flavor. Research has shown that poor mastication can result in issues with subsequent stages of digestion, with the large particles of food not being sufficiently accessible to digestive enzymes. Further, the texture and consistency of food manipulated with mastication also contribute significantly to the satiety signals sent to the brain, hence contributing to the regulation of appetite. While scientists investigate the implications of mastication, more interest is shown in mimicking the physiological conditions of this oral processing step through various in vitro models.

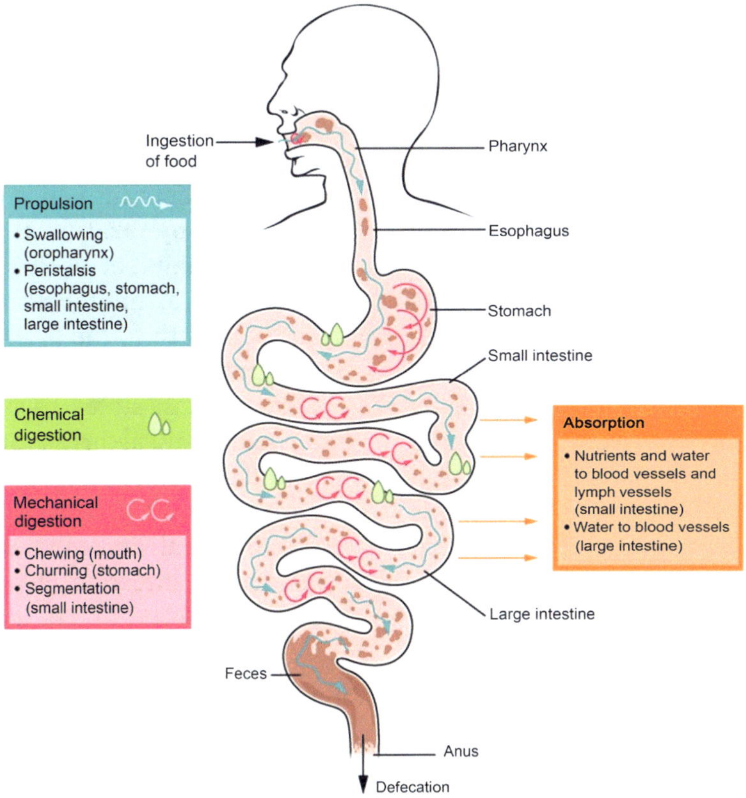

Figure 4.6. The digestive processes are ingestion, propulsion, mechanical digestion, chemical digestion, absorption, and defecation.

Source: https://s3-us-west-2.amazonaws.com/courses-images-archive-read-only/wp-content/uploads/sites/403/2015/04/21031707/2405_Digestive_Process.jpg

These models are designed to replicate oral digestion and, for a better understanding of how physically manipulated food interacts with digestive enzymes and other physiological processes, may achieve a broader understanding of human digestion (Adlercreutz et al., 2014). Finally, a broad understanding of the mechanics of mastication uncovers its pivotal position in the master plan of the digestive process. Data from areas like nutrition, medicine, and food technology can greatly contribute to a greater understanding of mastication and its health importance. Understanding its function in digestibility and nutrient absorption, future research can address dietary interventions more effectively to enhance digestive health and general well-being. Researchers and food technologists are encouraged to take note of the complexity of oral processing in their research, since this process is fundamental to maximizing food formulations and attaining nutritional necessities. As the research continues, strategies that closely mimic in vivo conditions will shed light on the complexity of mechanical digestion and its far-reaching repercussions on human health (Arvisenet et al., 2014).

4.2.2. Chemical Digestion With Saliva

Chemical digestion in the mouth is begun primarily by the activity of saliva, a biologically complex fluid secreted by salivary glands. Though the saliva not only moistens food during preparation for swallowing, it also begins macromolecule digestion. Salivary amylase in the saliva begins carbohydrate digestion by breaking down starches into simpler sugars. The enzymatic action is significant because it prepares the food for digestion in the digestive tract and maximizes nutrient uptake efficiency. Saliva also contains antibacterial compounds, which maintain the mouth free of potential pathogens without inhibiting healthy oral microbiota. The biochemical composition of saliva thus focuses on the numerous aspects of the role of saliva in digestion and oral health and illustrates how digestion and immune protection mechanisms are inextricably intertwined at the critical initial phase of food processing. The biochemical composition of saliva also illustrates how critical saliva is to chemical digestion. Saliva consists of water, electrolytes, enzymes, and other organic molecules that, in combination, constitute a digestive fluid. Enzyme possession, such as lipase, which is less significant compared to amylase, provides for the initial digestion of fats as well, illustrating the multifaceted function of salivary functions in digestion. Salivary gland secretion also adds mucins, which provide additional lubrication to facilitate the passage of the food bolus in the mouth as well as into the esophagus. Activation of these salivary components not only assures mechanical facilitation of digestion but also speeds up the chemical processes involved. This is to highlight the mutually dependent functioning of chemical and physical digestion in the oral cavity as the foundation for the successful passage of food to further stages of digestion, and of oral cavity health. Although chemical digestion in the mouth is a process mostly of saliva, of interest here is the implications on wider gastrointestinal health in general, in that it has been found that the oral cavity is a reservoir for microbial populations, expressing their influence on gastrointestinal microbiota by oral-fecal transmission, for example (Schmidt et al., 2019). More specifically, examination of microbial strains translocated from the mouth to the intestine is enlightening of the intricate interplay of oral health and systemic disease states, such as colorectal cancer and rheumatoid arthritis (Schmidt et al., 2019). The initial chemical digestion by saliva is thus more than food processing; it is inseparable from microbial dynamics of such tremendous influence on intestinal health and the disease process. Incorporation of these aspects into our understanding of chemical digestion brings us to an appreciation of how the oral cavity is not merely a digestive portal but a fundamental mediator of health *en masse* through its chemical and microbial dynamics (Hillman et al., 2017).

4.2.3. Role in Taste Perception

The intricate role of the oral cavity in the experience of taste is the very foundation of human life, dictating food preference and nutritional level. The tongue and other oral mucosa carry taste buds that carry special cells that respond to sweet, sour, salty, bitter, and umami tastes. These trigger unique pathways that transmit information to the brain, ultimately dictating dietary preference so essential to optimal health. The genetic variation, for example, with the TAS2R38 bitter receptor, demonstrates how variation among individuals in taste sensitivity can affect food intake and eating behavior. Through detection of the bitter molecules, individuals are able to naturally avoid potentially toxic compounds, demonstrating the protective role of taste perception within the gastrointestinal tract. Such sensitivities do not just affect immediate choice but have the potential to affect longer-term consequences on energy metabolism and eating behavior, such as demonstrated in perception of PROP sensitivity (Banni et al., 2014). The function of the salivary glands, of which the exocrine glands, such as Von Ebner's glands, are of specific significance, is a very important function in the process of taste perception. The salivary glands secrete digestive enzymes and condition the environment for the effective functioning of the taste buds. Strategically located in close proximity to the major taste structures, they drain the stimuli so that taste buds are able to continuously sample new flavors. It appears saliva's composition is capable of modulating taste receptor activation and hence modulating perceived taste. In addition, retromolar chemosensory structures of recent identification contribute to our information on gustatory perception of the human oral cavity. The structures contain taste buds that potentially contribute subtle sensory effects, particularly to the perception of flavor and texture. This demonstrates the complexity of the oral environment, going beyond ancient appreciation of the surface of the tongue alone, to flavor processing (Coburn et al., 2019). Furthermore, the link between taste perception and eating habits extends to the fields of diet and health. Variability in taste sensitivity can generate differential patterns of food and drink that can affect one's diet and thus affect metabolic health. Since these taste preferences are determined by genetic design and experience, they can predispose one to particular diets, demonstrating the psychological aspect of taste. For instance, heightened sensitivity to bitterness can lead to the avoidance of certain vegetables, potentially limiting their consumption of essential nutrients, while preference for sweeter food can lead them to move towards less healthy food. Thus, the physiological and biochemical determinants of taste perception are not only involved in immediate survival but also determine long-term health outcomes, demonstrating the oral cavity's critical role in the digestive process (Banni et al., 2014; Coburn et al., 2019).

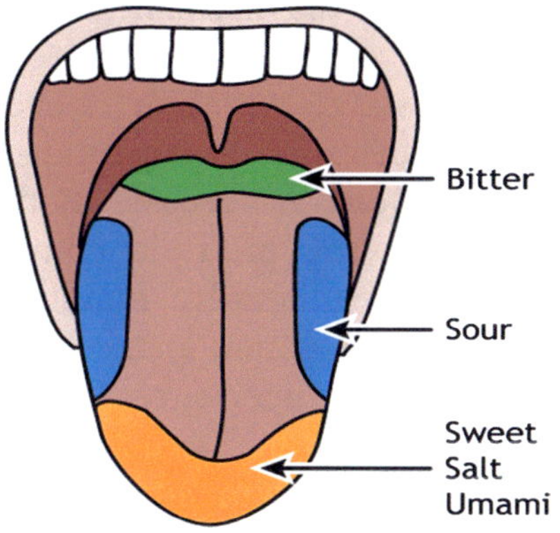

Figure 4.7. Although all tastes can be perceived across the entire tongue, sensitivity levels vary for each taste. The front of the tongue has the lowest threshold for sweet, salt, and umami tastes; the side of the tongue has the lowest threshold for sour tastes, and the back of the tongue has the lowest threshold for bitter tastes.

Source: https://openbooks.lib.msu.edu/app/uploads/sites/6/2021/04/TasteMap.png

Test Your Knowledge

1. What is the chemical digestion in oral cavity?
2. What is the role of the oral cavity in taste perception?

4.3. Salivary Glands

Learning Outcome

1. Describe the types of salivary glands
2. Describe the functions of saliva
3. Understand the regulation of salivary secretion

The salivary glands play a central role in the digestive process, with a structural role in the oral cavity. The exocrine glands, such as the parotid, submandibular, and sublingual glands, are responsible for the first step of digestion. The saliva produced by the glands contains enzymes such as amylase, initiating carbohydrate breakdown, allowing for chemical digestion. Beyond enzyme function, saliva acts as a lubricant to allow the mechanical breakdown of food during mastication. Moreover, the stimulation of saliva secretion is evoked by the perception of taste, thus creating a close association between the process of digestion and perception. The multiple contribution demonstrates the integrative function of the salivary glands in digestion and, consequently, the sensory eating experience. The salivary glands also have other crucial functions besides digestion. Saliva maintains oral health through control of pH and protection of the oral mucosa against infections. The antibacterial constituents in saliva, such as lysozyme, stabilize the microbial environment, thus preventing infection. The pathological disruption of the functioning of the salivary glands can have a profound impact on oral health, leading to disorders such as xerostomia or dry mouth. This reduction in saliva can be utilized as a clinical indicator of systemic disorders, reflecting on the interconnectedness of the salivary glands with overall well-being. Alteration of the salivary glands may often be the first sign of metabolic disturbances, as noted by researchers who emphasize the effect of systemic disorders on oral cavity well-being, e.g., diabetes and iron deficiency anemia (Kotionova-Ovod et al., 2023). Moreover, the functioning of the salivary glands is engaged in the regulation of dietary intake through the interaction of the salivary glands with nitrate-reducing bacteria in the oral cavity. These bacteria convert salivary nitrate to nitrite, with both health and preventive significance. This process not only enhances vasodilation and enhances blood supply but also protects oral microecology by halting the development of caries through metabolic processes. The balance achieved by these bacteria can be significant in the prevention of dental caries, underlining the function of the salivary glands in digestive health as well as in the prevention of oral disease (Feng et al., 2023). These glands therefore show the complexity and importance of understanding the oral cavity's function within the greater human digestive system.

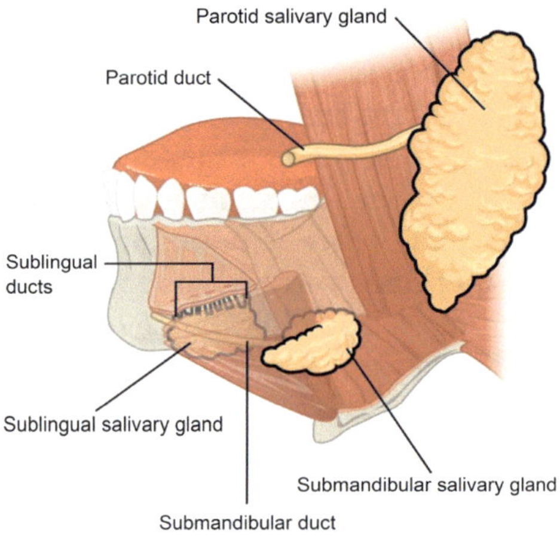

Figure 4.8. The major salivary glands are located outside the oral mucosa and deliver saliva into the mouth through ducts.

Source: https://s3-us-west-2.amazonaws.com/courses-images-archive-read-only/wp-content/uploads/sites/403/2015/04/21031712/2408_Salivary_Glands.jpg

4.3.1. Types of Salivary Glands

The human oral cavity holds three main types of salivary glands, each with its own function and secretions crucial to the early process of digestion. The parotid glands, located near the ear, are the largest and serve to produce a serous, enzyme-rich saliva critical to carbohydrate digestion. The parotid glands secrete mostly amylase, an enzyme that initiates the digestion process of starches, thereby facilitating the process of the digestive system. The parotid glands also affect the sense of taste directly by providing a medium where the food particles can be dissolved, thereby increasing the sense of taste. This enzymatic function illustrates the cooperation of taste and digestion, proving that the salivary glands are more than accessory organs but an active part of the digestive process, conditioning food for the process of further digestion as it travels on into the gastrointestinal tract. Beneath the parotid glands are the submandibular glands, which secrete both the mucous and serous components of saliva. These glands' secretions facilitate the lubrication of food, providing ease of swallowing and allowing for the process of mechanical digestion. The submandibular glands are critical to the process of the digestive system as they secrete a higher percentage of mucin, providing for the conservation of moisture and protection of oral cavity tissues from the abrasive qualities of food. In addition to their function in digestion, the glands also afford the pleasure of taste, as saliva facilitates the transfer of molecules of taste to the taste receptors. The blending of mucous and serous fluid thus affords an ideal composition of saliva critical to optimal oral and digestive health, proving the versatility of the salivary gland in the oral cavity. Lastly, the sublingual glands, located below the tongue, secrete a mucus-rich secretion that aids in the formation of a food bolus, hence easier swallowing. This type of saliva plays an important role in the quick digestion of food because it provides immediate lubrication and also supports oral taste. The composition of salivary content from the sublingual gland involves a mix of various proteins and antibacterial chemicals that support the defense of the oral cavity against the establishment of unwanted bacteria. The role of these salivary components collectively not only contributes to the role of digestion but also contributes to oral health and oral hygiene. The role of all three salivary gland sources collectively contributes to pointing out their role in the digestion process and shows the sophisticated ways in which the oral cavity prepares food for digestion and nutrient uptake (Baptista et al., 2012; Coburn et al., 2019).

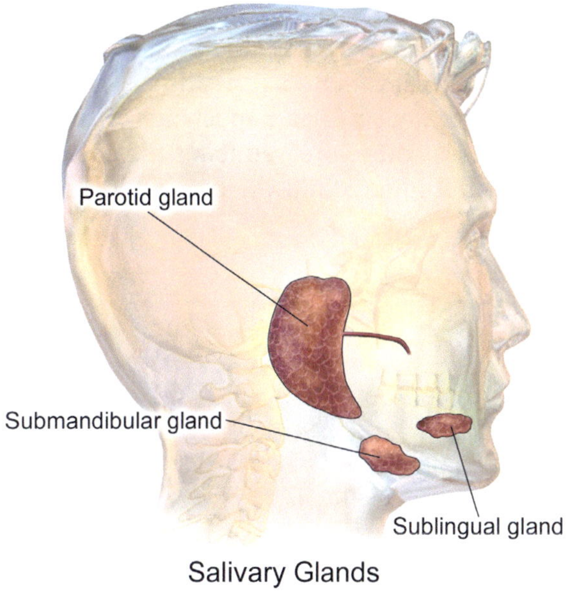

Figure 4.9. The three main paired salivary glands.

Source: https://upload.wikimedia.org/wikipedia/commons/d/df/Blausen_0780_SalivaryGlands.png

4.3.2. Functions of Saliva

Saliva has a number of key roles in the human digestive process, primarily in the oral cavity, as an early facilitator of digestion and oral tissue protector. Comprising water, electrolytes, enzymes, and antimicrobial agents, saliva is secreted by salivary glands, specifically the parotid, submandibular, and sublingual glands, secreting about 750–1500 ml of saliva daily, varying with food intake consumed and states of body physiology. The enzymes involved, such as amylase, initiate carbohydrate digestion, hydrolyzing complex starches to simpler carbohydrates even before food is ingested into the stomach. This enzymatic process is a typical example of saliva's fundamental contribution to digestion, indicating its function in nutrient absorption and overall digestion. Besides its function in digestion, saliva also has a significant function in oral health by serving as an early defense against pathogens and maintaining oral tissue integrity. Saliva consists of antimicrobial agents, including defensins and cationic antimicrobial peptides, which are effective against a broad spectrum of bacteria and viruses, therefore reducing the incidence of potential infection in the oral cavity (Huang et al., 2021).

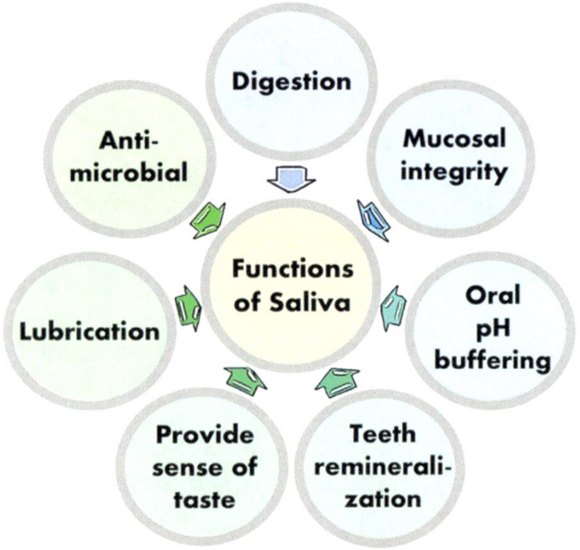

Figure 4.10. The main functions of saliva in the oral cavity.

Source: https://www.researchgate.net/publication/355761245/figure/fig1/AS:11431281180294101@1691552803029/Main-functions-of-saliva-in-oral-cavity.png

Saliva also helps to clear food particles and debris, reducing the incidence of plaque formation and subsequent dental caries. Saliva's buffering capacity also ensures oral pH stability, critical in the prevention of enamel erosion and acid-induced injury. Saliva, thus, is not only a digestive fluid but also a critical component in oral health as well as oral hygiene. Saliva also helps to maintain the sensation of taste and is involved in the creation of boluses, aiding in swallowing. The salivary solubilization helps break down food materials, making it possible for taste buds to properly sense flavors, which is integral to the human feeding process. Salivary lubrication also helps in mechanically conveying food from the mouth to the esophagus, making it possible to swallow and digest food efficiently (Huang et al., 2021). Therefore, the versatility of the functions of saliva from digestive aid to immune defense and sensory facilitation underscores its significance in the overall oral cavity and overall digestive system function. Through an appreciation of the diversity of the roles of saliva, we can realize its pivotal role in human health and the importance of salivary gland function.

4.3.3. Regulation of Salivary Secretion

Control of salivary secretion is a complex process involving neural and hormonal control, a reflection of the complex nature of the human digestive system. Salivary glands like the parotid, submandibular, and sublingual glands react to stimuli, possibly through the autonomic nervous system. Both sympathetic and parasympathetic branches are involved; for instance, parasympathetic stimulation results in a copious watery secretion, and sympathetic stimulation results in a thicker secretion. Double control results in a highly regulated response to a specific stimulus, for instance, sight or smell of food, that can result in a cephalic phase of salivation even before food enters the mouth, a reflection of the anticipatory nature of digestion. Apart from this, local control, like the type of microbiota of the oral cavity, has a grand role in the regulation of salivary secretion. The presence of bacterial biofilms in the oral microbiome seems to stimulate salivary flow and regulation of composition to oral health. The relationship between saliva and biofilms is of great significance since saliva not only results in the removal of pathogenic bacteria but also aids in the creation of a balanced microbial environment. Disturbances in the balance could result in oral disease, a reflection of the significance of the regulation of saliva in the preservation of health and prevention of disease and oral hygiene. Insofar as this is true, an understanding of the control mechanisms of the output of saliva becomes of great significance to the design of effective therapy for diseases that affect the functioning of salivary secretions, for instance, dryness of mouth or dysphagia. Besides, saliva secretions are controlled by enormous systemic factors such as stress, diet, and drugs. Stress, for example, can cause changes in salivary composition and flow, leading to xerostomia, which impacts oral health and digestion adversely. Certain drugs, for example, anticholinergics, similarly disturb salivary gland secretions and decrease the production of saliva, further destabilizing oral health. Such multi-factor interaction is thus creating the multi-dimensional regulation of salivary secretion. Additional research on the subject, therefore, is amply justified, especially on how disturbance of salivary secretion can be involved in chronic oral disease or systemic disease, for which evidence indicates that salivary change can be an indicator of more complicated health pathology (Lene K Vestby et al., 2020; Pedersen AML et al., 2018).

Test Your Knowledge

1. What are the three types of salivary glands?
2. What are the functions of saliva?

4.4. The Process of Digestion in the Oral Cavity

Learning Outcome

1. Know the ingestion of food
2. Describe the formation of the bolus
3. Understand the swallowing process

Digestion initially takes place in the oral cavity, with food being mechanically digested through mastication or chewing. This is an initial process required for increasing the surface area of food particles and paving the way for enzymatic action later on in digestion. Teeth play an important role in this process of mechanical digestion, with incisors designed for cutting and molars for grinding. Saliva, secreted from the salivary glands, is also important, and it contains enzymes such as amylase, which initiates carbohydrate digestion. The enzyme action is the beginning of separating complex carbohydrates into simple sugars, an initial process that occurs much earlier than food entering the stomach. The co-action of chemical and mechanical processes in the oral cavity serves to accentuate the critical preparatory processes that occur prior to swallowing, serving to further highlight the significance of proper chewing and salivation in the overall digestive process (Adlercreutz et al., 2014). Apart from mechanical breakdown, the oral cavity is also a vital sensory organ, where perception of taste influences the digestive process. The presence of food activates the cephalic phase of digestion by stimulating the vagus nerve and prompting various physiological responses in anticipation of nutrient intake. Not only does sensory stimulation prepare the body for digestive readiness, but it also maximizes salivary gland secretions, making digestive enzymes more readily available. In addition, the taste stimuli perceived within the oral cavity aid the brain in its assessment of the food consumed, facilitating the selection of energy-dense foods and rejection of suboptimal ones. This interaction suggests an interactive role of sensation and digestive efficiency, demonstrating how the oral cavity plays a multifaceted role in optimizing nutrient absorption (Mahía et al., 2019). Following the first stages of digestion, there is the formation of a bolus, which involves masticated food mixed with saliva being shaped into a unified mass ready to be swallowed. This is an important process because it enables the easy passage of food from the oral cavity to the pharynx and then on to the esophagus, opening the way from the oral stage to the pharyngeal stage of swallowing. The muscular coordination in the oral cavity plays a crucial role at this stage, as the tongue carries out precise motions that force the bolus to the posterior part of the throat. Furthermore, saliva's function extends beyond lubrication, as it contains antimicrobial components that help defend the oral cavity against pathogens. Hence, the digestive process of the oral cavity is not only fundamental in pre-digesting food prior to other digestion but critical in ensuring the health and integrity of the digestive system as a whole (Adlercreutz et al., 2014).

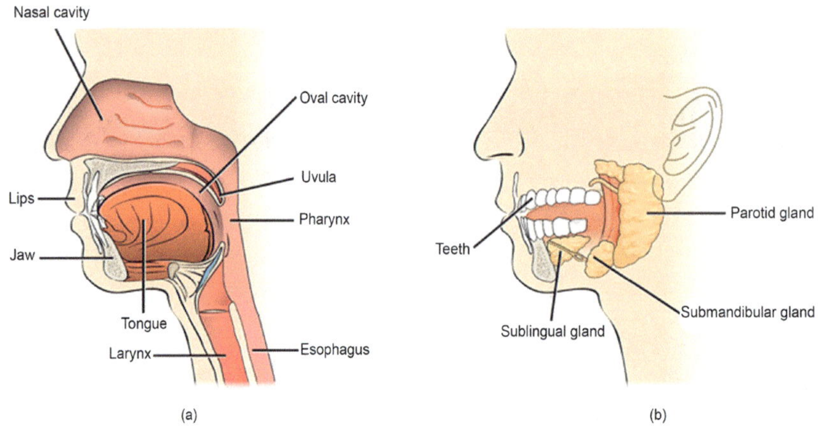

Figure 4.11. Digestion begins in the oral cavity: Digestion of food begins in the (a) oral cavity. Food is masticated by teeth and moistened by saliva secreted from the (b) salivary glands. Enzymes in the saliva begin to digest starches and fats. With the help of the tongue, the resulting bolus is moved into the esophagus by swallowing.

Source: https://bio.libretexts.org/@api/deki/files/77994/figure-34-01-08ab.jpeg?revision=1

4.4.1. Ingestion of Food

Food consumption sets the complex process of digestion underway and begins in the oral cavity, where the essential contact between food and sensory receptors occurs. In addition to being the oral cavity through which food enters the body, the oral cavity is also the site of taste, which has an important role to play in determining eating behavior. The tongue, which is covered with taste buds, senses different flavors such as sweetness, bitterness, and umami, guiding people on the right nutrition decisions to take. Some newly emerging findings have shown that identifying fats as a specific taste adds an additional dimension to such sensing beyond the traditional definitions, broadening our knowledge of taste. Unique receptors in taste bud cells sense fatty acids and trigger a series of neural responses transmitting taste messages to the brain and thus affect food intake and perception, and the resulting swallowing or spitting out of some of the food (Costanzo and Keast, 2015). The oral cavity is not just a passive tube but an active participant in the act of ingestion because of its mechanical and chemical action. Mastication or chewing breaks food up mechanically into smaller pieces so that there are more surface areas for digestive enzymes to act on during the rest of the processes. Besides, saliva, a major secretion of the salivary glands, plays a key role in the initial breakdown of carbohydrates. Saliva contains enzymes such as amylase that begin the breakdown of starches into sugar, and thus, chewing cannot be overemphasized in digestion. Saliva is also a lubricant, aiding in swallowing and the passage of food to the esophagus. The interaction between chemical and mechanical functions in the mouth, therefore, maximizes ingestion efficiency and forms the foundation for nutrient absorption (Baptista et al., 2012). In addition, the intricate interplay between taste perception and dietary preference extends from short-term sensory perception to long-term health outcomes.

Understanding the sensory mechanisms of ingestion can render diets and their significance in public health in obesity and metabolic disorders accessible. Cumulative data indicate that individuals with impaired detection capacity for fatty acids will overconsume fat-rich foods, which can result in weight gain and resultant disease. The oral cavity, in this regard, is an important meeting place where sensory processing not only influences short-term feeding behavior but also total dietary intake. The resolution of these determinants can be used to inform nutrition education and interventions that will lead to improved dietary practices, ultimately culminating in improved health outcomes in the population (Costanzo and Keast, 2015).

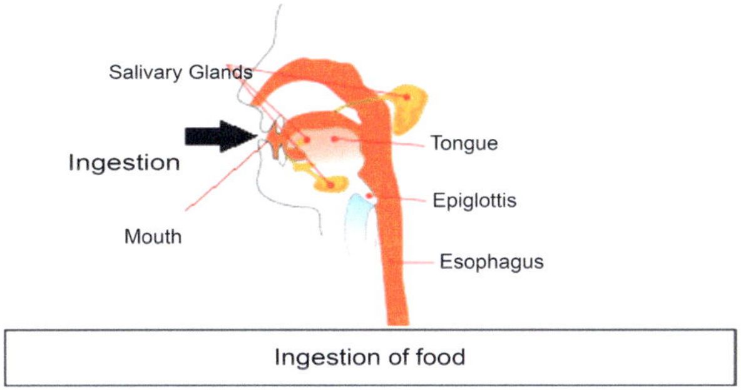

Figure 4.12. Ingestion of food.

Source: https://www.vedantu.com/question-sets/67c6e93d-46a8-4caf-8fab-0b2c6dd8e7c11348973926474993160.png

4.4.2. Formation of the Bolus

The bolus formation is a critical initial process of human digestion and is primarily accomplished in the mouth. It begins when one swallows food into the mouth, where it is subjected to mechanical fragmentation through chewing or mastication. Teeth play an extremely crucial role in this process, while the tongue assists in directing the food in a way that it gets fragmented in an even way. Salivary glands secrete saliva with digestive enzymes and lubricants following food stimulation to help mix food particles. The mixing of such ingredients is crucial during bolus formation so that it becomes more efficient and swallowable. The mechanical and enzymatic treatment used during this phase prepares the bolus for the next stages of digestion, emphasizing the importance of chewing in the entire digestion process. Having been well chewed and moistened with saliva, the bolus is ready to be swallowed, the act that is controlled by complicated neural mechanisms. The bolus is propelled to the back of the oral cavity, where it collides against pharyngeal walls, initiating the swallowing reflex. These reflexes need precise coordination among the muscles of the tongue, pharynx, and esophagus so that entry of the esophagus is permitted safely and aspiration from the trachea is prevented. Bolus formation and swallowing are mechanical movements, but also bring about the initiation of the process of digestion, leading to a cascade of physiological responses. The controlling role of the bolus in the digestion process serves to underscore co-action among the oral cavity and all the systems of digestion in establishing a foundation for enzymatic digestion in the stomach and beyond. In addition, the role of saliva in the formation of a bolus is not merely lubrication but the transmission of essential enzymes, such as amylase, that initiate the chemical digestion of carbohydrates.

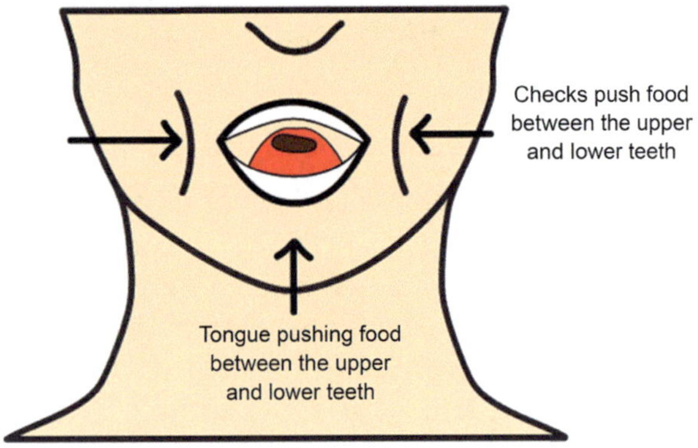

Figure 4.13. The main control features during the oral preparation phase in forming and placing a bolus.

Source: https://maxfacts.uk/help-selfhelp-oral-food-swallowing-anatomy-physiology-level2-figure1.png

This enzymatic activity initiates digestion prior to its entrance into the stomach, proof of this multifaceted role of the oral cavity as not simply a preparation room but as an active participant in the process of digestion. Additionally, the presence of some secondary plant metabolites in foods influences the digestion process, with emphasis laid on oral processing. According to studies, different in vitro models have been designed to simulate digestion in the mouth, an indication of the significance of bolus formation when evaluating nutrient bioavailability and health implications (Adlercreutz et al., 2014). Such a study is important in explaining how the bolus conditions the nutrients for absorption and toward a critical interface of nutritional content and digestive capability. Studying, therefore, how the bolus is formed is enlightening about both the physiological process and its importance for health and nutrition, demonstrating the critical role of the oral cavity in human digestion (Valls-Bellés, 2024).

4.4.3. Swallowing Process

Swallowing is a complex physiological mechanism that is the transition between the oral cavity and the esophagus, or the passage from voluntary to involuntary digestive function. Initiated by the voluntary process of mastication, food is molded into a solid bolus that progresses towards the back of the mouth. The role of the tongue becomes important in this phase, as it molds the bolus and forces it towards the pharynx through a series of coordinated muscle contractions. The soft palate also elevates to shut off the nasal cavities so that food does not flow into the nasal cavity. This intricate coordination between muscle motions not only facilitates the swallowing of food but also protects the airway by automatically closing the epiglottis, illustrating the importance of interaction between swallowing and the anatomy of the oral cavity. Following the initial voluntary phase, the act of swallowing transitions into an involuntary phase with intricate neural control. When the bolus enters the pharynx, sensory receptors cause a complex reflex action that coordinates the pharyngeal and esophageal movements. The reflex action prescribes closure of the airway passage to prevent aspiration, yet simultaneously initiates peristaltic movements in the esophagus to enable the bolus to move downwards. Muscles in the esophagus participate in rhythmic contractions that move the food downwards towards the stomach. Saliva, secreted by the salivary glands, plays a complementary function here and helps to lubricate the bolus and smooth swallowing. Saliva's component elements, including enzymes, also prepare the digestive process, contributing to the initiation of food destruction, which emphasizes the intricate interaction between saliva and swallowing (Maddu, 2019). Moreover, the process of swallowing is not just physical; it is also sensory and cognitive, allowing for additional efficiency in digestion. Stimulation of taste receptors in the mouth influences salivation, making swallowing even easier and further enhancing the digestive process. Disruptions to this very complex process could lead to dysphagia, or the ease of swallowing, which typically suggests the existence of underlying health issues. Continued advances in pharmaceutical approaches highlight the importance of investigating the mechanism of swallowing, especially for oral transmucosal drug delivery systems (Brown et al., 2011). The convergence of drug delivery on physiological processes highlights the position of the oral cavity as a vital component of digestion and therapeutic intervention, further consolidating the intricate relationship between the structure and function of the human gastrointestinal system.

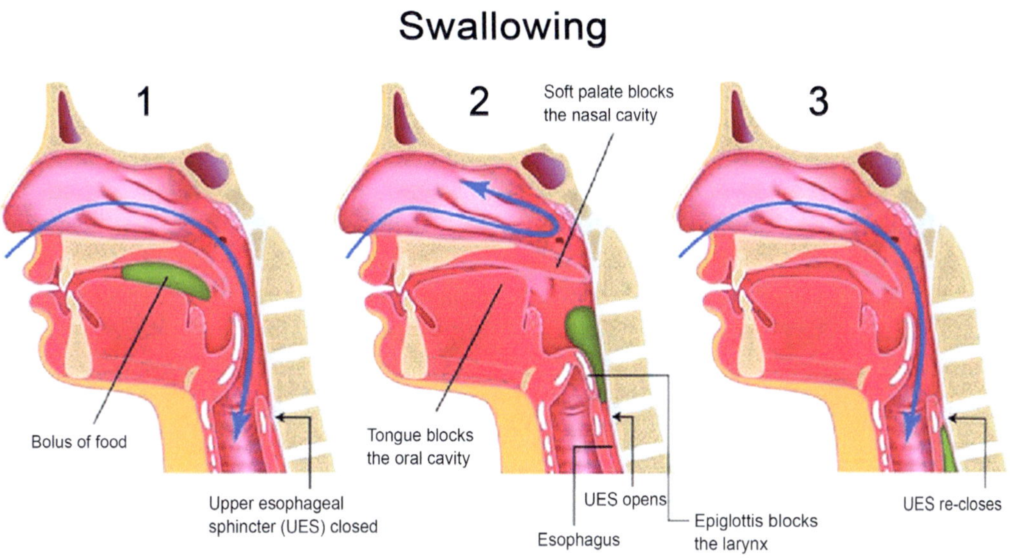

Figure 4.14. Swallowing process.

Source: https://www.researchgate.net/profile/Lauren-Tabor-Gray-2/publication/325908837/figure/fig1/AS:640059514572818@1529613488810/Swallowing-process.png

Test Your Knowledge

1. What is the ingestion of food?
2. What is the formation of a bolus?

4.5. Common Disorders of the Oral Cavity

Learning Outcome

1. Know the dental caries
2. Describe the gum disease
3. Describe the oral cancer

The oral cavity is an important part of the digestive system, acting not just as a means for food intake but also as an important part of overall health. Among the prevalent oral cavity disorders, halitosis or oral malodor is especially conspicuous. It has been established in studies that nearly 50% of the population suffers from halitosis, an affliction that is bound to affect one's social life and psychological condition to a great extent. While intra-oral causes such as periodontal disease and poor oral hygiene are prevalent, the etiology may be systemic in nature and thus necessitate assessment by a dentist to be treated properly. Additionally, such syndromes as pseudohalitosis, in which patients believe they have halitosis but have no physiological basis for such a belief, point out the importance of a strict clinical evaluation to avoid unnecessary treatment and to address any potential psychological condition, especially in special needs patients who are more likely to have such a condition given their complex health histories. Another common condition of the oral cavity is dental caries, which is due to bacterial infections producing destruction of tooth structure. Dental caries are created when plaque, a biofilm, binds to teeth and produces acids that dissolve enamel. This condition is most common in children and adolescents, but may be seen in adults too. Early treatment, typically including professional teeth cleaning, fluoridation, and attention to good oral hygiene, is necessary to prevent caries from advancing. Disregard for these can result in more severe issues, like the development of an abscess or dental extractions. As a preventable disease, public health intervention through education and regular dental visits should be done to reduce the incidence and prevalence of the common disorder among the general population. Oral cavity disorders have extended beyond the boundaries of halitosis and dental caries, with mucositis and oral cancers being highly risky disorders. Mucositis, which is mucous membrane inflammation and ulceration, can be caused by various factors such as chemotherapy, radiation, or infection. The condition, apart from being painful, also predisposes one to infection complications that complicate overall treatment plans. Oral cancers, further related to tobacco consumption and infection with human papillomavirus, are amongst the more severe disorders of the oral cavity. Since early diagnosis strongly improves treatment efficacy, education on risk factors and periodic screenings are necessary. Indeed, the complex relationship between oral and systemic health emphasizes the necessity for multifaceted approaches to treat these disorders and foster overall well-being in the framework of the gastrointestinal system (Blot et al., 2018).

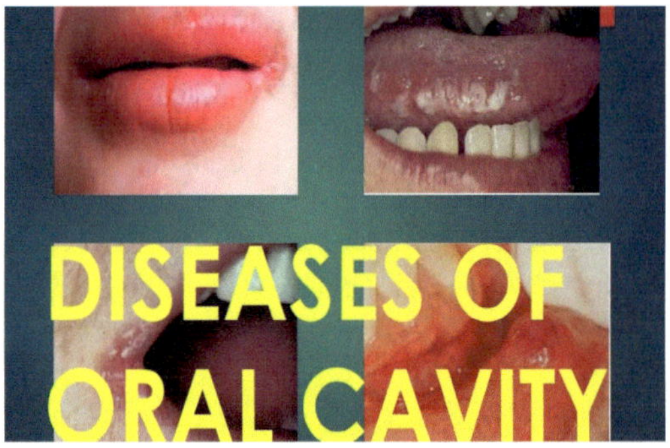

Figure 4.15. Common diseases of oral cavity.

Source: https://i.ytimg.com/vi/8-uz-O8Xpyk/maxresdefault.jpg

4.5.1. Dental Caries

Dental caries prevalence is a key oral cavity study concern because it not only affects oral health but also the general health of the digestive system. Dental caries or tooth decay results from the enamel on teeth dissolving as a result of acids that are produced when bacteria metabolize sugar. This process can create cavities, which are holes and pits that weaken the tooth. The intricacy that exists between the mouth and the digestive tract is the reason that the mouth needs to be cleaned. Lack of good oral hygiene can lead to an infection that will drastically weaken the digestive system, highlighting these systems' interdependencies. Preventive therapies, such as regular dental examinations and oral hygiene, are of paramount importance in managing the risk of dental caries and the overall health of the alimentary canal. Dental caries signs are extensive beyond tooth damage to a specific region, and the potential effect can extend to affect other physiological alimentary canal functions. The oral cavity is not merely the site of chewing but is also a part of the digestive process. As there are receptors present on the mucous membrane lining of the oral cavity, this site is a significant contributor to the motor and secretory process involved in digestion (et al., 2024). When oral tissue and tooth caries develop, they can alter the function of these reflexes, with impaired digestion and nutrient uptake as a consequence. This disturbance can then be expressed in broader syndromes of malnutrition and gastrointestinal dysfunction. The physiology of dental caries is therefore crucial to understand because it illustrates the broader context of oral disease influence upon body function and nutritional balance. Moreover, dental caries have also prompted public health agencies to develop programs whose objective is to educate individuals on oral hygiene and diet. The consumption of a diet contributes greatly to the etiology of dental caries, with acid- and sugar-rich diets being key perpetrators of tooth decay. Implementation of nutritional education programs targeting the importance of a diet that is high in calcium and phosphate has the potential to neutralize the effect of oral pathogens. Such interventions are consistent with the anatomical and physiological connection of the digestive system and the oral cavity, on which the incorporation of oral health as a component of general health is founded. Through the generation of awareness and promotion of preventive measures, public health interventions can make the prevalence of dental caries decline to foster a healthier populace, as well as improve the crucial interlinkages of the digestive system.

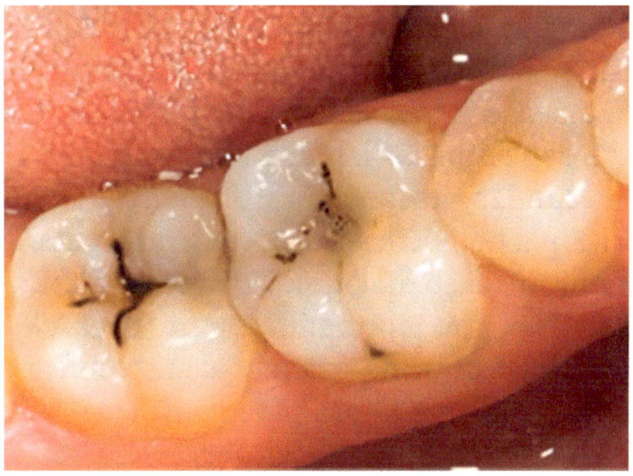

Figure 4.16. Dental caries.

Source: https://www.winningsmiletor.com/wp-content/uploads/2021/02/caries-dental-decay-dentist-mississauga-sferlazza.jpg

4.5.2. Gum Disease

Gum disease, or periodontal disease, is a serious oral health problem in the digestive system, if not more so in the oral cavity. A group of diseases that primarily affect the supporting tissues of the teeth, namely the gums. The course of gum disease begins with gingivitis, the inflammation of the gums caused by the accumulation of plaque, a sticky film of bacteria. Gingivitis, if left untreated, can evolve into periodontitis, which inflicts further damage through the loss of bone and tooth mobility. The process underscores the importance of early detection and treatment because untreated gum disease has systemic effects that extend beyond oral pathology to overall health and digestive effectiveness. Besides, gum disease is most commonly linked with bad breath or halitosis, which causes psychological distress and social impacts on individuals suffering from it (et al., 2018). Such a connection between gum disease and general health describes a bidirectional relationship between oral and bodily functions. It has been theorized that periodontal disease inflammation can be the etiologic factor for systemic conditions such as cardiovascular disease and diabetes. This connection is a result of how oral infecting agents and inflammatory markers may migrate into the bloodstream, causing inflammation in other body systems. Gum disease is also not an isolated occurrence; it is a reflection of larger oral conditions that are secondary to poor oral hygiene practices, nutritional deficiencies of certain nutrients, and systemic disease that impacts overall immunity. Given that the epithelia in the oral cavity serve as a front-line defense against infection, dysfunction or compromise in this area can have far-reaching implications, illustrative of the health of the mouth in maintaining digestive health (Angelov et al., 2021). As we proceed with the discussion of gum disease's implications, it is clear that prevention techniques are paramount in avoiding its impact on the oral cavity and, by extension, on the digestive system. Regular check-ups with a dentist and professional cleaning are important components of a preventive regimen for healthy gums. Further, people need to focus on rigorous oral hygiene practices that include brushing, flossing, and antimicrobial mouthwash. Education programs that make people aware of the importance of gum health can also prove to be of paramount significance in prevention. In particular, populations under systemic conditions stand to benefit from targeted interventions aimed at reducing disparities in oral health, thereby alleviating the broader interrelation among gum health, digestion, and overall physiological function. Such a holistic strategy places gum disease in its proper position as an issue of public health as part of the broader scheme of the digestive system (et al., 2018; Angelov et al., 2021).

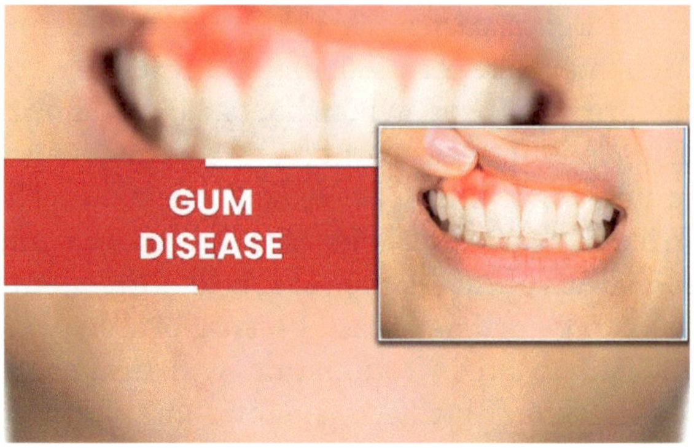

Figure 4.17. Gum disease.

Source: https://wilmotfamilydentistry.com/wp-content/uploads/2022/10/GUM-DISEASE-scaled.jpg

4.5.3. Oral Cancer

Oral cancer, such as lip, tongue, gum, and other mucosal neoplasms, is a serious health concern in the gastrointestinal field. Oral cancer has significant correlations with risk factors like tobacco use, alcohol consumption, and human papillomavirus (HPV). The oral cavity is a weak portal of entry for carcinogens and pathogens and, therefore, susceptible to cancers. As a surface-exposed body area in a permanent state, the intricate cellular structure of the oral cavity is prone to damage, which may result in pathologic overgrowth of cells. The clinicopathologic behavior of oral cancer takes an asymptomatic character during the initial stages of its development, which hinders diagnosis and treatment in a timely fashion. Therefore, one needs to be cognizant of the signs and risk factors so that preventive therapy can be promoted and oral cancer results can be improved. The ramifications of oral cancer also reach beyond local effects, playing an important role in the entire digestive system function. Since the mouth is an important location for initial digestion, i.e., salivation and mastication, the presence of tumors in the oral cavity is liable to interrupt the process of nutrient intake and alter normal physiological function. For example, lesions may cause oropharyngeal pain during chewing and swallowing and lead to malnutrition and systemic disease. Additionally, oral cancer patients also undergo the following oral cancer complications that are all contributing to diminished quality of life: change in taste, xerostomia, and infectivity. Given these multifaceted effects, it is apparent that treatment for oral cancer must be multidisciplinary in scope and utilize medical, nutritional, and psychological interventions to enable holistic patient healing and rehabilitation. Current comprehension has also heightened awareness of the intricate interaction between oral cancer and overall health, such as developing correlations with systemic disease. Studies have posited the theory that the oral cavity plays a role in the pathogenesis of certain diseases, such as cardiovascular disease and respiratory infections, particularly under immunocompromised states.

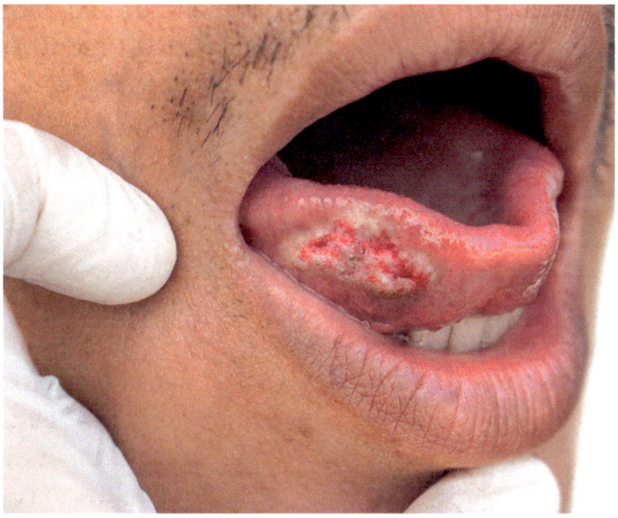

Figure 4.18. Oral cancer.

Source: https://my.clevelandclinic.org/-/scassets/Images/org/health/articles/tongue-cancer

Particularly, recent research reveals possible correlations between the microbiome dynamics and oral health and the susceptibility towards viral infection like SARS-CoV-2. This underscores the importance of maintaining oral health as a means of protecting against long-term health problems. Thus, awareness of the fundamental biological process of oral cancers interacting with other disorders makes room for new treatment models and public health practice towards early detection and integrative care, enhancing patient outcomes in the field of digestion and overall health (N/A, 2024; Chen et al., 2021).

Test Your Knowledge

1. What is dental caries?
2. What is oral cancer?

4.6. The Role of the Oral Cavity in Overall Health

Learning Outcome

1. Understand the connection between oral health and systemic health
2. Describe the impact of diet on oral cavity health
3. Understand the importance of oral hygiene

The oral cavity is a significant entry point into the digestive tract, playing a crucial role not only in digestion but also in the broader picture of overall health. Primary mechanical breakdown of food is facilitated by the teeth, which break up and tear consumed material into more manageable pieces for enzymatic activity. Saliva secreted by the salivary glands contains enzymes like amylase, which begin to break down carbohydrates. Also, saliva is a lubricant, which helps with swallowing.

This function emphasizes the mouth's purpose of delivering food smoothly into the esophagus, conditioning the digestive system for subsequent processing phases. This implies that any dysfunction of the oral cavity will have an effect on digestion, and oral health is therefore integral to overall health. Moreover, the oral cavity is not merely a digestive machine; it is inhabited by a diverse microbiome that has a substantial impact on overall health. The oral microbiota can influence systemic health, and their imbalance can predispose patients to various health conditions such as oral disease and systemic disorders like cardiovascular disease. Specifically, research has shown that periodontal infections are able to release inflammatory mediators into the circulatory system, which can exacerbate a priori diseases. Kushnirenko (2016) implied that the presence of fungal infection, such as oropharyngeal candidiasis, has the potential to compromise oral and general health by disrupting the balance of the microbiome. This illustrates the correlation between oral health and systemic physiological functions, emphasizing the significance of oral hygiene in achieving microbial homeostasis and overall resilience of health. In addition to its mechanical and microbiological functions, the oral cavity also plays a vital role in sensory perception, which is important in nutritional evaluation and the regulation of ingestion. Taste is a multifaceted sense that gives individuals information regarding the nutritional content and tastiness of food. The recent discovery that the tongue can detect fat as a unique taste has enhanced knowledge of the mechanisms of taste and their health implications. (Costanzo and Keast, 2015) note that fatty acids stimulate specific receptors on the taste buds, giving the body information regarding nutrient content. The ability to taste improves the enjoyment of eating and impacts food choice, with long-term implications for health. Furthermore, accurate taste perception is linked to mechanisms of satiation that act to regulate energy intake. This emphasizes the oral cavity's key role in the inter-relation of digestion, sensory experience, and nutritional health.

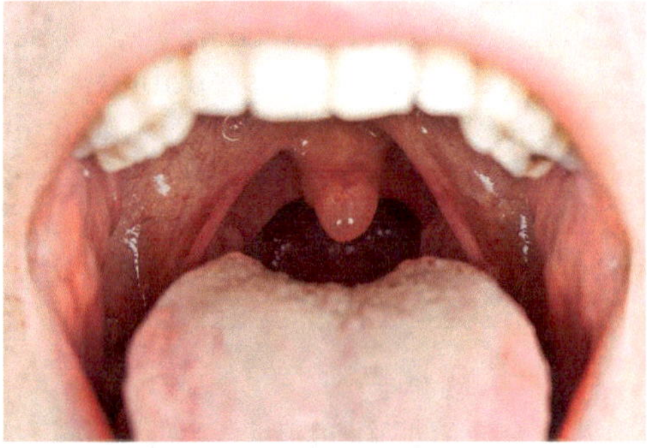

Figure 4.19. Your mouth is part of your digestive and respiratory systems. It supports many daily functions.

Source: https://my.clevelandclinic.org/-/scassets/Images/org/health/articles/21765-parts-of-the-mouth

4.6.1. Connection Between Oral Health and Systemic Health

The interconnection of oral health and systemic health is increasingly considered an important area of research, and the number of diseases, beyond those of the mouth, that can be explained. The mouth is a portal of entry for microorganisms that can become transported into the bloodstream and travel throughout the body, offering pathways of systemic disease, including cardiovascular disease, diabetes, and respiratory infection. Literature indicates that periodontal disease, a condition of chronic inflammation of the gums, is linked with inflammatory processes in the body that improve such health conditions. Oral infection and inflammatory mediators can affect systemic health and, hence, favor oral hygiene preservation in holistic healthcare modalities. Furthermore, co-communication between oral and systemic health accentuates the role of microbiota in both realms. The oral cavity harbors a highly concentrated biofilm of microbes, which may affect metabolism and digestion. Disruption of oral microbiota homeostasis may trigger dysbiosis to cause extrinsic factors like obesity and metabolic syndrome. Increasing evidence suggests that inflammation from disrupted oral health affects disease pathways involved in obesity-related disease, including tumorigenesis. For instance, more recent theories propose that long-standing oral bacterial inflammation is capable of initiating carcinogenesis pathways, providing considerable proof of causality between oral health and systemic disease risk and deserving the worth of healthy oral environments to overall well-being. In addition to these direct links, lifestyle and nutrition have primary functions in deciding oral and systemic health. Diet, particularly a diet high in sweets and processed foods, may promote pathogenic oral bacteria growth and initiate systemic inflammation. Meanwhile, whole-food diets high in fruits, vegetables, and probiotics can benefit oral health by being beneficial to the oral microbiome. Therefore, diet-focused public health interventions to improve diets are needed not only to avoid disease in the mouth but also to reduce their systemic effects. Controlling such interdependent aspects of health can yield more integrated healthcare solutions with greatly improved individual and community levels of health.

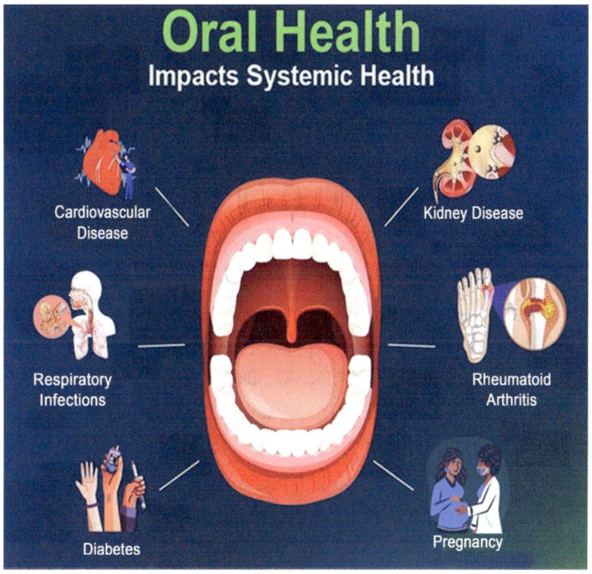

Figure 4.20. The Surprising Link Between Oral Health and Systemic Disease.

Source: https://www.agapedental.ca/wp-content/uploads/2024/11/the-surprising-link-between-oral-health-and-systemic-disease.png

4.6.2. Impact of Diet on Oral Cavity Health

Diet is a fundamental factor in oral cavity health and has a direct influence on the composition of the oral microbiota and the integrity of oral tissues. Sugar and processed carbohydrate intake must be avoided, particularly. These foods provide substrates for disease-causing bacteria, inducing enamel demineralization and dental caries (cavities) formation. When bacteria in the oral cavity ferment sugars, acids are released that dissolve tooth enamel, with the ensuing possibility of decay. On the other hand, a diet of whole foods, consisting of whole grains, vegetables, and fruits, maintains the oral microbiome in health and diversity. These foods not only stimulate the production of saliva, which is beneficial in the neutralization of poisonous acids, but also contain significant vitamins and minerals needed in the maintenance of oral tissues' health. Lastly, diet significantly influences the oral cavity status, thus necessitating public health policy promoting healthy diets for prevention against oral disease. Diet also plays a greater role than its effect on the teeth; diet influences the condition of gums as well, which is also key to preventing periodontal disease. Consuming excessive processed food and sugars can lead to even more inflammation within the oral cavity, setting the stage for gingivitis and, if not treated, continuing on to periodontitis. These are diseases associated with gum tissue and supporting structure destruction, with potential loss of teeth. On the other hand, an antioxidant-rich diet, which is abundant in pigmented fruits and vegetables, can decrease gum inflammation and oxidative stress. Green tea and foods with high levels of omega-3 fatty acids have been promising in modulating inflammatory reactions within periodontal tissues. Therefore, nutrition therapy with nutrient-dense diets can be harnessed as a preventive strategy for gum disease, a pointer to the dual role of nutrition towards managing oral health. The recent postbiotics studies also add more complexity to the diet's contribution to oral cavity health. Postbiotics—byproducts of the probiotic metabolism—also have additional systemic health benefits in addition to oral health. These viably non-existent microbial fractions are able to modulate the microbial population in the oral cavity and bring about an equilibrium between pathogenic and health-supporting strains. Some dietary habits favoring gut well-being, such as dietary fiber and fermented foods supplementation, among them, may be responsible for postbiotic formation. As gut microbiota cross-talks with the gut-brain axis, it has also been found to influence oral health in addition to affecting the gut in inflammatory and immune response-mediated pathways (Salminen et al., 2021). All these intricate interactions among oral cavity health, gut microbiota, and diet ensure that the overall vision of nutrition and its extensive influence on the gastrointestinal tract, particularly the oral cavity, is essential (Silva et al., 2020).

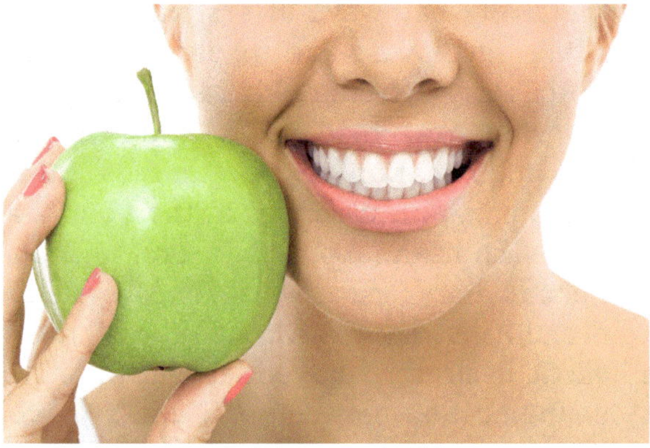

Figure 4.21. The impact of diet on oral health.

Source: https://www.andrewhousedental.com/wp-content/uploads/2024/02/Capture152-1.png

4.6.3. Importance of Oral Hygiene

Proper oral hygiene is vital to the general well-being of the digestive system, starting from the oral cavity. The mouth plays not only the role of food entry but also that of a complex environment where there are varying microorganisms that inhabit it. Regular oral hygiene procedures, such as brushing and flossing, control the number of pathogenic bacteria, which otherwise lead to dental disorders such as caries and periodontitis. The results of ignoring these practices may spill over into the rest of the body since pathogenic bacteria can become systemic in the bloodstream, potentially impacting far-distant organ systems. For example, research has shown that inadequate oral hygiene greatly increases the likelihood of developing conditions such as heart disease and diabetes, highlighting the interdependence of oral health and systemic health (Annibali et al., 2017). Thus, the creation of a habit of good oral hygiene not just keeps teeth and gums healthy but also safeguards one's overall health. Good oral hygiene is also important in avoiding diseases of the oral cavity, which can result from the accumulation of bacterial plaque. Such accumulation can cause inflammation, leading to gingivitis and more severe conditions like periodontitis, characterized by the breakdown of the supporting structures of the teeth. Periodontal disease has an association with various health complications, such as the induction of other systemic diseases due to the transmission of periodontal pathogens via the circulatory system. Of particular note are certain oral bacteria implicated in chronic inflammatory diseases, thus establishing a link between oral health and decreasing cognition, such as Alzheimer's disease (Crean et al., 2014). Thus, appreciation of oral hygiene is more than a mere cosmetic concern; it is a key factor in the prevention of inflammatory disorders that impact the whole body. In addition, oral hygiene is significant because it aids digestion and absorption of nutrients. The mouth is the initiation site of the digestive process, where food breakdown starts through enzymes. When oral hygiene is neglected, food residue and pathogenic bacteria can compromise the oral environment, causing improper chewing and digestion. The production of saliva that contains digestive enzymes also suffers from the state of the oral cavity. Saliva is required to cover food and initiate digestion, but inflammation and infection caused by poor oral hygiene can disrupt salivary flow and structure. Complications due to such neglect may lead to digestive issues, altering nutrient absorption and overall health (Crean et al., 2014). In all, good oral hygiene is an integral part of the digestive process, influencing not only oral but also overall digestive and systemic health outcomes.

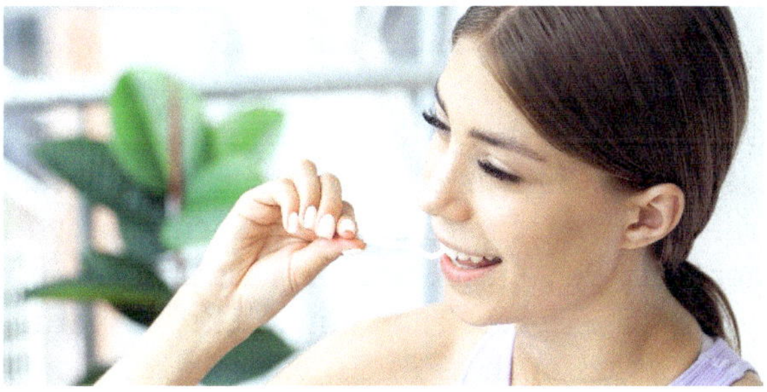

Figure 4.22. The importance of oral hygiene in daily routine.

Source: https://jamaicaplaindental.com/wp-content/uploads/2024/04/The-Importance-of-Oral-Hygiene-in-Daily-Life.jpg

Test Your Knowledge

1. What is the impact of diet on oral cavity health?
2. Why is oral hygiene important?

SUMMARY

In building the oral cavity's essential roles in the grand scheme of the human digestive process, it is apparent that this initial phase of digestion plays an overarching role in general health and well-being. The oral cavity not only provides for the mechanical breakdown of food by chewing but for the activation of the biochemical processes necessary for nutrient absorption. Salivary enzymes, in the form of amylase, begin carbohydrate digestion, and the oral cavity thus becomes the first site of contact where mechanical and enzymic activity begin concurrently. This initial processing is critical, as it sets the quality of what ensues in the digestive process and places oral health on center stage as a determinant of the maintenance of systemic health. In addition, the oral cavity is a portal to microbial communities and also actively participates in the modulation of gut microbiota. The nascent science of the microbiome and its implications for health has already begun to reveal how oral microbiota can affect processes in the gastrointestinal tract as well as systemic functions from immune status to neurological health. The oral microbiome's interaction with systemic physiology, which is mediated through multiple metabolites, is a complex process and should be considered. Notably, the inter-relationship of the gastrointestinal system means that disruption of oral microbiota can go up to influencing the gut-brain axis as well as other physiological functions, as seen in recent revelations regarding the role of gut microbiota in neuro-immunoendocrine regulation (Silva et al., 2020). Finally, the perception of the role of the oral cavity in digestion and general health has substantial clinical and public health intervention consequences. With increased awareness of oral health mechanisms and associations with disease, systemic and preventive procedures and therapy intervention must be restructured as a step towards accordination of oral health and oral hygiene measures. The vulnerability to pathogens, as evidenced by the oral mucosa's possession of receptors such as ACE2, emphasizes the urgency for an effective prevention method in dental wellness to suppress infection (Xu et al., 2020). Ultimately, the function of the oral cavity extends beyond digestion and represents a complete spectrum of health concerns warranting an in-depth investigation and active management both in the clinical and social environments.

The oral cavity is the initial segment of the human gastrointestinal system, beginning the complex process of food digestion. It is not just a pipe where food enters, but an area of importance where mechanical and chemical digestion begins. Teeth, assisted by the musculature of the jaws, initiate the mechanical breakdown of food, while saliva that is secreted by the salivary glands primes the food for the introduction of enzymes to initiate carbohydrate digestion. Saliva also provides lubrication, making swallowing easy, so that food can be directed to the esophagus next. OraCavity also has a resident population of microorganisms, which form part of an active oral ecology of significance to oral as well as digestive health. An understanding of the function and role of these is a foundation for understanding how the oral cavity prepares the entire digestive process. Having multiple bacterial populations in the oral cavity is crucial for general health and digestion. Oral microbiota were divided based on their respective habitats, i.e., buccal mucosa, tongue, and saliva, each of which had its own populations of distinct bacteria. Besides the function of digesting the constituents of food, these microbial flora also defend against pathogenic bacteria by competing for scarce space and resources. The relationship among these bacteria can produce metabolic activities that influence health on an international scale, such as the production of short-chain fatty acids and other beneficial compounds. Imbalances in the delicate balance of these microbial populations can result in oral disease and highlight the importance of maintaining a healthy oral microbiome in order to optimize digestive function (Gevers et al., 2012). Moreover, its incorporation with the rest of the gastrointestinal tract solidifies its importance in global health. As food is transferred from the mouth to the stomach, initial chemical breakdown still characterizes digestive efficiency and nutrient absorption. Disruptions during this phase, such as dental issues or microbiota disturbances, can indirectly cause more intrinsic gastrointestinal problems downstream. An understanding of the major factors is essential to clinicians and researchers since it points out the need for convergent care that considers both oral and systemic health. Focusing on oral health can therefore avert overall health problems as well as improve the quality of life, proving that the entrance of the gastrointestinal tract is also important enough (Bochsler et al., 2007).

KEY TERMS FROM THIS CHAPTER

Amylase	Antimicrobial resistance
Chemical digestion	Chewing
Dental caries	Digestive system
EnamelFlavor perception	Immune systems
Mastication	Microorganisms
Oral cavity	Saliva
Salivary glands	Taste buds

CRITICAL THINKING QUESTIONS

1. **The oral cavity is part of which organ system?**
   a. Respiratory system
   b. Nervous system
   c. Digestive system
   d. Endocrine system
2. **The main function of the oral cavity in digestion is:**
   a. Chemical digestion of proteins
   b. Mechanical and chemical breakdown of food
   c. Absorption of nutrients
   d. Production of bile
3. **The roof of the oral cavity is formed by:**
   a. Tongue
   b. Hard and soft palate
   c. Pharynx
   d. Teeth
4. **The floor of the oral cavity is mainly formed by:**
   a. Palate
   b. Tongue
   c. Teeth
   d. Salivary glands
5. **Which of the following are the major salivary glands?**
   a. Parotid, submandibular, and sublingual glands
   b. Parotid, thyroid, and adrenal glands
   c. Submandibular, adrenal, and thymus glands
   d. Sublingual, pancreas, and liver

Short Answer Questions

1. What is the digestive system?
2. What is the importance of the oral cavity in digestion?
3. Describe the functions of the oral cavity.
4. What are the salivary glands?
5. What are the common disorders of the oral cavity?

Answer to Critical Thinking Questions

1. (c) 2. (b) 3. (b) 4. (b) 5. (a)

REFERENCES

1. Adams, J., Aidara-Kane, A., Alvarez, L., Amidon, G., Andersson, D. I., Andremont, A., et al. (2016). Veterinary medicine needs new green antimicrobial drugs. 3
2. Adlercreutz, H., Aherne, S., Aps, J. K. M., Armand, M., Armand, M., Armand, M., et al. (2014). *In vitro* models for studying secondary plant metabolite digestion and bio accessibility. https://core.ac.uk/download/pdf/70607414.pdf (accessed on 15th June 2025).
3. Alekseyenko, A. V., Beiting, D. P., Curtis, J. L., He, X., et al. (2019). OHMI: The ontology of host-microbiome interactions. https://core.ac.uk/download/286357479.pdf (accessed on 15th June 2025).
4. Allocca, G., Menozzi, G., Grossi, G. B., & M. F., et al. (2018). Oral malodor in special care patients: Current knowledge. https://core.ac.uk/download/159636738.pdf (accessed on 15th June 2025).
5. Angelov, N., Arboleda, S., Arce, R. M., Suárez, L. J., et al. (2021). Oral versus gastrointestinal mucosal immune niches in homeostasis and allostasis. https://core.ac.uk/download/604668404.pdf (accessed on 15th June 2025).
6. Annibali, S., Biagi, M., Cristalli, M. P., D'Ambrini, A., et al. (2017). Prevention and early diagnosis of oral carcinoma in construction workers in Italy: A pilot project. https://core.ac.uk/download/54537924.pdf (accessed on 15th June 2025).
7. Arvisenet, G., Björklund, M., Bongaerts, J., Bornhorst, G. M., Boyar, A., Buettner, A., et al. (2014). Understanding the relevance of in-mouth food processing: A review of *in vitro* techniques. https://riunet.upv.es:443/bitstream/handle/10251/63046/Revised%20Manuscript.pdf?sequence=3&isAllowed=y (accessed on 15th June 2025).
8. Banni, S., Crnjar, R., Melis, M., Tepper, B. J., & Tomassini Barbarossa, I. (2014). Genetic sensitivity to the bitter taste of 6-n-propylthiouracil (PROP) and its association with physiological mechanisms controlling body mass index (BMI). https://core.ac.uk/download/pdf/54598551.pdf (accessed on 15th June 2025).
9. Baptista, E. S., Capela e Silva, F., Ferreira, A., Lamy, E., et al. (2012). The influence of oral environment on diet choices in goats: A focus on saliva protein composition. https://core.ac.uk/download/62453121.pdf (accessed on 15th June 2025).
10. Beck Coburn, G., Karabucak, B., Nguyen, Q., Tizzano, M., et al. (2019). Gingival taste bud papillae associated with retromolar salivary gland. https://core.ac.uk/download/237179005.pdf (accessed on 15th June 2025).
11. Bekish, V. J., & Zorina, V. V. (2014). *Biology*. https://core.ac.uk/download/80152204.pdf (accessed on 15th June 2025).
12. Blot, S., Deschepper, M., Eeckloo, K., Vogelaers, D., et al. (2018). Effects of chlorhexidine gluconate oral care on hospital mortality: A hospital-wide, observational cohort study. https://core.ac.uk/download/158345560.pdf (accessed on 15th June 2025).
13. Bochsler, V. S., Galloway, S. B., Harley, R. A., Kramarsky-Winters, E., et al. (2007). Coral disease and health workshop: Coral histopathology II. https://core.ac.uk/download/11017972.pdf (accessed on 15th June 2025).

14. Brown, M., Liu, F., & Patel, V. F. (2011). Advances in oral transmucosal drug delivery. https://core.ac.uk/download/1641789.pdf (accessed on 15th June 2025).

15. Chatra, L., Dandekeri, S., Prabhu, R. V., Prabhu, V. M., et al. (2014). Areca nut and its role in oral submucous fibrosis. https://core.ac.uk/download/71035750.pdf (accessed on 15th June 2025).

16. Chen, Q., Koo, H., Liu, Y., Simón-Soro, A., et al. (2021). Potential implications of SARS-CoV-2 oral infection in the host microbiota. https://core.ac.uk/download/560388745.pdf (accessed on 15th June 2025).

17. Costanzo, A., & Keast, R. (2015). Is fat the sixth taste primary? Evidence and implications. https://core.ac.uk/download/pdf/30672828.pdf (accessed on 15th June 2025).

18. Crean, S., Harding, A., Kesavalu, L., Robinson, C., et al. (2014). Oral inflammation, tooth loss, risk factors, and association with progression of Alzheimer's disease. https://core.ac.uk/download/42137086.pdf (accessed on 15th June 2025).

19. Dallas, D. C., German, J. B., Underwood, M. A., & Zivkovic, A. M. (2012). Digestion of protein in premature and term infants. https://core.ac.uk/download/323070580.pdf (accessed on 15th June 2025).

20. Darlington, L. G., McPherson, M., & Stone, T. W. (2018). Obesity and cancer: Existing and new hypotheses for a causal connection. https://core.ac.uk/download/153444767.pdf (accessed on 15th June 2025).

21. Dynowska, M., Góralska, K., & Rosłon, M. (2013). *Saccharomyces cerevisiae* in the respiratory system, digestive system and on the skin in humans. https://core.ac.uk/download/236959388.pdf (accessed on 15th June 2025).

22. Feng, J., Liu, J., Jiang, M., Chen, Q., Zhang, Y., Yang, M., & Zhai, Y. (2023). The role of oral nitrate-reducing bacteria in the prevention of caries: A review related to caries and nitrate metabolism. *Caries Research, 57*, 119–132. https://www.semanticscholar.org/paper/ba7fabb91060a3fc9f2361994d56e427df8bccea (accessed on 15th June 2025).

23. Gevers, D., Haake, S. K., Huttenhower, C., Izard, J., et al. (2012). Composition of the adult digestive tract bacterial microbiome based on seven mouth surfaces, tonsils, throat and stool samples. https://core.ac.uk/download/28941105.pdf (accessed on 15th June 2025).

24. Hillman, E. T., Lu, H., Yao, T., & Nakatsu, C. H. (2017). Microbial ecology along the gastrointestinal tract. *Microbes and Environments, 32*, 300–313. https://doi.org/10.1264/jsme2.me17017 (accessed on 15th June 2025).

25. Huang, K., Wu, L., & Yang, Y. (2021). Gut microbiota: An emerging biological diagnostic and treatment approach for gastrointestinal diseases. *JGH Open: An Open Access Journal of Gastroenterology and Hepatology, 5*, 973–975. https://www.semanticscholar.org/paper/3ab1a27e126034b241d21eba30f8dbf1cf2d27fc (accessed on 15th June 2025).

26. Kotionova-Ovod, I. A., Simanovskaya, O. E., Postnikov, M., & Mokshin, A. K. (2023). The condition of the oral mucosa and salivary glands against the background of systemic diseases. *Journal of Volgograd State Medical University*. https://www.semanticscholar.org/paper/50d40a3ffdd17911d9948dd4fadc65b75db61124 (accessed on 15th June 2025).

27. Kushnirenko, I. (2016). Iodine deficiency and pathology of thyroid gland as a background state of candidiasis of mucosa of the upper part of digestive tract. https://media.neliti.com/

media/publications/298174-iodine-deficiency-and-pathology-of-thyro-4623355a.pdf (accessed on 15th June 2025).

28. Maddu, N. (2019). Functions of saliva. https://core.ac.uk/download/322441800.pdf (accessed on 15th June 2025).

29. Mahía, J., Molina, F., Puerto, A., Simón, F., et al. (2019). Enteral feeding: Brain-visceral interactions in the processing of nutrients. https://core.ac.uk/download/322440690.pdf (accessed on 15th June 2025).

30. Murray, C. J. L., Ikuta, K. S., Sharara, F., Swetschinski, L. R., Robles Aguilar, G., Gray, A. P., Han, C., et al. (2022). Global burden of bacterial antimicrobial resistance in 2019: A systematic analysis. *The Lancet, 399*, 629–655. https://doi.org/10.1016/s0140-6736(21)02724-0 (accessed on 15th June 2025).

31. N/A. (2024). Full issue: Volume 17, Number 2, Spring 2024. https://core.ac.uk/download/621745508.pdf (accessed on 15th June 2025).

32. Patwardhan, K. (2008). Concepts of human physiology in Ayurveda. https://core.ac.uk/download/pdf/87482.pdf (accessed on 15th June 2025).

33. Pedersen, A. M. L., Sørensen, C. E., Proctor, G., Carpenter, G. H., & Ekström, J. (2018). Salivary secretion in health and disease. *Journal of Oral Rehabilitation, 45*, 730–746. https://doi.org/10.1111/joor.12664 (accessed on 15th June 2025).

34. Salminen, S., Collado, M. C., Endo, A., Hill, C., Lebeer, S., Quigley, E. M. M., Sanders, M. E., et al. (2021). The International Scientific Association of Probiotics and Prebiotics (ISAPP) consensus statement on the definition and scope of postbiotics. *Nature Reviews Gastroenterology & Hepatology, 18*, 649–667. https://doi.org/10.1038/s41575-021-00440-6 (accessed on 15th June 2025).

35. Schmidt, T., Hayward, M. R., Coelho, L. P., Li, S. S., Costea, P. I., Voigt, A. Y., Wirbel, J., et al. (2019). Extensive transmission of microbes along the gastrointestinal tract. *eLife, 8*. https://doi.org/10.7554/elife.42693 (accessed on 15th June 2025).

36. Silva, Y. P., Bernardi, A., & Frozza, R. L. (2020). The role of short-chain fatty acids from gut microbiota in gut-brain communication. *Frontiers in Endocrinology, 11*. https://doi.org/10.3389/fendo.2020.00025 (accessed on 15th June 2025).

37. Valls-Bellés, V. (2024). The biochemistry of digestion. https://core.ac.uk/download/614526814.pdf (accessed on 15th June 2025).

38. Vestby, L. K., Grønseth, T., Simm, R., & Nesse, L. L. (2020). Bacterial biofilm and its role in the pathogenesis of disease. *Antibiotics, 9*, 59–59. https://doi.org/10.3390/antibiotics9020059 (accessed on 15th June 2025).

39. Xu, H., Zhong, L., Deng, J. S., Peng, J., Dan, H., Zeng, X., Li, T., et al. (2020). High expression of ACE2 receptor of 2019-nCoV on the epithelial cells of oral mucosa. *International Journal of Oral Science, 12*. https://doi.org/10.1038/s41368-020-0074-x (accessed on 15th June 2025).

ESOPHAGUS AND STOMACH

5

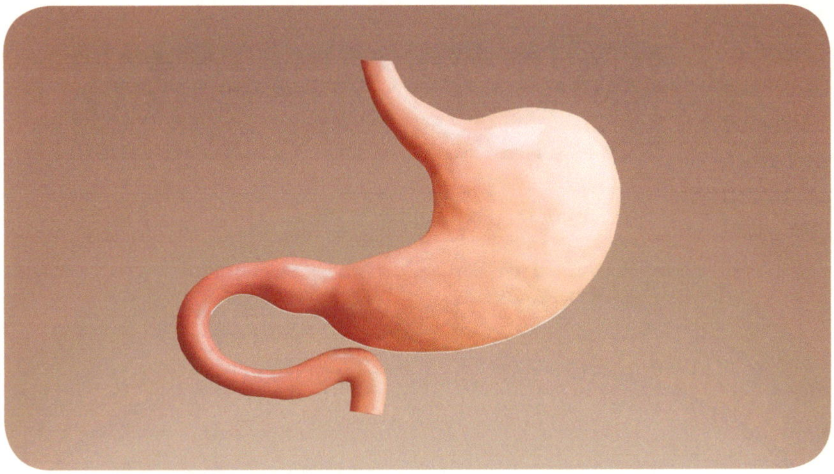

LEARNING OBJECTIVES

After studying this chapter, you will be able to:

1. Understand the anatomy of the esophagus
2. Describe the function of the esophagus
3. Understand the anatomy of the stomach
4. Describe the function of the stomach
5. Describe the common disorders of the esophagus
6. Explain the common disorders of the stomach

Introduction

Esophagus and stomach are the essential parts of the human digestive system, both playing important roles in the sophisticated process of food consumption and nutritional absorption. The esophagus is a muscular tube that transports food from the mouth into the stomach, a sophisticated network of musculature and nervous supply ensuring the efficacy of peristalsis. This oscillatory contraction is necessary to move boluses of individualized size along the gastrointestinal tract, reducing the risk of aspiration and optimizing the delivery efficiency of nutrients. The same applies to the anatomical structure of the esophagus, its multilayered tissue construction, which provides both strength and elasticity needed in an active process of digestion. Knowledge of these fundamental aspects of esophageal anatomy serves as a basis for the study of more specialized relationships between the stomach and esophagus and their mutual application to human health and nutrition. In addition to the esophagus, the stomach is also a transit chamber that participates in mechanical and chemical digestion of the food. As a muscle organ, its unique structure permits considerable enlargement to accommodate variable quantities of ingested material. Its mucosa contains specialized secretory cells that secrete gastric juice, which is responsible for protein digestion and the absorption of some nutrients. The cooperation between esophageal transport activities and gastric processing is a highly cooperative process to ensure effective digestion. Careful analysis of these interactions is intended to portray not only the physiologic mechanisms involved but also the relevance to a variety of disorders resulting from malfunction of either organ. Abnormalities in esophageal motility, for instance, may lead to gastroesophageal reflux disease (GERD), highlighting the value of an integrated perspective of the esophagus and stomachs function.

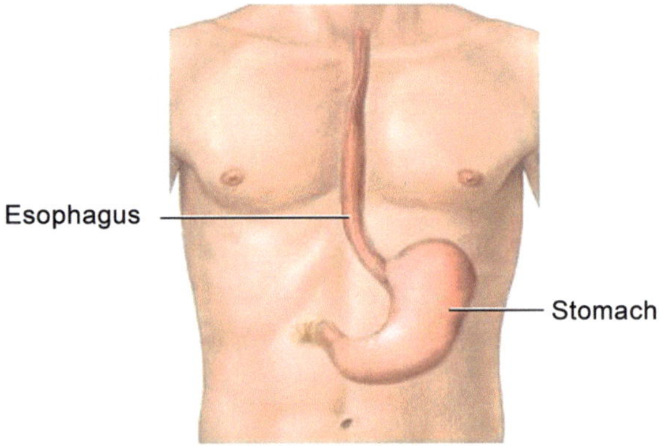

Figure 5.1. Esophagus and stomach anatomy.

Source: https://medlineplus.gov/ency/images/ency/fullsize/8756.jpg

For a fuller understanding of the esophagus and stomach complexities, this chapter will explore anatomical and functional interrelations that enable their functioning in the human body. Drawing on a critical research that goes beyond descriptive narration, it seeks to provide an extensive explanation of the role these organs play in overall digestive health. The situation of modern biomedical ontologies, with a more refined mechanism for expressing anatomical relationships, enables them to describe interactions in a better way (Mejino and Rosse, 2004). Further exploration of vascular structures, e.g., between gastric capillary beds and the esophageal submucosal venous plexus, will reveal transport systems in support of their physiological function (Aharinejad et al., 1991). All these discussions will focus on how important the esophagus and the stomach are not only in each individual's digestive system but also in overall human health.

5.1. Anatomy of the Esophagus

Learning Outcome

1. Describe the structure and length of the esophagus
2. Describe the layers of the esophageal wall
3. Understand the location and connection to other digestive organs

The esophagus is a vital component of the human body's digestive system, which links the throat and stomach through a muscular tube. The anatomy of the esophagus measures approximately 25 centimeters in length and is, in turn, divided into three segments: the cervical, thoracic, and abdominal segments. Each segment has a specific role in transferring food from the mouth to the stomach. The inner lining of the esophagus is made of stratified squamous epithelium, which protects against food abrasion of a mechanical nature. Muscle layers external to the lumen, skeletal and smooth, provide peristaltic movement, required for food propulsion. Additionally, the esophagus has sphincters at both ends: the upper esophageal sphincter, to prevent swallowing of air, and the lower esophageal sphincter to prevent backflow of stomach contents into the esophagus (Jain et al., 2018). Esophageal function is achieved by a series of coordinated muscular contractions known as peristalsis. The rhythmic contractions are initiated by the action of swallowing and are maintained even after food reaches the stomach. This mechanism guides ingested food through the esophagus and into the digestive system with maximum efficiency. Notably, the esophagus is also provided with a number of mechanisms for reflexes that assist in preserving its integrity against noxious substances like gastric acids. The fact that mucous glands are present all over the lining of the esophagus lubricates food so that it slips down easily. Besides, the lower esophageal sphincter has a defensive role against GERD by maintaining an effective barrier to acid gastric secretions that otherwise might lead to injury of the epithelial lining of the esophagus (Jain et al., 2018).

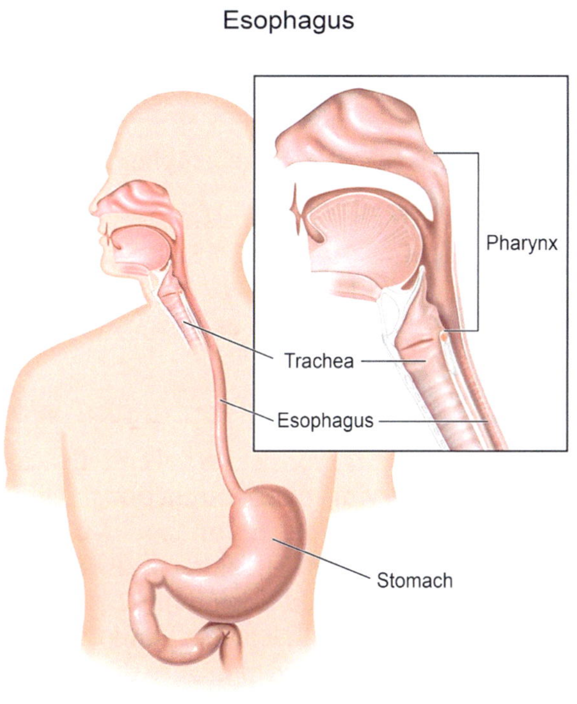

Figure 5.2. Anatomy of the esophagus.

Source: https://my.clevelandclinic.org/-/scassets/images/org/health/articles/21728-esophagus

Anatomical variations of the esophagus can dramatically influence its function and susceptibility to various disorders. For instance, variations in the length and diameter of the esophagus may occur among individuals, altering the effectiveness of swallowing and the passage rate of food. Moreover, alterations in esophageal motility due to changes with age can predispose to dysphagia or difficulty in swallowing. Disease conditions like esophagitis, malignancies, or strictures may impair motility and lead to food blockage complications. Understanding of the anatomy of the esophagus and its interfacing with surrounding structures is pivotal in the handling of such clinical conditions. As researchers explore deeper into the microbiological setting that envelops the esophagus, new information on how microbial interactions are able to impact digestive health is emerging, pointing towards the need for integrative research studies on esophageal function and anatomy (Kastl et al., 2019).

5.1.1. Structure and Length of the Esophagus

The esophagus, a part of the human digestive system, is a muscular tube roughly 25 centimeters (10 inches) long that transports food from the pharynx to the stomach. Its multi-layered structure consists of a mucosal lining inside, a submucosa, and outer muscular layers to allow food to be propelled through. This structure allows the esophagus to perform peristaltic movements—coordinated muscle contractions that propel swallowed food downwards towards the stomach. The mucosal lining stratified squamous epithelium protects from chemical and mechanical injury, and the peculiar arrangement of the muscular layers helps in easy movement and pressure regulation, which is essential in allowing the food to flow smoothly from the throat to the gastric cavity. The immeasurable flexibility of the esophagus, both in width and length, is a testimony to its role in human physiology, where various food textures and quantities can be easily accommodated. The lower esophageal sphincter (LES), anatomically positioned where the stomach interfaces with the esophagus, is a significant structure for maintaining gastrointestinal integrity. Though science has not yet fully defined the anatomical structure of the LES, its role in preventing gastric reflux is widely understood. The LES functions by virtue of a complex arrangement of muscle fascicles that encircle the esophagus to create a natural protective barrier against stomach contents. As has been described in research, the unique myo-architectural arrangement of the LES and the adjacent crural diaphragm resembles a noose that exerts circumferential pressure, thus controlling the passage of the bolus into the stomach and preventing backflow (Cheng et al., 2017). Such a highly controlled mechanism is vital not only for digestion but for the homeostatic esophageal environment as well. Hence, understanding of the LES and its geometry helps in attaining worthwhile information on conditions such as GERD and dysphagia. Peristalsis, the coordinated muscular contractions within the esophagus, is responsible for the successful transport of food swallowed to the stomach. This physiological process is the interaction between the dynamic stimulation of the esophageal muscles and the food bolus, enabling a smooth passage. The musculature of the esophagus, as a multi-layered tube, allows for this subtle interaction, and mucosal layers play critical functions in the mechanics of bolus movement. Recent simulations have shed light on pressure dynamics generated as peristaltic waves travel along the esophagus and emphasized the subtle interaction among muscle activation, pressure peaks, and bolus progression (Bhalla et al., 2015). These findings highlight the esophagus's crucial position in mechanical digestion and have significant clinical implications concerning esophageal dysfunctions. These studies of timing and coordination of esophageal contractions reiterate the significance of its structure and length, illustrating how these aspects impinge on anatomical as well as functional outcomes in human digestion.

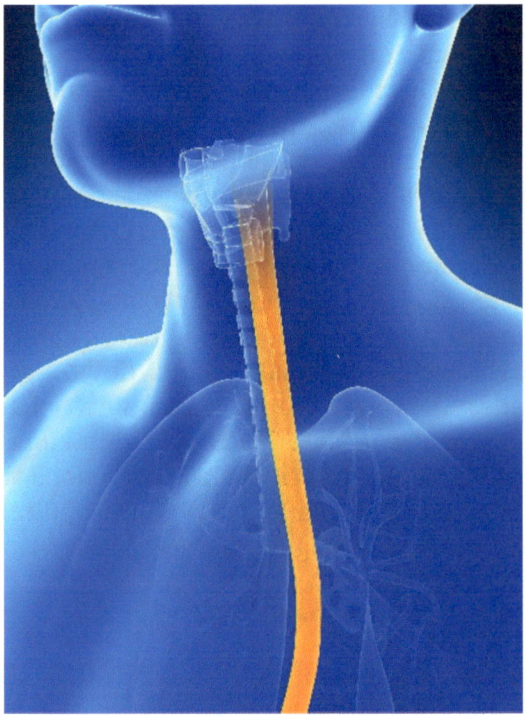

Figure 5.3. Structure of the esophagus.

Source: https://images.squarespace-cdn.com/content/v1/5935dd1515cf7db7aa9ed120/1497362720675-9F8IK4AGMHEFSY4SY2NO/esophagus-structure

5.1.2. Layers of the Esophageal Wall

The esophageal wall consists of several intricate layers, each serving distinct functions critical to the organs' movement of food from the mouth to the stomach. The inner wall, mucosa, consists of a stratified squamous epithelium that protects against mechanical and chemical injuries throughout food passage. Underneath the epithelium is the lamina propria, upon which the epithelium lies and in which some glands that secrete mucus are embedded, so that the food passes freely. The muscularis mucosae is a very thin muscle layer that assists in forcing the food into the esophagus and assists in glandular secretion regulation so that the mucosal surface is well maintained and moistened during peristalsis. Submucosa is a second one, filled with rich connective tissue, blood vessels, and lymphatics, and is a very important one in the structural support of the esophagus. Submucosal glands, in this layer, also assist in lubrication by secreting mucus, giving smooth flow without friction for bolus movement. It is also governing the presence of the submucosal nerve plexus, or Meissner's plexus, which controls the secretory function of the glands and muscularis mucosae contractions, thereby controlling the motility of the esophagus.

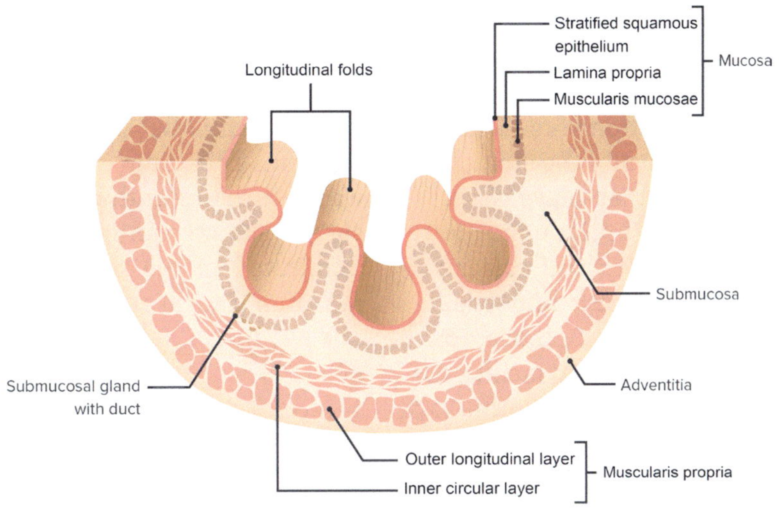

Figure 5.4. Layers of the esophageal wall.

Source: https://cdn.lecturio.com/assets/Layers-of-the-esophageal-wall.jpg

The submucosal layer occupies a pivotal role in enteric nervous system signal integration and is of concern to esophageal motility disorders like Parkinson's disease, where the dysfunction of motility results from intrinsic pathology of neurons (Cersósimo and Benarroch, 2008). Externally, the muscularis propria is beneath the submucosa and made up mainly of smooth muscle fibers that are in two layers: an internal circular and an external longitudinal layer. The double structure allows for concomitant contraction during peristalsis to propel the food bolus downwards into the stomach. In the upper esophagus, the muscle must be striated to have voluntary control with swallowing, and smooth muscle in the lower portion to have involuntary control. The outer covering, or adventitia, holds the esophagus to surrounding structures and provides yet another barrier. Researchers and clinicians must be able to recognize these layers' unique features and function, particularly in relation to emerging diagnostic tools under development, such as endoscopic optical coherence tomography, offering new insights into the status of the esophageal walls and potential disease (Michalina J Gora et al., 2017).

5.1.3. Location and Connection to Other Digestive Organs

The esophagus is a critical passageway within the digestive system of the human body, linking the mouth to the stomach. Geographically, it starts at the pharynx in the posterior part of the throat, moving downwards through the thorax and neck before piercing through the diaphragm to gain access to the abdominal cavity. Its location in the anatomy is crucial for ensuring the smooth passage of boluses (chewed food) into the stomach for further digestion. The esophagus's relationship with surrounding structures is also noteworthy; it runs adjacent to the trachea, with the two being separated by connective tissue, thereby minimizing any potential interference during the swallowing process. Moreover, there are significant sphincters of the esophagus, including the upper esophageal sphincter (UES) and lower esophageal sphincter, that regulate food passage and prevent reflux, and allow easy passage into the stomach while protecting the superior airway against aspiration of food. Food moves through the esophagus into the stomach, which is a muscular organ that plays a very critical role during digestion. In the upper left region of the abdominal cavity, the stomach is located in a position to digest and break down food through the actions of gastric acid and enzymes. The pyloric sphincter facilitates its connection to other gastrointestinal organs, particularly the small intestine, by managing the release of chyme into the duodenum. This is important for effective absorption and digestion of nutrients after preliminary degradation in the stomach. In addition, the stomach also interacts with the pancreas and liver through the secretion of bile and digestive enzymes, further proving that it is a central organ in the body's digestive system. Coordination of these organs is important to ensure that overall digestion is effective. When food is transported from the stomach to the small intestine, it undergoes complex interactions not only with the surrounding environment but also with other components of the gut. Due to the acidic properties of the stomach, protein digestion is catalytic while also helping to absorb some nutrients, and the subsequent release of chyme into the small intestine is highly regulated by hormonal signals. This process also serves to highlight the significance of the gut-brain axis, through which feedback from the stomach in the form of ghrelin and gastric inhibitory peptide is relayed back to appetite management and digestive readiness. The connection between the stomach and the other organs is also facilitated via the microbiome, with evidence indicating that the development of gut flora can be manipulated by the release of gastric contents and their interaction with intestinal walls. Understanding these interactions is significant in comprehending the complexity implicated in the regulation of digestion and nutrition (Indrio et al., 2022; Keller et al., 2021).

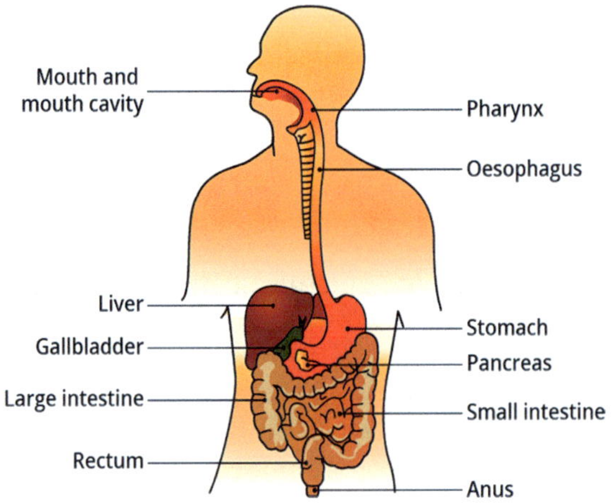

Figure 5.5. Illustration showing some of the main organs that form the digestive system.

Source: https://media.healthdirect.org.au/images/inline/original/digestive-system-2257b1.png

Test Your Knowledge

1. What is the structure of the esophagus?
2. What are the 4 layers of the esophageal wall?

5.2. Function of the Esophagus

Learning Outcome

1. Understand the role of the esophagus in food transportation
2. Know the mechanism of peristalsis
3. Describe the esophageal sphincters and their functions

The esophagus is a significant channel in the digestive system, primarily tasked with transferring food from the mouth to the stomach. The nearly 10-inch-long muscular tube employs a type of synchronous series of muscle contractions known as peristalsis. This is an automatic movement that allows the esophagus to thrust food downwards against the force of gravity. Interestingly, the esophagus also has structural mechanisms, such as a sphincter at its upper and lower ends, which regulate the intake and expulsion of food. The functioning of the esophagus is not only vital for the mechanical movement of food but also to avoid aspiration of the airway. This key pathway's dysfunction can lead to significant complications, such as GERD or dysphagia, and hence underscores its importance in human digestive physiology. The esophagus's anatomy reveals its functional adaptation as a channel and not a site for digestion. Stratified squamous epithelium covering the esophagus makes it resistant to the mechanical abrasion caused by the movement of food. Interestingly, this bodily organization also makes the esophagus susceptible to various stimuli that enable reflex action, such as swallowing. Besides simple transport, recent research has discovered that the esophagus participates in sensing nutrients during early stages. For instance, on the arrival of food in the esophagus, it stimulates the release of salivary enzymes to initiate the process of digestion. These interactions highlight the peripheral status of the esophagus in digestive signaling, linking it in close association with the physiological activities of both stomach and intestines, indicating its position within the broader metabolic scheme of digestion (Wojtunik K-Kulesza et al., 2020). New developments in the field of metabolomics have opened new avenues for the investigation of the multigenerational functions of the esophagus in digestion as well as the absorption of nutrients. This emerging field uses analytical techniques to examine metabolite profiles of diet and digestion. These examinations have revealed the influence of metabolites on organ function and between the elements of the gastrointestinal tract. For example, the hydrolysis and bioavailability of plant diet polyphenols during digestion, initiated in the esophagus, have attracted considerable scholarly attention. These metabolites possess different health-giving properties but require an understanding of the way that they are modified during digestion in order to ascertain their functional activity. The esophagus, therefore, is more than a mere physical channel; it is centrally involved in nutrient bioavailability and gut health. By continued research into these interactions, scientists hope to come to a greater understanding of the synergetic interactions between metabolites, proteins, and genes in human physiology (David S Wishart, 2019).

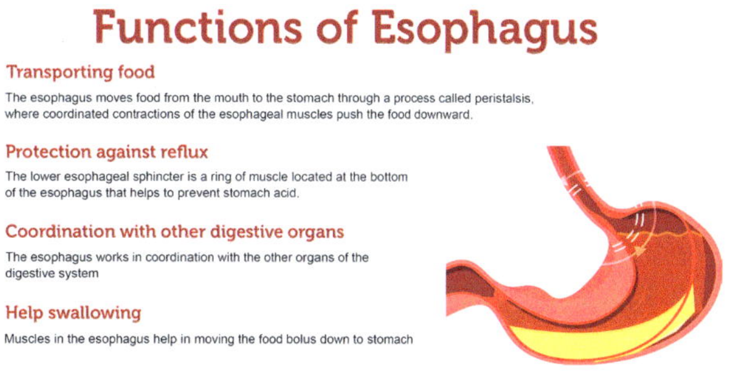

Figure 5.6. Function of the esophagus.

Source: https://assets.lybrate.com/imgs/tic/enadp/functions-of-esophagus.jpg

5.2.1. Role in Food Transportation

The esophagus has a crucial function in the complex process of human digestion, primarily by ensuring the passage of food from the mouth to the stomach. The muscular tube is made such that it keeps food in effective flow through the thoracic region by synchronized muscle contraction, peristalsis. Peristalsis generates waves that push the swallowed food mass downward, as far as possible without backflow and regurgitation. The esophagus has a significant role not only in the mechanical transport of food but also in the timely coordination in the process of digestion. Disturbance or obstruction of the esophagus may lead to many complications, and even its involvement in providing a smooth passage of food through the gastrointestinal tract is vital. Apart from its mechanical role, the esophagus also plays a part in the chemical process of digestion. The esophagus does not directly play any role in chemical digestion, but has a significant role to play in propelling food towards the stomach in preparation for food particle breakdown brought about by gastric juice. The efficiency of transport is governed by a myriad of dietary factors, including the food consumed. For instance, too much processed food can be capable of affecting the gastric motility and, therefore, the overall process of digestion. Research has proven that the type of diet can aggravate the esophageal disorder, therefore impacting the movement of food and leading to non-communicable diseases (NCDs) stemming from poor digestion and metabolism (Clemente VJ-Suárez et al., 2023). This is a crucial point to note when dealing with and preventing it. Food, after being swallowed into the stomach, enters a completely different world, one being hugely acidic and enzyme-filled, for digestion. The muscular walls of the stomach also help grind and mix food so that it is a semi-fluid food called chyme. This is proof of how the stomach and the esophagus depend upon each other in food transportation; the esophagus must be able to deliver food at the appropriate rate so that the stomach can perform its functions. Additionally, patterns and tendencies of consumption of nutrition can create a lasting effect on how efficient this system of transportation works, affecting metabolic well-being and disease susceptibility (Budrevi Ačiūtė et al., 2020). Therefore, an understanding of the intricate mechanisms of the esophagus and stomach not only provides greater insight into how human digestion occurs but also underscores the need for making the appropriate dietary choices to ensure optimal digestive health.

5.2.2. Mechanism of Peristalsis

Peristalsis, which is now recognized as a significant function to establish gastrointestinal motility, is a rhythmic relaxation and contraction of the smooth muscle layers of the stomach and the esophagus. With the coordinated effort of smooth muscles, one moves food along the digestive tract with effective transport and digestion of ingested material. Peristalsis is initiated through voluntary swallowing, which initiates a wave of involuntary muscle contractions of the esophageal muscle. These peristalses are under the control of the enteric nervous system, a sophisticated network of neurons in the wall of the gastrointestinal tract. In this way, peristalsis not only allows the passage of food along but also helps to break up and mix food particles, assisting effective digestion. One should understand the complexity of this mechanism, particularly in the case of most of the gastrointestinal illnesses disrupting the normal flow patterns of motility. Peristalsis mechanisms rely on the coordination among different types of muscle contractions in the gastrointestinal tract. In the case of the esophagus, circular muscles contract at the rear of the bolus of food, and longitudinal muscles relax at the front, creating a push force that moves the bolus into the stomach. In the case of the area of the stomach, churning movements assist peristalsis and help to further digest and mix food with stomach juices. This coordinated movement of muscle contractions is regulated by neural input and hormonal factors that modulate motility in relation to physiological needs. Interruptions of this intricate system give rise to various motility disorders, such as achalasia and gastroparesis, that can affect nutrient uptake and GI health substantially, emphasizing the role played by peristalsis in maintaining homeostasis in the GI tract. It has recently been established that gut microbiota, a complex microbial association of the gastrointestinal tract that is diverse, is also a permissive determinant for peristaltic function.

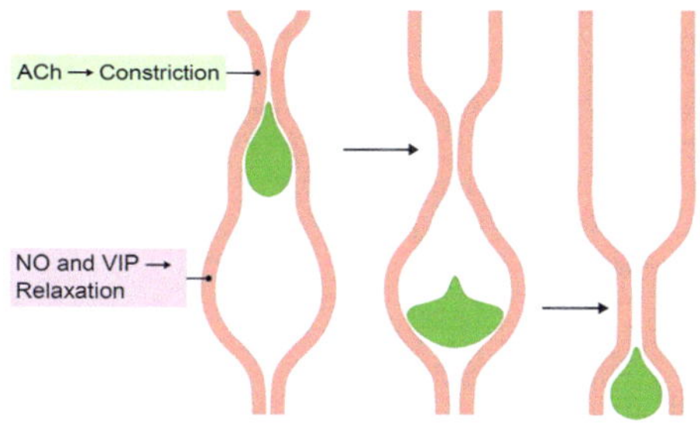

Figure 5.7. Mechanism of peristalsis.

Source: https://cdn-ildfibj.nitrocdn.com/qaWeLntkRcyxNUcEoWbLpZLQkcgLFsiJ/assets/images/optimized/www.biologyonline.com/wp-content/uploads/2019/10/Mechanism-of-peristalsis.png

Host physiology interaction with gut flora and the microbiota, being accountable for nutrient metabolism and local immunity, is challenging to explain. Microbial imbalance can influence the gut flora community and lead to gastrointestinal disorders, which in turn can influence peristaltic movement. For instance, dysbiosis or alteration of microbial composition worsens irritable bowel syndrome and leads to variable motility of the intestine. Moreover, the influence of diet and antibiotics on gut microbiota demonstrates the delicate balance that ensures maximum digestive efficiency and peristalsis. By using research, scientists attempt to explain these connections, noting the necessity of an equilibrium intestinal microbiome for normal peristalsis and overall gut well-being (John B Miller et al., 2017; Jandhyala, 2015).

5.2.3. Esophageal Sphincters and Their Functions

The esophagus, a muscle tube connecting the throat to the stomach, is equipped with two essential structures referred to as esophageal sphincters: the UES and the lower esophageal sphincter (LES). The UES is located at the junction level of the pharynx and the esophagus and serves to prevent air from entering the esophagus during breathing and to prevent backflow of contents from the esophagus into the throat. Functionally, the UES closes in response to swallowing, permitting food passage while simultaneously sealing off the respiratory tract. This two-way function is meant to help keep the airway intact, highlighting the importance of the sphincter in organizing complex physiological processes during digestion and respiration. The lower esophageal sphincter is an important barrier between the esophagus and the stomach. Positioned at the gastroesophageal junction, the LES prevents reflux of gastric content and thus protects the esophagus from the acidic environment of the stomach. Under usual conditions, the LES maintains a high resting tone, which is crucial to preventing GERD. Abnormalities of this sphincter may lead to reflux of stomach acid that induces inflammation and even damage to the lining of the esophagus. Therefore, LES integrity is important for gastrointestinal comfort and health because its failure would result in morbid complications of heartburn or esophagitis. The functioning of the UES and LES is influenced by several factors, including diet, body position, and physiological status, that interact to control their overall functioning. The operation of such sphincters can also be enhanced by some gastroretentive drug delivery systems (GRDDS), which have been explored as an approach for maximizing the therapeutic effect of drugs that need a stable gastric environment (Tripathi et al., 2019). Knowledge of the functional dynamics of such esophageal sphincters is not only significant for understanding digestion, but also for detecting pathological conditions resulting from their malfunction. Furthermore, ongoing studies on these structures continue to reveal a complex ecosystem that is shaped by environmental and dietary forces, echoing results in larger gastrointestinal contexts (Ethan T Hillman et al., 2017).

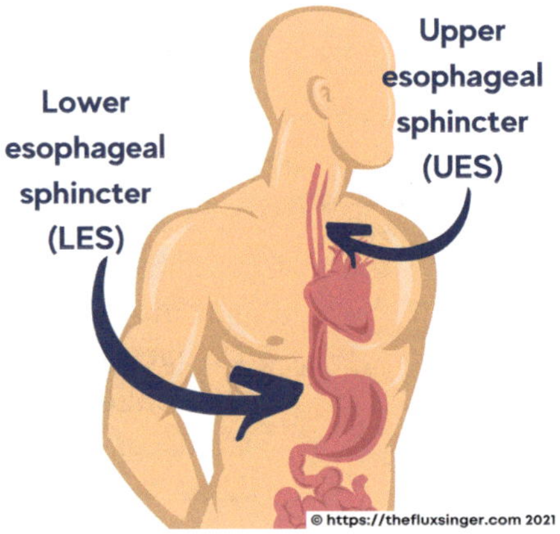

Figure 5.8. Upper and Lower Esophageal Sphincters.

Source: https://i0.wp.com/thefluxsinger.com/wp-content/uploads/2021/10/10-w-copyright.png?resize=768%2C768&ssl=1

Test Your Knowledge

1. What is the mechanism of action of peristalsis?
2. What are the functions of the esophageal sphincter?

5.3. Anatomy of the Stomach

Learning Outcome

1. Know the structure and regions of the stomach
2. Describe the layers of the stomach wall
3. Know the connection between the esophagus, stomach, and small intestine for the digestive process in humans

The stomach is a crucial organ in the human digestive system and performs several key functions that support the overall digestive process. The stomach is anatomically segmented into four major areas, namely the cardia, fundus, body, and pylorus. Each of these areas has a distinct function in food processing. The cardia, nearest to the esophagus, provides a passageway for food into the stomach, and the fundus is used as a holding compartment. The body of the stomach churns and grinds ingested food and slowly moves it toward the pylorus, where the ingested food, now called chyme, is further acted upon and released into the small intestine. Thus, understanding the gross anatomical structures of the stomach presents aspects of its complex functions within the human gastrointestinal system. Anatomy of the stomach, as homologous in most human groups, could, however, differ based on genetics and physiology. For example, as it appears in research evidence of non-human mammals, e.g., white-breasted rats, there exist certain structural characteristics whose importance lies in comparison with the anatomy of human beings. The rat stomach has common sections with other vertebrates that exhibit a sac-like configuration with digestive implications. In human beings, the sac-like character of the stomach provides for storage capacity for large quantities of food and enzymatic digestion over a period of time with the assistance of special cells that secrete digestive enzymes and gastric acids. Identifying these differences helps to put into focus the evolutionary developments that the human stomach has undergone in order to allow it to be adequately flexible to a range of diets. Moreover, the relationship between the stomach and the surrounding organs is a significant factor in the digestive system anatomy. As an organ located close to the liver, the stomach benefits from the liver's ability to produce bile, which is crucial for fat emulsification in the process of digestion. The anatomical location of the stomach, with its greater and lesser curvatures, is critical not only in mechanical digestion but also in the correct absorption of nutrients in the subsequent digestive tract. The intricate anatomical location suggests the coordination that is required between the organs of the digestive system. Comparing the anatomy of the human stomach to comparative analyses of other organisms, such as rats, can yield vast information regarding its functionality and evolutionary importance (ST, 2023; Complementary and Medicine, 2023).

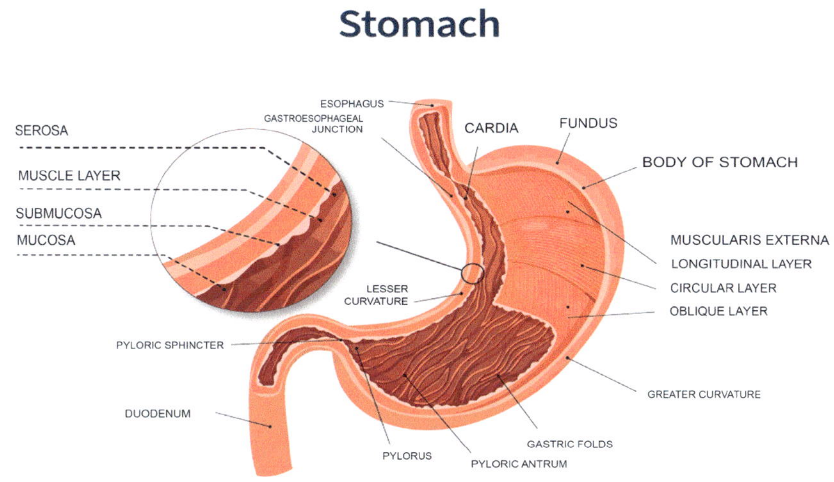

Figure 5.9. Diagram of Stomach.

Source: https://media.geeksforgeeks.org/wp-content/uploads/20240326172454/Layers-of-Stomach.png

5.3.1. Structure and Regions of the Stomach

The stomach is a muscular organ that is primarily part of the digestive system, with its principal role being to mechanically and chemically digest food. Anatomically, the stomach consists of four largest regions known as the cardia, fundus, body, and pylorus. Cardia is the region of the stomach where the esophagus discharges its contents into the stomach and plays a part in admitting the bolus of food. Outside of the cardia is the fundus, a holding compartment in which food swallowed can accumulate and become preliminarily digested. The fundus is particularly important when speaking about secretions that are gastric because there are specialized cells that secrete digestive acids and enzymes that participate in the digestion of swallowed materials. Knowledge of the stomach's structure is fundamental to knowledge of its role in disease processes, specifically gastric ulcers and cancers, which remain significant health concerns globally, with 4.9% of 2022 new cancer diagnoses being stomach cancer (Bray et al., 2024). The corpus, which is the largest part of the stomach, continues the digestion that has already begun within the cardia and fundus. This central portion is innervated by numerous gastric glands that secrete hydrochloric acid and digestive enzymes, such as pepsin, involved in protein digestion. Its secretion is regulated via neural and hormonal mechanisms, with the vagus nerve playing a primary role. As a component of the parasympathetic nervous system, the vagus nerve links the stomach to the central nervous system and communicates information about states of the stomach at the same time that it causes gastric secretion and motility (Breit et al., 2018). Coordination between the muscular contractions of the stomach and the nervous system makes food mixing and propulsion highly effective, a classic demonstration of how structural features come to enable greater functional performance. The final region, the pylorus, is a junction between the stomach and the small intestine. It is subdivided into the pyloric antrum and the pyloric canal, the latter of which drains into the duodenum. The pylorus has a muscular sphincter that regulates the entry of the partly digested food mixture, the chyme, into the small intestine. This control system is necessary to ensure that the process of digestion is properly timed so that complete disintegration and absorption of nutrients can take place. Structure and function of the pylorus are also involved when considering gastrointestinal diseases, especially where pyloric stenosis may cause major complications. Effective digestion relies on the symbiotic activities of all parts of the stomach; therefore, understanding their structure and interrelationships in the broader scheme of human digestion is important (Bray et al., 2024).

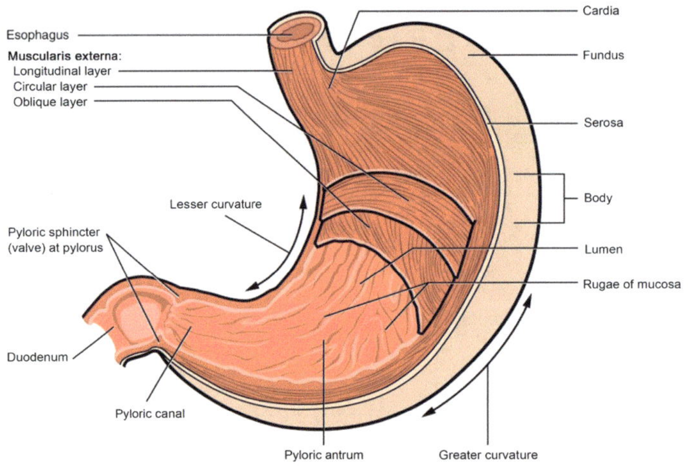

Figure 5.10. The stomach has four major regions: the cardia, fundus, body, and pylorus. The addition of an inner oblique smooth muscle layer gives the muscularis the ability to vigorously churn and mix food.

Source: https://s3-us-west-2.amazonaws.com/courses-images-archive-read-only/wp-content/uploads/sites/403/2015/04/21031722/2414_Stomach.jpg

5.3.2. Layers of the Stomach Wall

The wall of the stomach comprises four distinct layers that contribute to its multifaceted nature. From the inner layer towards the outside, the mucosa is primarily the barrier and secreting layer. The function is to secrete gastric juice that contains hydrochloric acid as well as digestive enzymes accountable for the breakdown of food. The mucosa is lined with specialized epithelial cells that have gastric pits open to gastric glands as part of the secretion of compounds needed. The meticulous organization of structures in the mucosa not only inhibits efficient digestion but also protects against infection and mechanical damage, facilitating a favorable condition for food processing. Ringing the mucosa is the layer of submucosa, which contains connective tissue that protects blood vessels, nerves, and lymphatics to enable the exchange of nutrients and messages throughout the stomach. The layer plays a crucial role in maintaining the stomach's structural integrity while providing it with the means that enable it to be an effective digestive organ. The submucosa also allows the functioning of the mucosa by delivering oxygen and nutrients to sustain cell repair and regeneration for the maintenance of stomach lining health. Through this layer mechanism, the submucosa offers a firm bonding between the stomach's internal functions and its external governing mechanisms, emphasizing its role in the entire gastrointestinal tract. The muscularis layer, made up of smooth muscle tissue, permits churning and mixing of stomach contents, an action essential for effective digestion. The layer is formed of a three-sub-layer structure: the inner oblique, middle circular, and outer longitudinal muscles. The arrangement provides complex movement, such as peristalsis and segmentation, which propel food into the small intestine. Additionally, the muscularis regulates gastric motility and the release of gastric contents. The most external covering, the serosa, is a structural support for the stomach, binds the stomach to nearby organs, and protects the stomach from damage. This stomach wall, with its intricate structure, thus triggers the significant interaction of the layers to maximize digestion and protective roles within the gastrointestinal tract (Homayun et al., 2019; Jain et al., 2018).

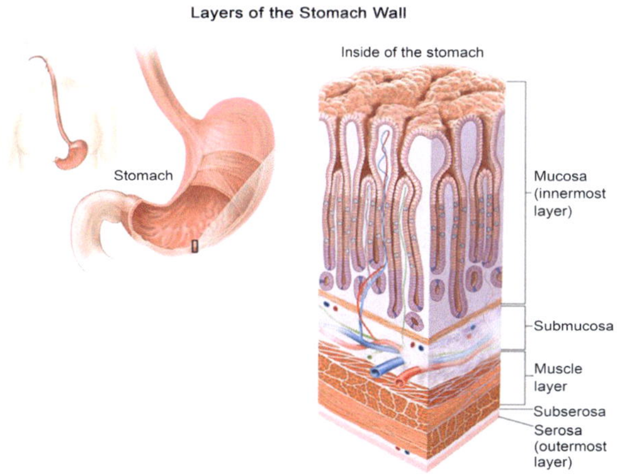

Figure 5.11. Layers of the stomach wall.

Source: https://visualsonline.cancer.gov/retrieve.cfm?imageid=12051&dpi=72&fileformat=jpg&disposition=attachment

5.3.3. Connection to the Small Intestine

The connection between the esophagus, stomach, and small intestine is central to the human digestive process. The esophagus serves as a conduit through which food passes from the oral cavity to the stomach, where initial enzymatic digestion begins. This is carried out by churning food within gastric juices, which enable the process of transformation into a semi-liquid chyme. When the chyme is in the small intestine, it is where most of the absorption of nutrients occurs, which emphasizes coordination between these digestive organs. These interactions are critical not just for physical food movement but also for digestive enzyme regulation and hormones, which direct the timing and release of digestive secretions. Therefore, the comprehension of how these organs relate becomes a critical element in explaining the intricate mechanisms that provide overall digestive efficacy and health. In the small intestine, some signaling pathways, such as the Neuregulin 1 (NRG1) and its corresponding ErbB receptors, play a pivotal role in the growth and functioning of the enteric nervous system (ENS) that regulates intestinal functions. These systems are critical to make sure that the small intestine is able to digest the chyme from the stomach effectively, allowing precise regulation of intestinal secretion and motility. NRG1 signaling dysregulation may cause a wide range of gastrointestinal disorders, which is why it is important in maintaining gut health. (Gonkowski, 2024) describes where NRG1 and ErbB receptors exist throughout the gastrointestinal tract, including important sites in the esophagus and stomach, thereby emphasizing the presence of an integrated network of regulatory activities extending into the small intestine. The link emphasizes the importance of the ENS in coordinating the functioning of these digestive segments. Moreover, the cultural and philosophical dimension of ingestion and digestion present in ancient literature can also have relevance to our contemporary perception of the esophagus, stomach, and small intestine. For instance, the symbolism present in the Palestinian Midrash Leviticus Rabbah with regards to sacrifice and ingestion offers a larger introspection concerning the act of eating as bestial action against the sacrificial offering for a higher purpose. (Albeck et al., 2014) creates a dichotomy where consumption can symbolize lower-order desires and sacrifice higher-order moral and spiritual ends. Such rich cultural understanding is reflective of the physiological functions of these organs, which not only digest food but also become symbols of the intricacy of life's issues and ethical dimensions of sustenance. This ongoing interplay of physiological process and cultural narrative illustrates how the human body and its functioning are typically represented in broader cultural debates concerning consumption, ethics, and spirituality.

Test Your Knowledge

1. Name the 4 layers of the stomach wall.
2. What is the connection between the stomach and the small intestine?

5.4. Function of the Stomach

Learning Outcome

1. Understand the role of esophagus in food storage
2. Describe the role of digestive processes in the stomach
3. Know the production of gastric juices

The stomach is a digestive organ that is crucial primarily because of its ability to digest and store food prior to being transferred to the intestines. The stomach is an organ that is muscular in constitution and aids in mechanical and chemical digestion of food. The walls of the stomach are lined with gastric mucosa, which secretes gastric juices containing hydrochloric acid and enzymes such as pepsin, which aid in protein digestion. The acidic environment assists not only in the digestion of food material but also assists in carrying out the function of a defense mechanism against pathogenic microbes. As it breaks down its contents, the stomach breaks up food eaten into a semi-fluid state, chyme, and then drains it into the small intestine in a managed process. The process repeats the function of the stomach as an essential go-between between the esophagus and more distal areas of the gastrointestinal tract. Aside from the digestion function, the stomach has a pivotal position in the regulation of the pace at which food is moved to the intestines, a function that is essential to optimum nutrient absorption. The pyloric sphincter, which is where the stomach joins with the small intestine, controls the flow of chyme to make it egress gradually and in manageable amounts. It ensures that nutrients, vitamins, and minerals are properly absorbed by the small intestine and, consequently, provides the body with proper nutrition. Furthermore, the ability of the stomach to recognize the chemical composition of content regulates some of the gastrointestinal hormones that synchronize digestive processes. This stomach role as a connection to the hormones highlights not only its status as a digestive organ, but also as a necessary controller of overall metabolic regulation of the gastrointestinal tract.

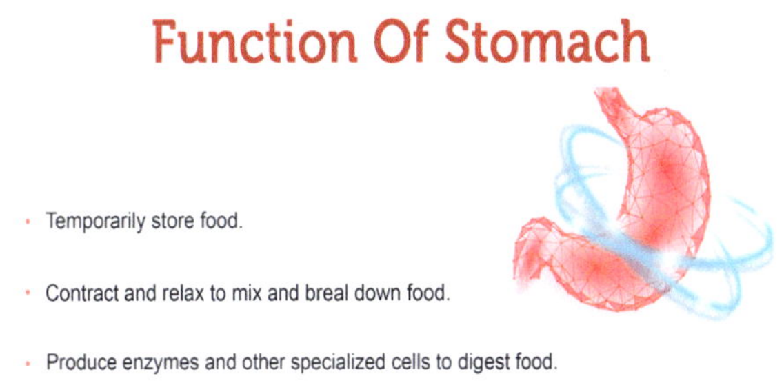

Figure 5.12. Function of the Stomach.

Source: https://assets.lybrate.com/imgs/tic/enadp/function-of-stomach.jpg

Stomach pathological conditions will probably affect overall health more radically, highlighting the significance of the organ during digestion. Diseases such as ulcers, gastritis, and gastric cancer can impair its effectiveness, leading to a series of digestive problems and nutrient deficiencies. New evidence suggests a promising correlation between stomach cancers and molecular processes, whereby tetraspanin takes part in cancer formation in the gastrointestinal system. Elevated expression of certain tetraspanins has been linked with gastric cancer invasion and migration, with implications for treatment strategies and patient prognosis (Shao et al., 2024). Further, technological advancements in surgical technique, e.g., the development of LED retractors allowing enhanced lighting during surgery within the stomach and esophagus, reflect the importance of maintaining function in these critical organs (Kolesnikov et al., 2024). Therefore, proper comprehension of the stomach's functions is essential not just for health maintenance but also for the development of therapeutic approaches for gastrointestinal pathology.

5.4.1. Role in Food Storage

The human esophagus is a significant component of the initial stages of digestion, serving not only as a pipeline for food but also as an element of food storage. The food, having been swallowed, is transported down the esophagus by peristaltic movements to reach the stomach. The muscular tube, primarily a transport conduit, provides space for food for short durations, which could be considered as temporary storage. This generates effectiveness by preventing undue stress on the stomach so that it can receive and digest food within a managed state. The mucous-studded lining of the esophagus facilitates this process through lubrication, further increasing the smoothness of food movement and storage until it reaches the stomach, where proper digestion begins and the biochemistry of nutrient absorption is triggered (Mohammed S Alqahtani et al., 2021). The food, upon reaching the stomach, undergoes radical modification facilitated by gastric secretions and mechanical action. The stomach serves as a principal storage site, retaining food and maintaining it in a moist state so that it can become commingled with gastric juices, necessary for food digestion. The food capacity of the stomach differs, but is typically up to one liter, with the most favorable setting where enzymatic breakdown can be initiated. The stomach's rhythmic contractions, together with the release of enzymes and acids regulate this storage phase, dictating the rate at which chyme ends up in the small intestine. As a key process, this storage function maximizes the absorption of nutrients through ensuring the food is optimally processed before it is subjected to further digestion and absorption in the gastrointestinal tract (Mohammed S Alqahtani et al., 2021). Moreover, the digestive process itself, as defined by the stomach's storage ability, has repercussions that go beyond mere nutrient acquisition; it also impinges on the overall metabolic status. Smooth storage and controlled release of nutrients play a significant role in the modulation of hunger stimuli and satiety, which are neural-mediated mechanisms related to the vagus nerve. This interaction puts forward the way the stomach contributes to body function as well as psychological health in relation to hunger and satiety (Breit et al., 2018). A healthy stomach, therefore, not only aids in digestion but also helps with homeostasis in the body, which points to its importance in digestive wellness as well as physiological equilibrium. This dynamism illustrates the interactive nature between storage, digestion, and nutrient absorption in human physiology.

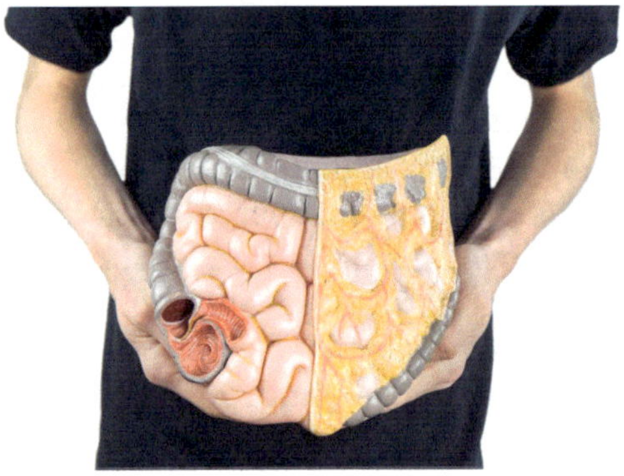

Figure 5.13. On average, food takes 6 to 8 hours to pass from the stomach and small intestine to the large intestine. From there, it may take over a day to digest further.

Source: https://cdn-prod.medicalnewstoday.com/content/images/articles/319/319583/model-of-human-digestive-system-being-held-up-over-where-it-is-in-the-body-by-man-in-black-shirt.jpg

5.4.2. Digestive Processes in the Stomach

The stomach plays a critical role during the process of digestion, primarily by mechanical and chemical breakdown of food. Once the food has been delivered from the esophagus into the stomach, churning movements occur. Contractions are helpful in blending the food with gastric juice, which contains hydrochloric acid and enzymes like pepsin. The acidic environment not only helps in the breakdown of protein structures but also activates pepsinogen to pepsin, which is a functional enzyme needed for protein digestion. The mechanical process, along with the chemical degradation, makes the food into a liquid-or semi-liquid known as chyme. The acidic environment of the stomach also protects the body from pathogens because it serves as a barrier against noxious microbes that are consumed with food. Also, the role of the stomach does not end at mere digestion; it is also involved in the regulation of the digestive process through hormonal signaling. Gastrin is one such critical hormone secreted upon food intake and functions to stimulate gastric acid secretion. This helps maintain the stomach environment in its best form for digestion. Secretion of gastric juice is not merely a response to food intake; it can also be provoked by sensory stimuli such as vision, smell, and taste, which prepare the stomach to receive food in the queue. Such an organized response says a lot about the stomach's pivotal role in the digestive apparatus, linking it with neural and hormonal pathways directly, and thus plays an important part in maintaining homeostasis within the digestive tract. Moreover, the composition of gut microbiota is also vital in gastrointestinal health, as it specifies metabolic processes and overall health. The study has revealed that certain bacteria in the stomach, particularly those with the ability to perform nitrate reductase, play a role in various physiological processes, including the reduction of nitrates from the diet into bioactive compounds like nitric oxide (NO). This substance has been utilized for its vasodilating action and potential in enhancing gut health and function. Additionally, the existence of these microbes will also help modulate the acidity of the stomach and hence affect digestion. An understanding of the complex interactions between these bacteria and host processes can create new therapeutic approaches to digestive disease, underscoring the need for a well-balanced microbiota for optimal digestive function (Song et al., 2023; Liu et al., 2023).

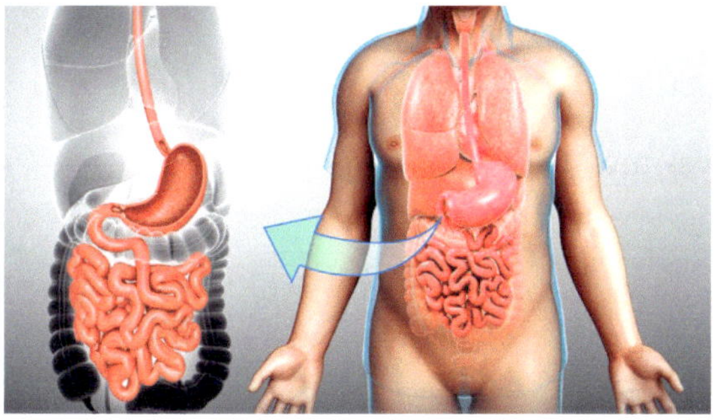

Figure 5.14. The Stomach's Role in Digestion.

Source: https://renewbariatrics.com/wp-content/uploads/2017/09/Stomach-Digestion.png

5.4.3. Production of Gastric Juices

Production of gastric juices is an important aspect of the digestion process that begins once food is inside the stomach. Gastric juice, primarily composed of hydrochloric acid, pepsinogen, intrinsic factor, and mucous, plays an essential role in the digestion of food material and the process of nutrient absorption. Gastric epithelium secretes this mixture, essential to ensure an acidic pH for the activation of digestive enzymes. When it arrives at the stomach, the physiological processes trigger the release of gastric juices to cue digestive action. The coordination of the neural and hormonal system is present in precipitating this response, highlighting the complexity of gastric function. Proper pH level is also crucial, as this helps guard against pathogens, thereby enhancing the intrinsic function of gastric juices as digestive agents as well as immune protectants. Pepsinogen, the enzyme precursor, is one of the most significant gastric juice components. Pepsinogen is converted to its active form, pepsin, when it mixes with the acidic environment created by hydrochloric acid. Pepsin plays a key role in protein digestion. This enzyme activation characterizes the astounding flexibility of the stomach system to enable protein degradation from the diet, a process that breaks down large proteins into smaller peptides, which are broken down further in the intestine. Further, regulation of pepsinogen secretion is regulated by factors such as gastric pH and food presence, exhibiting the fine equilibrium in the stomach's environment. Understanding these mechanisms not only allows for the appreciation of the stomach's vital role in digestion but also contributes to knowledge regarding gastrointestinal health and the significance of imbalances that may lead to disorders of gastric secretion. The intrinsic factor, which is another vital component of gastric juice, plays a role in the absorption of nutrients, specifically the absorption of vitamin B12. This glycoprotein is secreted by gastric lining specialized cells and makes intestinal absorption of vitamin B12, essential in red blood cell development and nerve function, possible. A deficiency in intrinsic factor may lead to fatal anemia and neurological illness, showing its role in overall health. Additionally, studies have shown that the interaction between some of these factors, including gastric secretions and microbial environment in the stomach, could have functional effects on the production of intrinsic factor and, consequently, vitamin B12 absorption. With the examination of such aspects, one is able to appreciate how the intricate mechanism behind gastric juice production not only facilitates digestion but also reflects the interconnectedness of the digestive and overall physiological processes in human beings.

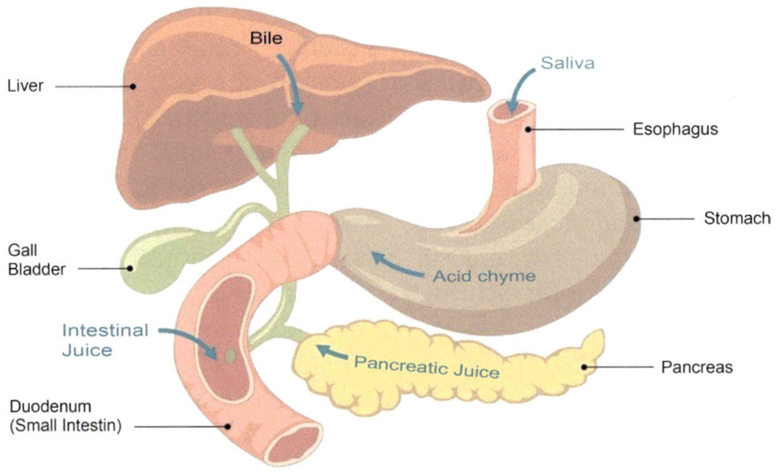

Figure 5.15. Organs Involved in Digestive Juice Production.

Source: https://old-ib.bioninja.com.au/_Media/digestive-juice-organs_med.jpeg

Test Your Knowledge

1. What digestive processes occur in the stomach?
2. What is the role of esophagus in food storage?

5.5. Common Disorders of the Esophagus

Learning Outcome

1. Describe the gastroesophageal reflux disease (GERD)
2. Describe the esophageal cancer
3. Know the esophagitis and its causes

Disorders of the esophagus are relatively common and can significantly impact both physical health and well-being. One of the most frequent disorders is GERD, involving retrograde flow of stomach contents into the esophagus, leading to symptoms such as heartburn, regurgitation, and dysphagia. Reflux occurring chronically can cause esophagitis, or painful esophagitis of the esophageal lining, and expose to Barrett's esophagus, a precancerous lesion secondary to chronic exposure to acidic content. GERD is becoming increasingly prevalent all around the globe, and hence, information about its pathophysiology, risk factors, and optimal management to avoid potential complications of the disorder is required. Achalasia is another significant disorder of the esophagus. Achalasia is a debilitating disorder that ruins the normal peristalsis of the esophagus and prevents food from progressing further in the stomach. Patients with achalasia typically present with dysphagia, regurgitation of food that is not digested, and chest pain. This condition results from degeneration of the esophageal nerve cells, creating a hypertonic lower esophageal sphincter. The pathophysiology of achalasia is unknown, but autoimmune and genetic causes have been postulated. Treatment is symptomatic relief and may be via endoscopic treatments such as balloon dilatation or surgery to relax the sphincter. Achalasia requires treatment due to the risk of esophageal dilation and potential malignancy of untreated long-standing conditions. Esophagitis, resulting from a myriad of causes such as infections, drugs, or hypersensitivity reactions, plays a pivotal role in esophageal pathology. Infectious esophagitis occurs frequently in immunocompromised hosts, with Candida, herpes simplex virus, and cytomegalovirus being frequent pathogens. Drug-induced esophagitis is most often the result of ingesting some oral drugs without sufficient water intake, leading to local irritation and mucosal ulceration of the esophagus. In addition, eosinophilic esophagitis, characterized by a characteristic predominant eosinophilic inflammation in the esophagus, has become a significant allergic disorder, particularly among children and adolescents. The fact that it's linked to food allergy underscores the importance of dietary management of the condition. Overall, understanding the disorders and their causative mechanisms is crucial not only for proper control but also for prevention of potential complications due to chronic esophageal disorders (Xu et al., 2020; Rawla and Barsouk, 2019).

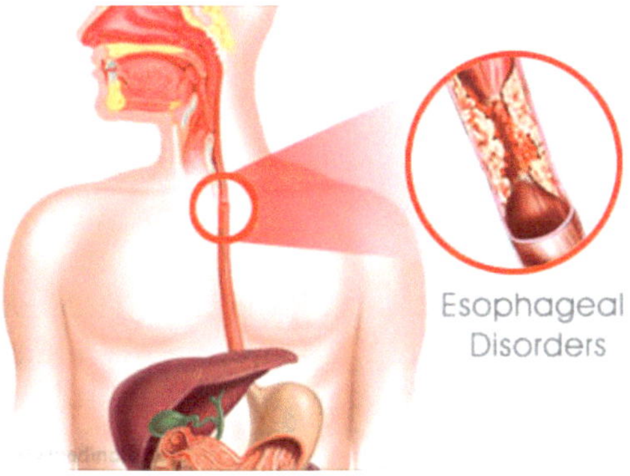

Figure 5.16. Esophageal Disorders.

Source: https://images.medindia.net/patientinfo/950_400/esophageal-disorders.jpg

5.5.1. Gastroesophageal Reflux Disease

Gastroesophageal reflux disease (GERD) is a common and multifactorial disorder that involves the retrogression of contents from the stomach into the esophagus, producing pain and potential complications. The disease is characterized by typical symptoms of heartburn, regurgitation, and dysphagia, which can have a significant effect on the quality of life. It is important to appreciate the pathophysiology behind inducing GERD, which includes lower esophageal sphincter dysfunction, excessive acid production within the stomach, and anatomical abnormalities such as hiatal hernias. All these are significant contributing factors in causing esophageal mucosal injury frequently observed in patients, and therefore treatment becomes a multifactorial process, including symptomatic control as well as treatment of the pathophysiology of the disease. The prevalence of GERD is influenced by a number of risk factors, most notably obesity, which is a rapidly expanding global health condition. Obesity worsens the symptoms of GERD by means such as increased intra-abdominal pressure, which could impair the functioning of the lower esophageal sphincter. Therefore, weight management emerges as a valuable intervention in avoiding GERD symptoms and maximizing patient outcomes. Recent studies have found that the valuable benefits of weight reduction in obese patients with GERD are that even minimal reductions in body mass index can result in meaningful symptom relief. Notably, bariatric surgery has come to be widely accepted as an efficient therapeutic option for this population of patients, with the dual benefits of weight loss and resolution of GERD frequency and severity, particularly with procedures such as Roux-en-Y gastric bypass, with which satisfactory results have been achieved in clinical practice (Khan, 2016). GERD calls for a correct comprehension of the functional interaction of the stomach and esophagus, and sensory functions engaged in such a process. The vagus nerve, central to the autonomic function of the gastrointestinal tract, has been suggested to be involved in esophageal sensation and motility. Advances in neuroanatomy in recent times emphasize the heterogeneity of vagal neurons whose various forms are involved in monitoring different physiological conditions, including those of the gastrointestinal tract (Kupari et al., 2019). Such complexity emphasizes the importance of maintaining both neurological and mechanistic factors while approaching GERD, as the therapeutic landscape continues to evolve. Overall, the integration of an understanding of both the anatomical organs and the newly developed research into the nervous system can lead to better treatment protocols for those suffering from this disabling disease.

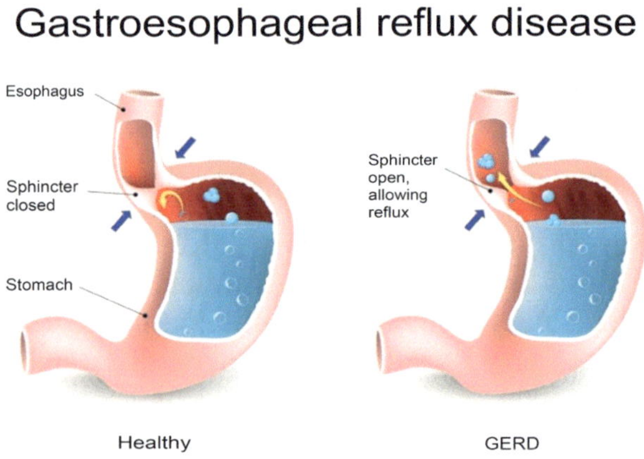

Figure 5.17. Gastroesophageal reflux disease.

Source: https://www.eatright.org/-/media/images/eatright-articles/eatright-article-feature-images/gastroesophagealreflux_600x450.jpg?as=0&w=967&rev=2aebbfc74fa249ae9134e0fc3c28c5cd&hash=26F3F6995B54A7DF301FFE0B14259251

5.5.2. Esophageal Cancer

The esophagus is an important tube of the human digestive system, but it is susceptible to malignant change causing esophageal cancer. The majority of this cancer is in the form of adenocarcinoma and squamous cell carcinoma with varying risk factors and population profiles. Adenocarcinoma is most strongly associated with GERD and Barrett's esophagus, which are complications of chronic irritation and dysplasia of esophageal mucosa. On the other hand, squamous cell carcinoma is more intensely linked with lifestyle factors such as smoking and excessive alcohol consumption. Elucidation of the etiology of cancer of the esophagus is essential to developing preventive strategies. As progress is made towards unravelling the environmental and genetic factors, similarly, it is imperative to implement specially designed interventions that can check the rising incidence of this aggressive neoplasm. Esophageal cancer diagnosis is frequently delayed to a later stage because the early symptoms, while often nonspecific, may involve dysphagia and weight loss. Endoscopic methods play a central role in detecting the disease early and staging it. Endoscopic ultrasound (EUS) and esophagogastroduodenoscopy (EGD) are diagnostic techniques through which visible lesions within the esophagus can be visualized and biopsied. In addition, advances in imaging modalities like computed tomography (CT) and positron emission tomography (PET) are crucial in establishing the disease spread. Prompt treatment significantly improves treatment success; hence, identification of the physiological changes in the esophagus can stimulate the development of screening algorithms. Early detection not only enhances prognosis but also allows for an increased number of therapeutic modalities, including surgical resection, chemotherapy, and radiotherapy. Therapeutic management of esophageal cancer is a function of stage, location, and overall condition of the patient. Surgical resection remains the treatment of choice for local disease and, in a high percentage, provides a good chance for long-term survival. Advanced disease, on the other hand, requires further management with a multimodal regimen such as concurrent chemoradiation therapy to palliate symptoms and improve quality of life. New advances in targeted therapy and immunotherapies are on the horizon with very promising lines of treatment, particularly if traditional modalities fail. Current research gives utmost importance to treatments specific to an individual patient's own special biological characteristics of the tumor in addition to individual preference. Moreover, the inclusion of new drug delivery systems, as discussed in existing literature, may yield more effective efficacy for therapeutic drugs, particularly for patients in need of treatments with high side effects or low therapeutic ratios (Hua et al., 2023). What is learned from existing research may reshape the extent of esophageal cancer treatment.

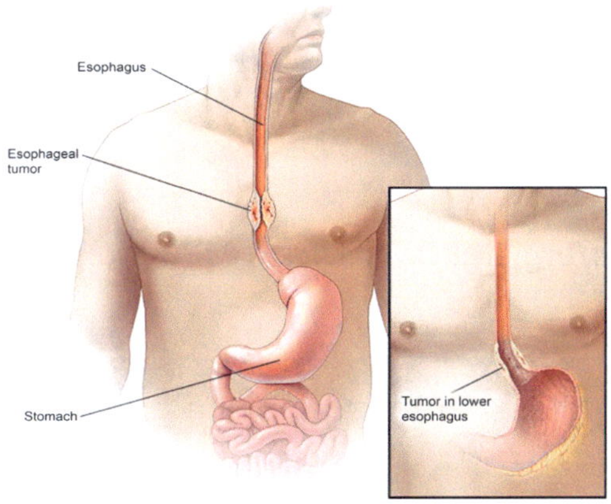

Figure 5.18. Esophageal Cancer.

Source: https://www.mayoclinic.org/-/media/kcms/gbs/patient-consumer/images/2013/08/26/10/06/ds00500_hq00312_im03991_c7_esophagealcancerthu_jpg.jpg

5.5.3. Esophagitis and Its Causes

Esophagitis, or inflammation of the esophagus, occurs with symptoms of throat pain on swallowing, chest pain, and midepigastric pain. There is more than one etiological cause behind the formation of the condition. The most frequent cause is GERD, in which acidic content from the stomach refluxes into the esophagus and causes irritation. Repeated exposure to acid in the stomach induces inflammation and, if not treated, may lead to severe damage, such as strictures and esophageal ulcers. Infection by fungi like Candida or viruses like herpes simplex may also induce esophagitis, especially in immunocompromised patients. Also, certain medications have the tendency to further complicate the disease by inflaming the lining of the esophagus when there is a lack of adequate water or when taken in high amounts, which attests to the complexity of esophagitis because it occurs in different patients (Shields and Lightdale, 2018). Also, eosinophilic esophagitis has been a leading cause of esophagitis, particularly in children. The disease is characterized by a pathological deposition of eosinophils, a type of white blood cell, in the esophagus in response to food allergy or response to environmental allergens. The presentation includes dysphagia, food impaction, and chronic vomiting in the patients. In the majority of the cases of eosinophilic esophagitis, there is comorbidity with other atopic diseases such as asthma or allergic rhinitis, setting up an indistinguishable immunologic characteristic of the disease. Diagnosis is commonly made by endoscopy and biopsy, and eosinophilia can be identified in tissue samples. It subsequently suggests that there is a necessity to diagnose eosinophilic esophagitis as not only an esophageal problem but as part of an allergic reaction involving the whole system in such patients, which requires special care that may involve changes in diet and medication to reduce inflammation (Scarpignato et al., 2016). Apart from the aforementioned causes, lifestyle is also the prime cause of esophagitis. Smoking and alcohol consumption have been found to induce inflammation of the lining of the esophagus, hence inducing susceptibility to reflux. Weight control and modification of diet can be vital in preventing and managing esophagitis. For instance, patients with GERD are usually advised against such symptom-provoking foods as spicy foods, caffeine, and carbonated beverages. Inappropriate long-term proton pump inhibitor (PPI) use is also dangerous. While the drug effectively cures acid sickness, it may be accompanied by side effects such as malabsorption of nutrients and gut dysbiosis. Hence, identification of the quantity of causes and way of life determinants of esophagitis is significant in management and prevention procedures in the framework of esophageal health (Shields and Lightdale, 2018).

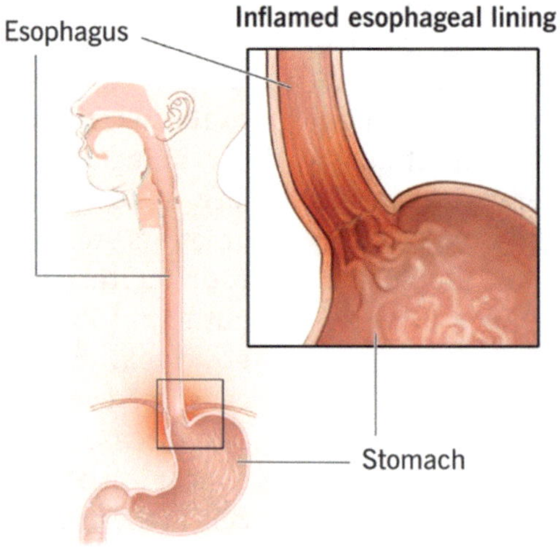

Figure 5.19. Esophagitis.

Source: https://my.clevelandclinic.org/-/scassets/images/org/health/articles/10138-esophagitis

Test Your Knowledge

1. What is esophageal cancer?
2. What are the main causes of esophagitis?

5.6. Common Disorders of the Stomach

Learning Outcome

1. Describe the pathophysiology of peptic ulcers
2. Understand the gastritis
3. Describe the stomach cancer

Disorders of the stomach are not uncommon and can consist of several gastrointestinal conditions that profoundly impact the quality of a person's life. The most common disorder is the GERD, where the stomach acid prefers to reflux into the esophagus on a regular basis, resulting in heartburn and regurgitation. It is due to the failure of the functioning of the lower esophageal sphincter, which should otherwise close to prevent backflow. As per studies, GERD has been found to be controlled by lifestyle changes and medication that decreases gastric acidity. For instance, omeprazole proton pump inhibitor therapy was found to raise gastric pH significantly and therefore relieve symptoms.

Nonetheless, the complexity of GERD demands a more in-depth understanding regarding physiological pathways as well as complications like esophagitis or Barrett's esophagus that can lead to more severe gastrointestinal diseases (Belafsky et al., 2017). Another common ailment is gastritis, inflammation of the gastric mucosa, generally secondary to causes such as bacterial infection, chronic alcohol consumption, or prolonged use of nonsteroidal anti-inflammatory drugs (NSAIDs). Gastritis can be acute or chronic in nature with varying severity. Clinical presentation of gastritis can be abdominal pain, nausea, and indigestion. The interesting association is that chronic gastritis is associated with a risk of gastric ulcer or gastric carcinoma. Treatment of gastritis is the removal of the cause, e.g., certain antibiotic therapy for *Helicobacter pylori* infection. Notably, the fine dynamic interactions of gastric physiology and inflammation can be enhanced. therapeutic approaches. In recent gastrointestinal disease reviews, the presence of growth factors in the NRG1/ErbB signaling pathway also suggests complex dynamics in regulatory processes in the stomach (Gonkowski, 2024). Peptic ulcers is yet another threatening gastric mucosa disease because of an imbalance between gastric acid and mucosal protection synthesis. They can happen in the stomach (gastric ulcers) or duodenum (duodenal ulcers). Symptoms of peptic ulcers are typically associated with gnawing abdominal pain, bloating, and potential complications such as bleeding. Treatment strategies can involve proton pump inhibitors to decrease acid production and facilitate healing, and antibiotics in those etiologies with *H. pylori*. The etiology of peptic ulcers in the majority can be traced back to chronic NSAID use or chronic alcohol use. Both of these must be discovered for prevention and treatment to be effective. Moreover, breakthroughs in more recent research of the molecular events attached to gastric health continue to uncover more information about the peptic ulcer mechanism and treatment, so that integrative modalities are required in relieving such common gastrointestinal ailments (Belafsky et al., 2017).

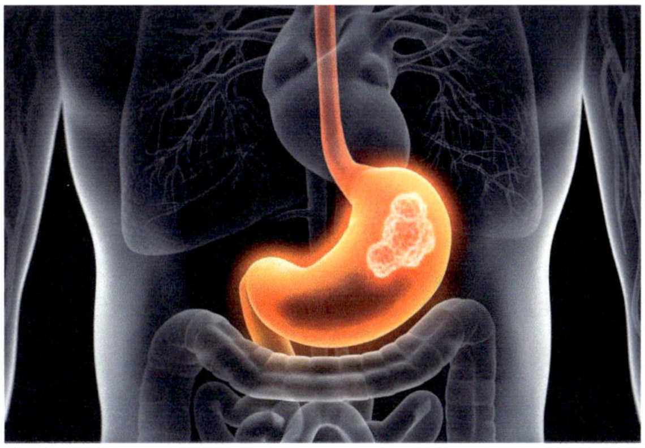

Source: https://www.gastropune.com/wp-content/uploads/2022/08/Stomach-Problem.jpg

5.6.1. Peptic Ulcers

The pathophysiology of peptic ulcers is one of the most important areas of study in the human esophagus and stomach research, connecting multiple pathological conditions to gastric and duodenal health. Peptic ulcers are observed when there is an imbalance between the injurious factors, i.e., gastric acid and pepsin, and the protective elements ensuring the security of the gastric mucosa. This imbalance may be added to by several such reasons, like *H. pylori* infection, nonsteroidal anti-inflammatory drugs (NSAIDs), and daily habits like smoking and alcohol consumption. These ulcers may present themselves in an immense range of symptoms from inharmonious discomfort to agonizing pain, which may severely restrict the life of an individual. It is of essential importance to study the etiologic pathways and pathogenic mechanisms of peptic ulcers in order to create effective prevention and treatment methods in clinical practice on the basis of the world's gastric health. The recent years saw a recognition of *H. pylori* as a causative agent of peptic ulcers that transformed the disease's treatment, leading to diagnosis and management. This pathogen causes inflammation and injury in the gastric epithelium by releasing virulence factors upon infecting it. As has been debated in recent literature, with the high prevalence of *H. pylori* infection, some eradication therapy is needed, and it is a combination of antibiotics and PPIs. The evolving understanding of the disease role of this pathogen strengthens the interface between microbiology and gastrointestinal pathophysiology, demonstrating how advances in research can lead to better therapeutic regimens.

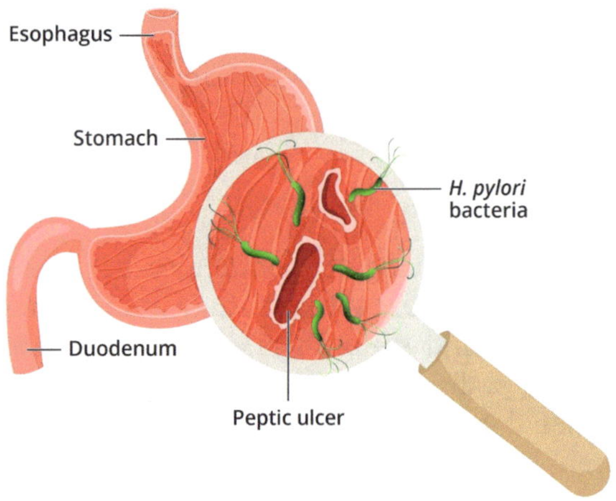

Figure 5.20. People are more likely to develop peptic ulcers if they are infected with *H. pylori* bacteria.

Source: https://www.niddk.nih.gov/-/media/Images/Health-Information/Digestive-Diseases/Peptic-Ulcers-English-FINAL_7-18-23_1200x1040.jpg

In addition, ongoing research into the interface between psychosomatic factors and peptic ulcers demonstrates the relevance of an integrative model of care for the disease, such as the notion that available treatments are capable of curing symptoms while eradicating psychological causatives. Subsequent studies have further investigated more general gastrointestinal implications of peptic ulcers, linking them to such sequelae as gastric cancer and hemorrhage. Of particular note, untreated chronic ulcers can lead to severe morbidity from potential perforation and bleeding that may be life-threatening. Therefore, mathematical and computational modeling of the stomach is an extremely promising area of research that offers an understanding of the biomechanical responses of the stomach under conditions apt to predispose them to ulcer generation. Such models contribute to an improved understanding of gastric physiology by enabling researchers to predict and simulate results of interest in relation to ulcer generation and development. They also point out the commonality of gastric anatomy, physiology, and pathology that validates the necessity of continuous peptic ulcer disease research as an essential field of gastrointestinal health that opens up possibilities for novel approaches to treatment in clinical practice in the future (Chen and Pan, 2021; Brandstaeter et al., 2019).

5.6.2. Gastritis

Gastritis, or inflammation of the stomach lining, is a significant matter of interest as far as dealing with the esophagus-stomach relationship in man is concerned. It has several causes like infection by *H. pylori*, stress, alcoholism, and prolonged NSAID usage. The acute form of gastritis usually sees sudden inflammation from irritants, while chronic gastritis is progressive, causing progressive degeneration of the gastric mucosa. Patients with gastritis may have abdominal pain due to the interaction between the stomach and esophagus, nausea, vomiting, and bloating, as the inflammatory processes can provoke reflux symptoms in the esophagus. Last but not least, gastritis makes it easy to treat generalized gastrointestinal disorders. Chronic gastritis may transform into other, more dangerous gastrointestinal conditions, all of which attest to the relationship between the digestive system and gastric cancer in particular. Chronic gastritis of the stomach, which is triggered by *H. pylori* in the first place, has been discovered in studies to precede gastric cancer and represent a serious global health issue. The linkage of gastritis and gastric cancers can be observed in the fact that chronic gastritis tends to preclude other pathologies of the stomach and, hence, becomes increasingly difficult to diagnose and treat. Moreover, the effect of chronic gastritis is not limited to the stomach alone; it is linked to gastric motility and the process of digestion, which affects diseases such as GERD.

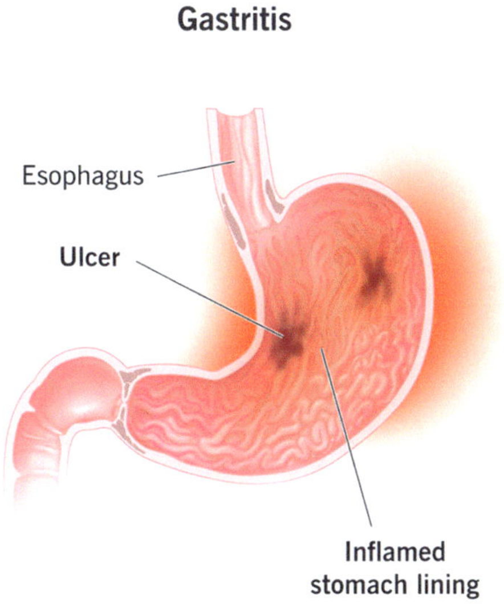

Figure 5.21. Gastritis is inflammation in your stomach lining.

Source: https://my.clevelandclinic.org/-/scassets/images/org/health/articles/10349-gastritis

This observation highlights the importance of early diagnosis and effective management of gastritis to prevent disease progression. Early interventions and preventive strategies are extremely crucial in the management of gastritis and the avoidance of possible evolution to more advanced disease states, including gastric cancer. These include dietary changes and the avoidance of offending drugs, among other life changes, and potential pharmacologic intervention that involves inhibition of gastric acid secretion or eradication of *H. pylori* infections. New findings bring to the forefront the function of such preventive interventions, demonstrating that their treatment of gastritis as an inappropriate development has the potential to lower the risk for gastric cancers significantly, these being among the major causes of cancer-related death worldwide. Chronic inflammation, such as gastritis, has been discovered to lead to the formation of malignancies, including adenocarcinomas as developed from the gastric mucosa (Complementary and Medicine, 2023; Sadiq, 2022). An integrative treatment for gastritis, therefore, not only maintains gastrointestinal tract health but also has long-term implications for the prevention of gastric cancer initiation.

5.6.3. Stomach Cancer

Gastric cancer or stomach cancer is a serious global health problem with an etiology of multifactorial genetic, environmental, and microbiological causes. Notably, *H. pylori* infection, a bacterium that resides in the stomach mucous lining, has been identified as a significant risk factor for this neoplastic disease. Chronic gastritis and ultimately gastric atrophy can be caused by prolonged exposure to these bacteria, which renders the subject susceptible to malignant transformation. Moreover, nutritional factors, such as high salt intake and consumption of processed or smoked food, are bound to augment this risk. An understanding of the mechanism of stomach cancer is crucial as it helps in drawing up potential preventive strategies aimed at minimizing incidence rates and improving survival in patients by way of early detection strategies, thereby pointing towards the importance of huge research work in this field. The role of the gastrointestinal microbiome in gastric cancer is an emerging area of research, with particular interest being focused on a variety of bacterial genera, of which Prevotella is one. While traditionally found to be associated with the oral environment, Prevotella also secures a niche within the gastrointestinal tract. Certain species of Prevotella have been implicated as playing a role in inflammation and other processes that may contribute to gastric tumorigenesis. For instance, shifts in the composition of the microbiome, such as the increased frequency of specific bacterial communities, can lead to dysbiosis that is associated with carcinogenic pathways. Investigating the interactions between microbial communities and gastric cancer are important, not only for disease mechanism learning, but also for engineering future therapeutic approaches that may incorporate microbiome modulation to enhance gastrointestinal health and reduce cancer risk, paving the way for novel preventive interventions in clinical practice. Lastly, stomach cancer is especially difficult to treat, particularly regarding nutritional support through enteral nutrition (EN).

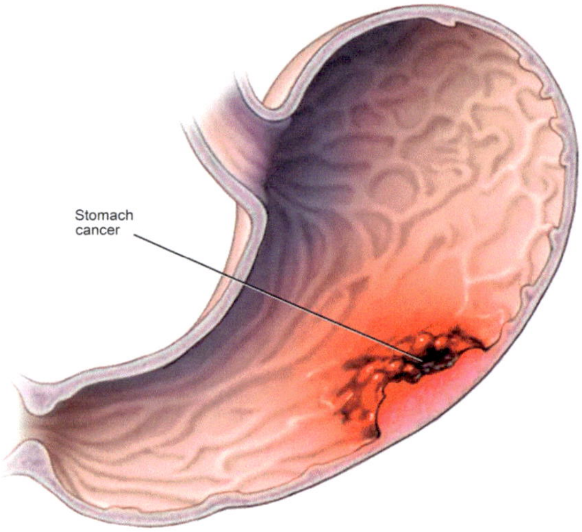

Figure 5.22. Stomach cancer.

Source: https://www.mayoclinic.org/-/media/kcms/gbs/patient-consumer/images/2016/05/02/14/07/c7_stomachcancer-8col.jpg

It is usual for patients undergoing treatment to suffer complications that affect their nutritional status, and hence, proper dietary intervention is the solution to sustaining strength and diminishing the effects of the therapy. Enteral nutrition is a significant clinical intervention that can support patients through the infusion of nutrients directly into the gastrointestinal system. Administration of EN is not risk-free, however, as wrong care may lead to serious side effects. There is a need to utilize an open communication program with the application of best practices to safely provide nutritional therapy to stomach cancer patients. Inclusive approaches can enhance treatment outcomes and aid in improved overall patient care in the arduous battle of combating the disease (Joseph I Boullata et al., 2016).

Test Your Knowledge

1. What is gastritis?
2. What is stomach cancer?

SUMMARY

Finally, the intricate structure and functioning of the stomach and esophagus reveal their fundamental roles in human digestion. The esophagus is a critical pipe that facilitates food travel from the oral cavity to the stomach by synchronized muscle contractions known as peristalsis. The mechanical process not only ensures continuous food movement but also prevents backflow, thus providing a one-way digestive path. By the time the food reaches the stomach, it has been exposed to an environment maximally conducive to digestion, with specialized anatomical structures such as rugae that facilitate expansion. These adaptive structures highlight the evolutionary significance of the gastrointestinal apparatus for dealing with varying sources of food, highlighting the sophistication of human physiology. Furthermore, the interface of the esophagus and the stomach extends into the domains of vascular architecture as well as mucosal functions. Evidence confirms the presence of a well-developed vascular system under which perforating esophageal vessels retain both structural integrity and functional capability as found in other animals, including humans (Aharinejad et al., 1991). Awareness of blood supply architecture and blood supply junctions contributes to the admiration for the manner in which such organs respond to physiological changes and stressors, such as inflammation or disease. The interplay between the muscular and circulatory systems supports the significance of a balanced perspective of digestive well-being, with a focus on interdependence in all gastrointestinal organs. Lastly, a comprehensive understanding of the esophagus and stomach can help direct approaches in treating prevalent gastrointestinal diseases in today's society. New trends in medical research provide insights into GERD and ulcers that profoundly impact the quality of life. As research in the contemporary era continues to enhance our understanding of these organs, therapeutic planning implications follow, with potential for enhanced management of digestive tract diseases and patient well-being. With continued research and integration of technological advancement, as evidenced in pedagogy (Krebs et al., 2015), we may further our understanding of the esophagus and stomach, placing them at the center of human health.

The stomach and esophagus are both essential components of the digestive system, both serving distinct but complementary functions in food digestion and nutrient absorption. The esophagus is a muscular tube through which food passes from the throat to the stomach through a series of peristaltic contractions. Dysfunction in this area can lead to various conditions, one of which is dysphagia, which is commonly present in patients with neurological disorders, such as Parkinson's disease. (Warnecke et al., 2022) refers to the manner in which the motility of the esophagus can be impaired by early pathophysiological changes characteristic of this disease, thus exacerbating swallowing impairment and affecting overall nutrition. Thus, studying the function and disease of the esophagus is a fundamental starting point for an appreciation of more complex gastrointestinal pathology and its systemic impact. From the esophagus, the stomach's role in digestion is dual, encompassing mechanical and chemical functions. The organ not only stores food temporarily but also mixes it with gastric juices to form chyme, enabling primary protein digestion by enzymatic and hydrochloric acid activity. The stomach possesses a highly regulated mechanism for emptying, releasing chyme into the small intestine at a set rate. It is a critical regulation because instability can lead to gastroparesis or gastric outlet obstruction and greatly impact nutrient absorption. Recent research, as quoted in Warnecke et al., (2022), indicates that gastric failure can lead to severe consequences like malnutrition and dehydration, emphasizing the functioning of the stomach in maintaining metabolic health. The fine balance of digestive processes in the stomach is pivotal in guaranteeing the supply of required nutrients to the body effectively. Moreover, the interaction between the esophagus and stomach is not exclusive to the movement of food and digestion but also involves the greater gastrointestinal tract and interactions with general health. The latest figures emphasize that gastrointestinal dysfunction is prevalent in conditions such as Parkinsons disease, whose symptoms range from constipation to severe malnutrition due to impaired motility. (Warnecke et al., 2022) reaffirms that immediate correction of these dysfunctions is critical in the care of patients. Importantly, there is also development in diagnostic tools and treatment methods in the pipeline, with promises of better management of these diseases. Also, the introduction of AI technology in healthcare centers has a promise of enhancing diagnostic accuracy and efficacy of treatments, as discussed. These innovations are needed to address the diverse challenges posed by esophageal and gastric dysfunction, thereby encouraging multidisciplinary recognition of their significance to human health.

KEY TERMS FROM THIS CHAPTER

- Cancers
- Digestive tract
- Dysphagia
- Enteric nervous system
- Esophageal sphincter
- Esophagus
- Gastric ulcers
- Gastroesophageal reflux disease
- Lamina propria
- Meissners plexus
- Nutrient absorption
- Peristalsis
- Pylorus
- Stomach
- Submucosa

CRITICAL THINKING QUESTIONS

1. **The esophagus is a part of the:**
   a. Respiratory system
   b. Digestive system
   c. Endocrine system
   d. Nervous system
2. **The esophagus connects the:**
   a. Mouth to the stomach
   b. Pharynx to the stomach
   c. Larynx to the trachea
   d. Mouth to the duodenum
3. **The movement of food through the esophagus is facilitated by:**
   a. Gravity
   b. Peristalsis
   c. Diffusion
   d. Osmosis
4. **The esophageal sphincter that prevents reflux of stomach contents into the esophagus is called the:**
   a. Upper esophageal sphincter
   b. Lower esophageal sphincter
   c. Pyloric sphincter
   d. Duodenal sphincter
5. **The primary function of the stomach is:**
   a. Absorption of nutrients
   b. Mechanical and chemical digestion of food
   c. Production of bile
   d. Elimination of waste

Short Answer Questions

1. What is the length of an esophagus?
2. What is the function of the esophagus?
3. What is the anatomy of the stomach?
4. What is the function of the stomach?
5. Describe the common disorders of the stomach.

Answer to Critical Thinking Questions

1. (b) 2. (b) 3. (b) 4. (b) 5. (b)

REFERENCES

1. Abell, C., Castell, D. O., von Ritter, C., Jüngst, D., Fiske, W., Gallinger, S., et al. (1991). Role of high total protein in gallbladder bile in the formation of cholesterol gallstones. https://core.ac.uk/download/12167349.pdf (accessed on 15th June 2025).
2. Agnisola, C., Alexandrowicz, Z., Altman, J., Altman, S., Anadon, R., Andrews, P., et al. (2020). Can cephalopods vomit? Hypothesis based on a review of circumstantial evidence and preliminary experimental observations. https://core.ac.uk/download/481438031.pdf (accessed on 15th June 2025).
3. Aharinejad, S., Firbas, W., Franz, P., & Lametschwandtner, A. (1991). The vascularization of the digestive tract studied by scanning electron microscopy with special emphasis on the teeth, esophagus, stomach, small and large intestine, pancreas, and liver. https://core.ac.uk/download/427316097.pdf (accessed on 15th June 2025).
4. Albeck, D., Brakke, S., Brown, J., Burton-Christie, D., Bynum, J., Coveney, J., Detienne, K., et al. (2014). The animalistic gullet and the godlike soul: Reframing sacrifice in Midrash Leviticus Rabbah. https://core.ac.uk/download/288432952.pdf (accessed on 15th June 2025).
5. Alqahtani, M. S., Kazi, M., Alsenaidy, M. A., & Ahmad, M. Z. (2021). Advances in oral drug delivery. *Frontiers in Pharmacology, 12*. https://doi.org/10.3389/fphar.2021.618411 (accessed on 15th June 2025).
6. Belafsky, P. C., Della Maggiore, A., Fulton, A., Garcia, J., et al. (2017). Prevalence of gastroesophageal reflux in cats during anesthesia and effect of omeprazole on gastric pH. https://core.ac.uk/download/323069592.pdf (accessed on 15th June 2025).
7. Bhalla, A. P. S., Griffith, B. E., Kahrilas, P. J., Kou, W., et al. (2015). A fully resolved active musculo-mechanical model for esophageal transport. http://arxiv.org/abs/1501.02010 (accessed on 15th June 2025).
8. Boullata, J. I., Carrera, A. L., Harvey, L. P., Escuro, A. A., Hudson, L., Mays, A., McGinnis, C., et al. (2016). ASPEN safe practices for enteral nutrition therapy. *Journal of Parenteral and Enteral Nutrition, 41*, 15–103. https://doi.org/10.1177/0148607116673053 (accessed on 15th June 2025).
9. Brandstaeter, S., Fuchs, S. L., Aydin, R. C., & Cyron, C. J. (2019). Mechanics of the stomach: A review of an emerging field of biomechanics. *GAMM-Mitteilungen, 42*. https://doi.org/10.1002/gamm.201900001 (accessed on 15th June 2025).
10. Bray, F., Laversanne, M., Sung, H., Ferlay, J., Siegel, R. L., Soerjomataram, I., & Jemal, A. (2024). Global cancer statistics 2022: GLOBOCAN estimates of incidence and mortality worldwide for 36 cancers in 185 countries. *CA: A Cancer Journal for Clinicians, 74*, 229–263. https://doi.org/10.3322/caac.21834 (accessed on 15th June 2025).
11. Breit, S., Kupferberg, A., Rogler, G., & Hasler, G. (2018). Vigus nerve as modulator of the brain–gut axis in psychiatric and inflammatory disorders. *Frontiers in Psychiatry, 9*. https://doi.org/10.3389/fpsyt.2018.00044 (accessed on 15th June 2025).
12. Budrevičiūtė, A., Damiati, S., Sabir, D. K., Önder, K., Schuller-Goetzburg, P., Plakys, G., Katileviciute, A., et al. (2020). Management and prevention strategies for non-communicable diseases (NCDs) and their risk factors. *Frontiers in Public Health, 8*. https://doi.org/10.3389/fpubh.2020.574111 (accessed on 15th June 2025).

13. Cersósimo, M. G., & Benarroch, E. E. (2008). Neural control of the gastrointestinal tract: Implications for Parkinson disease. *Movement Disorders, 23*, 1065–1075. https://doi.org/10.1002/mds.22051 (accessed on 15th June 2025).

14. Chen, W., & Pan, J. Y. (2021). Anatomical and pathological observation and analysis of SARS and COVID-19: Microthrombus's is the main cause of death. *Biological Procedures Online, 23*. https://doi.org/10.1186/s12575-021-00142-y (accessed on 15th June 2025).

15. Cheng, L. K., Kumar, D., Mittal, R. K., Zifan, A., et al. (2017). Three-dimensional myoarchitecture of the lower esophageal sphincter and esophageal hiatus using optical sectioning microscopy. https://core.ac.uk/download/323064197.pdf (accessed on 15th June 2025).

16. Clemente-Suárez, V. J., Beltrán-Velasco, A. I., Redondo-Flórez, L., Martín-Rodríguez, A., & Tornero-Aguilera, J. F. (2023). Global impacts of Western diet and its effects on metabolism and health: A narrative review. *Nutrients, 15*, 2749–2749. https://doi.org/10.3390/nu15122749 (accessed on 15th June 2025).

17. Evidence-Based Complementary and Alternative Medicine. (2023). Retracted: Expression and possible significance of ACE2 in the human liver, esophagus, stomach, and colon. *Evidence-Based Complementary and Alternative Medicine: eCAM, 2023*. https://www.semanticscholar.org/paper/4d308da1363732e761682d48eae178603238393d (accessed on 15th June 2025).

18. Gonkowski, S. (2024). Neuregulin 1 (NRG1) and its receptors in the enteric nervous system and other parts of the gastrointestinal wall. https://core.ac.uk/download/619656530.pdf (accessed on 15th June 2025).

19. Gora, M. J., Suter, M. J., Tearney, G. J., & Li, X. (2017). Endoscopic optical coherence tomography: Technologies and clinical applications [Invited]. *Biomedical Optics Express, 8*, 2405–2405. https://doi.org/10.1364/boe.8.002405 (accessed on 15th June 2025).

20. Hillman, E. T., Lu, H., Yao, T., & Nakatsu, C. H. (2017). Microbial ecology along the gastrointestinal tract. *Microbes and Environments, 32*, 300–313. https://doi.org/10.1264/jsme2.me17017 (accessed on 15th June 2025).

21. Homayun, B., Lin, X., & Choi, H. J. (2019). Challenges and recent progress in oral drug delivery systems for biopharmaceuticals. *Pharmaceutics, 11*, 129–129. https://doi.org/10.3390/pharmaceutics11030129 (accessed on 15th June 2025).

22. Hua, S., Lim, A. W., Storm, G., Talley, N. J., et al. (2023). Current status and advances in esophageal drug delivery technology: Influence of physiological, pathophysiological and pharmaceutical factors. https://core.ac.uk/download/604657655.pdf (accessed on 15th June 2025).

23. Indrio, F., Neu, J., Pettoello-Mantovani, M., Marchese, F., Martini, S., Salatto, A., & Aceti, A. (2022). Development of the gastrointestinal tract in newborns as a challenge for an appropriate nutrition: A narrative review. *Nutrients, 14*, 1405–1405. https://doi.org/10.3390/nu14071405 (accessed on 15th June 2025).

24. Jain, M., Mann, T., Stulić, M., Rao, S., Kirsch, A., Pullirsch, D., Strobl, X., et al. (2018). RNA editing of Filamin A pre-mRNA regulates vascular contraction and diastolic blood pressure. *The EMBO Journal, 37*. https://doi.org/10.15252/embj.201694813 (accessed on 15th June 2025).

25. Jandhyala, S. M. (2015). Role of the normal gut microbiota. *World Journal of Gastroenterology, 21*, 8787–8787. https://doi.org/10.3748/wjg.v21.i29.8787 (accessed on 15th June 2025).
26. Kastl, A., Terry, N. A., Wu, G. D., & Albenberg, L. (2019). The structure and function of the human small intestinal microbiota: Current understanding and future directions. *Cellular and Molecular Gastroenterology and Hepatology, 9*, 33–45. https://doi.org/10.1016/j.jcmgh.2019.07.006 (accessed on 15th June 2025).
27. Keller, A., Gröger, L., Tschernig, T., Solomon, J., Laham, O., Schaum, N., Wagner, V., et al. (2021). miRNATissueAtlas2: An update to the human miRNA tissue atlas. *Nucleic Acids Research, 50*, D211–D221. https://doi.org/10.1093/nar/gkab808 (accessed on 15th June 2025).
28. Khan, A. (2016). Impact of obesity treatment on gastroesophageal reflux disease. *World Journal of Gastroenterology, 22*, 1627–1627. https://doi.org/10.3748/wjg.v22.i4.1627 (accessed on 15th June 2025).
29. Kolesnikov, S. A., Bugaeva, S. R., & Bugaev, V. V. (2024). Lighting innovations in open surgery of the esophagus, stomach and diaphragm. *Journal of Experimental and Clinical Surgery*. https://www.semanticscholar.org/paper/b4ab8d6786addad5f4b69f9e22d2e6ed8e62ad1d (accessed on 15th June 2025).
30. Krebs, D. J. (2015). Implementing blended classroom pedagogy to deepen student understanding in high school biology. https://core.ac.uk/download/638982211.pdf (accessed on 15th June 2025).
31. Kupari, J., Häring, M., Agirre, E., Castelo-Branco, G., & Ernfors, P. (2019). An atlas of vagal sensory neurons and their molecular specialization. *Cell Reports, 27*, 2508–2523.e4. https://doi.org/10.1016/j.celrep.2019.04.096 (accessed on 15th June 2025).
32. Liu, H., Huang, Y., Huang, M., Wang, M., Ming, Y., Chen, W., Chen, Y., et al. (2023). From nitrate to NO: Potential effects of nitrate-reducing bacteria on systemic health and disease. *European Journal of Medical Research, 28*. https://www.semanticscholar.org/paper/c450a4150007cdc5b08d27cdc57327cd7e70beb7 (accessed on 15th June 2025).
33. Liu, P., Lu, L., Zhang, J., Huo, T., Liu, S., & Ye, Z. (2021). Application of artificial intelligence in medicine: An overview. *Current Medical Science, 41*, 1105–1115. https://doi.org/10.1007/s11596-021-2474-3 (accessed on 15th June 2025).
34. Mejino, J. L. V., & Rosse, C. (2004). Symbolic modeling of structural relationships in the Foundational Model of Anatomy. https://core.ac.uk/download/pdf/9412298.pdf (accessed on 15th June 2025).
35. Miller, J. B., Gandhi, N., Clarke, J. O., & McMahan, Z. H. (2017). Gastrointestinal involvement in systemic sclerosis. *JCR: Journal of Clinical Rheumatology, 24*, 328–337. https://doi.org/10.1097/rhu.0000000000000626 (accessed on 15th June 2025).
36. Osugi, T., Sasakura, Y., & Satake, H. (2020). The ventral peptidergic system of the adult ascidian *Ciona robusta* (*Ciona intestinalis* Type A): Insights from a transgenic animal model. https://core.ac.uk/download/639052645.pdf (accessed on 15th June 2025).
37. Rawla, P., & Barsouk, A. (2019). Epidemiology of gastric cancer: Global trends, risk factors and prevention. *Gastroenterology Review, 14*, 26–38. https://doi.org/10.5114/pg.2018.80001 (accessed on 15th June 2025).
38.

39. Sadiq, I. Z. (2022). Nutraceuticals as potential therapeutic agents for preventing gastric cancer: Towards targeting chronic inflammation. *Revita Española de Nutrition Humana y Dietetical.* https://www.semanticscholar.org/paper/58e3a5a18bfb57272e477095e3e20e57 23f381f5 (accessed on 15th June 2025).

40. Scarpignato, C., Gatta, L., Zullo, A., & Blandizzi, C. (2016). Effective and safe proton pump inhibitor therapy in acid-related diseases–A position paper addressing benefits and potential harms of acid suppression. *BMC Medicine, 14.* https://doi.org/10.1186/s12916-016-0718-z (accessed on 15th June 2025).

41. Shao, S., Bu, Z., Xiang, J., Liu, J., Tan, R., Sun, H., Hu, Y., et al. (2024). The role of tetraspanins in digestive system tumor development: Update and emerging evidence. *Frontiers in Cell and Developmental Biology, 12.* https://www.semanticscholar.org/paper/ca76f47389a4d08f084a3dabc18c6016190db756 (accessed on 15th June 2025).

42. Shields, T. M., & Lightdale, J. R. (2018). Vomiting in children. *Pediatrics in Review, 39*, 342–358. https://doi.org/10.1542/pir.2017-0053 (accessed on 15th June 2025).

43. Song, Q., Mao, X., Jing, M., Fu, Y., & Yan, W. (2023). Pathophysiological role of BACH transcription factors in digestive system diseases. *Frontiers in Physiology, 14.* https://www.semanticscholar.org/paper/be52539428ea2f15d5ae96d3e98a77875249d686 (accessed on 15th June 2025).

44. Teshaev, Sh. (2023). Similarities between morphological indicators of the stomach of humans and white-breadless rats. *European Journal of Medical Genetics and Clinical Biology.* https://www.semanticscholar.org/paper/9436dba013f698cee6ac9f0c9394976197cd8f38 (accessed on 15th June 2025).

45. Tripathi, J., Thapa, P., Maharjan, R., & Jeong, S. H. (2019). Current state and future perspectives on gastroprotective drug delivery systems. *Pharmaceutics, 11*, 193–193. https://doi.org/10.3390/pharmaceutics11040193 (accessed on 15th June 2025).

46. Warnecke, T., Schäfer, K. H., Claus, I., Del Tredici, K., & Jost, W. H. (2022). Gastrointestinal involvement in Parkinson's disease: Pathophysiology, diagnosis, and management. *npj Parkinson's Disease, 8.* https://doi.org/10.1038/s41531-022-00295-x (accessed on 15th June 2025).

47. Wishart, D. S. (2019). Metabolomics for investigating physiological and pathophysiological processes. *Physiological Reviews, 99*, 1819–1875. https://doi.org/10.1152/physrev.00035.2018 (accessed on 15th June 2025).

48. Wojtunik-Kulesza, K., Oniszczuk, A., Oniszczuk, T., Combrzyński, M., Nowakowska, D., & Matwijczuk, A. (2020). Influence of *in vitro* digestion on composition, bio accessibility and antioxidant activity of food polyphenols—A non-systematic review. *Nutrients, 12*, 1401–1401. https://doi.org/10.3390/nu12051401 (accessed on 15th June 2025).

49. Wurm, P., Dörner, E., Kremer, C., Spranger, J., Maddox, C., Halwachs, B., Harrison, U., et al. (2018). Qualitative and quantitative DNA- and RNA-based analysis of the bacterial stomach microbiota in humans, mice, and gerbils. *mSystems, 3.* https://doi.org/10.1128/msystems.00262-18 (accessed on 15th June 2025).

50. Xu, H., Zhong, L., Deng, J. S., Peng, J., Dan, H., Zeng, X., Li, T., et al. (2020). High expression of ACE2 receptor of 2019-nCoV on the epithelial cells of oral mucosa. *International Journal of Oral Science, 12.* https://doi.org/10.1038/s41368-020-0074-x (accessed on 15th June 2025).

SMALL AND LARGE INTESTINE

6

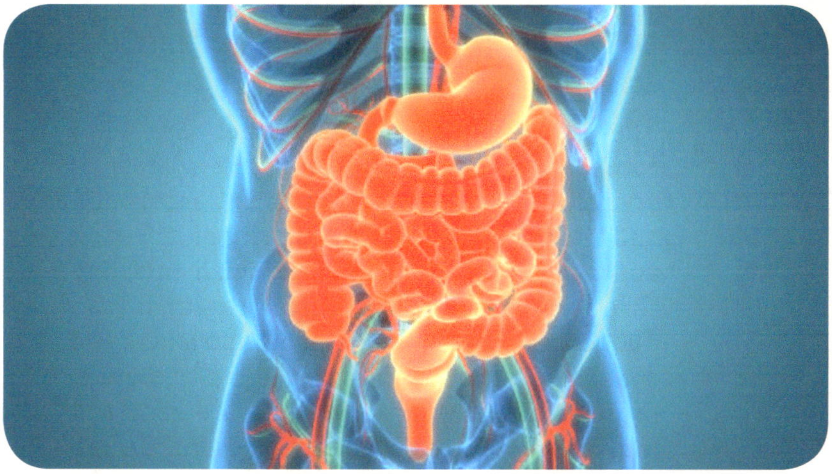

LEARNING OBJECTIVES

After studying this chapter, you will be able to:

1. Understand the anatomy of the small intestine
2. Describe the function of the small intestine
3. Understand the anatomy of the large intestine
4. Describe the function of the large intestine
5. Explain the common disorders of the small intestine
6. Explain the common disorders of the large intestine

Introduction

The human digestive system is a highly choreographed set of organs that work harmoniously within an incredibly complex process to process food, absorb nutrients, and eliminate waste. The small intestine and large intestine are two vital components of this incredibly choreographed system with complementary functions that are required for health. The duodenum, jejunum, and ileum consist of the small intestine, whose primary purpose is to digest food and route nutrients into the body through the circulatory system. Its enormous surface area, through specialized mechanisms like villi and microvilli, is helpful in nutrient absorption, which is necessary for retaining body function and energy levels. An understanding of the anatomy and physiology of the small intestine gives some indication of its function in digestion and how gastrointestinal health impacts people and populations. The large intestine, or colon, is, nonetheless, a vital site for water and electrolyte absorption and the creation and movement of feces. This organ is also crucial in maintaining the body's electrolyte and water balance through the reabsorption of water from undigested substances and ensuring hydration. The large intestine is also home to a vast microbiome that aids digestion and the fermentation of dietary fiber to produce short-chain fatty acids, which have numerous health-promoting effects. These symbiotic, diverse microbes also play roles in immune function and resistance to disease, and show us the importance of considering gut health within overall health.

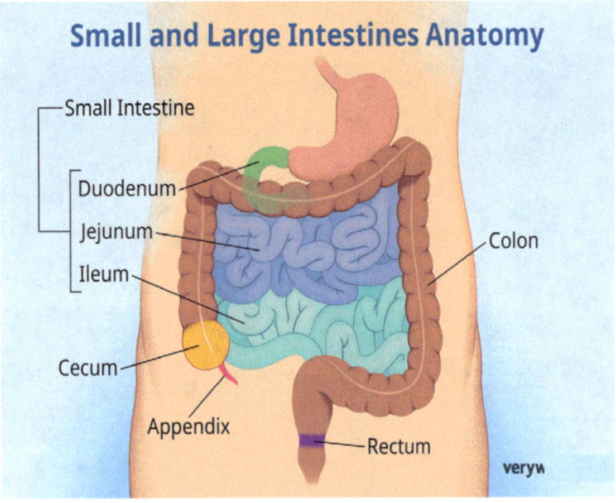

Figure 6.1. Small and large intestines anatomy.

Source: https://www.verywellhealth.com/thmb/pb_0HsAkSBH3m9NXhNUXRvs4IzU=/1500x0/filters:no_upscale():max_bytes(150000):strip_icc()/TheIntestines-LabeledDiagramFunctionConditions-v1-e2d44170a8d246b3a92adcede86a63cd.png

The science of the large intestine teaches us about dietary and lifestyle influences on health, and the importance of holistic strategies toward gastrointestinal health. Small and large intestines are both vital to human health, and their roles have a direct link to nutrition, metabolism, and the prevention of diseases. Understanding the complex interaction between the intestinal segments yields valuable information about malabsorption syndromes, inflammatory bowel disease, and colorectal cancer. Additionally, information gained from studies on the organs is directly transferable to public health policy for better digestive health and healthy eating. With subsequent scientific advances and the unveiling of the roles of the small and large intestines, creating individual therapies and diets becomes increasingly possible. What may be achieved through this much-needed integration can lead to novel strategies for deriving optimal health benefits and disease control in forthcoming years that can contribute further to human health and nutrition knowledge globally.

Definition and Importance of the Intestines

The small and large intestines are vital components of the human body's system of digestion, with the role of nutrient absorption and waste expulsion. The majority of digestion and absorption occurs in the small intestine through three consecutive regions: the duodenum, jejunum, and ileum. Nutrients from consumed food, such as vitamins, minerals, proteins, fat, and carbohydrates, are absorbed into the bloodstream at this juncture. On the other hand, the large intestine, consisting of the cecum, colon, and rectum, primarily serves to absorb water and electrolytes while forming and discharging feces. The health of the intestines directly influences overall health and well-being, where dietary disorders lead to nutritional deficiencies and various gastrointestinal diseases. The function of the intestines is more than mere digestion and involves critical functions of metabolic regulation and immune system modulation. The intestines host a diverse microbiota that is accountable for the breakdown of complex carbohydrates and the production of vital SCFAs such as butyrate, propionate, and acetate. SCFAs aid in intestinal homeostasis and have systemic impacts, such as energy metabolism and regulation of the immune system, crucial for health maintenance and disease prevention (Hee, 2021). Besides, recent findings put the gut-brain axis in the limelight, highlighting the interaction between the intestines and the central nervous system.

The axis suggests that the well-being of the intestine is at the core of the well-being of the mind and cognitive functions, and therefore opening up yet another aspect of the significance of intestines to humanity's overall well-being (John F Cryan et al., 2019). It is important to understand the role and significance of the intestines in addressing contemporary health problems, particularly low-fiber and high-processing food diets. With the shifts in present dietary habits towards forsaking traditional high-fiber-type diets, the influence on intestinal function and microbiota composition has become increasingly significant. Decreased fiber consumption is related to rising gastrointestinal disease, such as inflammatory bowel disease and metabolic syndrome. This change underscores the importance of dietary changes that promote intestinal health, e.g., supplementing non-digestible fiber essential for SCFA production and microbiome homeostasis. These food changes, not only promoting digestive health, maximize systemic outcome benefits, exemplifying the key position the intestines have in the general human status.

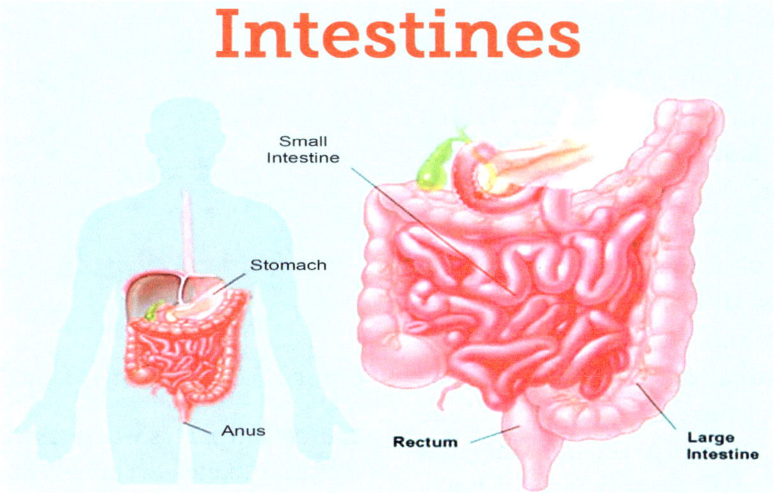

Figure 6.2. Intestines.

Source: https://assets.lybrate.com/imgs/tic/enadp/image-of-the-intestines.jpg

6.1. Anatomy of the Small Intestine

Learning Outcome

1. Describe the structure and length of the small intestine
2. Understand the division of the small intestine
3. Describe the role of villi and microvilli in nutrient absorption

Small intestine anatomy is part of its role in the digestive process because it is the primary site for nutrient absorption. It consists of three parts of differing function—the duodenum, jejunum, and ileum. There are specialized functions within each segment that collectively serve to enhance the digestion process. The duodenum, the first segment, primarily houses the mixing of chyme with pancreatic and bile juices in preparation for initial enzyme action on foodstuffs. The jejunum's long villi and microvilli maximize nutrient absorption, and the ileum continues the process and absorbs bile acids and vitamin B12. The functionally divided structure maximizes the efficiency with which nutrients are processed and utilized by the body and shows the evolutionary adaptation of the small intestine to its critical contribution to human digestion. The intricate structure of the walls of the small intestines is essential to its absorptive role. Composed of four layers—mucosa, submucosa, muscularis externa, and serosa—the wall possesses specialized characteristics for enhancing its purpose. The mucous layer is overlaid by villi and microvilli, which give an enormous boost to the surface area for absorption. Moreover, enterocytes, the villous epithelial cells, possess numerous transport proteins and enzymes that enable nutrient absorption.

The submucosa is comprised of connective tissue, blood vessels, and lymphatics, which play a vital role in moving absorbed nutrients from the intestine. The kind of structural specialization that exists in this case points to the efficiency of the small intestine in absorbing nutrients, affirming its status as the central location for nutrient processing in the human gastrointestinal tract. Delving deeper into the dynamics of the small intestine sheds light on the coordination between anatomy and physiological function. Current research shows that alterations, for instance, resulting from procedures such as gastric bypass surgery, can influence intestinal adaptation and pancreatic function. Studies show that alterations in nutrient delivery by surgical procedures cause changes in pancreatic islet size and function, showing the intricate interrelationship of digestive tract adjustment and hormonal response within the endocrine system (Aguilar Diosdado et al., 2015). Furthermore, technological advancement, such as the development of wireless sensors to monitor gastrointestinal conditions, emphasizes understanding the structure and dynamics of the small intestines. Such innovations have the promise to develop less invasive diagnostic procedures with more comfortable patients while uncovering essential information on gastrointestinal health (Chirwa et al., 2003). This meeting of anatomy and physiology and technology sheds light on the continuous research into the function of the small intestines in the grand scheme of human health.

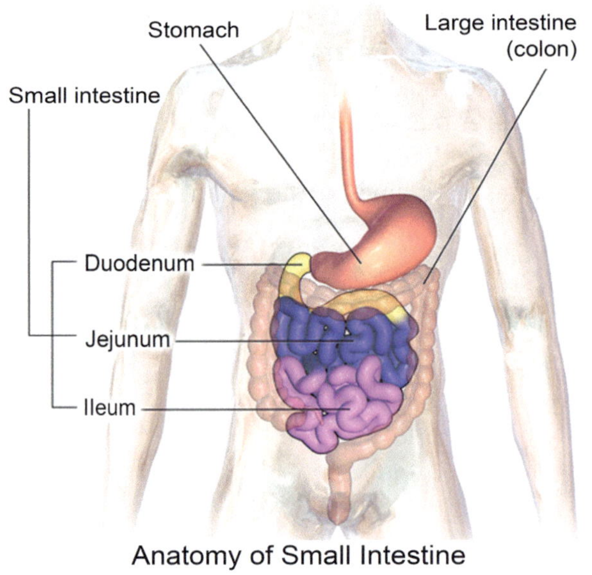

Figure 6.3. Anatomy of the Small Intestine.

Source: https://s3-us-west-2.amazonaws.com/courses-images-archive-read-only/wp-content/uploads/sites/1470/2015/11/04064736/480px-Blausen_0817_SmallIntestine_Anatomy.png

6.1.1. Structure and Length of the Small Intestine

The small intestine is a critical component of the human digestive system since most nutrient absorption happens here. The duodenum, jejunum, and ileum are three highly differentiated components that make up the anatomy, each performing a specialized role throughout digestion. The total length of the small intestine measures about 20 feet in adults, but it can be very inconsistent between individuals. The large surface area, courtesy of microvilli and villi, allows it to absorb a wide variety of nutrients from digested food. Structural protections like this are required as the body must be able to have a good system for receiving and absorbing vital vitamins, minerals, and macronutrients required for health and metabolism. Aside from size, the intricate small intestine structure is key to optimal functioning and intestinal well-being. Intestinal wall microanatomy includes several layers that house an inner mucosal layer of closely packed epithelial cells that produce digestive enzymes and mucus.

A network of enterocytes and specialized cells that have critical roles in immune protection and intestinal microbiome maintenance is found interposed between epithelial cells. The importance of the small intestinal microbiome (SIM) with a rich diversity of microorganisms, e.g., bacteria and archaea, was underscored in recent research. In such cases, the microbiome is responsible for the host's health by facilitating nutrient absorption and providing a protective barrier against pathogens, indicating an interdependence between the host's structural and microbial inhabitants of the small intestine (Brimberry et al., 2024). Furthermore, defensins reinforce the immunological defense of the small intestine, and human defensin 6 (HD6) is pivotal in the protection against microbial invasion of the epithelial lining. HD6 has been observed as filamentous structures, or, more simply, nanonets, which ensnare and disable pathogenic bacteria so they cannot cross the epithelial barrier.

This novel mechanism of defense highlights the interplay between the structural elements and functional capacity of the small intestine, since it contrasts nutrient absorption with the need for defense of the host. Smooth control of the structural configuration and the microbiome attests to the plasticity and importance of the small intestine in the physiology of the human body and a key area to aim future research and clinical study (Kamyshinsky et al., 2024).

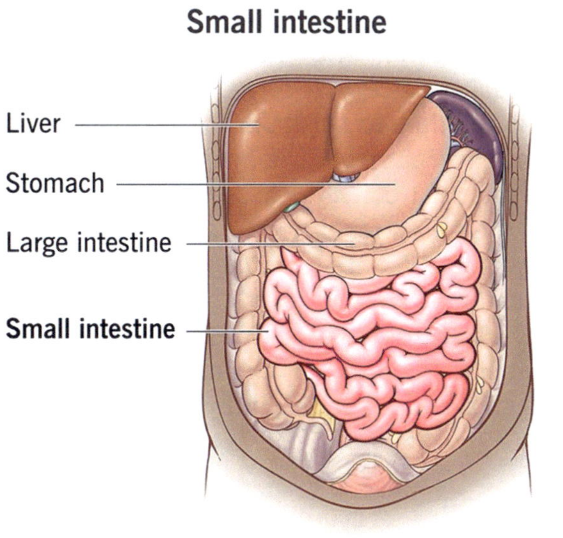

Figure 6.4. The small intestine sits under the stomach.

Source: https://my.clevelandclinic.org/-/scassets/images/org/health/articles/22135-small-intestine-illustration-final.ashx

6.1.2. Division Into Duodenum, Jejunum, and Ileum

The division of the small intestine into three distinct portions—duodenum, jejunum, and ileum—has crucial physiological functions in the digestion and absorption of nutrients. The duodenum is the initial part that receives chyme from the stomach and also combines it with bile from the gallbladder and pancreatic secretions. This combination has an ideal alkaline medium for enzymatic digestion. The duodenum's lining, rich in absorptive cells and specialized glands, plays a significant role in carbohydrate, protein, and fat breakdown into absorbable units. The small intestine's sectional anatomy is an example of how structural differences are related to functional specialization to ensure digestion occurs effectively as food is transported from one segment to another. The jejunum, second after the duodenum, is primarily engaged in nutrient absorption. Its unique morphology is defined by extensive vascularization and the enormously folded mucosal surface that forms a maximum area for absorption. The jejunum is optimally adapted to the absorption of carbohydrates, amino acids, and fats and conveys these nutrients directly into the blood for distribution throughout the body. The jejunum's physiological significance is underscored by noting that a healthy jejunum is essential to overall nutritional well-being; a number of diseases impacting its function can lead to malabsorption syndromes.

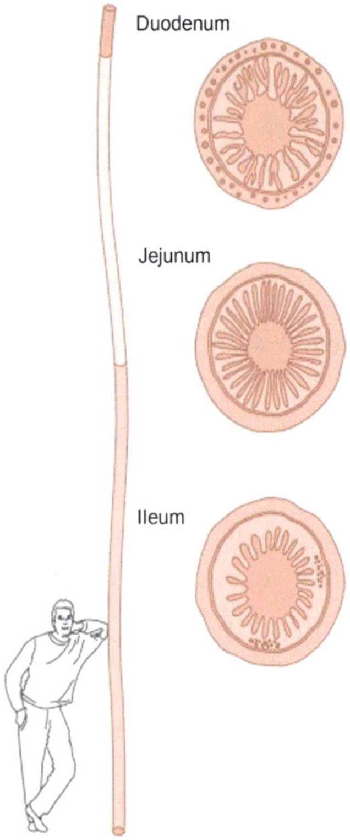

Figure 6.5. The three portions of small intestine.

Source: https://www.pharmacy180.com/media/imgph04/MJg17PO.jpg

The comprehension of the jejunum's role in the anatomy of the intestine gives insight into the relationship between gastrointestinal health and dietary input, and underscores the importance of this section to human nutrition and metabolism. The ileum, the terminal part of the small intestine, has a unique role in absorbing certain nutrients, notably vitamin B12 and bile salts, which are critical to digestion and health. It has fewer villi and a thinner lining than the jejunum but is adapted for effective absorption under its own distinct biochemical conditions. With the issue of digestion transported from the ileum to the large intestine, there is bulk electrolyte and water absorption, which is critical for body fluid balance. The ileum also hosts a diverse microbiota that commutes with the host immune system and provides metabolic functions, reflecting the segment's importance beyond just nutrient uptake. The dialogue between the ileum and gut microbiome is demonstrated in research, as spatial gradients of microbial species along the intestinal tract lie at the foundation of many disease mechanisms, testifying to the interconnectedness of intestinal structure and function (Yang et al., 2025; Thelin, 2024).

6.1.3. Role of Villi and Microvilli in Nutrient Absorption

The intricate structure of the small intestine plays a crucial role in nutrient digestion, primarily due to the presence of villi and microvilli. The finger-like protrusions of the intestinal lining that branch into multiple segments increase the surface area for digestion immensely. Microvilli are present in all villi, further increasing the area for absorption, and are referred to as the "brush border" in common language. This brilliant spatial arrangement permits efficient absorption of nutrients such as amino acids, fatty acids, and monosaccharides into the blood. The added surface area provided by the projections enables the intestine to be able to absorb sufficient nutrients that are necessary in order to meet the metabolic demands of the body, hence making the villi and microvilli necessary structures in the whole digestive process. The morphological adaptation of villi and microvilli in their varied response to various physiological conditions, such as feeding and fasting, is a reflection of their plastic nature. Experiments have shown that after oral ingestion, the enterocytes that line the intestine hypertrophy, lengthening and packing the microvilli more tightly, thereby enhancing nutrient uptake. For instance, in the Burmese python, villus length and height of microvilli were increased hours postfeeding, and this established the capacity of intestines to adjust to the nutritional state of the organism within a very short duration (Aldewachi et al., 2006). This more rapid postprandial response illustrates the importance of villi and microvilli not only for nutrient absorption but also for the efficiency of organisms in consuming nutrients and energy at the right time. Further, structural variation of villi and microvilli may affect the overall function of the gut and adaptive response during different stages of life, as also emphasized by research in young pigs. Villi development begins robustly at birth, followed by a significant suckling-related increase in height and surface area that declines as weaning commences. The adaptive mechanism can be described by the 18-fold enhancement of villi absorptive capacity that gets further augmented a staggering 400-fold by microvilli, ultimately supporting digestion and absorption as the young animals acclimatize to food (Elefson, 2019). These changes in development emphasize the strategic value of villi and microvilli in maintaining the intestines in functional capacity of nutrient absorption at any given time during an organism's life, in homeostasis, and in development.

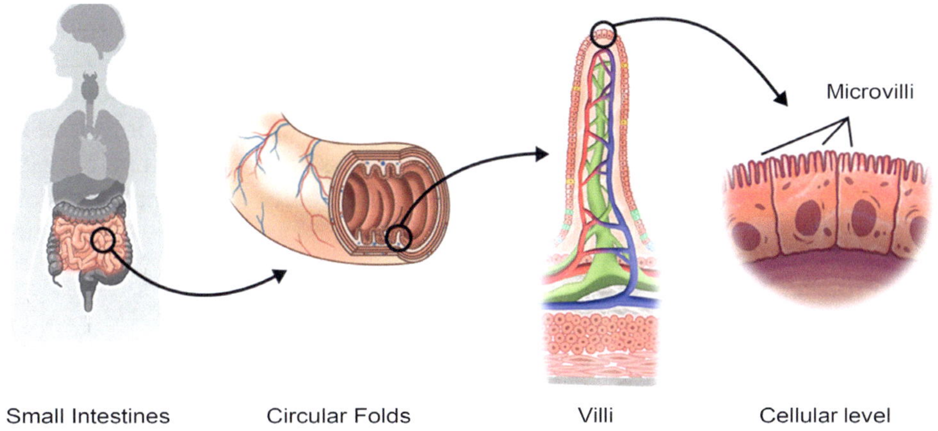

Figure 6.6. Three levels of complexity of the structure of the small intestine. The lining of the small intestine has circular folds, which are rich in villi. Each villus has absorptive cells that contain microvilli. All structures increase absorption surface area of the intestine.

Source: https://images.my.labster.com/v2/GIA/bfad5e1e-a35c-44b9-bd31-d8a93315f8c3/GIA_SmallIntestine_ComplexStructure.en.x1024.png

Test Your Knowledge

1. Describe the three main parts of the small intestine in order from proximal to distal, and explain one key anatomical feature that distinguishes each part.
2. What structural modifications of the small intestine increase its surface area for absorption, and how does each modification contribute to efficient nutrient absorption?

6.2. Function of the Small Intestine

Learning Outcome

1. Learn about digestion of macronutrients
2. Understand the absorption of vitamins and minerals
3. Describe the interaction with digestive enzymes and bile

The small intestine is a crucial part of the digestive system, serving solely as the site of nutrient absorption. Formed of three sections—the duodenum, jejunum, and ileum—it enables food to be digested by enzymatic activities as well as mechanical mixing. Upon entry of the chyme into the duodenum, bile from the liver and pancreatic fluids facilitate lipid and carbohydrate digestion. In the jejunum, the highly folded mucosal surface, with the occurrence of villi and microvilli, highly enhances the absorptive surface to enable effective uptake of nutrients like amino acids, fatty acids, and monosaccharides. Such an intricate structure not only maximizes nutrient extraction but also covers and protects enterocytes, forming a barrier against pathogen invasion, which is necessary to maintain gut health. Its appreciation underscores the importance of the small intestine in nutritional homeostasis and overall health. The interaction between the small intestine and the gut microbiome underscores its role in metabolic regulation. The gut microbiota, within which trillions of microbes are housed, assists in the breakdown of complex carbohydrates and in the synthesis of vitamins. These microbial activities produce short-chain fatty acids (SCFAs), which are significant energy sources for colonic epithelial cells and are involved in metabolic and immune homeostasis within the body. New research finds the role of SCFAs within the framework of the gut-brain axis, where they influence neurochemical processes and are involved in mental health and wellness. The balance of the small intestine's beneficial and pathogenic microorganisms is, therefore, important not only for efficient digestion but also for preventing dysbiosis that can contribute to a range of gastrointestinal diseases and even systemic diseases reported in literature (Silva et al., 2020). The capacity of the small intestines to cope with adverse external factors, i.e., heavy metal exposure, is also increasingly recognized. Long-term exposure to heavy metals, which are available in water, air, and certain foods, is harmful and can cause toxicity and cell damage. Though the primary function of the small intestine is the absorption of nutrients, it is also an exclusion barrier to toxic substances. Any type of disturbance in its absorptive function will lead to serious health risks, including impaired metabolism as well as increased oxidative stress (Balali M-Mood et al., 2021). This necessitates the maintenance of the integrity of the intestinal lining and its liaison with the gut microbiota in resisting the toxic effects of environmental pollutants. Thus, the varied roles of the small intestine not only shed light on its critical functions but also accentuate its vulnerability to the challenges of present-day environments.

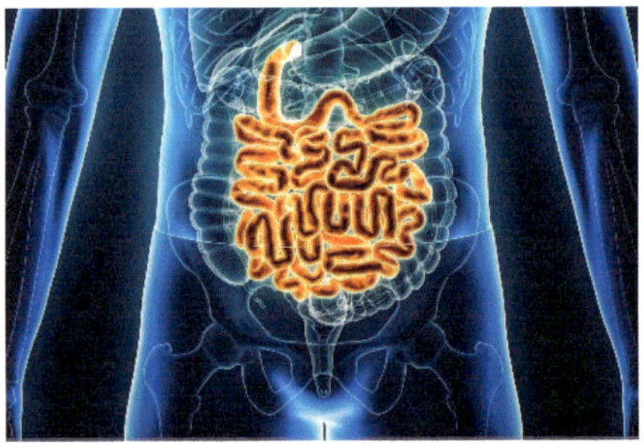

Source: https://www.verywellhealth.com/thmb/ZvMLihJtO00pbDiOIDsZDFyws6M=/1500x0/filters:no_upscale():max_bytes(150000):strip_icc()/VWH-GettyImages-1435918094-48e2c5ec776d4ae8a938ba6338801846.jpg

6.2.1. Digestion of Macronutrients

Macronutrient digestion is a complex process with the initiation in the oral cavity but eventual completion in the small intestine. Carbohydrates, proteins, and lipids are digested by distinctive enzymic processes with the participation of different secretions of the digestive tract. Salivary amylase facilitates the initiation of carbohydrate digestion, while pepsin released from gastric glands of the stomach initiates protein digestion. But the majority of digestion takes place in the small intestine, in which pancreatic enzymes, such as amylase, lipase, and proteases, break down macronutrients into absorbable units: monosaccharides, fatty acids, and amino acids.

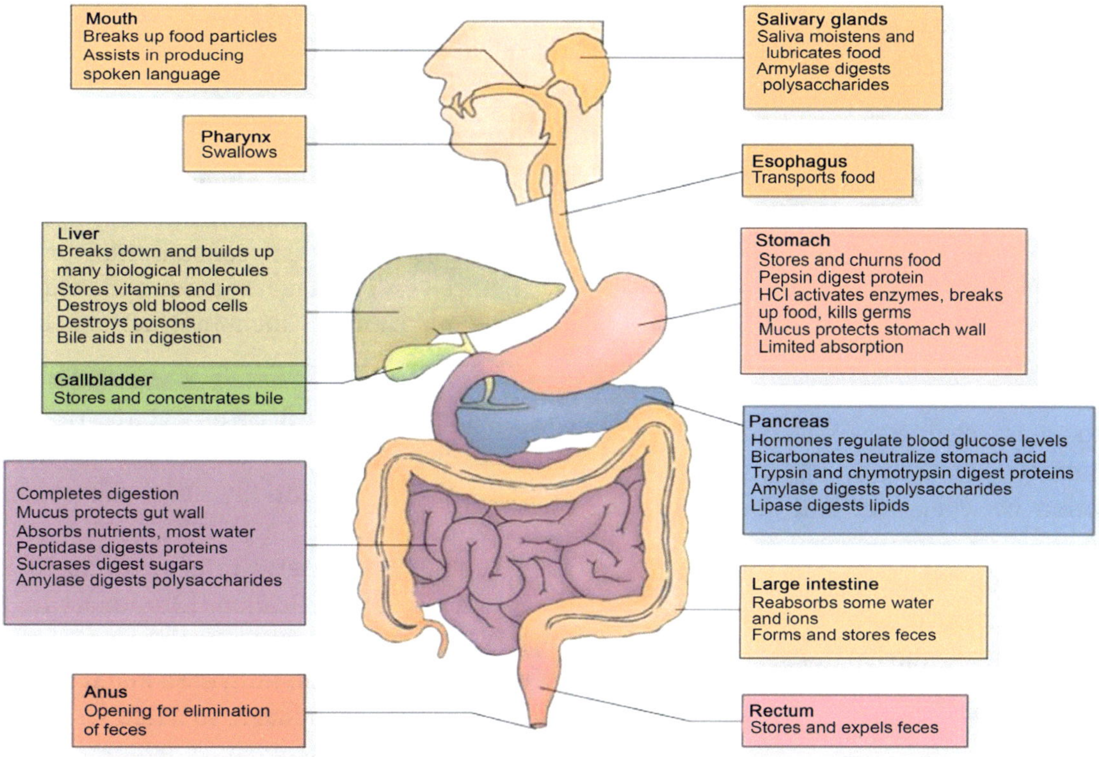

Figure 6.7. Digesting Macronutrients.

Source: https://blogger.googleusercontent.com/img/b/R29vZ2xl/AVvXsEgP7YmF-3pkkDySqc_8lZe0CbLZHu7iWHKoSzRZz3iVLSMQxBHO1vIIGQh2FBnDmoqRxZrrzoIzejifVdJtzzo-zPGbmBZU0wD1td3dJ_bVSW9-XlAakEtVlR4e8mWNdmvcOazKt_aoYKg/s1600/macro-diagram.jpg

The highly regulated process that extracts as much as possible of nutrients is needed to sustain metabolic homeostasis. These nutrients are then absorbed primarily by the intestinal mucosa villi and microvilli, which display the interconnectedness of digestion and absorption activities of macronutrient assimilation. The small intestine contains specialized regions with specific functions in digestion and macronutrient absorption. It is the site where chyme from the stomach is admitted with bile and pancreatic secretions, which provide emulsification as well as enzymatic hydrolysis of fat. Vitamin E is taken as an example here for a lipophilic nutrient whose availability in the body can be regulated by gut mechanisms in the small intestine. Stability and bioaccessibility studies of vitamin E, particularly when vitamin E is encapsulated in Pickering emulsions that are stabilized with nano-hydroxyapatite, demonstrate how nutrient uptake is influenced by mechanical and physiological interactions within the gut. Food macronutrient intake can also influence the absorption of compounds such as vitamin E, with research indicating differences in bioaccessibility based on emulsified fat droplet size, which can significantly modify nutrient absorption kinetics (Ribeiro et al., 2021). In addition, the gut microbiota also plays a very important role in macronutrient digestion and metabolism and impacts health and disease. Some families of bacteria, including Lachnospiraceae, are known to be centrally involved in the fermentation of undigested carbohydrates to yield short-chain fatty acids that are beneficial in a variety of ways. These metabolites are less easily discerned in their contribution to energy homeostasis, but also in modulating colonic health and systemic inflammation. Interestingly, the dietary regimens are also able to change the size and behavior of such microbial populations, suggesting symbiotic interaction between diet and gut microbiota with an effect on macronutrient digestion. Thus, the capacity for understanding how the gut microbiome interacts with dietary intake in a way to maximize nutrient absorption speaks volumes about the complexity of digestive processes and their additional value to overall human health (Vacca et al., 2020).

6.2.2. Absorption of Vitamins and Minerals

The uptake of minerals and vitamins in the body is a critical process that, to a large extent, occurs in the small intestine. The process of food breaking down to simpler compounds releases the required nutrients like vitamins and minerals, making them available for absorption. The large surface area of the small intestine, also aided by the presence of villi and microvilli, is crucial in facilitating this uptake. Particular transport mechanisms—such as passive diffusion and active transport—allow these nutrients to pass through the intestinal wall and enter the bloodstream. Such absorption not only contributes to general well-being but also equips the body with enough reserves to maintain metabolic processes in the long term. The small intestine's vitamin and mineral absorption modifiers are varied and often related to one another. One such important factor is the presence of specific dietary components, either facilitators or inhibitors of nutrient consumption. Certain fats, for instance, are facilitators of the absorption of fat-soluble vitamins (A, D, E, and K), while phytates in cereals inhibit the absorption of essential minerals like zinc and iron. With age-related problems in nutrient consumption presenting themselves, particularly among the elderly, the determination of such interactions becomes increasingly important.

Evidence indicates that the aging gastrointestinal tract undergoes physiological changes that potentially delay the absorption of vital nutrients, highlighting the need for personalized dietetic interventions to lower malnutrition complications (Bordoni et al., 2015). In addition to changes in the gastrointestinal tract's structure, malnutrition might complicate the existing problems associated with nutrient absorption, particularly in older individuals. Loss of chemical and mechanical digestion may lead to ineffective nutrient absorption, thereby worsening health issues such as vitamin deficiencies and mineral deficiencies. One should understand the interconnection between the functioning of the aging gastrointestinal tract and nutrient availability. The strategies used to address the issues should focus on identifying biomarkers to accurately measure food intake and nutrient absorption. By utilizing knowledge of the intricate relationship between gut function and nutrition status, medical professionals are better able to design diets with a focus on optimizing nutrient absorption, hence enhancing the health status and well-being of the elderly (Kline, 1988).

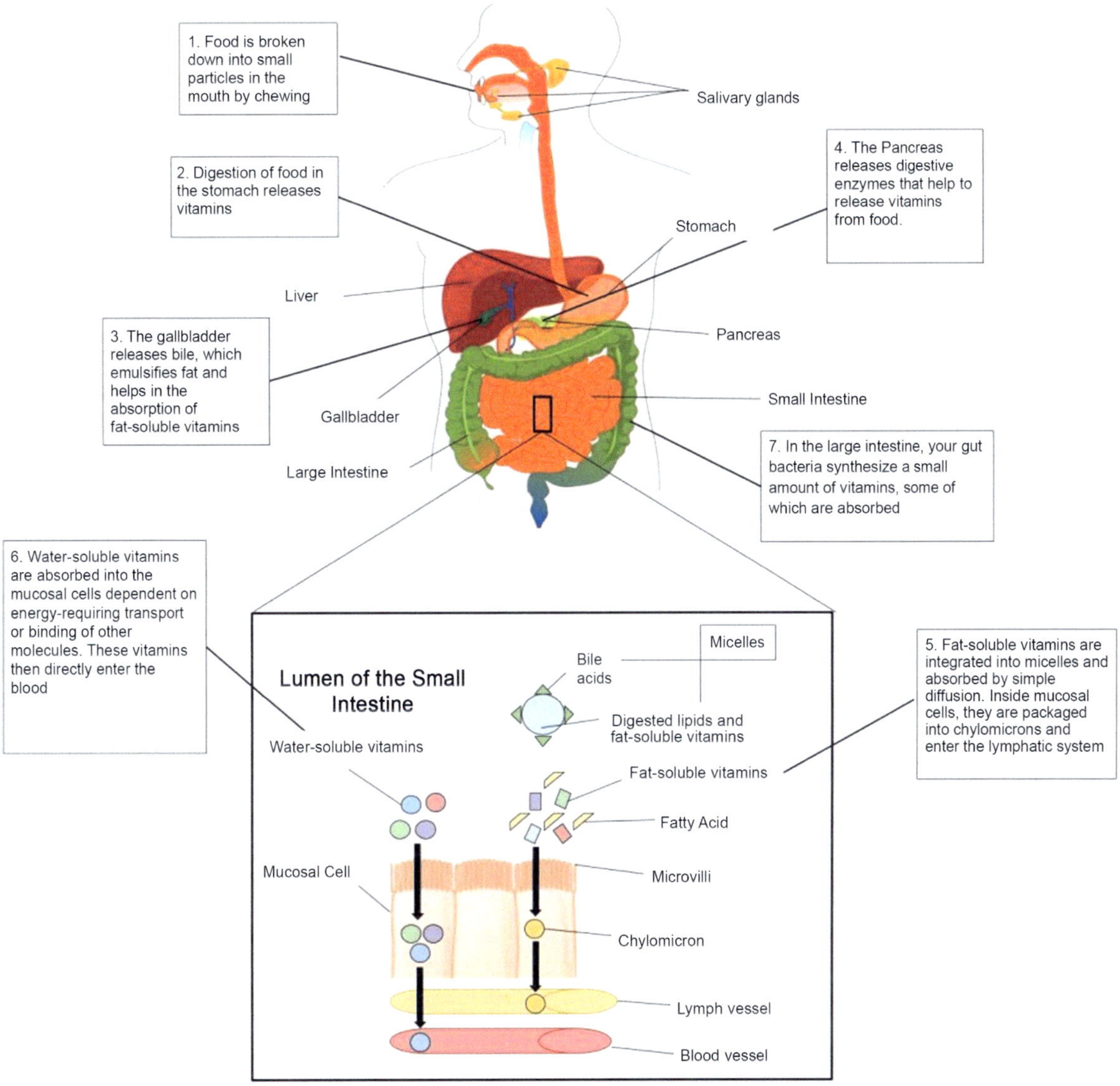

Figure 6.8. Absorption of Fat-Soluble and Water-Soluble Vitamins.

Source: https://openoregon.pressbooks.pub/app/uploads/sites/282/2022/06/image1-1-6.png

6.2.3. Interaction With Digestive Enzymes and Bile

The small intestine is a crucial site for nutrient absorption, where digestive enzymes and bile cooperate to play a critical role in making this possible. The pancreas secretes a variety of enzymes that target macronutrients, including carbohydrates, proteins, and fats. These enzymes, for instance, amylases, lipases, and proteases, disintegrate the large molecules into absorbable units. Concomitantly, bile produced in the liver and stored within the gallbladder is emptied into the small intestine, primarily to emulsify the dietary lipids, increasing the surface area available for lipid digestion. Emulsification is essential since it allows for the lipases to hydrolyze triglycerides effectively into fatty acids and monoglycerides, allowing for maximal absorption by the intestinal epithelial cells.

Pancreatic enzyme-bile interaction thus points towards the importance of a concerted digestive response to nutrient uptake in the small intestine. Structural elements of plant cell walls also determine the interaction with pancreatic enzymes and bile. The complexity of such cell walls, composed of cellulose, hemicellulosic, and pectic polysaccharides determines the bioaccessibility of nutrients encapsulated in plant tissues. Based on the structure and organization, plant cell walls either limit or allow the activity of digestive enzymes. Effective digestion is reliant on mechanical disruption of these barriers, which are controlled to a significant degree by mechanical and enzymatic forces during digestion. Accordingly, nutrient release efficiency is controlled, and the importance of digestive enzyme activity and bile in overcoming such structural barriers of plant foods is brought to the fore (Edwards et al., 2020). Such interaction ultimately decides the profile of nutrients made available for absorption in the small intestine. In addition to the enzymatic and mechanical activities, the bioavailability of secondary metabolites, such as carotenoids and polyphenols, further reflects the complex dynamics of nutrient interaction in the gut. They are health-improving secondary metabolites, but their release on digestion can vary immensely due to varying models and conditions of digestion. In vitro digestion studies have served to simulate the gastrointestinal environment to enable scientists to be in a position to predict the bioaccessibility of these compounds. Variations in variables such as enzyme concentration, pH, and the sequence of digestion contribute to the complexity of nutrient release and absorption (Adlercreutz et al., 2014). Understanding these forces is crucial to maximizing nutritional value because it uncovers the strong interaction between digestive enzymes and bile in enhancing the bioavailability of major phytochemicals, thereby affecting the final effect on human health outcomes.

Test Your Knowledge

1. How are vitamins and minerals absorbed?
2. What do digestive enzymes interact with?

6.3. Anatomy of the Large Intestine

Learning Outcome

1. Describe the structure and length of the large intestine
2. Describe the components of the large intestine
3. Differentiate between the large and small intestines

The large intestine or large bowel, a vital component of the human gut, has various roles like absorption of water, electrolyte regulation, and fermentation of what cannot be digested. The large intestine anatomically contains a number of sections, including the cecum, colon, rectum, and anal canal. The cecum or pouch is the one that receives chyme from the ileum and is the beginning of the colon. The colon is further divided into four regions: ascending, transverse, descending, and sigmoid. Each part plays a crucial role: metabolizing waste products, facilitating the absorption of residual nutrients, and forming stools. The internal structure of the colon is characterized by a mucosal layer with a dense microbiome that is diverse, involved in fermentation processes for the synthesis of short-chain fatty acids that coat the colonic epithelial cells and contribute to the maintenance of gut health (Irıs D Nagtegaal et al., 2019). Other than its composition, the physiology of the large intestine is essential for digestive efficacy. There are four layers in the wall of the large intestine: mucosa, submucosa, muscularis, and serosa. The muscularis contains two layers of muscle that facilitate peristaltic motion, leading to the transportation of fecal material towards the rectum. During the movement through the colon, water is absorbed, essentially transforming liquid chyme into more solid feces.

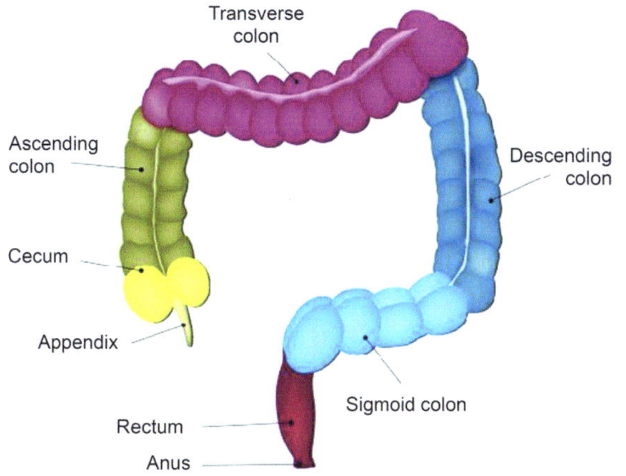

Figure 6.9. Anatomy of the large intestine.

Source: https://www.researchgate.net/profile/Ravindra-Kale-5/publication/364954411/figure/fig1/AS:11431281093787770@1667276984221/Anatomy-of-the-large-intestine.png

This process is largely governed by specialized nerve reflexes that drive locomotion. Finally, the large intestine microbiota is also important in modulating digestion and immune function, illustrating the interrelation of anatomical structure and physiological function to enable homeostasis (Irıs D Nagtegaal et al., 2019). The anatomy of the large intestine is also central to the understanding of various pathologies of digestive wellness. Diseases such as colorectal cancer, inflammatory bowel diseases, and diverticulitis illustrate the clinical relevance of having a healthy large intestine. The development of effective screening technologies, including colonoscopies, makes it possible for early neoplastic mucosal changes of the colon to be recognized, ultimately leading to more favorable patient outcomes. Similarly, elucidated correlations between gut microbiota dysbiosis and inflammatory illnesses, as detailed in recent studies, underscore the importance of understanding the large intestine beyond anatomy. Further studies into the genetic and epigenetic determinants of gastrointestinal wellness are crucial, as it informs therapeutic interventions and prevention strategies crucial in controlling diseases common to the colon (Kastl et al., 2019).

6.3.1. Structure and Length of the Large Intestine

The colon or large intestine is one of the parts of the human gut, measuring approximately 1.5 meters in length, with its special structure. Unlike the small intestine, which consists of highly folded inner lining for optimal absorption of nutrients, the large intestine consists of a smoother surface with a wider lumen for fecal storage and compaction. The large intestine consists of different segments: the cecum, the ascending colon, the transverse colon, the descending colon, and the sigmoid colon. This segmentation is not only the result of functional differentiation but is also of crucial importance in the overall digestive process for water absorption as well as fermentation of unabsorbed nutrients by gut microbiota. The anatomy of the large intestine is suited to its primary function of reabsorbing water and salt from non-absorbable food content to avoid dehydration and to create solid wastes for excretion. Physiologically, the length of the large intestine constitutes a significant portion of the human gastrointestinal tract. The duration of the colon is long enough to absorb water and minerals from the rest of the contents that pass through it. In numerous studies, the colon has been shown to have extremely high numbers of microbial communities that aid in nutrient fermentation as well as synthesis of certain vitamins, like vitamin K. Fermentation is more obviously observed in the large intestine where transit time is slow enough to permit some extensive microbial contact with the substrate, and digestion and short-chain fatty acid production that is beneficial to the host. Gut microbiome balance between various microbial populations in the colon is necessary for which dysbiosis will lead to pathologic impacts on health, and hence optimum gut microbiome is a must (Kastl et al., 2019). Further, morphological characteristics of the large intestine, such as its typical *haustra* and *teniae coli*, enable it to satisfy its functional requirements. The *haustra* are pouch-like areas that allow segmentation contractions, which increase the migration and blending of material in the colon. The unique architecture maximizes the colon's ability to process waste products by peristalsis and storage. The *teniae coli* also—have three different bands of muscle, longitudinal—contribute to the colon's contractile activities and having a wider luminal diameter than the small intestine. This anatomic formation not only gives the large intestines a storage function but also ensures the removal of feces slowly, since the colon has a significant role in the human digestive process. Having this information regarding the structural and functional elements is important for the purpose of understanding the complex relationships of the gastrointestinal tract, particularly on the overall human health and nutrition (Hedvig E Jakobsson et al., 2014).

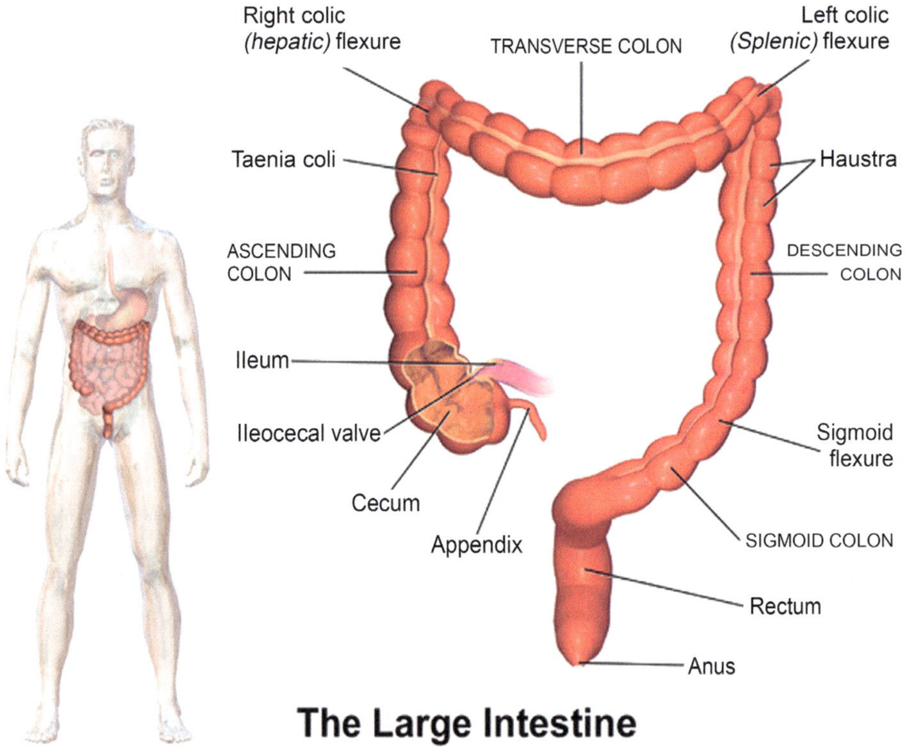

Figure 6.10. Structure of the large intestine.

Source: https://s3-us-west-2.amazonaws.com/courses-images-archive-read-only/wp-content/uploads/sites/1470/2015/11/04064738/600px-Blausen_0604_LargeIntestine2-1.png

6.3.2. Components: Cecum, Colon, Rectum, and Anus

The cecum is the initial section of the large intestine and is very important in digestion as it acts to connect the ileum, which is the terminal part of the small intestine, to the colon. The cecum is found at the bottom right part of the abdomen and is a reservoir of the chyme so that it can be passed on to further phases of digestion. It also includes an array of microorganisms that allow the fermentation of the unutilized food, particularly fiber. The appendix is a pouch that suspends from the cecum and has been the subject of considerable controversy regarding its function, even though newer research suggests that it may have some involvement in the immune system in providing a location for friendly gut bacteria to thrive. Conceptualizations of the cecum's various functions in immunity and digestion shed light on its various but underappreciated roles in the human gastrointestinal tract. Following on from the cecum, the colon is a highly structured and significant component of the large intestine, and consists of four major sections: the ascending, transverse, descending, and sigmoid colon. The overall function of the colon is to reabsorb water and electrolytes from undigested food residue left behind, thereby turning liquid waste into stool. The colon also plays a critical role in maintaining a healthy microbiome that enables fermentation, which produces some of the various short-chain fatty acids that benefit the health of the colon. As this region deals with waste, peristaltic movements allow sequential movement of contents, hence resulting in storage of fecal material until it is eliminated. Integrity of the colon is important because any change in function has the potential to result in constipation, inflammatory bowel disease, or colorectal cancer. Therefore, proper knowledge of the structure and operation of the colon is essential to deal with gastrointestinal health. Finally, the anus and rectum are the terminal digestive system organs responsible for the elimination of wastes from the body. The muscle tube, the rectum, stores feces, and the walls contain stretch receptors responsible for inducing a desire to have a bowel movement. Once the rectum is filled, the brain receives a signal to initiate the defecation reflex, which includes coordinated contraction of the rectal and abdominal muscles and relaxation of the anal sphincter. Control of fecal ejection and continence is managed by the anus, which is endowed with specific sphincter muscles. This fine control mechanism highlights the concordance between nervous messages and anatomy in intestinal health. Rectal and anal function abnormalities, such as one finds in conditions of hemorrhoids or fecal incontinence, reflect the significance of this system to one's health and demand further investigation into treatments that minimize these problems.

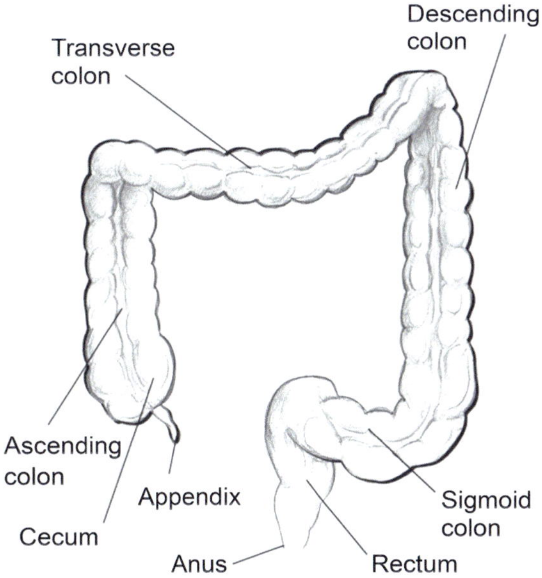

Figure 6.11. Large intestine with labels for the appendix, cecum, ascending colon, transverse colon, descending colon, sigmoid colon, rectum, and anus.

Source: https://www.niddk.nih.gov/media-assets/18248/N01651-H_thumbnail.jpg?imbypass=true

6.3.3. Differences Between the Large and Small Intestines

Anatomical variations of the small and large intestines form the foundation of understanding their varied physiological functions in human digestion. The small intestine, subdivided into three parts—duodenum, jejunum, and ileum—is roughly 20 feet in length and smaller in diameter compared to the large intestine. The main function of the small intestine is nutrient absorption, facilitated by a highly folded inner lining composed of villi and microvilli that greatly expand its surface area. Conversely, the 5-foot-long, wider-diameter large intestine is tasked with the absorption of water and electrolytes, and the formation and expulsion of feces. The specially designed shapes of such intestines support their respective functions and point to how intestinal shape is suitable for its digestive purpose in the human body. Histological differences also point to the functional differences of the small and large intestines.

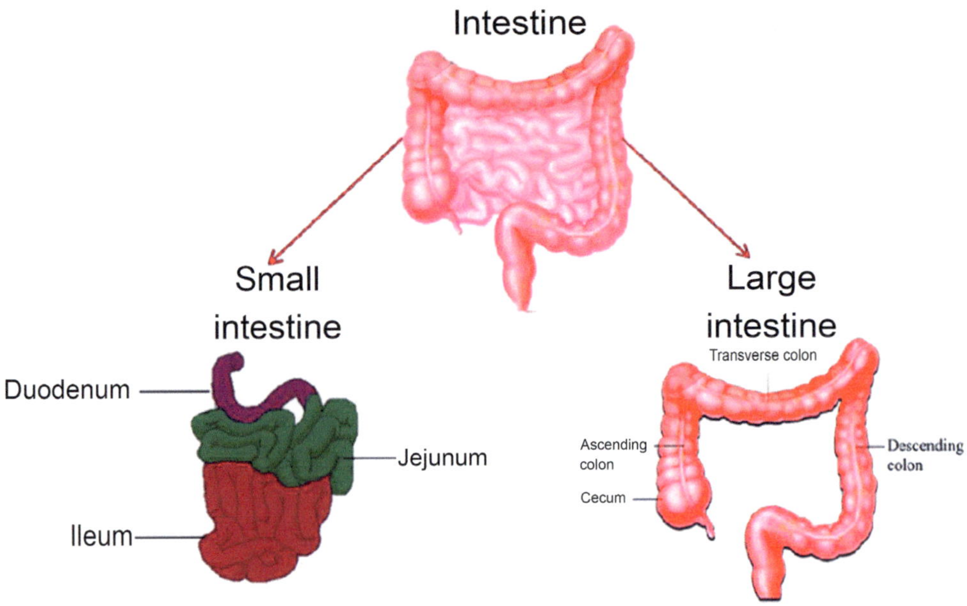

Figure 6.12. Difference Between Small Intestine and Large Intestine.

Source: https://www.careerpower.in/blog/wp-content/uploads/sites/2/2023/09/11101703/instestines.png

The mucosa of the small intestine contains numerous crypts of Lieberkühn and intestinal villi, enhancing the absorption of nutrients by increasing the surface area and the efficiency of the surface. The small intestine also accommodates specialized cells, such as enterocytes and goblet cells, for the absorption of nutrients and the secretion of mucus. Conversely, the large intestine is a less complex structure with fewer villi, and its mucosa has numerous goblet cells that secrete mucus to lubricate fecal matter. This structural adaptation is efficient in the reabsorption of water, and the constitution of waste as food residues are transformed into solid waste. The histological characteristics of each segment are such that they are tailored to optimize their respective digestive process, effectively connecting the structure and function of the intestines. When people get older, different physiological processes may affect the functioning of the intestines, especially in the large intestine. Studies have shown that neuromuscular processes in the colon can decrease with age, particularly in the ascending colon, leading to altered muscle contractions and relaxation responses (Ahmed et al., 2018). This is an important point to highlight since it may have the potential to affect digestive efficiency and bowel health among older populations. Also, operations on the intestines, such as resection, can highlight the nuanced differences in how the large and small intestines adapt. Short bowel syndrome, because of extensive intestine removal, for instance, highlights the vital roles these intestines play in nutrient absorption and metabolic support (Aguilar Diosdado et al., 2015). Knowledge about age-related and surgical effects on intestinal function is vital for creating guidelines to meet gastrointestinal health in heterogeneous patient populations.

Test Your Knowledge

1. What is the length of the large intestine?
2. What are the components of the large intestine?

6.4. Function of the Large Intestine

Learning Outcome

1. Describe the role of small intestine in water absorption and electrolyte balance
2. Describe the formation and storage of feces
3. Understand the role of gut microbiota in digestion

The large intestine, or colon, is an important component of the digestive system that primarily performs water absorption and stool formation. The terminal segment of the gastrointestinal tract, it breaks down the remnants of digested food that are delivered to it from the small intestine. The small intestine absorbs the majority of nutrients, leaving behind undigested matter and liquids. The large intestine absorbs approximately 1.5 liters of water per day, ensuring the body has the required fluids. This reaction is also essential since dehydration can cause significant complications. Furthermore, colon mucus lubricates the stool, allowing it to move through the digestive system. The functioning of the large intestine is hence key to maintaining homeostasis within the human body and making its contribution to health vital. Other than absorption, the large intestine also harbors gut microbiota that are responsible for a number of physiological processes. The trillions of microbes that make up the gut microbiome are responsible for the fermentation of unabsorbed carbohydrates, with the short-chain fatty acids being beneficial to the colon. Fatty acids can provide energy to colonic cells and support immune function. The equilibrium of these microbial communities is essential, with dysbiosis—gut flora imbalance—possibly resulting in diseases such as inflammatory bowel disease and irritable bowel syndrome. The interaction of food components and gut microbiota reflects the complexity of gastrointestinal health, that is, specialized functions of the large intestine beyond waste elimination. The intricate interaction of gut health and the large intestine highlights its vital role in human health. Besides, the large intestine plays a part in regulating inflammatory processes, albeit more towards chronic stress and diseases like colorectal cancer. Recent research highlights the interconnections between stress, inflammation, and cancer development, which suggest that neuropeptide signaling pathways play a significant role in regulating these interactions. Chronic stress can induce inflammatory responses with the capacity to stimulate the development of colorectal cancer, the large intestine is not only a passive waste reservoir but actively participates in systemic signaling and disease resistance.

These kinds of discoveries regarding immunological functions of the large intestines enhance avenues for targeted therapies. Through the understanding of these mechanisms, it may become possible to develop tailored strategies for disease prevention and treatment related to the large intestine's function, such as learning how conditions are treated as explained in Baritaki et al. (2019) and Linson (2013).

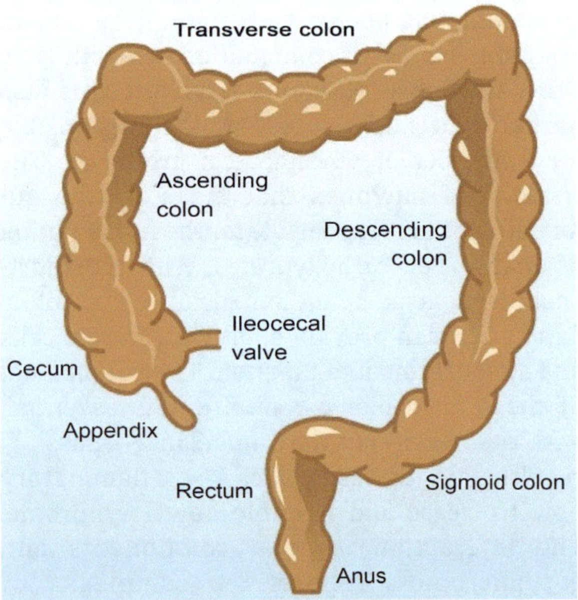

Figure 6.13. Large intestine function.

Source: https://www.sciencelearn.org.nz/_next/image?url=https%3A%2F%2Fwww.datocms-assets.com%2F117510%2F1722387142-the-large-intestine20161028-31233-ta0k1b.jpg%3Fw%3D1840%26h%3D1226.6666666666665&w=1920&q=85&dpl=dpl_4n9pVfrF4H6vbtWLHqt8okXU1ahu

6.4.1. Water Absorption and Electrolyte Balance

The small intestine is a key location of water reabsorption and electrolyte homeostasis, a dynamic site where approximately 90% of fluid ingested is reabsorbed. This extensive reabsorption occurs through various mechanisms, predominantly active transport and osmosis of specialized epithelial cells, including enterocytes. These transporters contain multiple transporters, which selectively reabsorb sodium, chloride, and potassium ions, which are crucial for the body's electrolyte balance. Proper hydration and proper balance of these electrolytes not only sustain cellular processes but are also essential to the organism's overall physiological homeostasis. Disruptions in this balance can result in disorders like dehydration or electrolyte imbalance, which have a dramatic effect on one's health. The process of absorption of these is increasingly found to be controlled by gut microbiota and their metabolites, which can potentiate or modulate active transport systems, outlining the intricate relationship between microbiota and gut functions, as observed by Ghosh et al. (2021). As the process of digestion proceeds to the large intestine, water continues to be absorbed, though less intensely than in the small intestine. The principal function of the large intestine is the recovery of water and electrolytes from undigested food material and the formation of solid waste as a consequence. Through the action of colon cells, specifically those lining the large intestinal lumen, much water is recovered into the blood by osmosis. It is a function that must be carefully regulated to see that the body has sufficient fluid and electrolytes and removes waste. Moreover, the secretion of potassium, hydrogen ions, and bicarbonate by colonic epithelium is of vital significance in acid-base balance, an element of homeostasis. The interaction between the absorption function of the large intestine and electrolyte regulation is therefore fundamental to digestive health, impacting constipation and diarrhea, and hence of utmost clinical significance. There is increasing evidence to indicate that gut microbiota is involved in the mechanisms that regulate water and electrolyte balance in the small and large intestine. The gut microbiome impacts both gut barrier function and intestinal motility, influencing the manner in which water and electrolytes are absorbed. Other microbial products, such as short-chain fatty acids produced by fiber fermentation, have been shown to enhance intestinal epithelial well-being and to play a role in water absorption. Dysbiosis—abnormality of normal microbial flora—can also disrupt these functions and lead to disease states of inflammatory bowel disease or irritable bowel syndrome, both of which have a significant impact on water and electrolyte homeostasis. Understanding these microbial interactions contributes to explaining the potential therapeutic interventions directed towards gut health restoration and, thus, enhanced water and electrolyte balance within the body, as elaborated in Cryan et al., (2019).

6.4.2. Formation and Storage of Feces

The construction of feces is one of the critical functions of the large intestine, particularly in human digestion. Upon arrival of chyme, the moist bulk of undigested food in the large intestine, it comes under forced alteration due to both absorption and microbial activity. Water absorption becomes essential at this stage because almost 90% of the water present in the chyme gets absorbed and thereby hardens the material. This dehydration process is aided by the various components of the large intestine, which include the cecum, colon, and rectum. The complex relationship between the gut microbiota and the host also aids in the fermentation of undigested carbohydrate, producing gases and short-chain fatty acids that play critical roles in intestinal health. Being aware of all these mechanisms describes the necessity of an equilibrium gut flora to provide optimal fecal formation along with avoidance of gastrointestinal diseases, sounding familiar with information from (Brinkman et al., 2015). Fecal material is stored mainly in the rectum, which serves as a reservoir before elimination. The rectum is structured so that it can accommodate expanding volumes without impairing bowel function. Sensory stimuli sent by the rectal wall trigger defecation when the storage capacity is reached, which indicates the strong communication between the central nervous system and the gastrointestinal tract. The neural feedback system is vital for the regulation of the timing of defecation so that the expulsion of feces happens at socially acceptable times and in an individual's comfort. Effective storage and subsequent disposal also rely on the unimpaired working of the anal sphincters, which are voluntarily responsible for letting feces out. The ideal balance in such physiological processes is important for digestive health and overall well-being because any dysfunction can lead to conditions such as constipation or fecal incontinence. Apart from the physiological process of feces formation and storage, lifestyle and diet are also crucial determinants of these processes. The nature of the diet taken directly affects the properties of feces, including bulk and consistency. Having a high-fiber diet is not only beneficial for free defecation but also maintains the gut microbiota healthy, which in turn strengthens the fermentative activities involved in fecal production. Conversely, excessive consumption of processed foods can reduce fecal bulk and even result in gastrointestinal issues. Recent studies emphasize the importance of holistic nutrition approaches that take into consideration these dynamics, with the potential implication being that interventions directed towards the gut may have impacts transcending the digestive realm. The intersection between diet, microbiome function, and fecal creation suggests the interrelatedness of body systems, as described in texts on nutrition and gastrointestinal anatomy, e.g., as reported by Cherian (2020).

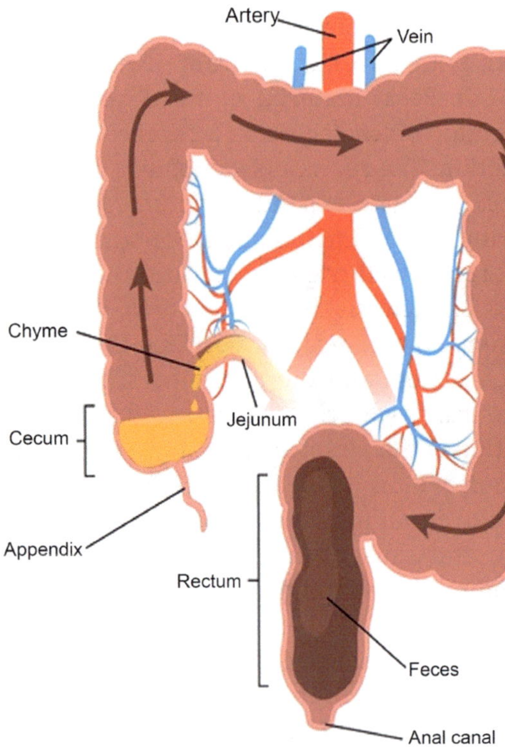

Figure 6.14. Formation of feces and defecation.

Source: https://www.shutterstock.com/image-vector/digestive-process-formation-feces-defecation-600nw-492260707.jpg

6.4.3. Role of Gut Microbiota in Digestion

The intricate interplay between gut microbiota and digestion is a prominent function of the human gastrointestinal system, particularly in the small and large intestines. Microbiota, composed of trillions of microorganisms, collaborates with the host to increase nutrient absorption and metabolic processes. In the small intestine, for instance, they assist in the breakdown of food complex carbohydrates by fermentation to give rise to short-chain fatty acids that are used as a source of energy by intestinal epithelial cells. Besides augmenting nutrient assimilation, the process further aids in intestinal lining integrity. Furthermore, the microbiota is capable of influencing digestive enzymes and the metabolism of bile acids to ensure that fat in the diet is emulsified and absorbed appropriately, thus resulting in maximum energy derived from food substrates. The gut microbiota's multifunctions highlight its pivotal role in ensuring digestive competence and metabolic homeostasis. While food transits to the large intestine, the function of the gut microbiota becomes still more critical. Here, the microbial group assists in the fermentation of unabsorbable fiber and defends against pathogens to develop a balanced microbiome that prevents gastrointestinal disorder. Dysbiosis, or any imbalance of the balance among this microbial population, may lead to many health problems, such as inflammatory bowel disease, obesity, and irritable bowel syndrome. It is critical to identify the individual microbial populations residing in the large intestine, as they synthesize vitamins needed by the host, such as vitamin K and certain B vitamins, thereby supporting the host's nutritional status. Furthermore, the circadian fluctuation in daily dietary intake significantly influences microbial populations, proving that food choices play a direct part in dictating gut function and overall well-being. An exploration of such interactions can provide insight into therapeutics aimed at the gut microbiome to improve digestion and health outcomes. Gut microbiota impact digestion through interaction with the immune system and hormone responses. Microbiota have been found to interact with the host through a plethora of routes, including the production of microbial metabolites, which possess the capacity to modulate immune status as well as impact appetite control. For instance, certain short-chain fatty acids originating from microbiota have been reported to enhance the release of gut hormones that play a role in satiety, hence regulating weight. In addition, the microbiota-gut-brain axis is a fascinating area of research, as new findings indicate that gut microbiota can influence mood and cognitive processes by influencing the central nervous system.

This bidirectional communication highlights the importance of an ideal microbiome in not only gut health but also overall physiological processes. Therefore, the health of gut microbiota becomes essential for digestive efficiency as well as overall homeostasis of the human body (John F Cryan et al., 2019; Kastl et al., 2019).

Test Your Knowledge

1. What is water and electrolyte absorption in the small intestine?
2. What is role of gut microbiota in digestion?

6.5. Common Disorders of the Small Intestine

Learning Outcome

1. Know the celiac disease and its impact on absorption
2. Describe the Crohn's disease and inflammation
3. Describe the intestinal infections and their effects

The small intestine is a common organ for digestion and nutrient uptake, but it is susceptible to a variety of disorders that can play a significant role in overall health. The most common disorders of the small intestine are celiac disease, Crohn's disease, and irritable bowel syndrome (IBS). Celiac disease is an autoimmune illness in which the ingestion of gluten leads to inflammation and injury to the intestinal lining, malabsorption of nutrients, and a broad array of symptoms, including diarrhea, weight loss, and weakness. Crohn's disease, a type of inflammatory bowel disease (IBD), can affect any part of the gastrointestinal tract but most commonly affects the small intestine. This chronic condition is mediated by inflammation that can lead to dangerous complications, including strictures and fistulas, which require close management by the physician. Understanding of these conditions is essential for adequate treatment and a favorable long-term outcome. In addition to autoimmune and inflammatory diseases, the small intestine can also be affected by functional disorders such as irritable bowel syndrome (IBS), manifested by abdominal pain, bloating, and altered bowel habits. Unlike Crohn's disease and celiac disease, IBS does not cause primary injury of the intestine but is believed to be linked with dysregulation of gut-brain interactions and modulation of gut motility. The pathophysiology of IBS is still unclear, but evidence in recent times suggests that the gut microbiota could be central in the pathogenesis of symptoms. The host-microbiota interactions have the potential to influence immunity, metabolism, and even psychological health, emphasizing the complexity of gut function (Willem M de Vos et al., 2022). Other conditions with a functional basis, such as small intestinal bacterial overgrowth (SIBO), potentially complicate clinical presentation by causing symptoms that can simulate IBS and once more emphasize the value of an integrated diagnostic approach. Moreover, nutritional practices and external environment exposures are also involved in the causation of small intestine illnesses. For instance, regular consumption of processed meals containing heavy metals like toxins cadmium and lead has been linked with gastrointestinal disturbances and can aggravate diseases like IBS and IBD (Balali M-Mood et al., 2021). The metal body burden can inhibit cellular function in the small intestine, leading to oxidative stress and chronic health problems. Hence, knowledge of the intricate interplay of diet, exposures, and gut health is necessary to formulate prevention strategies and targeted treatment. This integrated model for small intestine disorders will ultimately result in improved patient outcomes and an increased quality of life for individuals with these disorders.

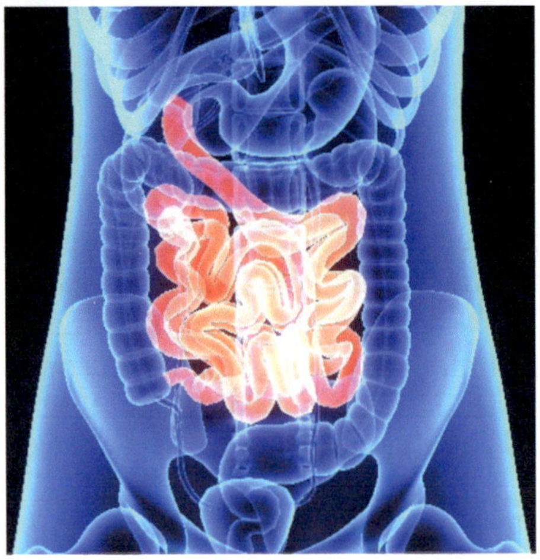

Source: https://medlineplus.gov/images/Malabsorption Syndromesand SmallIntestine Diseases_share.jpg

6.5.1. Celiac Disease and Its Impact on Absorption

Celiac disease, a condition where the immune system of the body responds to gluten, a protein found in wheat, barley, and rye, significantly transforms the usual function of the small intestine. When the immune system comes in contact with gluten, upon consumption, it leads to inflammation in the intestinal lining. Inflammation flattens and damages the villi, finger-shaped structures responsible for nutrient absorption. Therefore, the small intestine is severely hampered in the uptake of nutrients, and a variety of deficiencies like iron, calcium, and vitamins D and B12 result. The abnormal absorption also manifests its clinical presence in presentations of anemia, osteoporosis, and retardation of growth in children, proving the core role of the small intestine in nutrition. With the need for proper intake of nutrients for overall well-being, the damaging effects of celiac disease validate the physiological function of the small intestine (Borgen, 2020). In addition to disrupting celiac disease's pathophysiology and causing faulty nutrient intake, the pharmacokinetics of oral drugs are also affected. Anatomy that has been disrupted by celiac disease in the intestines can affect drug absorption such that the bioavailability of therapeutic drugs becomes unreliable. This instability creates a question of the effectiveness of medication, as delivery of active constituents can be impaired by reduced surface area for absorption. Drug metabolism variability can even occur with untreated celiac disease due to malabsorption-related deficiencies of intestinal enzymes and transport.

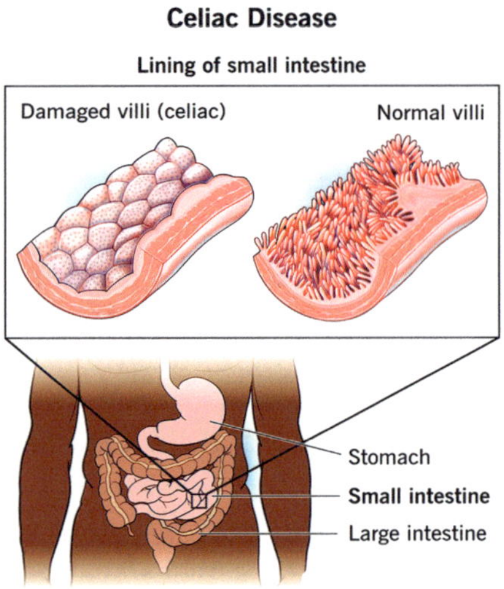

Figure 6.15. Celiac disease erodes the lining of your small intestine.

Source: https://my.clevelandclinic.org/-/scassets/Images/org/health/articles/14240-celiac-disease

Therefore, those prescribing medication to this group should have knowledge of the effect of celiac disease on drug absorption since individualized therapeutic effects might be required (Basit et al., 2018). Secondly, management of celiac disease by adherence to a gluten-free diet highlights the significance of knowledge on nutritional aspects of the autoimmune condition. Though the following diet significantly lessens symptoms and regularizes bowel function, the long-term impact on absorption and nutritional levels should be carefully monitored. Patients must learn to find safe sources of food that are compatible with dietary restrictions but also facilitate securing adequate levels of essential nutrients. Health care professionals also should offer nutrition supplementation as necessary to prevent deficiency, especially in basic nutrients that are usually absorbed in the intestine. The intricate impact of celiac disease on absorption thus necessitates stringent management programs that consider both nutritional compliance and counseling (Borgen, 2020).

6.5.2. Crohn's Disease and Inflammation

Crohn's disease is an idiopathic chronic inflammatory bowel disease (IBD) predominantly affecting the gastrointestinal tract, with particular predilection for the terminal ileum and areas of colon. It is a disease that can have intermittent periods of inflammation, causing symptoms such as abdominal pain, diarrhea, and malnutrition. The pathophysiology of Crohn's disease is multifactorial in nature with complex interaction between environmental factors and genetic predispositions, eventually leading to an immune system imbalance. This exaggerated immune reaction finally destroys the integrity of the intestinal barrier, resulting in increased intestinal permeability, which is otherwise referred to as leaky gut. Not only do these alterations allow for toxin and pathogen translocation into systemic flow, but they also induce chronic inflammation, which may increase the disease symptoms and complications (Camilleri, 2019). To the clinical management of Crohn's disease is also added the requirement of correcting the nutritional deficit that often results from the malabsorption associated with chronic inflammation. Inflammatory injury to mucosal integrity interferes with the absorption of nutrients. Additionally, the role of lifestyle and dietary factors in modulating inflammatory responses has gained more attention among scientists and researchers. Certain dietary interventions, such as the incorporation of anti-inflammatory foods and probiotics, can reverse barrier function and decrease inflammation. How effective these interventions are remains controversial. Because Crohn's disease can present differently in various individuals, personalized dietary approaches could be valuable as adjunct therapy for inflammation and overall gut health management (Vancamelbeke and Vermeire, 2017).

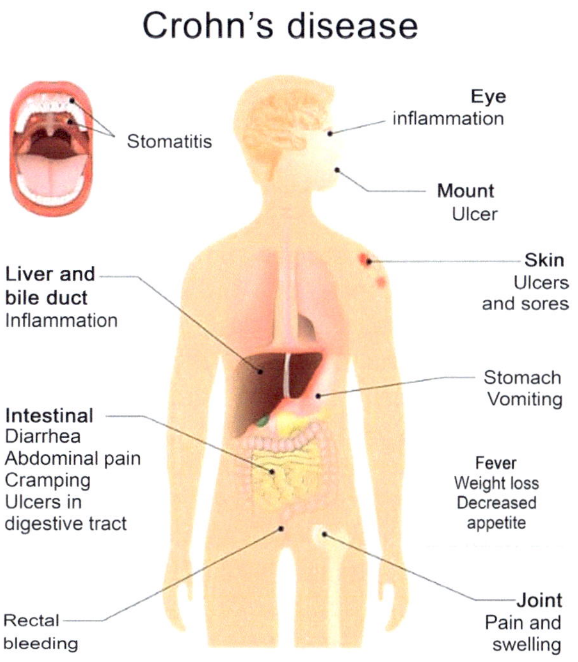

Figure 6.16. Crohn's disease.

Source: https://www.gastrolondon.co.uk/wp-content/uploads/crohns-disease.jpg

The relationship between inflammation and Crohn's disease extends beyond the gut, in the sense that systemic effects may result from chronic low-grade inflammation. It has been demonstrated that Crohn's patients may exhibit extra-intestinal manifestations, including arthritis, dermatologic conditions, and even an increased risk of colorectal cancer. Such systemic phenomena need more integrated treatment modalities than focal treatments. Current therapies, i.e., biologics, target the inhibition of single inflammatory pathways, thereby inhibiting intestinal and systemic inflammation. Yet the question is how to fully restore the integrity of the intestinal barrier, as normalization of barrier function has not yet been demonstrated to enhance the overall clinical manifestations of Crohn's disease (Camilleri, 2019). Consequently, further research into new therapeutic strategies focused on barrier repair and overall health is crucial to optimizing patient care in this disabling condition.

6.5.3. Intestinal Infections and Their Effects

Intestinal infections are an important component of gastrointestinal illness pathophysiology, with severe consequences for the integrity of the large and small intestines. Intestinal infections can be caused by a wide variety of pathogens, such as bacteria, viruses, and parasites, each capable of disrupting the normal functioning of the gut. The intestinal mucosal barrier, created by the strongly junctioned epithelial cells, offers a first line of defense against infection by microorganisms. However, once such pathogens breach this barrier, they induce increased permeability, also known as leaky gut, facilitating the translocation of harmful contents into the systemic circulation. The host is thus exposed to systemic inflammatory responses and a myriad of complications. Recent research suggests that the altered gut microbiota is primarily responsible for deciding the severity of infection and subsequent immune response, developing a complex interaction between the host, microbial flora, and disease severity (Ghosh et al., 2021). Intestinal infection has consequences extending beyond localized symptoms such as diarrhea and abdominal pain. Chronic infection may lead to chronic disease like inflammatory bowel disease (IBD), thereby expanding the already tenuous margin of gut microbiota and immune homeostasis. Infections produced by pathogenic strains like *Clostridium difficile*, for instance, can be most notorious for disrupting intestinal flora and leading to antibiotic-associated diarrhea and life-threatening colitis. By linking microbial composition to gut health, researchers have learned that dysbiosis, the imbalance between pathogenic and beneficial microorganisms, can complicate the course of various gastrointestinal infections. Understanding how infections manipulate microbial communities is central to the development of specific therapy to restore gut health and prevent long-term sequelae. A comprehensive management of intestinal infections can thus involve not only antimicrobial medication but also strategies for restoring microbiota (Willers et al., 2020). Host immune reactions are also very important during intestinal infections in determining the progress of the disease. The gut-associated lymphoid tissue (GALT) is very important in regulating immune reactions to pathogens without causing intolerance against harmless microbes and food antigens. In infections, gut immune cells, including macrophages and T regulatory cells, exhibit complex signaling networks that either lead to effective pathogen clearance or initiate intestinal inflammation and tissue damage. Interestingly, disturbances in immune regulation by maternal diet, infant microbial exposure, and genetics greatly influence susceptibility to infections as well as the magnitude of immune responses. Research has shown that dietary constituents, such as the S100 calcium-binding proteins present in the breast milk, are key in the development of the gut microbiota and immune system maturation, implying potential intervention pathways in high-risk groups (Ghosh et al., 2021).

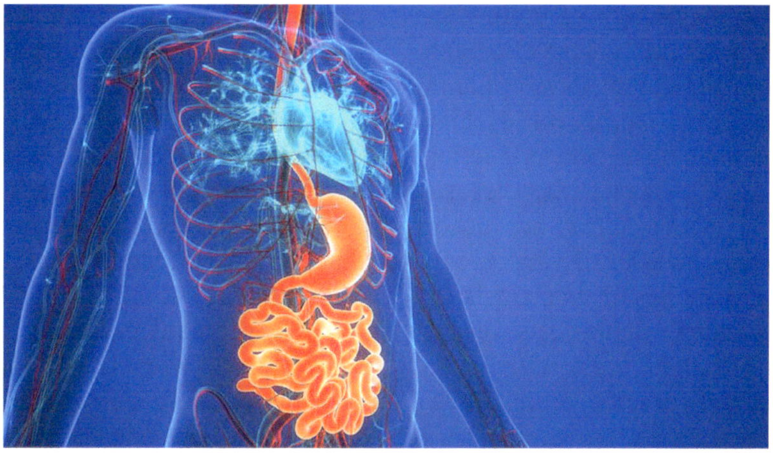

Figure 6.17. Intestinal infection.

Source: https://www.koruhastanesi.com/images/haber/main/10-intestinal-infection-symptoms-you-must-know-about-3086.jpg

Test Your Knowledge

1. How does celiac disease affect absorption?
2. What is Crohn's disease?

6.6. Common Disorders of the Large Intestine

Learning Outcome

1. Understand the irritable bowel syndrome (IBS)
2. Describe the colorectal cancer and risk factors
3. Know the diverticulitis and its complications

The large intestine, or colon, is a vital part of the human gut system whose prime function is the absorption of water and electrolytes and the fermentation of unabsorbed food material. It is nevertheless susceptible to a very broad spectrum of disorders, which can have very dire consequences for overall well-being and health. Among the most common illnesses are inflammatory bowel diseases (IBD), like Crohn's disease and ulcerative colitis, and irritable bowel syndrome (IBS). IBS is a disease of inflammation of the bowel with abdominal pain, bloating, and change of bowel habits, while IBD is a chronic inflammatory gastrointestinal tract disease. Such disorders are generally related to complex interactions of environmental, genetic, and microbial components and may result in over-inflammation and intestinal wall damage, like obstruction in the intestine or increased cancer risk in subsequent phases (Willem M de Vos et al., 2022). Colorectal cancer is another prevalent large intestine disorder, which has become a prominent global public health concern. It is most likely to be caused by adenomatous polyps, which become malignant if they remain undetected and unresected. Risk factors include age, genetic predisposition, nutrition, and inflammatory bowel conditions like IBD. Frequency and modality of screening, including colonoscopy, also have a role to play in achieving early diagnosis and survival. The gut-microbiome interface is progressively being identified in the etiology of colorectal cancer. Changes in gut microbiota have also been shown to be an element in tumor development, showing the part microbial communities play in maintaining gut homeostasis and impacting disease (Tilg et al., 2020). Diverticular disease, or diverticulosis and diverticulitis, are other common large intestine diseases. Diverticulosis is the growth of small pouches or diverticula on the colonic wall, a condition that affects a large percentage of elderly people. Most individuals are asymptomatic, but if infected or inflamed, diverticula cause diverticulitis, which can lead to abdominal pain, fever, and a change in bowel habit. Diverticular disease may be treated with dietary modification, including a high-fiber diet to make stool bulkier and prevent recurrence. Fresh information also indicates that gut microbiota may potentially influence the development and severity of diverticular disease, and it is possible to gain more knowledge about microbial interactions, which could be exploited in guiding therapeutic interventions in these common large intestine diseases (Willem M de Vos et al., 2022).

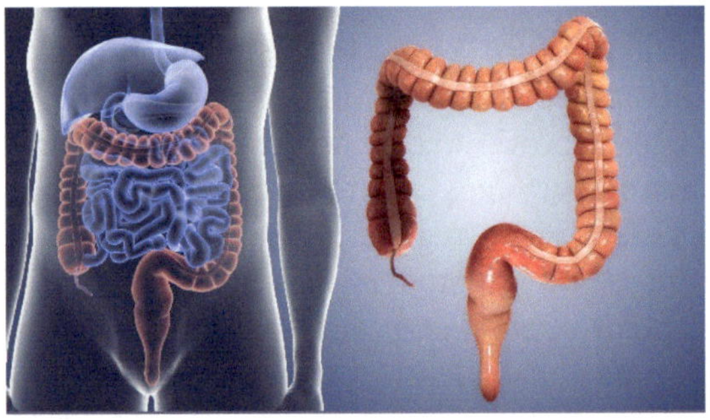

Figure 6.18. Large Intestine Disorders.

Source: https://www.scientificanimations.com/wp-content/uploads/2019/04/Large-Interstine.jpg

6.6.1. Irritable Bowel Syndrome (IBS)

The complexity of the human GI tract extends beyond anatomical features, as it also supports an enormous number of microorganisms whose function plays an important role in intestinal regulation. IBS is just one of those ailments whose dynamics are extremely entangled with gut microbiota and intestinal physiology. IBS patients typically report symptoms of abdominal pain, bloating, and altered bowel habits, which can be triggered or exacerbated by diet and stress. With reference to microbial imbalance, or dysbiosis, newer findings indicate that changes in the microbial communities within the gut can cause or worsen symptoms of IBS. This is in support of a requirement to understand the intricate interaction between host physiology and intestinal microbiome, agreeing with the data that intestinal microbial community participates in numerous gastrointestinal diseases, such as IBS, indicating the importance of gut health in overall well-being (Willem M de Vos et al., 2022). Gut barrier integrity is crucial in maintaining healthy digestive function and immune protection against pathogenic impact. In IBS patients, dysfunctional intestinal barrier function can be involved in increased intestinal permeability, so that pathologic substances can translocate to systemic circulation and cause inflammation. Through research, it has been determined that gut dysbiosis can amplify this barrier dysfunction, which increases the clinical presentation of IBS. Of particular interest, certain microbial metabolites produced during gut production can reinforce or compromise epithelial barrier integrity, engendering an inflammatory-dysfunction vicious cycle (Ghosh et al., 2021). As a result, this finding implies that therapeutic options for gut microbiota stabilization and improved barrier integrity may be key to controlling IBS symptoms, providing a more holistic solution for both microbial well-being and intestinal function. IBS treatment success is revealed by a multidimensional interaction between microbiological and physiological understanding. As gut conditions are better explained and transferred to IBS, new therapies such as dietary modification, probiotics, and fecal microbiota transplantation (FMT) are becoming increasingly popular. These would restore microbial balance and allow for improvement of gut barrier function, with hope for bettering IBS pathogenesis and symptoms. In addition, the recognition of individual gut-derived metabolites has provided further insight into the mechanisms through which diet and microbiome interactions impact IBS presentations. By taking an integrative approach to treatment with the interaction among gut microbiota, diet, and the physical integrity of intestinal barrier in mind, the scientists and doctors can develop more optimal treatment strategies for their patients suffering from this chronic condition (Willem M de Vos et al., 2022).

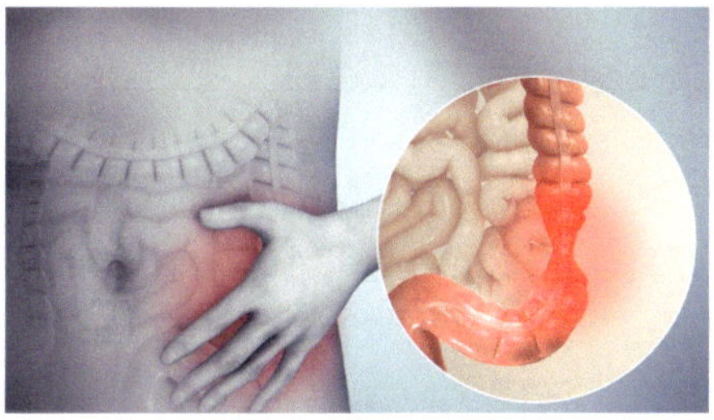

Figure 6.19. Irritable bowel syndrome.

Source: https://upload.wikimedia.org/wikipedia/commons/1/1a/Irritable_bowel_syndrome.jpg

6.6.2. Colorectal Cancer and Risk Factors

Colorectal cancer, or CRC, is a severe health concern whose development is influenced by a range of variables in today's society. Lifestyle, that is, diet and physical activity, is one of the most significant. Eating habits, such as high consumption of red and processed foods and low consumption of fruits and vegetables, respectively, have been reported to enhance the risk of developing colorectal cancers. Moreover, overweight and obesity indirectly lead to a higher risk of CRC by altering metabolic functions and promoting inflammation in the intestinal niche. They not only facilitate tumorigenesis but also initiate a dynamic interaction with the body's physiological response, which requires prevention strategies that promote a well-balanced diet and exercise to reduce the incidence of colorectal cancer. Chronic stress is more and more realized to play a role in disease development and progression in many diseases, including colorectal cancer. The pathophysiology of stress, inflammation, and cancer development is complex and not yet fully realized, but recent research suggests chronic stress may be an enhancer for inflammatory mechanisms that promote oncogenesis within the colorectal tract. Key modulators of stress responses, such as the corticotropin-releasing hormone family, influence cellular signaling pathways implicated in cancer development and inflammation. This connection underscores the importance of psychological and behavioral interventions as adjuncts to standard medical management, through the provision of a holistic approach to colorectal cancer prevention and treatment. Through such psychosocial determinants, there is a chance to enhance the effectiveness of CRC treatment protocols and overall patient outcome (Baritaki et al., 2019). Gut microbiota is also important in the risk for colorectal cancer, showcasing the intricate relationship between the kind of diet intake and the intestinal microbial makeup. Some bacteria within the intestines, along with some of the food processing methods, have the ability to cause toxins, leading to carcinogenesis. For instance, proteins such as chymotrypsin and subtilisin are involved in the breakdown of tumor suppressor proteins, and this offers a biochemical link between diet, risk of cancer, and tumor growth. In return, gut microbiota imbalance—typically due to excessive meat consumption—can evoke a microenvironment conducive to tumor growth. Conversely, a high intake of vegetables has protective effects, perhaps due to natural compounds that prevent harmful interactions triggered by gut bacteria. Understanding such non-genetic mechanisms of CRC susceptibility informs us of the best dietary interventions for cancer prevention (Darlington and Stone, 2017).

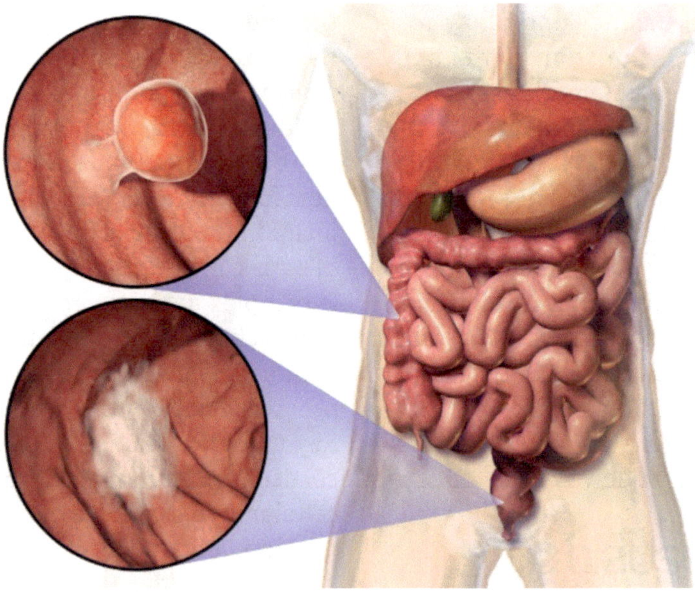

Figure 6.20. Colorectal cancer.

Source: https://upload.wikimedia.org/wikipedia/commons/1/12/Blausen_0246_ColorectalCancer.png

6.6.3. Diverticulitis and Its Complications

Diverticulitis is a consequence of the formation of diverticula—small pouches that develop in the wall of the colon, with the majority occurring in the sigmoid colon. The pouches are a direct consequence of elevated pressure within the colon, typically supplemented by factors such as low dietary fiber, obesity, and physical inactivity. When these diverticula become infected or inflamed, diverticulitis is established, which may lead to abdominal pain, fever, and irregular bowel movements. Diverticulitis's significance extends beyond its direct symptoms, as it may precipitate a number of complications that impair patients' overall well-being. It is significant to be aware of these associated risks because they are responsible for the morbidity and healthcare costs related to patients with this gastrointestinal condition. Complications of diverticulitis can range from mild to severe, one of the most concerning of which is the risk of abscess. An abscess occurs when localized infections that happen in the inflamed diverticula result in pus formation in the surrounding tissue. It is extremely painful and may require drainage or surgical drainage to address. Furthermore, diverticulitis may lead to fistulas, abnormally formed channels between the colon and neighboring organs, e.g., bladder or vagina, which further complicate treatment and worsen the condition of the patients. In severe cases, the perforation of the colon leads to the leakage of intestinal contents in the abdominal cavity, causing peritonitis—a sudden, life-threatening infection that requires prompt medical care. Chronic diverticulitis, such as recurrent episodes of inflammation, is a special problem in itself because it will often develop complications such as strictures or bowel obstruction. Inflammation may lead to narrowing of the bowel and blockage of the passage of stool, with resultant severe pain and necessitating surgical intervention, such as resection of the involved portions of bowel. Additionally, patients with a history of diverticulitis are at increased risk for colorectal cancer, thus the need for careful surveillance and preventive measures. The association of diverticulitis with such major complications once more underscores the need for healthcare professionals to enforce effective dietary and lifestyle changes, encouraging high-fiber consumption and physical exercise to ward off such diverticulitis-associated risks and maintain general gastrointestinal welfare (Tsung-Lee et al., 2023; Fahed et al., 2022).

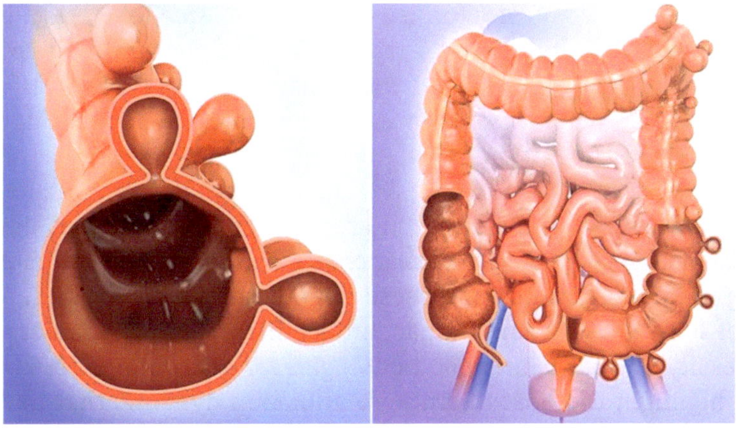

Figure 6.21. Diverticulitis complications.

Source: https://images.everydayhealth.com/images/digestive-health/diverticulitis/diverticulitis-progression-and-potential-complications-722x406.jpg?sfvrsn=21f5d58f_3

Test Your Knowledge

1. What is irritable bowel syndrome (IBS)?
2. What are the risk factors for colorectal cancer?

SUMMARY

Briefly, the intricate movements of the small and large intestines are significant to the sustenance of human health and to the passage of critical physiological processes. The small intestine, being the primary site for nutrient absorption and enzymatic digestion, plays a significant role in the immune system as well, best characterized perhaps in the field of scientific research into eosinophilic responses in the gastrointestinal tract. For example, research confirms the superior role of eosinophils as an anti-parasitic defense mechanism by showing the efficacy of their ability to destroy *Ascaris suum* larvae when administered with some antibodies (Chiers et al., 2013). This lends credibility to the central role of the small intestine not only in digestion but also in immune defense, attributing it a superior-level function beyond nutrient processing alone. Besides that, the large intestine is also important in intestinal microbiota modulation that directly relates to the health outcome. Increasingly, it is understood that changes in the gut microbiota can lead to a range of diseases, including inflammatory bowel disease and metabolic syndromes. Notably, conclusions from rodent models of self-reinoculation's impact on the microbiota contradict previous hypotheses and highlight the necessity of well-defined methodologies for microbiome research (Bogatyrev et al., 2019). Such findings highlight the host-microbe relationship dynamic that necessitates continued research in these dynamics in order to most effectively understand gastrointestinal health. It is partly true that the shared perception of the small and large intestines explains much about human physiology and disease processes. Both intestines have specific but interdependent functions that explain why gut health is important. The interplay between nutrient uptake, immune function, and microbiota equilibrium indicates the complexity of the gastrointestinal tract, thus inviting further study. Fill the loopholes in our understanding, especially those of the small intestine microbiome and their effects on human health, and it will lay the foundation for enhanced therapeutic practice and interventions. In the long run, it will contribute towards advancing our approach method towards understanding and treating a wide spectrum of gastrointestinal diseases.

The small intestine is a highly significant organ of digestion, particularly for nutrient assimilation. The 20-foot-long organ consists of three sections: the duodenum, jejunum, and ileum. To begin with, the liver bile and pancreatic digestive juices in the duodenum break down the food so that subsequently the food is absorbed as carbohydrates, proteins, and fats. The extensive surface area of the small intestine, through the development of villi and microvilli, enables it to maximize its capacity to be an effective transferor of these macronutrients and micronutrients into the bloodstream. Not only does this functional purpose alleviate the small intestine's involvement in nutrient integration, but it also illustrates how its wellness is directly linked to overall wellness. Any malfunction in this part can lead to malabsorption syndromes, stressing the importance of a healthy small intestine by adopting the right dietary and lifestyle choices. On the other hand, the large intestine or colon has a distinct yet very crucial role in human digestion. The primary role of water and electrolyte absorption is that the large intestine breaks down liquid waste into solid waste, which can be eliminated. The colon itself contains a symbiotic group of microbes that aid in the fermentation of unused carbohydrates and the production of vital vitamins such as Vitamin K and some of the B vitamins. Furthermore, the large intestine is a reservoir of gut microbiota and a principal function is to ensure gut integrity and immune status. The interaction of diet, gut microbiota, and the water and nutrient absorption potential of the colon is reflected in the importance of the organ within the entire digestive system. Consequently, what is known about what happens in the large intestine can yield information that is beneficial for dietary management with respect to gut health. The small and the large intestines are highly interdependent on each other, and their malfunction will have critical effects on the other. For instance, an imbalance in gut microbiota in the large intestine may be triggered by poor eating habits to cause gastrointestinal symptoms, inflammation, or disease like irritable bowel syndrome. It has also begun to investigate the contribution of eating habits and regular food consumption, such as gastrophagy, to intestinal microbial diversity modulation. Studies have found that eating prey digestive content may be a widespread tradition among Arctic Indigenous peoples, resulting in a richer gut microbiota composition that optimizes gut health and immunity against most diseases (Bj Mørn Bjørnsen et al., 2024). Urbanization also affects the diet, and this is reflected in the gut microbiota of various species, including humans (Jason L Anders et al., 2021). Multidimensionality herein implies the need for a holistic understanding of both intestines to advance overall health and prevent gastrointestinal disease.

KEY TERMS FROM THIS CHAPTER

- Amino acids
- Anus
- Bloodstream
- Carbohydrates
- Cecum
- Colon
- Colorectal cancer
- Duodenum
- Fatty acids
- Ileum
- Jejunum
- Large intestine
- Microvilli
- Minerals
- Monosaccharides
- Proteins

CRITICAL THINKING QUESTIONS

1. **The small intestine is divided into which three segments?**
   a. Duodenum, jejunum, ileum
   b. Cecum, colon, rectum
   c. Esophagus, stomach, duodenum
   d. Pylorus, jejunum, colon
2. **The primary function of the small intestine is:**
   a. Water absorption
   b. Nutrient digestion and absorption
   c. Protein storage
   d. Fat emulsification
3. **The part of the small intestine where most chemical digestion occurs is:**
   a. Duodenum
   b. Jejunum
   c. Ileum
   d. Colon
4. **The primary function of the large intestine is:**
   a. Digestion of proteins
   b. Absorption of water and electrolytes
   c. Nutrient absorption
   d. Secretion of bile
5. **The first part of the large intestine is called the:**
   a. Cecum
   b. Colon
   c. Rectum
   d. Sigmoid

Short Answer Questions

1. What is the small intestine length?
2. What are the roles of villi and microvilli in nutrient absorption?
3. What are the functions of the small intestine?
4. What is the structure of the large intestine?
5. What is the difference between large and small intestines?

Answer to Critical Thinking Questions

1. (a) 2. (b) 3. (a) 4. (b) 5. (a)

REFERENCES

1. Adlercreutz, H., Aherne, S., Aps, J. K. M., Armand, M., Armand, M., Armand, M., et al. (2014). *In vitro* models for studying secondary plant metabolite digestion and bio accessibility. https://core.ac.uk/download/pdf/70607414.pdf (accessed on 15th June 2025).
2. Aguilar Diosdado, M., Camacho Ramírez, A., Lechuga Sancho, A. M., Prada Oliveira, D., et al. (2015). A surgical model of short bowel syndrome induces a long-lasting increase in pancreatic beta-cell mass. https://core.ac.uk/download/161360305.pdf (accessed on 15th June 2025).
3. Ahmed, S., Broad, J., Carroll, R., Chin-Aleong, J., et al. (2018). Changes in neuromuscular structure and functions of human colon during ageing are region-dependent. https://core.ac.uk/download/161396574.pdf (accessed on 15th June 2025).
4. Aldewachi, H., Carey, F. W., Carey, D., Cramp, C., Helmstetter, C., Diamond, J., Diaz, S., et al. (2006). Postprandial morphological response of the intestinal epithelium of the Burmese python (*Python molurus*). http://arxiv.org/abs/q-bio/0611019 (accessed on 15th June 2025).
5. Anders, J. L., Mychajliw, A., Moustafa, M. M., Mohamed, W., Hayakawa, T., Nakao, R., & Koizumi, I. (2021). Dietary niche breadth influences the effects of urbanization on the gut microbiota of sympatric rodents. *Ecology and Evolution, 12*. https://www.semanticscholar.org/paper/cc2879f2695b2e14b32eb5ee65fe86f61d299cd9 (accessed on 15th June 2025).
6. Balali-Mood, M., Naseri, K., Tahergorabi, Z., Khazdair, M. R., & Sadeghi, M. (2021). Toxic mechanisms of five heavy metals: Mercury, lead, chromium, cadmium, and arsenic. *Frontiers in Pharmacology, 12*. https://doi.org/10.3389/fphar.2021.643972 (accessed on 15th June 2025).
7. Ball, G. F. M. (2021). *Vitamins: Their Role in The Human Body.*
8. Baritaki, S., Chatzaki, E., de Bree, E., Pothoulakis, C., et al. (2019). Chronic stress, inflammation, and colon cancer: A CRH system-driven molecular crosstalk. https://core.ac.uk/download/323076588.pdf (accessed on 15th June 2025).
9. Basit, A. W., Hatton, G. B., Madla, C. M., Rabbie, S. C., et al. (2018). All disease begins in the gut: Influence of gastrointestinal disorders and surgery on oral drug performance. https://core.ac.uk/download/195304393.pdf (accessed on 15th June 2025).
10. Bjørnsen, M. B., Valerón, N. R., Vásquez, D. P., Velasco, E. M., Hansen, A. J., & Hauptmann, A. (2024). Microbiota in the ptarmigan intestine—An Inuit delicacy and its potential in popular cuisine. *PLOS ONE, 19*. https://www.semanticscholar.org/paper/59cb5cdaddfdb2874cbc62a9dc61b3ec4f028f9c (accessed on 15th June 2025).
11. Bogatyrev, S. R., Ismagilov, R. F., & Rolando, J. C. (2019). Self-reinoculation with fecal flora changes microbiota density and composition leading to an altered bile-acid profile in the mouse small intestine. https://core.ac.uk/download/287633428.pdf (accessed on 15th June 2025).
12. Bordoni, A., Dupont, D., Gille, D., Kachalova, M., et al. (2015). Understanding the gastrointestinal tract of the elderly to develop dietary solutions that prevent malnutrition. https://core.ac.uk/download/286575279.pdf (accessed on 15th June 2025).
13. Borgen, A. (2020). Health related effects of wheat varieties. https://core.ac.uk/download/323144679.pdf (accessed on 15th June 2025).

14. Brimberry, D., Leite, G., Pimentel, M., Barlow, G., & Mathur, R. (2024). Obesity and beyond: The novel technical standard to study the small bowel microbiome. *Archives of Gastroenterology Research*. https://www.semanticscholar.org/paper/6e57841aafd782728614ff1ef4dd5cb0805ca28e (accessed on 15th June 2025).

15. Brinkman, B., De Vos, M., Laukens, D., Raes, J., et al. (2015). Heterogeneity of the gut microbiome in mice: Guidelines for optimizing experimental design. https://core.ac.uk/download/55846318.pdf (accessed on 15th June 2025).

16. Camilleri, M. (2019). Leaky gut: Mechanisms, measurement and clinical implications in humans. *Gut, 68*, 1516–1526. https://doi.org/10.1136/gutjnl-2019-318427 (accessed on 15th June 2025).

17. Cherian, G. (2020). *A Guide to The Principles of Animal Nutrition*. https://core.ac.uk/download/622361034.pdf (accessed on 15th June 2025).

18. Chiers, K., Geldhof, P., Masure, D., Van Den Broeck, W., et al. (2013). A role for eosinophils in the intestinal immunity against infective *Ascaris suum* larvae. https://core.ac.uk/download/55807127.pdf (accessed on 15th June 2025).

19. Chirwa, L. C., Cumming, D. R. S., Hammond, P. A., Roy, S., et al. (2003). Electromagnetic radiation from ingested sources in the human intestine between 150 MHz and 1.2 GHz. https://core.ac.uk/download/1393541.pdf (accessed on 15th June 2025).

20. Cryan, J. F., O'Riordan, K. J., Cowan, C. S. M., Sandhu, K. V., Bastiaanssen, T. F. S., Boehme, M., Codagnone, M. G., et al. (2019). The microbiota-gut-brain axis. *Physiological Reviews, 99*, 1877–2013. https://doi.org/10.1152/physrev.00018.2018 (accessed on 15th June 2025).

21. Darlington, L. G., & Stone, T. W. (2017). Microbial carcinogenic toxins and dietary anti-cancer protectants. https://core.ac.uk/download/80696830.pdf (accessed on 15th June 2025).

22. de Vos, W. M., Tilg, H., Van Hul, M., & Cani, P. D. (2022). Gut microbiome and health: Mechanistic insights. *Gut, 71*, 1020–1032. https://doi.org/10.1136/gutjnl-2021-326789 (accessed on 15th June 2025).

23. Edwards, C. H., Grundy, M. M. L., Holland, C., Ryden, P., et al. (2020). Plant cell walls: Impact on nutrient bio accessibility and digestibility. https://core.ac.uk/download/287579488.pdf (accessed on 15th June 2025).

24. Elefson, S. K. (2019). *Developmental Changes in the Pig from Birth to 42 Days Post-Weaning (1.5–25 Kilograms Bodyweight)*. https://core.ac.uk/download/270036319.pdf (accessed on 15th June 2025).

25. Fahed, G., Aoun, L., Bou Zerdan, M., Allam, S., Bou Zerdan, M., Bouferraa, Y., & Assi, H. (2022). Metabolic syndrome: Updates on pathophysiology and management in 2021. *International Journal of Molecular Sciences, 23*, 786–786. https://doi.org/10.3390/ijms23020786 (accessed on 15th June 2025).

26. Ghosh, S., Whitley, C. S., Haribabu, B., & Jala, V. R. (2021). Regulation of intestinal barrier function by microbial metabolites. *Cellular and Molecular Gastroenterology and Hepatology, 11*, 1463–1482. https://doi.org/10.1016/j.jcmgh.2021.02.007 (accessed on 15th June 2025).

27. Homayun, B., Lin, X., & Choi, H. J. (2019). Challenges and recent progress in oral drug delivery systems for biopharmaceuticals. *Pharmaceutics, 11*, 129–129. https://doi.org/10.3390/pharmaceutics11030129 (accessed on 15th June 2025).

28. Jakobsson, H. E., Rodríguez-Piñeiro, A. M., Schutte, A. H., Ermund, A., Boysen, P., Bemark, M., Sommer, F., et al. (2014). The composition of the gut microbiota shapes the colon mucus barrier. *EMBO Reports, 16*, 164–177. https://doi.org/10.15252/embr.201439263 (accessed on 15th June 2025).

29. Kamyshinsky, R., Khmelnitsky, L., Kalepu, R., Elad, N., & Fass, D. (2024). Cryo-EM structure of the HD6 defensin helical assembly. *BIO Web of Conferences*. https://www.semanticscholar.org/paper/bf3ecdc29ffa7edbf317ab3412e7488e25d0befa (accessed on 15th June 2025).

30. Kastl, A., Terry, N. A., Wu, G. D., & Albenberg, L. (2019). The structure and function of the human small intestinal microbiota: Current understanding and future directions. *Cellular and Molecular Gastroenterology and Hepatology, 9*, 33–45. https://doi.org/10.1016/j.jcmgh.2019.07.006 (accessed on 15th June 2025).

31. Keckstein, J., Sarıdoğan, E., Ulrich, U., Sillem, M., Oppelt, P., Schweppe, K. W., Krentel, H., et al. (2021). The #Enzian classification: A comprehensive non-invasive and surgical description system for endometriosis. *Acta Obstetrician et Gynecological Scandinavica, 100*, 1165–1175. https://doi.org/10.1111/aogs.14099 (accessed on 15th June 2025).

32. Kline, R. C. (1988). *Horse Nutrition*. https://core.ac.uk/download/286359521.pdf (accessed on 15th June 2025).

33. Lee, T. C., Staller, K., Botoman, V., Pathipati, M. P., Varma, S., & Kuo, B. (2023). ChatGPT answers common patient questions about colonoscopy. *Gastroenterology, 165*, 509–511.e7. https://doi.org/10.1053/j.gastro.2023.04.033 (accessed on 15th June 2025).

34. Linson, E. A. (2013). *The Interplay Between Hormones and Irritable Bowel Disease*. https://open.bu.edu/bitstream/2144/12149/6/Linson_Elyse_2013_nosig_nocv.pdf (accessed on 15th June 2025).

35. Nagtegaal, I. D., Odze, R. D., Klimstra, D. S., Paradis, V., Rugge, M., Schirmacher, P., Washington, K., et al. (2019). The 2019 WHO classification of tumors of the digestive system. *Histopathology, 76*, 182–188. https://doi.org/10.1111/his.13975 (accessed on 15th June 2025).

36. Ribeiro, A., Gonçalves, R. F. S., Pinheiro, A. C., Manrique, Y. A., Barreiro, M. F., Lopes, J. C. B., & Dias, M. M. (2021). *In vitro* digestion and bio accessibility studies of vitamin E-loaded nanohydroxyapatite Pickering emulsions and derived fortified foods. *LWT, 154*, 112706–112706. https://doi.org/10.1016/j.lwt.2021.112706 (accessed on 15th June 2025).

37. Silva, Y. P., Bernardi, A., & Frozza, R. L. (2020). The role of short-chain fatty acids from gut microbiota in gut-brain communication. *Frontiers in Endocrinology, 11*. https://doi.org/10.3389/fendo.2020.00025 (accessed on 15th June 2025).

38. Thelin, W. (2024). The development of human primary culture models to model inflammatory signaling in Crohn's disease and ulcerative colitis. *Inflammatory Bowel Diseases*. https://www.semanticscholar.org/paper/1408802230105e26ecb829c017b456a03963304f (accessed on 15th June 2025).

39. Tilg, H., Adolph, T. E., & Moschen, A. R. (2020). Multiple parallel hits hypothesis in nonalcoholic fatty liver disease: Revisited after a decade. *Hepatology, 73*, 833–842. https://doi.org/10.1002/hep.31518 (accessed on 15th June 2025).

40. V'kovski, P., Kratzel, A., Steiner, S., Stalder, H., & Thiel, V. (2020). Coronavirus biology and replication: Implications for SARS-CoV-2. *Nature Reviews Microbiology, 19*, 155–170. https://doi.org/10.1038/s41579-020-00468-6 (accessed on 15th June 2025).

41. Vacca, M., Celano, G., Calabrese, F. M., Portincasa, P., Gobbetti, M., & De Angelis, M. (2020). The controversial role of human gut *Lachnospiraceae*. *Microorganisms, 8*, 573–573. https://doi.org/10.3390/microorganisms8040573 (accessed on 15th June 2025).

42. van der Hee, B., & Wells, J. M. (2021). Microbial regulation of host physiology by short-chain fatty acids. *Trends in Microbiology, 29*, 700–712. https://doi.org/10.1016/j.tim.2021.02.001 (accessed on 15th June 2025).

43. Vancamelbeke, M., & Vermeire, S. (2017). The intestinal barrier: A fundamental role in health and disease. *Expert Review of Gastroenterology & Hepatology, 11*, 821–834. https://doi.org/10.1080/17474124.2017.1343143 (accessed on 15th June 2025).

44. Willers, M., Ulas, T., Völlger, L., Vogl, T., Heinemann, A. S., Pirr, S., Pagel, J., et al. (2020). S100A8 and S100A9 are important for postnatal development of gut microbiota and immune system in mice and infants. *Gastroenterology, 159*, 2130–2145.e5. https://doi.org/10.1053/j.gastro.2020.08.019 (accessed on 15th June 2025).

45. Yang, K., Li, G., Li, Q., Wang, W., Zhao, X., Shao, N., Qiu, H., et al. (2025). Distribution of gut microbiota across intestinal segments and their impact on human physiological and pathological processes. *Cell & Bioscience, 15*. https://www.semanticscholar.org/paper/a9993a3b328f29d539e1a8246bc1a899f4e74dda (accessed on 15th June 2025).

LIVER

7

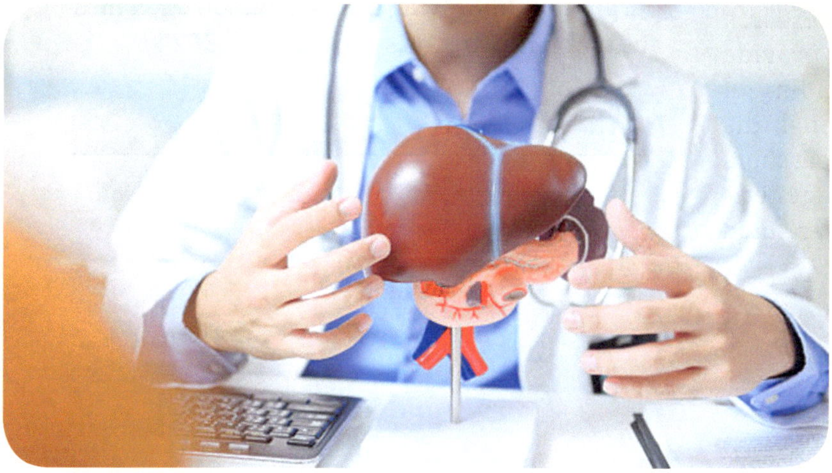

LEARNING OBJECTIVES

After studying this chapter, you will be able to:

1. Understand the anatomy of the liver
2. Describe the functions of the liver
3. Learn about liver diseases
4. Describe the liver health and maintenance
5. Learn about liver transplantation

Introduction

The liver is a critical organ of human biology, renowned for serving multiple functions including metabolic control, detoxification, and synthesis of proteins required. Its complex anatomy allows it to serve varied biochemical processes, and therefore, its health is critical for the general well-being of human health. The liver's job is to take the nutrients we take in from what we eat and process them into chemicals that our bodies use for energy and growth while simultaneously filtering out poisons that can settle in the bloodstream. Beyond basic biology, understanding how the liver works is essential to understanding how lifestyle, genetics, and the environment contribute to liver well-being. Therefore, an observational eye into the livers working can provide valuable information on disease prevention and control within the liver, as well as therapeutic innovations for diseases such as fatty liver disease and hepatitis that exert a significant influence on public health in aggregate. Research has provided insights into several aspects of liver health, including the dramatic prevalence of liver disorders throughout the world. Liver fat content changes, for instance, have been demonstrated to impair liver function, leading to conditions that are detrimental to human health. Recent investigations on Atlantic salmon have shed light on phenotypic, genetic, and transcriptomic shifts in liver fat deposition, a testament to the growing fascination with metabolic processes similar to those in human livers. It is important to understand that liver health is integrally connected to the way the body metabolizes fat and carbohydrate. This research is not only relevant to fish but can provide analogies that enhance our understanding of metabolic syndromes in humans. Through the identification of such relationships, researchers could potentially be able to detect genetic upgrades and treatments to resist liver-related illnesses (Horn et al., 2025).

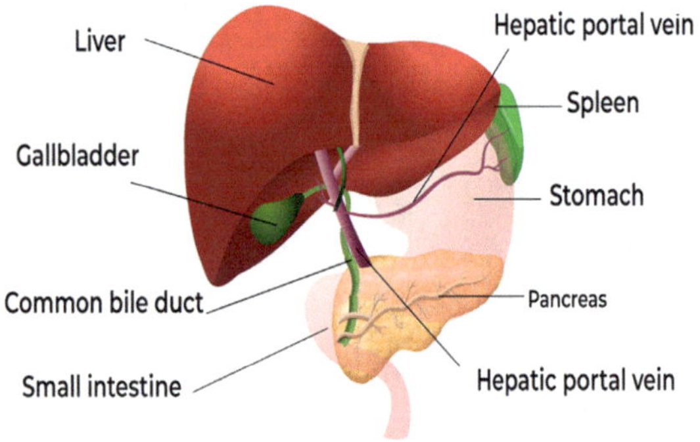

Figure 7.1. Diagram of Liver.

Source: https://media.geeksforgeeks.org/wp-content/uploads/20240305155402/diagram-of-live.png

The significance of early allograft function in liver transplantation is another key research area that points to the complexity of the liver. The link between anesthetic agents and early poor graft function (IPGF) has encouraged good studies towards strengthening better outcomes in pediatric liver transplants. It has been researched that the anesthetic agent applied during donor hepatectomy is responsible for the incidence of IPGF, and that preconditioning routines could advance graft survival rates. Conclusions from such research highlight the extent to which preoperative status can influence post-transplant liver function, establishing the need for greater examination of the surgical process and its impact. Lastly, the contribution of the liver to such a case once again establishes its position as a non-replaceable organ, as well as the worth of optimizing its function for the purposes of improving transplantation outcomes and patient prognosis (Dieu et al., 2024).

7.1. Anatomy of the Liver

Learning Outcome

1. Describe the location and size of the liver
2. Understand the lobular structure and blood supply
3. Know the livers relationship with other organs

The liver, located in the upper right part of the abdominal cavity, performs numerous basic functions integral to the mechanism of homeostasis maintenance. Its unique anatomical structure, with a double circulation from the hepatic artery and the portal vein, highlights its role in processing nutrients and detoxifying harmful substances.

The liver is divided into lobes, the largest of which is the right lobe, subdivided into smaller functional units known as lobules. The lobules are based around a central vein and consist of hepatocytes, the predominant cell involved in the organ's diverse functions, including protein synthesis, bile secretion, and carbohydrate and lipid metabolism. This complex anatomy not only permits its multi-dimensional functions but also illustrates the relevance of understanding liver diseases, which can interfere with these essential processes and lead to systemic disease. Within the liver's complex architecture, one of its most pervasive aspects is the biliary system, which has an important role in the transport of bile, a substance crucial for emulsification and absorption of fats. Bile is secreted by hepatocytes and is stored in bile canaliculi, which drain into larger bile ducts. The common bile duct results from the joining of these larger ducts and ultimately drains into the duodenum. This functional anatomy points not only to the liver's metabolic function but also to its contribution to digestion. Dysfunction of the biliary system, either by obstructions or liver diseases such as cholestasis, can give rise to severe complications, illustrating the liver's linkage with the overall condition in the body. Having a good understanding of the anatomy of the liver is thus important in the clinical setting, where the knowledge allows diagnosis and management of certain hepatic diseases. The liver's anatomical importance also extends to its unparalleled regenerative capacity among human organs. Whenever the liver is diminished by injury or resection to a portion of itself, the remaining hepatocytes possess the unique ability to grow and regenerate, replacing the organ's bulk and function. This has significant implications for liver surgery and liver transplantation, as partial hepatectomy can yield excellent outcomes due to the liver's ability to regenerate. This capacity is not indefinite, however; chronic liver damage from conditions such as cirrhosis or hepatitis can thwart this healing process with profound implications for the health of the organ. Therefore, identification of the anatomy of the liver's regenerative capacity is important in therapy planning and the management of liver pathologies. As we move into the liver within human health, it becomes clear that its anatomy is not merely a lifeless construct but a dynamic one mirroring the resilience and adaptability of the organ in the face of adversity (Smith et al., 2005) (Chaviano et al., 2017).

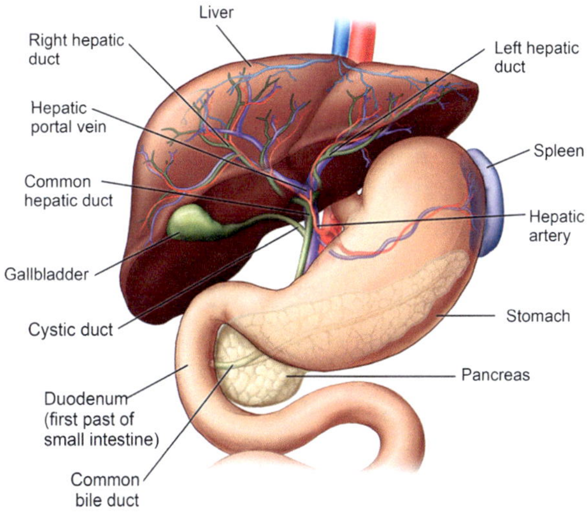

Figure 7.2. Anatomy of the Liver

Source: https://www.hopkinsmedicine.org/-/media/images/health/1_-conditions/liver-gallbladder-and-pancreas/liver-anatomy.png

7.1.1. Location and Size of the Liver

Within the human body, the liver is mostly situated within the right upper quadrant of the abdominal cavity, inferior to the diaphragm. It lies in front of the right kidney and is partially shielded by the rib cage. The location of the liver allows it to effectively process the intake of nutrients from the gastrointestinal tract, which enters in the hepatic portal vein. This positioning is vital because of its various metabolic functions, including the synthesis of plasma proteins and the detoxification of certain metabolites. The physiological positioning within the abdominal cavity is also imperative in the liver's accessibility to medical procedures, such as biopsies or imaging. A strong understanding of the positions of the livers is necessary for medical professionals to prevent complications in surgeries and provide efficient patient care (Bart van der Hee et al., 2021). In terms of size, the liver is one of the largest solid organs in the human body, weighing approximately 1.5 kilograms in adults. The liver is about 15 to 20 centimeters long and 20 to 25 centimeters in width, and roughly the same size as a football. Its enormous size is a reflection of the organ's complex metabolism, immune-related functions, and detoxification processes. Variability in the size of the liver is caused by factors such as age, sex, and possible internal disease conditions like liver disease or metabolic syndromes. For instance, patients with fatty liver disease may show enlargement of the liver (hepatomegaly), while in other ailments, there may be a reduction in size (atrophy) (Bart van der Hee et al., 2021). This great variability in the size of the liver is essential for its round-the-clock functioning and ability to adapt to evolving body physiological needs. Its location and size not only influence its physiological functions but also are of importance for disease mechanisms. Since liver tumors are one of the most prevalent forms of cancer, knowledge of their anatomy is of great importance to both the diagnosis and treatment regimen. Tumors can arise in various locations throughout the liver, and discrimination between abnormal and normal tissue is essential in treatment planning. The development of imaging technology, for example, the use of sophisticated convolutional neural networks (CNNs) for liver tumor segmentation from computed tomography (CT) scans, has improved the accuracy of liver diagnosis (Meng et al., 2019). As the liver's complex structure and location increase challenges in tumor detection, better segmentation techniques will lead to earlier diagnosis and improve patient care with early intervention, emphasizing the liver's inherent role in human well-being.

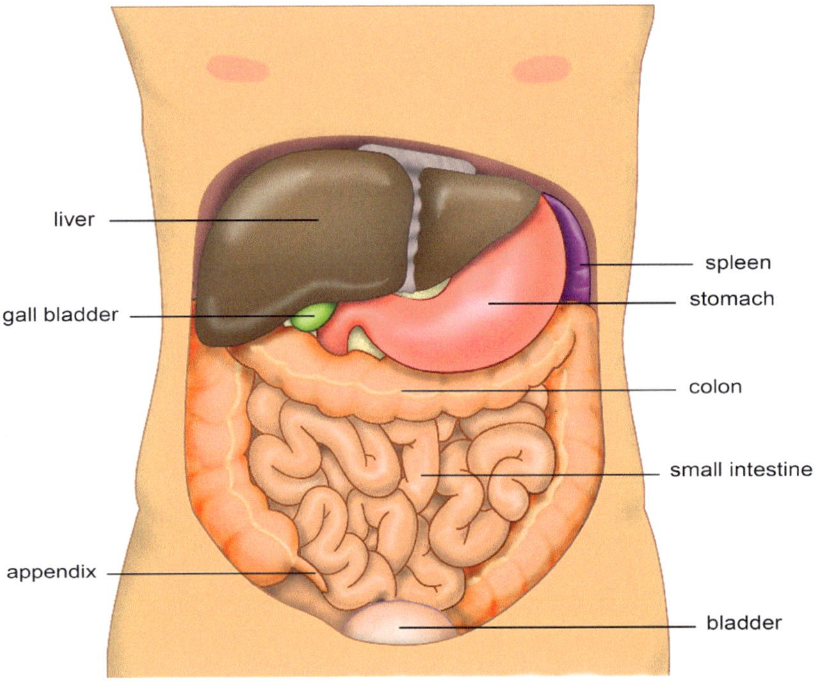

Figure 7.3. The human liver is located in the upper right abdomen.

Source: https://upload.wikimedia.org/wikipedia/commons/1/15/Anatomy_Abdomen_Tiesworks.jpg

7.1.2. Lobular Structure and Blood Supply

Lobular structure of the liver's anatomy plays a critical role to its processes of bile secretion, detoxification, and multi-functionality of metabolism. A liver lobule is created by a portal triad that includes a portal vein, hepatic artery, and bile ducts, and collectively plays a role in controlling the blood supply to the liver and bile secretion. The liver lobule is organized in hexagonal patterns with the hepatic cells or hepatocytes radiating from a central vein. This arrangement allows for effective exchange and processing of materials. The structure allows for oxygen and nutrient supply to hepatocytes and the removal of wastes. In addition, its unique lobular organization enables it to compartmentalize various metabolic functions, thereby ensuring optimal efficiency in liver function. Its perfusion is unique and recalls its role as a mid-point in ensuring metabolic homeostasis. Approximately 75% of the liver perfusion is through the portal vein with nutrient-supplied blood from the gastrointestinal tract, and the remaining 25% through the hepatic artery with oxygenated blood. This dual-blood circulation system is important because it allows the liver to metabolize absorbed toxins and nutrients before entering systemic circulation. The dual sources of blood talk to each other in liver sinusoids, fenestrated capillaries that form a route of material exchange between hepatocytes and blood. Due to the dual supply, the liver can regulate blood glucose appropriately, catering for the synthesis of proteins required, and detoxifying hazardous substances, which points to its central position in the human body. The importance of blood supply and lobular pattern is also given in pathological findings like cirrhosis or hepatitis, which can negatively affect healthy bloodstream and lobular pattern and lead to abnormal operation of the liver. For instance, fibrosis will replace normal liver tissue with fibrous tissue, which will then influence the gradient of blood flow and thus hinder nutrition processing as well as detoxification ability. Further, the severely distorted lobular structure can lead to complications like portal hypertension, in which increased pressure in the portal vein impedes blood supply and circulation. Understanding the sensitive interaction between the liver's vascular supply and the lobular structure is critical in diagnosing and treating liver disease since these components have a great role in maintaining liver's physiological integrity and overall health.

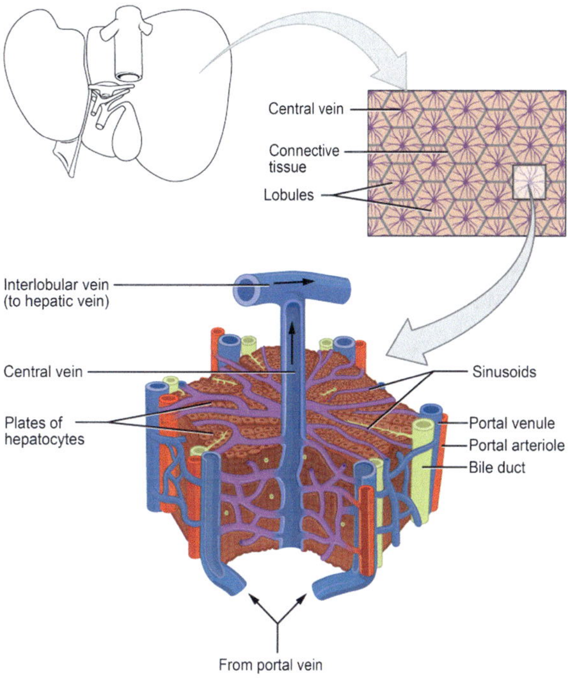

Figure 7.4. The structure of the liver's functional units or lobules. Blood enters the lobules through branches of the portal vein and hepatic artery proper, then flows through sinusoids.

Source: https://upload.wikimedia.org/wikipedia/commons/b/b7/2423_Microscopic_Anatomy_of_Liver.jpg

7.1.3. Relationship With Other Organs

The interaction of the liver with the other organs is essential in maintaining metabolic homeostasis within the human body. As the centralized organ for metabolic processes, the liver interacts with the gut and kidneys through a complex network of transporters and enzymes that are specialized in organ-to-organ communications. Synthesis and secretion of liver bile acids allow intestinal bacteria to hydrolyze fats, and bile acids are signaling molecules that regulate liver function and fat metabolism. Notably, gut microbiota influences the liver through the release of metabolites having the potential to influence liver disease and health and showing the intricate dependence of this organ on the gastrointestinal system. The coordinated harmony between the liver and the intestines enables optimal nutrient uptake and the release of toxic substances, an essential component of overall metabolic balance. Of course, in addition to its relationship with the gut, the complex communication of the livers with the kidneys is essential in order to maintain body fluid and electrolyte equilibrium. The gut-liver-kidney (GLK) network operates through a set of transporters known as SLC and ABC transporters, which are involved in the absorption, distribution, metabolism, and elimination (ADME) of endogenous and exogenous compounds. Besides this, regulation at the gene level through transcription factors such as HNF4α and PXR also plays an important role in modulating transporters and enzymes for proper inter-organ communication. As research has established, interference in this web of interconnectivity can lead to severe health issues, such as kidney disease and liver failure, which illustrate the importance of maintaining this relationship. Understanding the GLK network thus clarifies the processes underlying organ interactions and their influence on homeostasis. Its metabolic functions also extend to its interaction with other principal organs that handle the immune response. By synthesizing acute-phase proteins and regulating the metabolism of immune cells, the liver is central to the body's defense mechanism. Its interaction with lymph nodes and spleen is particularly vital because the liver cleanses blood by removing pathogens and dead cells, thus playing a critical role in immune surveillance. Also, the liver serves as a site for the activation and differentiation of immune cells, once more linking metabolic activity with the immune function. This demonstrates how the liver not only serves as a metabolic organ but also as a part of the immune system itself, and thus why global understanding of organ relationships is so essential to health and the prevention of disease.

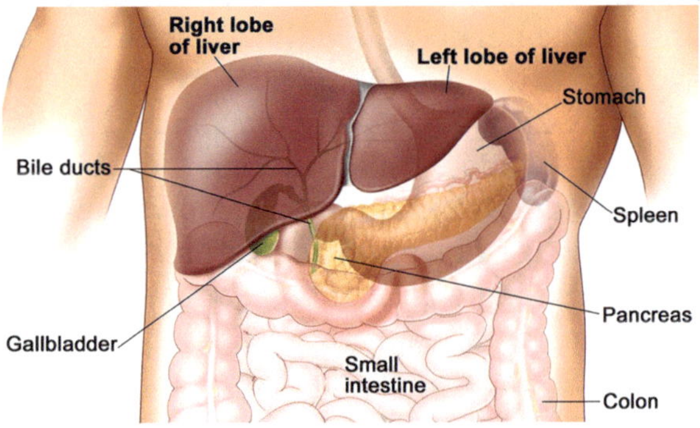

Figure 7.5. Liver anatomy: position of the liver and neighboring organs within the thoracic cage.

Source: https://www.researchgate.net/profile/Francois-Chung/publication/245002843/figure/fig1/AS:650038304862275@1531992617623/Liver-anatomy-a-position-of-the-liver-and-neighboring-organs-within-the-thoracic-cage.png

Test Your Knowledge

1. What is the blood supply of the liver lobule?
2. How is the liver connected to other organs?

7.2. Functions of the Liver

Learning Outcome

1. Describe the metabolism of carbohydrates, proteins, and fats
2. Know the detoxification of harmful substances
3. Understand the production of bile and its role in digestion

The liver is a versatile organ that plays a significant role in homeostasis in the human body. Detoxification of harmful substances such as metabolic waste, drugs, and toxins entering the blood is one basic function. Hepatocytes, the functional cells of the liver, have the special capacity to metabolize these substances, making them less toxic or to excrete them via bile or urine. In severe liver failure, an extracorporeal liver support device (ELSD) has the ability to replicate detoxifying functions, virtually serving as a substitute for the liver until recovery occurs or a transplant is required. This technology confirms the liver's immense regenerative capacity as its healing potential is the premise for such replacement therapy, and therefore it is critical to understand liver functions and therapies in modern medicine (Al-Chalabi et al., 2016). The liver also plays a pivotal role in regulating metabolic processes, particularly in carbohydrate and lipid metabolism. The liver plays an active role in glucose homeostasis by storing excess glucose as glycogen and releasing it into the bloodstream when the body needs it, a process regulated by hormones. This regulatory function becomes increasingly significant in the setting of metabolic disease, such as nonalcoholic fatty liver disease (NAFLD), where macrophages in the liver and other cell types experience robust changes that modulate insulin sensitivity and lipid metabolism. Derangements in normal liver physiology have the potential to lead to fat accumulation and eventually provide a mechanism for severe complications such as fibrosis and cirrhosis. Consequently, an integrated understanding of liver metabolism and its applicability to obesity disease is pivotal in developing effective interventions (Barreby, 2023). Also, the liver's critical role in protein synthesis impacts overall health. It produces essential proteins, such as albumin and clotting factors, which help maintain oncotic pressure and facilitate blood coagulation, respectively. Albumin is a vehicle for many compounds in the blood, facilitating the carrying of nutrients and fluids. In liver disease, decreased synthesis of these proteins may cause serious health problems, including swelling and increased susceptibility to bleeding. These functions indicate the liver's essential function in the body's normal processes and highlight the importance of maintaining the health of the liver through lifestyle and diet. Together, all these various functions illustrate the liver's complexity and important role in human physiology and therefore create the focal point of medical research and patient care strategy.

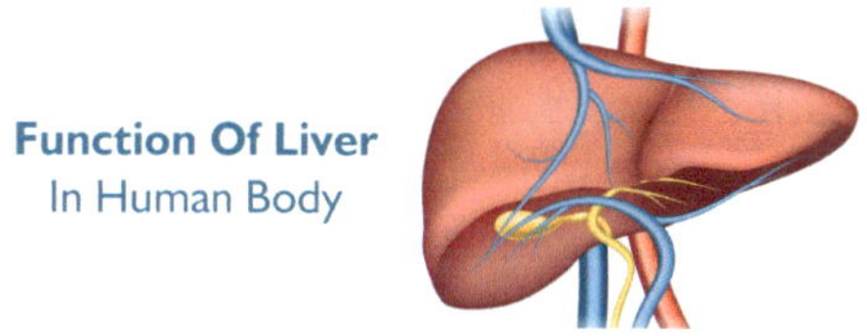

Figure 7.6. Function of the Liver in the Human Body.

Source: https://www.medicoverhospitals.in/images/articles/function-of-liver-in-human-body.webp

7.2.1. Metabolism of Carbohydrates, Proteins, and Fats

The liver is a metabolic hub for carbohydrates, lipids, and proteins, coordinating an intricate network of biochemical reactions to ensure energy homeostasis and regulate metabolic processes in the body. Most carbohydrates are metabolized glucose is converted to glycogen and stored in the liver to be used later. Glycogenolysis cleaves glucose into the bloodstream during fasting or increased energy demand. Apart from that, the liver is also involved in gluconeogenesis, where it makes glucose from non-carbohydrate precursors such as amino acids and glycerol. This bifunction ensures that the body tightly regulates blood glucose levels, with focus on the liver's essential function in carbohydrate metabolism and energy homeostasis, especially vital for metabolic well-being and disease avoidance, such as type 2 diabetes, which afflicts patients with nonalcoholic fatty liver disease (NAFLD; Rinella, 2023). Liver protein metabolism involves a range of processes that include nitrogenous amino acid synthesis and the urea cycle that eliminates ammonia derived during amino acid breakdown. The liver deaminates the surplus amino acids and metabolizes them to yield energy or glucose. This also highlights the liver's primary function of preventing waste accumulation of nitrogenous compounds because ammonia is converted to urea and then eliminated by the kidneys. The liver is also responsible for the production of numerous plasma proteins, such as albumin and coagulation factors, which help maintain oncotic pressure and hemostasis. Protein metabolic disturbances can have adverse effects on health, as seen through the concurrent presence of liver disease with nutritional alterations, muscle wasting, and immunodeficiency (Rinella, 2023). Liver fat metabolism is also important because it plays a role in the storage, synthesis, and degradation of fats. The liver also regulates oxidation of fatty acids and lipoprotein production, which are involved in lipid transport within the body. Under tight control, surplus proteins and carbohydrates are under the liver's ability to convert to fatty acids via de novo lipogenesis, the process most characteristically described in NAFLD and insulin resistance. Conversely, if the liver is subjected to an excess of fatty acids with obesity, this leads to steatosis and exacerbates lipid disorders. In addition, the liver centrally participates in the biosynthesis of crucial biochemicals such as cholesterol and bile acids that are important for fat digestion and dietary fatty food absorption. Therefore, it is critical to understand the liver's role in fat metabolism to improve the control of metabolic disorders and liver health(Tilg et al., 2020).

7.2.2. Detoxification of Harmful Substances

Human detoxification by the liver is a multifaceted and vital process, and its function is to rid the body of harmful substances. As the body's principal organ of detoxification, the liver is responsible for metabolizing toxins, drugs, and metabolic waste products of diverse kinds. This type of biotransformation is a two-step enzymatic process that metabolizes lipophilic substances into water-soluble, readily excretable forms via urine or bile. The efficacy of this detoxification is important against the backdrop of exposure of the liver to toxic agents, as this leads to damage of the liver and diseases such as cirrhosis. Thus, understanding the mechanisms of hepatic detoxication is important not only in an assessment of the probable effectiveness of drugs administered therapeutically but also in the planning of ways to oppose toxicity as a result of environmental poisons and other nasty chemicals, as highlighted in the instance of liver metabolism (Frojdenfal and Zuchowska, 2024). In addition, some toxins, such as ammonia, are especially challenging for the liver. Ammonia, a metabolic byproduct of protein, is of special importance as it is neurotoxic when it is sequestered in the blood. A necessary organ for the metabolism of ammonia into urea, which is then excreted harmlessly, is the liver. Recently developed information from animal models revealed that exposure to higher levels of ammonia triggers numerous pathological reactions in liver tissue. For instance, gene expression analysis has revealed massive upregulation of apoptotic and inflammatory genes, suggesting that hyperammonemia can compromise liver function through oxidative stress and cell death. The findings point to the livers vulnerability to toxic injury and merit further investigation into its protective detoxification processes (Li et al., 2022). Here, progress in research methods and liver modeling is needed to further illuminate our understanding of detoxification processes. New approaches, such as organ-on-a-chip technology, can be utilized to create in vivo-like conditions to study liver metabolism and detoxification. These models have the capability to mimic the liver's response to toxins and drugs accurately, and they provides new information regarding the efficacy and safety of pharmacologic drugs. Secondly, with a better understanding of how the liver's adaptation mechanisms in detoxifying toxins function, researchers are able to establish potential interventions that trigger healing or reduce harm. Not only do these methods predict improved therapeutic outcomes, but they also present opportunities for better strategies for dealing with the liver's role in detoxification and thus improving public safety and health (Frojdenfal and Zuchowska, 2024).

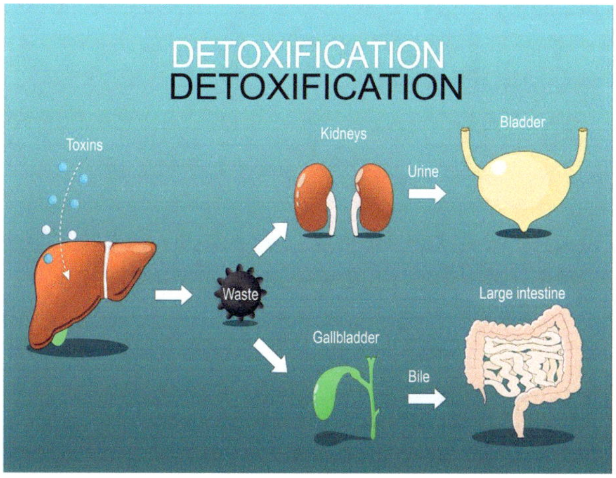

Figure 7.7. The liver detoxification process.

Source: https://www.detoxplusuk.com/wp-content/uploads/2024/10/detoxification-process-body-organs-diagram-1.jpg

7.2.3. Production of Bile and Its Role in Digestion

The liver plays a key role in bile production, a digestive fluid that is essential for the emulsification and absorption of dietary fats. Bile is comprised predominantly of bile acids, cholesterol, phospholipids, and bilirubin, which are synthesized by hepatocytes. During digestion, bile acids are excreted into the small intestine, where they induce lipids to break up into tiny micelles, becoming more easily absorbed into the intestinal lining. This function is important, since fats are a dense form of energy and essential fatty acids are necessary for various body functions. Also, the composition of bile is governed by dietary factors and intestinal flora, reflecting the liver's unifying function in digestion and metabolism beyond mere bile secretion. These interactions make the liver's role in overall digestive health and the intricate connection between the liver and other digestive organs more evident (Banerjee et al., 2023). Bile's role in digestion is not limited to emulsifying fat; it aids in the removal of body waste products. Bile is a vehicle for the removal of metabolic waste, drugs, and toxins like bilirubin, a product of heme catabolism. This is crucial in the context of liver function since an impaired liver will result in bile obstruction, resulting in toxic accumulation and liver failure. Interestingly, the enterohepatic cycle of bile acids, where they are reclaimed in the ileum and cycled back to the liver, shows the liver's capability to recycle such important molecules. Disruptions in this process can lead to conditions like cholestasis and other digestive disorders, demonstrating the importance of normal bile secretion and flow for digestive health and body homeostasis (Banerjee et al., 2023). Furthermore, bile production and excretion are stringently regulated by hormonal influences and neural mechanisms, a reflection of the liver's sensitivity to the body's physiological state. An example is the hormone cholecystokinin (CCK) released after food ingestion, which stimulates contraction of the gallbladder, allowing bile to be released into the small intestine. This type of control emphasizes bile production adaptability, which is extremely sensitive to the body's digestive needs. In addition, disturbances in bile production and circulation may have the capability to induce severe clinical implications, including the onset of liver disease and metabolic syndrome. The complexity of bile's involvement in digestion bolsters the multipurpose functions of the liver's in nutrient metabolism and expulsion of waste, reaffirming its central function in human physiology and health (Willem M de Vos et al., 2022).

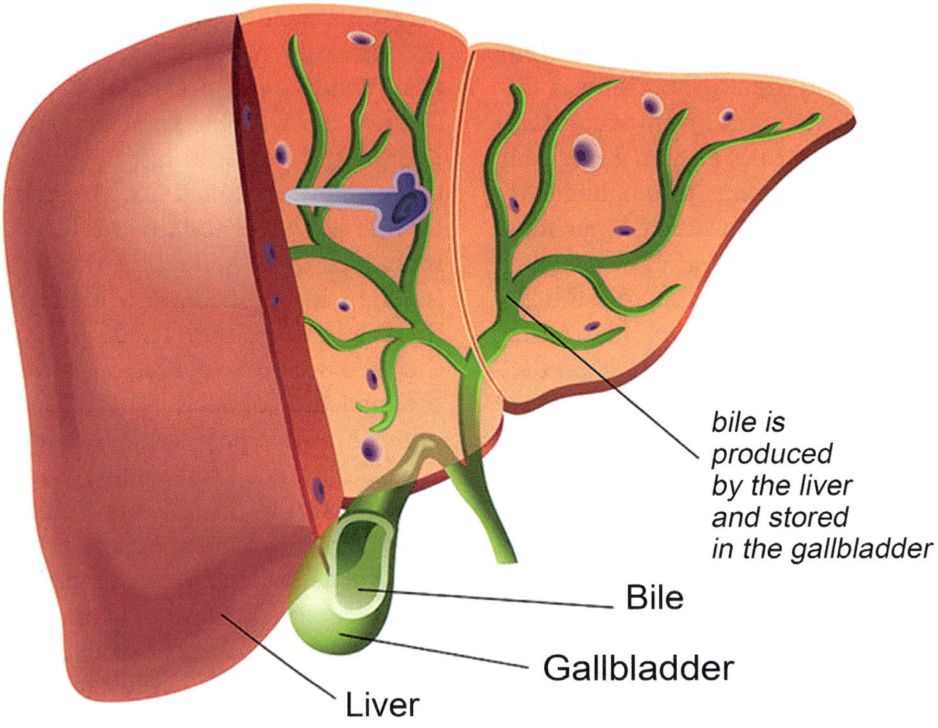

Figure 7.8. Role of bile in digestion.

Source: https://sp-ao.shortpixel.ai/client/to_auto,q_glossy,ret_img,w_1080,h_675/https://peacewithendo.com/wp-content/uploads/2013/07/role-of-bile-in-digestion-and-immunity.jpg

Test Your Knowledge

1. What is the metabolism of carbohydrates, proteins, and fats?
2. What is bile production and its role in digestion?

7.3. Liver Diseases

Learning Outcome

1. Describe the common liver diseases
2. Describe the causes and risk factors for liver diseases
3. Know the symptoms and diagnosis of liver conditions

The liver's role in homeostasis is underscored by its predisposition to a variety of diseases. Among them, liver disease is a significant worldwide public health issue. Hepatitis or inflammation of the liver may be caused by infectious agents, autoimmune diseases, or toxins. Clinical presentation of hepatitis is typically associated with jaundice, malaise, and abdominal pain that, if not treated, can result in severe systemic complications. Also, liver cirrhosis due to chronic liver damage includes substitution of the fibrotic tissue for the normal parenchyma and deranged hepatic architecture. In patients, portal hypertension and liver failure can result from loss of liver function, and thus early diagnosis and treatment are important to patient prognosis. It is in the comprehension of these diseases that not only does their complex etiology become clear, but the need for ongoing research into effective treatment modalities becomes essential to reduce their impact on human health. Alcoholic fatty liver disease (FALD) and non-alcoholic fatty liver disease (NAFLD) have emerged as leading causes of chronic liver disease. Both diseases are characterized by the abnormal deposition of lipids in the liver, which incites inflammation and fibrosis with a highly deleterious effect on the liver's functioning. The pathogenesis is multifactorial, involving dysregulation of lipid metabolism by the liver, and inflammation is now widely accepted as central to the disease. The cytochrome P450 (CYP450) enzyme system is of the utmost significance in this context, as these enzymes are responsible for metabolizing endogenous substrates and xenobiotics to a large extent. Alterations in CYP450 activity may result in pathologies observed in FALD and NAFLD. Even with extensive research, there is limited specific therapy that exists, and new means have to be discovered for the cure of these multifactorial ailments as well as to further improve the therapy of the patients (Jiang Y-J et al., 2024). There is also a deep comprehension of the immunological processes in liver disease required prior to successful treatment as well as management. For instance, visceral leishmaniasis (VL) is a significant challenge since it can either present as or overlie liver disease syndromes. The patients suffering from VL present with hepatosplenomegaly, pancytopenia, and increased liver enzymes, thus complicating diagnosis. Overlapping clinical presentation, for instance, the false positive hepatitis C virus antibody results in certain patients, indicates the intricate interdependence of infectious diseases and hepatic pathology (Liu, 2024). Misdiagnosis can lead to unjustified therapy or delayed appropriate therapy, and demonstrates the importance of careful epidemiologic assessment and diagnostic investigation with liver disease. Careful attention to such subtleties not only improves diagnostic accuracy but also calls to our attention the need for treatment regimens tailored to the individual based on the unique interaction between underlying disease and liver function.

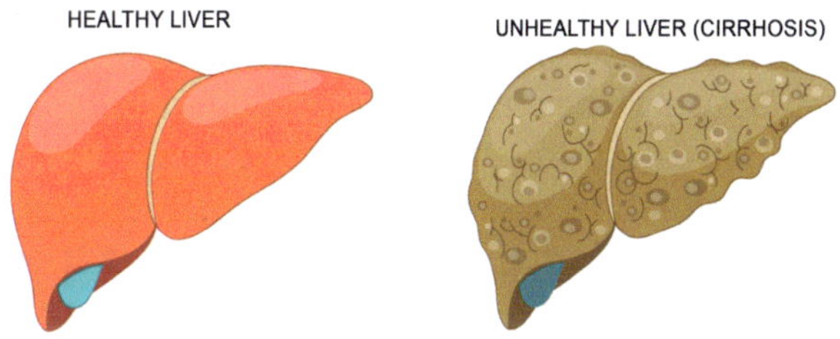

Figure 7.9. Liver disease.

Source: https://i0.wp.com/post.healthline.com/wp-content/uploads/2021/11/1684500-Liver-Problems-and-Their-Causes.png?w=1155&h=1436

7.3.1. Common Liver Diseases (e.g., Hepatitis, Cirrhosis)

The liver, being an extremely vital organ, performs many significant roles, and it is susceptible to many diseases, of which the most prevalent ones are hepatitis and cirrhosis. Hepatitis, usually the result of viral infections in hepatitis A, B, and C types, leads to inflammation of the liver. Hepatitis can lead to variable clinical presentations ranging from mild to advanced degrees of liver damage. Chronic infections of hepatitis B and C viruses are important for their capacity to progress to further severe liver diseases like cirrhosis and hepatocellular carcinoma. Complications of hepatitis also impact patients' quality of life greatly, and hence early diagnosis and treatment are needed to prevent long-term consequences. The importance of early diagnosis and treatment cannot be overstressed since today there are therapeutic interventions that can sufficiently alleviate morbidity due to chronic viral hepatitis (Keshavarzian et al., 2017). Cirrhosis, or the replacement of liver tissue with increasing amounts of scar tissue, is the end result of most chronic liver diseases, including hepatitis. The cirrhotic pathologic change predisposes the liver to failure in performing essential functions, leading to hepatic failure and portal hypertension. The etiology of cirrhosis is very heterogeneous and includes alcohol liver disease, non-alcoholic fatty liver disease (NAFLD), and type hepatitis chronic viral hepatitis infections. Patient outcomes improve through better early detection and treatment of cirrhosis, using more effective methods based on research correlating liver disease with liver function tests. In particular, studies have shown that altered liver function tests are also important indicators of disease early detection and, as such, provide a window of opportunity for therapeutic interventions prior to the progression of the disease to life-threatening complications (Butt et al., 2011). Effective management of common liver diseases such as hepatitis and cirrhosis largely rests on an early detection model, patient education, and newer therapeutic modalities within a multidisciplinary framework. Current guidelines for clinical practice suggest repeated screening, particularly in those with increased risk, so as to facilitate early detection of chronic viral hepatitis. New therapeutic developments, particularly direct-acting antivirals for hepatitis C and hepatitis A and B vaccines, have revolutionized the treatment area with hope of cure and prevention. Additionally, lifestyle modification—Weight reduction and alcohol decrease—is pivotal in the care of conditions such as NAFLD and alcoholic liver disease. In every stage of the cascade of liver diseases, a greater vigorous effort towards more awareness and access to care is critical in stemming the numbers and incidence of liver diseases worldwide (Keshavarzian et al., 2017).

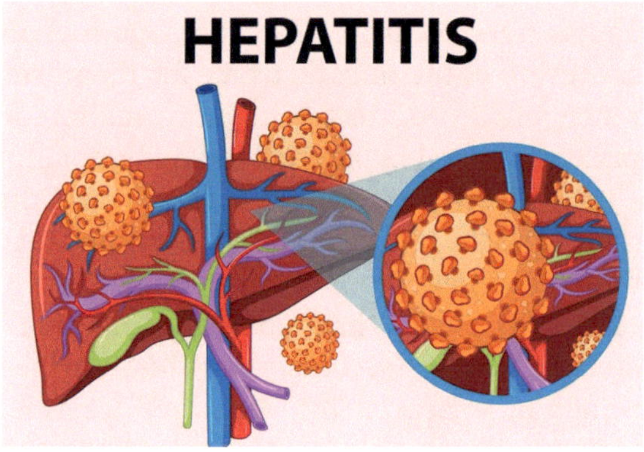

Figure 7.10. Hepatitis.

Source: https://images.onlymyhealth.com/imported/images/2024/July/23_Jul_2024/mn-hepatitis.jpg

7.3.2. Causes and Risk Factors For Liver Diseases

The liver plays a crucial role in the metabolism of nutrients and clearance of toxic substances, and thus is a susceptible organ for diseases. The single most universal cause of liver disease is chronic liver disease (CLD), which can in turn be caused by multiple etiologic factors, including chronic B and C hepatitis infection, alcohol use, and NAFLD. These diseases may eventually evolve into cirrhosis of the liver, which has been described as the final stage of CLD. The interference caused by cirrhosis profoundly damages the liver's homeostatic mechanisms in the body, which gives way to a chain of issues that may culminate in death. Furthermore, when cirrhosis becomes established, infection susceptibility like for *Clostridium difficile* Infection (CDI) is heightened, particularly as a result of the immunocompromised state typically present in cirrhotic patients, causing synergy of diseases that puts into prominence the weaknesses of the liver (Dumitru et al., 2019). NAFLD has emerged as the most common chronic liver disease globally, with millions affected and posing a significant public health concern. Pathogenesis of NAFLD is multi-factorial; it cannot be attributed to a single etiology but is rather influenced by several simultaneous physiological stressors—a phenomenon encapsulated by the multiple parallel hits theory. This model identifies that fat storage in hepatocytes and insulin resistance increase the liver's susceptibility to injury and inflammation. Additionally, malfunction in adipose tissue plays an important role by inducing chronic low-grade inflammation that is associated with causing liver injury (Barchetta et al., 2017). Vitamin D deficiency has also been associated with obesity and NAFLD, which indicates that its lack may further exacerbate liver pathology. Therefore, these interrelated risk factors are crucial to consider when designing preventive strategies and therapeutic interventions. Besides viral infections and metabolic syndrome, lifestyle also plays an important role in the etiology of liver diseases. Excessive alcohol consumption is also famously known to be the most frequent cause of liver damage, resulting in alcoholic liver disease (ALD) that can advance to cirrhosis and liver failure. Obesity has also been linked to many diseases of the liver, including NAFLD, which affects individuals across all age groups due to rising obesity rates globally. The remaining risk factors include certain drugs, exposure to toxins, and genetic conditions that predispose individuals to liver pathology. The intersection of these risk factors makes an integrative approach to liver well-being that involves lifestyle modification, detection of precursors to liver disease, and education regarding the impact of diet and drug use on liver function critical. As liver diseases become a ubiquitous health threat everywhere, addressing these multifaceted causes becomes a growing necessity.

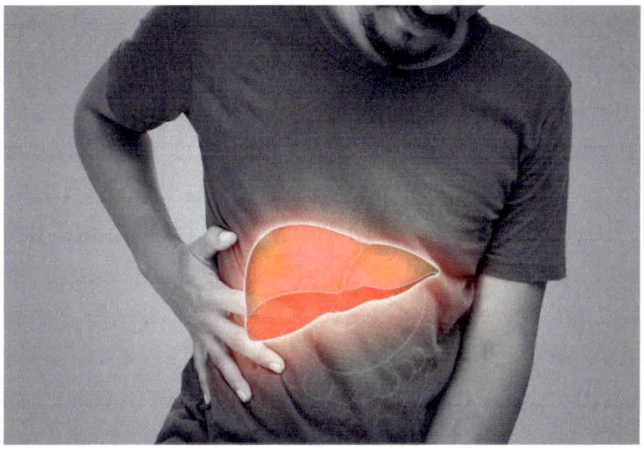

Source: https://www.omegahospitals.com/blog/storage/2025/03/illustration-liver-is-man-s-body-against-gray-background-men-with-hepatitis-fatty-liver-problem.jpg

7.3.3. Symptoms and Diagnosis of Liver Conditions

The liver is a vital organ that does many things, and its diseases can present themselves in nearly an unlimited variety of seemingly unrelated symptoms. The most commonly reported symptoms by patients are fatigue, pain in the abdomen, jaundice, and changes in weight or appetite. These presentations are not necessarily unique, which complicates diagnosis. Fatigue is just one such symptom that presents with many diseases of the liver, as well as other non-generalized illnesses. The symptoms' nonspecificity makes it possible for a "pandemic of diagnosis" when individuals are diagnosed with states of affairs that are not issues in their life. For this reason, there is a necessity to investigate liver symptoms instead of diagnosing them as illnesses. It is through Merleau-Ponty's embodied philosophy that both patient and clinician are sensitized to the nuance of illness and health, with particular experience overruling classifications (Sornsenee, 2025). In a liver diagnosis, methods are typically a combination of clinical assessment, imaging studies, and laboratory tests. The investigation typically begins with detailed patient histories and symptom- and risk factor-based physical examinations. Laboratory investigations using blood can also yield valuable information, such as liver enzyme levels to assess inflammation or damage, and the presence of certain viruses. Imaging investigations like ultrasound, CT scan, or MRI can find structural defects like tumors or cirrhosis complications. Diagnosis in conditions such as fascioliasis is not direct, since the infection may be presented with indigestion or fatigue, which are non-specific infection symptoms that can quickly lead to misdiagnosis. Imaging tests are, in such instances, able to detect diagnostic ultrasonographic findings, demonstratively indicating how optimal-fit diagnostic approaches enable us to accurately diagnose liver disease (Lee, 2024). Liver diseases can only be cured when they are diagnosed appropriately, and for that reason, future diseases have to be studied and worked on. For example, rising rates of fatty liver disease have driven the attention to the detection of its symptoms and application of diagnostic biomarkers in the first stage. The challenge is differentiation from other liver illnesses, like autoimmune hepatitis or cholestatic disease. In addition, increased awareness of diseases like fascioliasis places emphasis on accurate travel histories and eating habits among patients who may present symptoms of liver pain. Increased awareness of liver disease enables clinicians to provide greater assurance that care plans are well aligned with available data and patient experience, ultimately resulting in better health outcomes. The dynamic interaction among treatment, diagnosis, and liver health symptoms suggests the complexity of organs and the worth of care that is tailored in medicine (Lee, 2024).

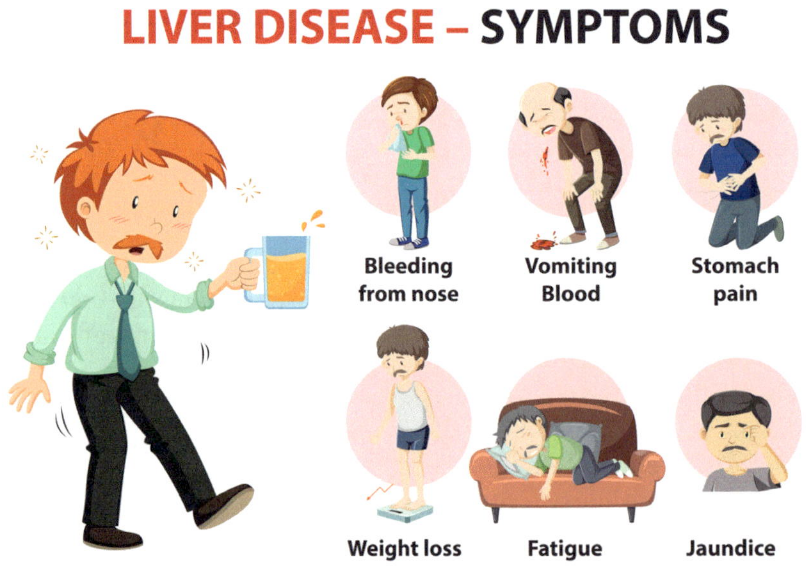

Figure 7.11. Symptoms of liver disease.

Source: https://drramchandrasoni.in/wp-content/uploads/2022/05/Liver-disease-Symptoms-scaled.jpg

Test Your Knowledge

1. What are the main causes of liver problems?
2. What are the symptoms of liver problems?

7.4. Liver Health and Maintenance

Learning Outcome

1. Know the importance of a balanced diet for liver health
2. Understand the role of exercise in maintaining liver function
3. Avoid harmful substances

Liver function is important to overall health because the organ performs tasks of metabolism, detoxification, and the storage of nutrients. Proper maintenance of the liver relies on a combination of lifestyle habits, including diet, exercise, and regular medical exams. A diet that is low in saturated fats but rich in fruits and vegetables is essential to the maintenance of liver function. Research has proven that frequent physical training can increase the liver's resistance, particularly for individuals prone to liver disease. Furthermore, monitoring liver enzyme levels with routine blood tests may lead to early identification of problems in progress. Including such routines not only supports the well-being of the liver but also eliminates complications associated with chronic illnesses, hence validating the necessity of active lifestyle habit management. Chronic liver injuries have the tendency to activate the liver's progenitor cells (LPCs) to contribute towards repairing tissue. Research has demonstrated that the liver microenvironment is most important to LPC function and injury responsiveness. In studying different models of chronic liver disease, including the CDE and TAA murine models, researchers have found that hepatocyte condition, as well as the development of inflammation and fibrosis, is critical for LPC responses. These findings enhance the understanding of hepatic regeneration and its limitations, demonstrating how multiple insults may hamper recovery and generate complications like hepatocellular carcinoma (HCC) in extreme cases, as studied in retrospective studies correlating LPCs with human disease progression (Köhn, 2016).

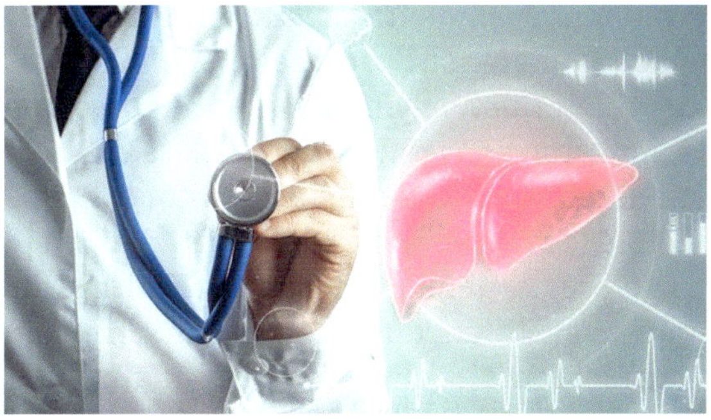

Figure 7.12. Liver Health.

Source: https://images.onlymyhealth.com/only-my-health-english/images/2025/04/21/article/image/mn-liver-health-1745234092630.jpg

This is why there is a continuous demand for monitoring and intervention strategies. It is required that an individual has an understanding of the social orientation of obesity and lifestyle in order to maintain their liver health successfully. The majority attribute obesity and its associated diseases to personal eating behaviors, yet studies have refuted this by indicating that calorie intake may not be the only factor determining obesity (Acheson et al.,

1990). Metabolic health, genetic predisposition, and socio-environmental determinants all play fundamentally important roles in the development of liver disease and overall health. Increased focus on comprehensive health education can help individuals make healthier decisions about diet and exercise and increase awareness of the complexity of liver disease. By addressing these intricate contributors, health programs can help individuals achieve sustainable changes that ensure liver health and enhance overall long-term health.

7.4.1. Importance of A Balanced Diet For Liver Health

Liver health is directly associated with adopting a well-balanced diet, which allows for adequate amounts of nutrients and well-controlled metabolic processes. The liver plays a key role in detoxifying poisons, metabolizing fats, and storing vitamins and minerals. A well-formulated diet consisting of high consumption of whole foods, such as fruits, vegetables, whole grain cereals, lean meats, and healthy fats, supports such functions through the provision of antioxidants as well as anti-inflammatory properties. Conversely, diets high in processed foods, saturated fats, and sugars overload the liver, leading to fatty liver disease and insulin resistance. Thus, awareness of the relationship between food intake and optimal liver function lies at the core of promoting general well-being. Such understanding points towards the need for equilibrated nutrition as a way of life, ultimately benefiting the liver and enhancing metabolic health. Dietary imbalances can enhance the risk of acquiring metabolic disorders, significantly influencing the liver's function. For instance, research indicates that the connection between nutrition and the development of Type 2 Diabetes Mellitus (T2DM) is intertwined with the liver health, as excessive caloric consumption may lead to insulin resistance and subsequent liver issues. Given that the liver is key in glucose control, adopting a balanced diet that stabilizes insulin is of significant importance. This means incorporating foods with fiber, which enhances glucose metabolism and reduces insulin spikes. Furthermore, the liver's function in fat metabolism brings focus to healthy fats such as omega-3 fatty acids contained in fish and nuts. Hence, food choices for the prevention of insulin resistance and maintaining liver strength and the body's metabolic equilibrium reinforce deliberate dietary choice. Additionally, the interplay between gut microbiota and liver disease illustrates the broader implications of a well-balanced diet. The microbiome greatly influences liver function as well as immune response, reinforcing the importance of nutritional diversity in promoting a healthy microbial community. Prebiotic- and probiotic-dense diets may promote healthy gut bacteria, which can enhance liver health by boosting immune function and reducing inflammation. Interestingly, disturbances in gut microbiota are also linked with increased metabolic syndromes, again highlighting the importance of diet. As these interactions between nutrition, microbiota, and liver function continue to unfold, further studies are required to explain these complex dynamics. Ultimately, a well-balanced diet is not only fuel but also a protective measure against liver disease, emphasizing its far-reaching worth in ensuring overall health and well-being in human physiology.

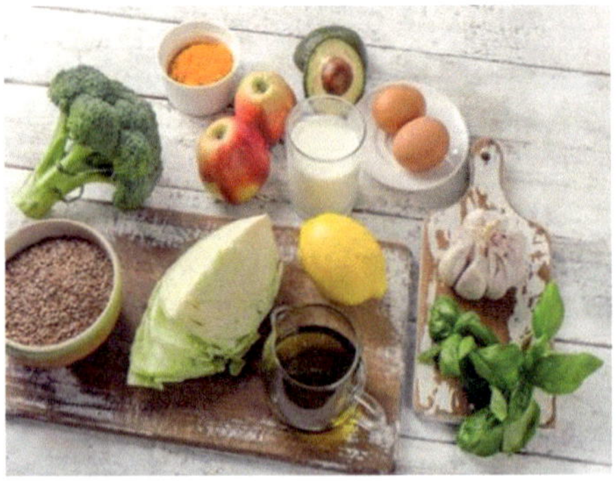

Figure 7.13. Diet to Keep the Liver Healthy.

Source: https://d35oenyzp35321.cloudfront.net/thumbnail_8bbfaec247.png

7.4.2. Role of Exercise in Maintaining Liver Function

Preservation of liver function by sustained physical activity is crucial through the regulation of multiple metabolic processes in the context of liver health. Preservation of sustained physical activity reduces the risk of risks associated with metabolic disorders, such as steatosis and inflammation, that may adversely affect liver physiology. Notably, exercise enhances insulin sensitivity and reduces systemic inflammation, thereby improving metabolic health. The crosstalk between muscle and liver tissue during exercise also amplifies the crosstalk, which is necessary for metabolic homeostasis. As indicated by studies, exercise interventions hold promising findings in terms of local anti-inflammation and boosting metabolic functions, thereby justifying the incorporation of physical activity as an essential aspect of liver health maintenance. Furthermore, the exercise-diet synergy can lead to extra benefits, particularly in individuals who are at risk of metabolic dysfunction-associated steatotic liver disease (MASLD) (Henin et al., 2024). In addition, recent studies focus on resistance training and endurance training for creating a robust hepatic environment, especially in the aging population. Exercise impact extends beyond weight loss; it directly affects liver cellular functions. As a case in point, senescence-accelerated mouse studies illustrate that exercise combination enhances liver tissue mitochondrial function, which usually declines with age. Such mitochondrial dynamic interventions may also reverse age-related deficits in hepatic function. Apart from this, the regulation of important transcriptomic expressions has been attributed to exercise, which illustrates its roles in regulating circadian rhythm and liver metabolism. These adaptations not only enhance liver health but also cellular longevity, pointing to a promising direction for therapeutic interventions to liver disease underlying age-related metabolic dysregulation (Pinto et al., 2024). The collective evidence for the role of exercise in the health of the liver also points towards its capacity to prevent and manage liver disease. Exercise regimens, including aerobic and resistance training, facilitate decreases in liver fat and improvements in liver histology. A well-structured exercise regimen significantly decreases the accumulation of lipid droplets in liver tissues that typically accompany hepatic steatosis. Maintenance of muscle is not merely beneficial to physical function but also indirectly safeguards liver function. Through enhanced muscle fat content and hepatic support, traditional exercise may be considered an interdisciplinary approach towards healthier liver function. Such an argument advocates growing public health initiatives towards establishing the role of physical activity as a central key to avoiding liver disease and maximizing overall metabolic status.

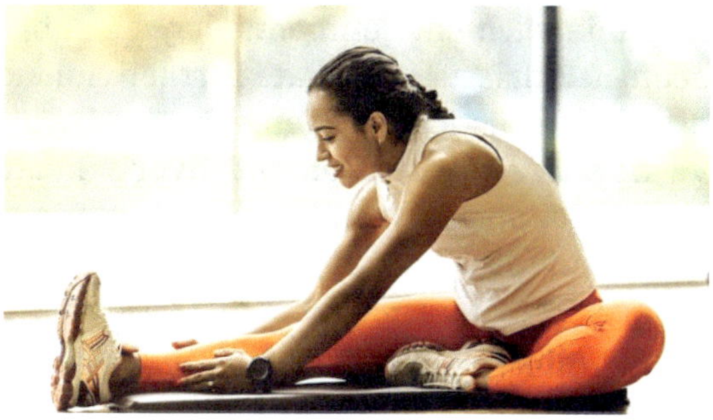

Source: https://images.moneycontrol.com/static-mcnews/2024/10/20241013054802_10.jpg?impolicy=website&width=770&height=431

7.4.3. Avoiding Harmful Substances (e.g., Alcohol, Drugs)

The liver is also crucial in detoxifying toxins and drug metabolism and is consequently vulnerable to the intoxicating effects of alcohol and drugs. Alcohol and drug abuse, particularly among young people, has attained epidemic proportions in that facts indicate that alcohol abuse accounts for approximately 3 million deaths annually and has a marked impact on the health of young adults. In 2018, almost 2.4 million adolescents experienced their first alcohol use, which is the most important awareness and prevention intervention during this age range. Of specific interest, psychoactive drug abuse can lead to acute liver injury, chronic illness, and even premature death, supporting the administration of protective substances against harmful substances for the health of this organ. Targeted interventions addressing the risks of alcohol and drug use are critical in the development of healthy lifestyles among young people (Ghelbash et al., 2022). Aside from the health implications to the individuals, substance abuse has extensive consequences to society, particularly in those areas that are semi-rural due to limited resources. Research indicates that geographical and social restrictions narrow down access to treatment and prevention services and compound the risks of alcohol and drug use among such populations. Persons who live in such environments may be subject to acute health issues, intimate partner violence, and criminal justice engagement, all of which have negative impacts on the liver's health. The interaction between local socioeconomic factors and patterns of substance abuse is unequivocal proof that must be tackled with multiple components to turn around these risks. By understanding the unique challenges in such environments, health policymakers will be able to create more effective systems for pro-social behavior modification, ultimately reducing unhealthy substance use and better liver health outcomes among communities. (Oliver, 2021).

Prevention and education at the level of young adulthood are of utmost priority in mitigating drug use and the resulting health complications. Young brain development, as it happens, is extremely susceptible to the negative effects of alcohol and drugs that interfere with cognitive skills and contribute to long-term health complications such as liver disease. Risk indicators such as peer pressure, psychiatric disorder, and poor self-esteem are also more prevalent in this category. Thus, developing resilience by creating supportive environments, parental involvement, and school-based interventions can play a powerful role in checking the excess of drug abuse. By increasing knowledge of the risks of harmful substances and promoting safe coping mechanisms, society can develop a culture in which healthier choices prevail, eventually influencing liver health and overall wellness (Ghelbash et al., 2022).

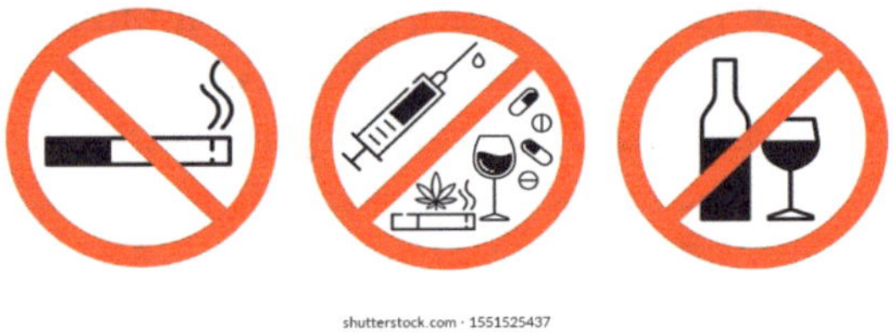

Source: https://www.shutterstock.com/image-vector/sign-forbidden-drugs-red-crossed-260nw-1551525437.jpg

Test Your Knowledge

1. What is the importance of a balanced diet for liver health?
2. What is the role of exercise in maintaining liver function?

7.5. Liver Transplantation

Learning Outcome

1. Know the indications for liver transplantation
2. Describe the transplantation process and criteria for the liver
3. Understand the liver post-transplant care and challenges

Liver transplantation (LT) remains an important medical intervention in patients with end-stage liver disease, a last resort for salvation when prior intervention has failed. Besides the surgical transplantation of an organizing liver with a donor liver, it encompasses careful assessment of numerous preoperative factors that have an impact on patient outcomes. With rising rates of metabolic diseases and age-related liver illnesses, LT cases grow exponentially more complex. For instance, some cardiovascular illnesses, including mitral annular calcification (MAC), have been reported to influence patient survival rate and postoperative complications, as seen in investigations of prevalence of MAC among LT recipients (Jang H-Y et al., 2024). These interconnected factors need to be understood to ensure optimum outcomes for liver transplantation. Patient care for patients with liver transplantation generally includes strict pretransplant evaluation procedures to determine their overall condition and potential fit for the surgery. Hepatorenal syndrome (HRS), which is a serious complication in the context of severe liver failure, poses significant challenges in patient management and pretransplantation planning. It is predominantly seen in those with elevated model for end-stage liver disease (MELD) scores, which are indicative of post-transplant survival and risk stratification (Park et al., 2020). Successful management strategies, including renal replacement therapy (RRT), are important for improving outcomes. Data show that use of pretransplant RRT has been associated with lower hospital mortality rates, which suggests the potential for intervention prior to transplantation to enhance the patient's resilience and recovery capability following transplantation. Outcomes following transplant are highly dependent on vigilant monitoring of patients and the treatment of potential complications emerging as the patients recover from the surgical procedure. Evidence has shown that the presence of cardiac diseases, such as MAC, adversely affects short- and long-term survival rates in liver transplant patients. Patients suffering from MAC have been reported to have a higher incidence of major adverse cardiac events 30 days after transplantation and poorer overall survival prospects, with an uneven effect on women (Jang H-Y et al., 2024). In addition, recent findings highlight the importance of managing complications like HRS and suggest the need for personalized treatment regimens based on each patient's unique health profile. Overall, careful understanding of all these factors is of utmost importance to maximize the success of liver transplantation and enhance recipients' quality of life.

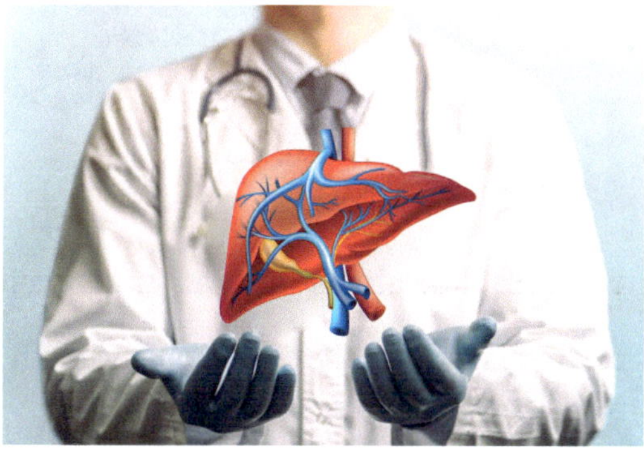

Figure 7.14. Liver Transplantation.

Source: https://eibfkobjiud.exactdn.com/wp-content/uploads/2022/04/liver-transplantation-02.jpg?strip=all&lossy=1&ssl=1

7.5.1. Indications For Liver Transplantation

The indication for liver transplant is normally based on various hepatic diseases that are extremely morbid and lethal. Chronic hepatitis

B and C infections are frequent causes that eventually result in cirrhosis and then hepatocellular carcinoma (HCC), which has emerged as a major indication for listing for transplant. In Poland, data in recent years show that a high percentage of liver transplants are done because of these viral infections and their resulting complications. Specifically, chronic hepatitis C was the reason for nearly 40% of liver transplants, underscoring the need for strong public health interventions to stem the influence of such diseases (Paweł Koczkodaj et al., 2019). Also, the treatment environment has evolved, as new antiviral therapies have shown promise in reducing the progression of liver disease and possibly reducing future transplant requirements. Liver transplantation is also indicated in patients with metabolic liver diseases, such as nonalcoholic fatty liver disease (NAFLD) and Wilson's disease.

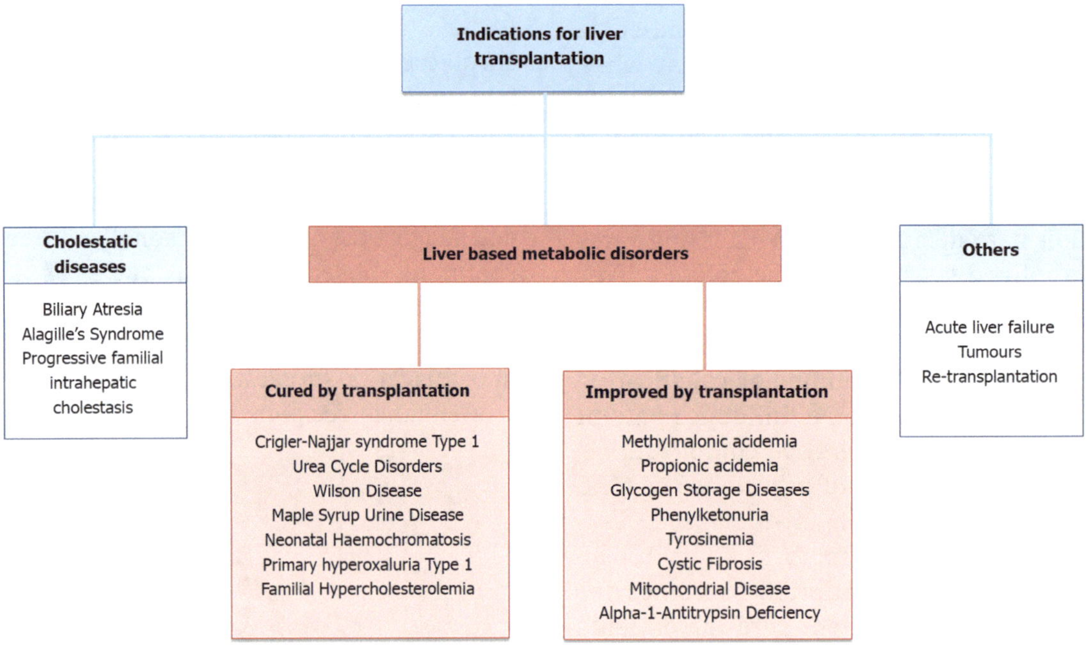

Figure 7.15. Indications for liver transplantation.

Source: https://f6publishing.blob.core.windows.net/3dcd2809-7d1b-49ce-9494-f79a3758f9cd/WJH-13-1351-g001.png

With an upsurge in obesity prevalence, NAFLD has emerged as a major cause of liver morbidity, elevating the prevalence of cirrhosis and the requirement for transplantation. This transformation in the disease profile calls for a redefinition of transplantation criteria to include the metabolic liver disorders in an effective manner. Moreover, autoimmune hepatitis is also a very important candidate for transplantation since it is likely to produce insurmountable liver damage if it remains untreated. The prudent selection of patients for liver transplant in these environments hinges on an adjustment of the underlying etiology and the extent of liver damage to yield the best post-transplant results. Cancer-related indications for liver transplantation present an interesting dilemma in this dynamic of a specialty. Specifically, HCC patients must meet very rigid criteria to qualify, with significant consideration given to staging and treatment of the cancer before transplant is undertaken. Increased concern regarding immunosuppression protocols tailored for oncological outcomes is imperative since these protocols are unlike typical liver transplant scenarios due to the potential risk of tumor recurrence. Recent studies show that individualized immunosuppression, such as strategies such as minimization or withdrawal of tacrolimus in favor of mTOR inhibitors, can improve oncological outcomes for specific tumor types, such as cholangiocarcinoma and colorectal liver metastases (Angelico et al., 2024). Finally, liver transplantation guidelines must adapt with advances in medical and surgical technology in order to optimally treat patients and maximize survival in this technologically demanding field.

7.5.2. The Transplantation Process and Criteria

The liver transplantation procedure consists of several critical procedures to confirm that a recipient's body successfully receives a donor organ. The initial procedure is to screen potential candidates with their medical history, the severity of their liver disease, and their health status. Laboratory tests such as blood tests, imaging tests, and sometimes liver biopsies are involved. The criteria for placement on a list for liver transplant generally align with objective measures, such as the Model for End-Stage Liver Disease (MELD) score, which rates the severity of liver disease and priority for transplant. Other factors, such as history of alcohol use, age, and comorbidities, are taken into account as well.

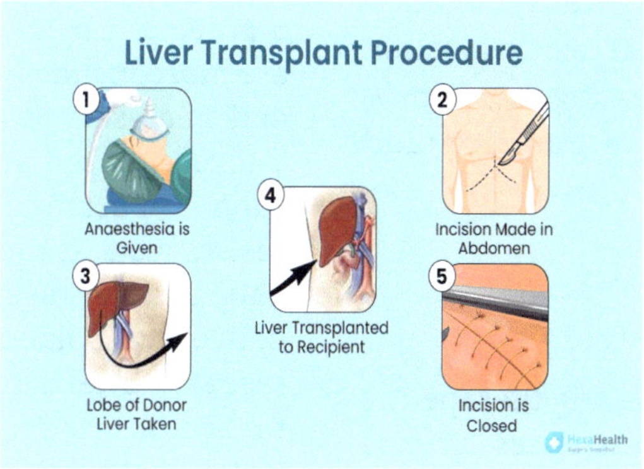

Figure 7.16. Liver Transplant Procedure.

Source: https://cdn.hexahealth.com/Image/1702357235415-377657803.webp

Together, these assessments provide for a fair and organized approach to sorting patients best suited to receive the surgery, addressing issues of ethics and feasibility that accompany transplantation. Once a patient has been deemed transplant eligible, procurement of a suitable donor begins. Both live and deceased donors can be utilized, but this is determined by several factors of compatibility, chief among them blood group and size. In addition, the human leukocyte antigen (HLA) characteristics of the donor and recipient must be compatible to reduce the risk of organ rejection. Transplantation itself is a risky surgical procedure that involves highly skilled medical professionals to provide anesthesia, perform the actual transplant, and look after the patient after surgery. With recent advancements, the role of natural killer (NK) cells has shown promising potential to enhance post-transplant results, particularly in recipients at risk of hepatocellular carcinoma (HCC). As evidenced by studies, NK cells from the donor liver hold potential to significantly improve prognosis when tailored to the recipient's KIR-HLA genotype, affirming the complexity of immunological compatibility in transplantation (Tanimine et al., 2024).

Lastly, the transplant procedure must be accompanied by ongoing research and technological development aimed at better outcomes and extended candidate suitability. An interesting area of inquiry is the design of bioartificial livers from decellularization technology to create scaffolds that mimic native liver structure. Such scaffold-engineered products hold out the prospect of addressing increasing liver transplantation demand with fewer human donor dependencies. Because the decellularization process preserves critical features of the liver but eliminates cellular components, it offers new possibilities for transplantation and recellularization (Primakova et al., 2024). Hence, enhancing transplantation necessitates the incorporation of tight evaluation standards, compatibility testing, and new approaches that bridge organ donation and replacement therapies.

7.5.3. Post-Transplant Care and Challenges

Liver transplantation is a lifesaving therapeutic intervention that significantly enhances survival for patients with end-stage liver disease. Care after transplant, however, is complex and multidimensional, encompassing a broad range of medical, psychological, and social concerns. Medication management, notably the administration of immunosuppressive agents such as tacrolimus, is one of the most important areas of concern. This medication is essential to organ rejection prophylaxis but has a narrow therapeutic index and is therefore liable to interaction with other medications. Novel evidence confirms that active components in marijuana block the cytochrome P-450 3A pathway used for tacrolimus metabolism, posing the risk of potentially harmful status in transplant patients (Chism and Moadel, 2019). Thus, physicians should be vigilant in monitoring drug interactions and patient adherence to treatment protocols in attempts to minimize risks of post-transplant complications. Beyond pharmacologic issues, the psychological condition of liver transplant patients also goes a long way towards their rehabilitation. The majority of patients are apprehensive about their outcomes and the resultant effects of the transplant, which affect their adherence to post-operative care protocols. Qualitative studies have indicated that religiosity and spiritual faith can be major coping mechanisms for patients who are faced with the austerity of terminal illness and the end-of-life concerns that accompany it. In particular, patients who are waiting for a liver transplant may be facing fear regarding death as well as their mortality. Research shows that patients who consider death to be a process rather than an irreversible endpoint are more inclined to accept their medical needs and necessary treatments (Cillo et al., 2017). Therefore, the integration of psychological support, such as spiritual therapy, can enhance resistance and the quality of care in transplant patients. Moreover, the social context involved in liver transplantation has profound effects on recovery after surgery. Family support, access to healthcare resources, and socio-economic status facilitate or hinder the complexities of post-transplantation care. Individuals lacking a supportive network usually have problems maintaining regular medical follow-up, adhering to regular medication, and leading healthy lifestyles post-surgery. Also, stigmatization of liver disease, particularly where alcohol is involved, may discourage open discussion within households or peer groups, which is so necessary for emotional support. For this reason, medical professionals ought to encourage holistic support systems that address both the medical and the social aspects of recovery. By taking a comprehensive approach to post-transplant management, such as education and community services, medical professionals can greatly enhance liver transplant patient outcomes.

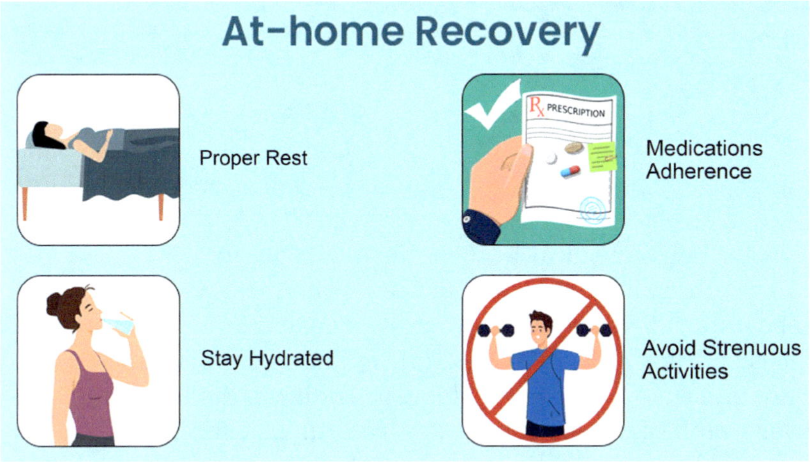

Figure 7.17. Home recovery after liver transplant.

Source: https://cdn.hexahealth.com/Image/1702356814309-757931735.webp

Test Your Knowledge

1. What are the indications for liver transplantation?
2. What is the process of liver transplant?

SUMMARY

In trying to downsize the liver's multifaceted role to human health, it is definite that this organ is a central metabolic, detoxifying, and immune organ. Its impact is outside the confines of the organ itself, with impacts reaching not only local systems but even the body's overall balance of physiology. It has been widely researched that the liver's sensitivity towards the intake of food and its connection with gut microbiota are the reasons why healthy habits should be formed to maintain the liver's proper functioning. Indeed, as argued, the liver's ability to regulate metabolism is crucial in preventing such conditions as nonalcoholic fatty liver disease (NAFLD) and other metabolic syndromes. The appeal for integrative models of liver health, encompassing internal and external physiology, is emphasized throughout the literature, and a multidimensional model is proposed for future research within the field of hepatology. In addition, the blending of the gastrointestinal system and the liver emphasizes the liver's key role in digestion and overall systemic health. Nutrient assimilation and hepatic metabolism of metabolic intakes reflect a continued conversation between such organs, which affects dietary impact as well as overall metabolic health. Recent evidence indicates that components derived from the mother, such as milk extracellular vesicles, can drastically modulate liver development and function by epigenetic mechanisms, and it has established the adaptability and biological complexity of the liver (Bodo C Melnik et al., 2021). This functional axis also emphasizes the ultimate importance of nutrition in early life and its long-term effects on liver health, suggesting that early nutritional intervention can prevent metabolic disorders in later adult life. Last but not least, the emergence of NAFLD as an epidemic has brought into perspective the important understanding of how inflammation and metabolic derangements might converge to compromise liver integrity (Tilg et al., 2020). More and more, investigations uncovers the liver's reaction to systemic inflammation from diet, lifestyle, and genetics as central areas of focus. Elucidating these interactions brings new therapy approaches for improving the liver above and beyond normal dietary strategies. Finally, the liver is the epic narrative of human health, characterized by its core role in metabolic control and by its intricate interactions with the systems of the body. With subsequent research being conducted, the future clinical practices will need to integrate these findings to promote improved prevention and treatment of liver ailments, vindicating the liver's important role in sustaining human existence.

The liver of humans has a pivotal role to play in many of the physiological functions, including metabolism, detoxification, and biomolecule synthesis for the organism. The liver contributes to blood glucose homeostasis by controlling gluconeogenesis and glycogenolysis, which ensure a long-term supply of energy to the organism. The liver has a role in lipid and protein metabolism, which testifies to its pivotal role in delivering overall metabolic homeostasis. By producing and secreting bile, the liver makes fat assimilation and digestion in the diet possible. The complexity of liver function underscores its intrinsic role in human health and therefore requires a comprehensive understanding of how it works and what stimulates its regulatory mechanisms. The liver's contribution to fetal development is also important, particularly as it pertains to neurodevelopment. The organ is a critical reservoir of necessary nutrients, including docosahexaenoic acid (DHA), which is critical in fetal brain development during pregnancy. Because of the inability of the human body to produce DHA, the efficiency of the liver in supplying this element to the developing fetus is critical. The quality and amount of these nutrients also count, and any disruption, as in disease states like pre-eclampsia, has far-reaching implications for fetal development and health. The liver, thus, is not only contributing to maternal well-being but is also charged with a basic function of facilitating proper fetal development. Lastly, the relationship between the liver and circadian rhythms further accounts for the intricacy of liver functions. Research has discovered that the internal biological clock of the body governs the liver, controlling hormonal and metabolic responses. The interaction validates that circadian dysregulation may result in severe disease, including metabolic disease, as well as disturbance of endocrine homeostasis. The interactions enhance the knowledge of how the liver function is entrained to the overall physiology and how rhythmicity plays a vital role in function. The results of such interactions can provide new avenues for treatment interventions aimed at liver disease and its systemic consequences (Freeman and Meyer, 2017; Bruscalupi and Gnocchi, 2017).

KEY TERMS FROM THIS CHAPTER

- Anxiety
- Biliary system
- Cirrhosis
- Computed tomography
- Depression
- Diabetes
- Dysbiosis
- Genetics
- Gluconeogenesis
- Gut microbiota
- Hepatitis
- Hepatocytes
- Liver
- Obesity
- Protein synthesis

CRITICAL THINKING QUESTIONS

1. **The liver is located in which abdominal quadrant?**
   a. Right upper quadrant
   b. Left upper quadrant
   c. Right lower quadrant
   d. Left lower quadrant
2. **The functional units of the liver are called:**
   a. Alveoli
   b. Nephrons
   c. Hepatocytes
   d. Lobules
3. **The liver receives blood from the:**
   a. Hepatic artery and portal vein
   b. Inferior vena cava and splenic vein
   c. Aorta and pulmonary vein
   d. Renal artery and mesenteric vein
4. **Which protein is primarily synthesized by the liver?**
   a. Hemoglobin
   b. Albumin
   c. Myoglobin
   d. Collagen
5. **The liver stores glucose in the form of:**
   a. Starch
   b. Glycogen
   c. Glucagon
   d. Insulin

Short Answer Questions

1. What is the size of a liver?
2. What is a lobular structure?
3. What are the main functions of the liver?
4. What are the common diseases of liver?
5. What is the diagnosis for liver disease?

Answer to Critical Thinking Questions

1. (a)   2. (d)   3. (a)   4. (b)   5. (b)

REFERENCES

1. Abduljalil, M., Aghazadeh-Habashi, A., Aigrain, J., Aitman, T., Al Za'abi, M., Alegre, S., Alnaqeeb, M., et al. (2019). Current trends in drug metabolism and pharmacokinetics. https://core.ac.uk/download/286361678.pdf (accessed on 15th June 2025).
2. Acheson, K. J., Benedict, F. G., Bennett, W., Bjorntorp, P., Borjeson, M., Bray, G. A., et al. (1990). Obesity: A biobehavioral point of view. https://digitalcommons.georgefox.edu/cgi/viewcontent.cgi?article=1280&context=gscp_fac (accessed on 15th June 2025).
3. Al-Chalabi, T., Antoniades, C., Arroyo, V., Bañares, R., Catalina, M. V., Chen, Y., Cisneros-Garza, L., et al. (2016). Extracorporeal liver support devices for listed patients. https://core.ac.uk/download/45467662.pdf (accessed on 15th June 2025).
4. Angelico, R., Bonaccorsi Riani, E., De Martin, E., Parente, A., Foguenne, M., Sensi, B., & Rodríguez-Perálvarez, M. (2024). Immunosuppression protocols for emerging oncological indications in liver transplantation: A systematic review and pooled analysis. *Liver Transplantation, 31*, 181–189. https://www.semanticscholar.org/paper/04647839b940ef24db39b81963d9d0efd6e81703 (accessed on 15th June 2025).
5. Banerjee, P., Gaddam, N., Chandler, V., & Chakraborty, S. (2023). Oxidative stress–induced liver damage and remodeling of the liver vasculature. *American Journal of Pathology, 193*, 1400–1414. https://doi.org/10.1016/j.ajpath.2023.06.002 (accessed on 15th June 2025).
6. Barchetta, I., Baroni, M. G., Bertoccini, L., Carotti, M., et al. (2017). Relationship between adipose tissue dysfunction, vitamin D deficiency and the pathogenesis of non-alcoholic fatty liver disease. https://core.ac.uk/download/98346849.pdf (accessed on 15th June 2025).
7. Barreby, E. (2023). The role of liver myeloid cells in obesity and metabolic disease. https://core.ac.uk/download/595407779.pdf (accessed on 15th June 2025).
8. Bruscalupi, G., & Gnocchi, D. (2017). Circadian rhythms and hormonal homeostasis: Pathophysiological implications. https://core.ac.uk/download/98342817.pdf (accessed on 15th June 2025).
9. Bush, K. T., Nigam, S. K., & Rosenthal, S. B. (2019). A network of SLC and ABC transporter and DME genes involved in remote sensing and signaling in the gut-liver-kidney axis. https://core.ac.uk/download/323064207.pdf (accessed on 15th June 2025).
10. Butt, A. A., Girling, A. J., Weber, B., Trepo, C., Wang, C. S., Lavanchy, D., Arnold, D. T., et al. (2011). Should patients with abnormal liver function tests in primary care be tested for chronic viral hepatitis: Cost minimization analysis based on a comprehensively tested cohort. https://core.ac.uk/download/pdf/1631226.pdf (accessed on 15th June 2025).
11. Chaviano, F., Orazi, A., Pizzi, M., Rugge, M., et al. (2017). A lucky mistake: The splenic glands of Marcello Malpighi. https://core.ac.uk/download/154325705.pdf (accessed on 15th June 2025).
12. Chism, K., & Moadel, D. (2019). Medical marijuana-induced tacrolimus toxicity. https://core.ac.uk/download/213445048.pdf (accessed on 15th June 2025).
13. Cillo, U., Feltrin, A., Germani, G., Milo, M., et al. (2017). Courage and representations of death in patients who are waiting for a liver transplantation. https://core.ac.uk/download/84920833.pdf (accessed on 15th June 2025).

14. Cryan, J. F., O'Riordan, K. J., Cowan, C. S. M., Sandhu, K. V., Bastiaanssen, T. F. S., Boehme, M., Codagnone, M. G., et al. (2019). The microbiota-gut-brain axis. *Physiological Reviews, 99*, 1877–2013. https://doi.org/10.1152/physrev.00018.2018 (accessed on 15th June 2025).

15. de Vos, W. M., Tilg, H., Van Hul, M., & Cani, P. D. (2022). Gut microbiome and health: Mechanistic insights. *Gut, 71*, 1020–1032. https://doi.org/10.1136/gutjnl-2021-326789 (accessed on 15th June 2025).

16. Dieu, A., Benoit, L., Dupont, C., de Magnée, C., Reding, R., Pirotte, T., & Steyaert, A. (2024). Sevoflurane preconditioning in living liver donation is associated with better initial graft function after pediatric transplantation: A retrospective study. *Perioperative Medicine, 13*. https://www.semanticscholar.org/paper/dd6c4174f7be521039f584f6a32d1b10ad52b533 (accessed on 15th June 2025).

17. Dolenšek, J., Pohorec, V., Rupnik, M. S., Stožer, H., et al. (2017). Pancreas physiology. https://core.ac.uk/download/322428900.pdf (accessed on 15th June 2025).

18. Dumitru, A., Popoiag, R. E., Micu, S. I., Moraru, M., et al. (2019). The burden of *Clostridium difficile* infection in patients with liver cirrhosis. https://core.ac.uk/download/232440323.pdf (accessed on 15th June 2025).

19. Freeman, D. J., & Meyer, B. J. (2017). Brain food for babies. https://core.ac.uk/download/78838098.pdf (accessed on 15th June 2025).

20. Frojdenfal, S., & Zuchowska, A. (2024). Advanced liver-on-a-chip model for evaluating drug metabolism and hepatotoxicity. *Biosensors, 14*. https://www.semanticscholar.org/paper/a5229e000a70b6002410dfea1813367f43d0069d (accessed on 15th June 2025).

21. Fulton, S., Décarie-Spain, L., Fioramonti, X., Guiard, B. P., & Nakajima, S. (2021). The menace of obesity to depression and anxiety prevalence. *Trends in Endocrinology and Metabolism, 33*, 18–35. https://doi.org/10.1016/j.tem.2021.10.005 (accessed on 15th June 2025).

22. Galicia-García, U., Benito-Vicente, A., Jebari, S., Larrea-Sebal, A., Siddiqi, H., Uribe, K. B., Ostolaza, H., et al. (2020). Pathophysiology of type 2 diabetes mellitus. *International Journal of Molecular Sciences, 21*, 6275–6275. https://doi.org/10.3390/ijms21176275 (accessed on 15th June 2025).

23. Ghelbash, Z., Alavi, M., West, S., Lees, D., & Cleary, M. (2022). A post-pandemic reset: Reversing the COVID-19 increase in substance use by adolescents and young adults. *Issues in Mental Health Nursing, 44*, 576–579. https://www.semanticscholar.org/paper/77a32e760679ec52f03bc574b83638da106de384 (accessed on 15th June 2025).

24. Henin, G., Loumaye, A., Deldicque, L., Leclercq, I. A., & Lanthier, N. (2024). Unlocking liver health: Can tackling myosteatosis spark remission in metabolic dysfunction-associated steatotic liver disease? *Liver International, 44*, 1781–1796. https://www.semanticscholar.org/paper/10a8d0745a338b5dadc49229065c30e3c1c2c076 (accessed on 15th June 2025).

25. Horn, S. S., Sonesson, A., Krasnov, A., Aslam, M. L., Hillestad, B., & Ruyter, B. (2025). Genetic and metabolic characterization of individual differences in liver fat accumulation in Atlantic salmon. *Frontiers in Genetics, 16*. https://www.semanticscholar.org/paper/c10ae48313a775570a37c82a453622beea31e74f (accessed on 15th June 2025).

26. Jang, H. Y., Han, S. B., Jeong, J. H., Kwon, H. M., Kim, K. S., Kim, J. H., Kim, S. H., et al. (2024). Prognostic value of mitral annular calcification in liver transplant patients: Implication in

posttransplant outcomes. *Transplantation, 108*, 1954–1961. https://www.semanticscholar.org/paper/f6480cc37d0b1bb0a89724a79ca2e1e845d41f30 (accessed on 15th June 2025).

27. Jiang, Y. J., Cao, Y. M., Cao, Y. B., Yan, T. H., Jia, C. L., & He, P. (2024). A review: Cytochrome P450 in alcoholic and non-alcoholic fatty liver disease. *Diabetes, Metabolic Syndrome and Obesity, 17*, 1511–1521. https://www.semanticscholar.org/paper/2d3b0e0e7d006aea103a842547e5a9ab2cd6f395 (accessed on 15th June 2025).

28. Keshavarzian, A., Yang, A. M., Schnabl, B., Bode, C., Chen, C. S., Hellerbrand, C., Llorente, C., et al. (2017). Intestinal fungi contribute to development of alcoholic liver disease. https://core.ac.uk/download/82969758.pdf (accessed on 15th June 2025).

29. Koczkodaj, P., Straś, W., Czerwiński, J., Małkowski, P., Pańczyk, M., & Gotlib, J. (2019). Evolution of indications for liver transplantation (LTx) in the years 2001–2017 in Poland. *Annals of Transplantation, 24*, 312–318. https://www.semanticscholar.org/paper/d4a44fca9609aee5e82cc28a2e460645e349611b (accessed on 15th June 2025).

30. Köhn, J. (2016). Characterization of liver progenitor cells and their microenvironment during chronic liver disease and hepatocarcinogenesis. https://core.ac.uk/download/195678148.pdf (accessed on 15th June 2025).

31. Kumar, P., Lee, S. S., Zhang, M., Tsang, Y. F., & Kim, K. H. (2019). Heavy metals in food crops: Health risks, fate, mechanisms, and management. *Environment International, 125*, 365–385. https://doi.org/10.1016/j.envint.2019.01.067 (accessed on 15th June 2025).

32. Lee, J. S. (2024). Fascioliasis: Image findings, diagnosis, and treatment. *Clinical Ultrasound*. https://www.semanticscholar.org/paper/5dd63fcd7b8bdd5b7f974a3207f2291d84658434 (accessed on 15th June 2025).

33. Li, D., Chen, S., Liu, C., Wei, B., & Li, X. (2022). Liver transcriptome analysis reveals biological pathways and transcription factors in response to high ammonia exposure. *Inhalation Toxicology, 34*, 219–229. https://www.semanticscholar.org/paper/1eac84b5666ba3a10ac35066217d6663e49faa45 (accessed on 15th June 2025).

34. Lim, S. Y. M., Chong, E. J., Mah, W. Y., Pan, Y., Fang, C. M., Murugaiah, C., & Alshagga, M. (2025). Exploring the anti-obesity effects of *Lactobacillus* in C57BL/6 mice: Mechanisms, interventions, and future directions. *Letters in Applied Microbiology*. https://www.semanticscholar.org/paper/459452b9b6aa90fdaeea9dc75dc3b2f36dbd868f (accessed on 15th June 2025).

35. Liu, Y., & Deng, C. (2024). Case report: Visceral leishmaniasis falsely diagnosed as viral hepatitis C without febrile symptoms. *Infection and Drug Resistance, 17*, 2009–2014. https://www.semanticscholar.org/paper/4c2732c43ebaff872807070aa8ca6a05028979c4 (accessed on 15th June 2025).

36. Lynch, S. V., Sharpton, S. R., Terrault, N. A., Yong, S. L., et al. (2019). Gut microbial metabolism and nonalcoholic fatty liver disease. https://core.ac.uk/download/323065660.pdf (accessed on 15th June 2025).

37. Melnik, B. C., Stremmel, W., Weiskirchen, R., John, S. M., & Schmitz, G. (2021). Exosome-derived microRNAs of human milk and their effects on infant health and development. *Biomolecules, 11*, 851–851. https://doi.org/10.3390/biom11060851 (accessed on 15th June 2025).

38. Meng, L., Tian, Y., & Bu, S. (2019). Liver tumor segmentation based on 3D convolutional neural network with dual scale. *Journal of Applied Clinical Medical Physics, 21*, 144–157. https://doi.org/10.1002/acm2.12784 (accessed on 15th June 2025).

39. Niu, L., Geyer, P. E., Wewer Albrechtsen, N. J., Gluud, L. L., Santos, A., Doll, S., Treit, P. V., et al. (2019). Plasma proteome profiling discovers novel proteins associated with non-alcoholic fatty liver disease. *Molecular Systems Biology, 15*. https://doi.org/10.15252/msb.20188793 (accessed on 15th June 2025).

40. Oliver, K. (2021). Pubs, pipes, pills and place: The experience of change in a semi-rural place. https://www.semanticscholar.org/paper/7b0ef8696b684e351db4912f87e2b0711aadea64 (accessed on 15th June 2025).

41. Park, G., Hwang, S., Jung, D., Song, G., Ahn, C., Kim, K. H., Moon, D., et al. (2020). Is renal replacement therapy necessary in deceased donor liver transplantation candidates with hepatorenal syndrome? A 2-year experience at a high-volume center. *Annals of Surgical Treatment and Research, 98*, 102–109. https://www.semanticscholar.org/paper/18e70e865ebc03d0da2eaddba2780767bdb1dff5 (accessed on 15th June 2025).

42. Pinto, A., Muñoz, V. R., Tavares, M. E. A., de Sousa Neto, I. V., Dos Santos, J. R., Rodrigues, G. S., Carolino, R., et al. (2024). Short-term exercise counteracts accelerated ageing impacts on physical performance and liver health in mice. *Clinical and Experimental Pharmacology and Physiology, 51*. https://www.semanticscholar.org/paper/01610bc5998e1033dff9c4ee432ea410a979475f (accessed on 15th June 2025).

43. Primakova, E. A., Efimov, D. Y., Sadouski, D. N., Nazarova, E. A., Symanovich, A. A., Yurkina, E. G., Romanova, I. A., et al. (2024). The quality and cytotoxicity assessment of the acellular human liver scaffold after decellularization. *Military Medicine*. https://www.semanticscholar.org/paper/eeb69f7c1e0a57a4add88cb6f9a3186d10cb678b (accessed on 15th June 2025).

44. Ren, H., Li, W., Liu, X., & Zhao, N. (2022). γδ T cells: The potential role in liver disease and implications for cancer immunotherapy. *Journal of Leukocyte Biology, 112*, 1663–1668. https://www.semanticscholar.org/paper/504a147a5c87b651ffb17d2c1a2861dd25338c68 (accessed on 15th June 2025).

45. Rinella, M. E., & Sookoian, S. (2023). From NAFLD to MASLD: Updated naming and diagnosis criteria for fatty liver disease. *Journal of Lipid Research, 65*, 100485–100485. https://doi.org/10.1016/j.jlr.2023.100485 (accessed on 15th June 2025).

46. Rinella, M. E., Neuschwander-Tetri, B. A., Siddiqui, M. S., Abdelmalek, M. F., Caldwell, S. H., Barb, D., Kleiner, D. E., et al. (2023). AASLD practice guidance on the clinical assessment and management of nonalcoholic fatty liver disease. *Hepatology, 77*, 1797–1835. https://doi.org/10.1097/hep.0000000000000323 (accessed on 15th June 2025).

47. Rowland, I., Gibson, G. R., Heinken, A., Scott, K. P., Swann, J. R., Thiele, I., & Tuohy, K. (2017). Gut microbiota functions: Metabolism of nutrients and other food components. *European Journal of Nutrition, 57*, 1–24. https://doi.org/10.1007/s00394-017-1445-8 (accessed on 15th June 2025).

48. Smith, B., Siebert, D., Ernst, D., Johansson, I., Munn, K., Elsner, K., & Tsikolia, N. (2005). Functional anatomy: A taxonomic proposal. https://core.ac.uk/download/131215354.pdf (accessed on 15th June 2025).

49. Sornsenee, P. (2025). From biopower to embodiment: Reconfiguring healthcare beyond the pandemic of medicalization. *PSU Medical Journal*. https://www.semanticscholar.org/paper/287e0821632297d24358788337590d38a3a518ba (accessed on 15th June 2025).

50. Swathi, K., Nehru, G., & Srihari, G. (2025). A review on current status and future directions on sesame phyllody. *Journal of Advances in Biology & Biotechnology*. https://www.semanticscholar.org/paper/2295e395d2f7a534782d2b3ae366658a58e499f0 (accessed on 15th June 2025).

51. Tanimine, N., Ohira, M., Kurita, E., Nakano, R., Sakai, H., Tahara, H., Ide, K., et al. (2024). Impact of KIR-HLA genotype on natural-killer-cell-based immunotherapy for preventing hepatocellular carcinoma after living-donor liver transplantation. *Cancers, 16*. https://www.semanticscholar.org/paper/d75fd0f8aaf25de699c2a575514cb761cc6c02f7 (accessed on 15th June 2025).

52. Tilg, H., Adolph, T. E., & Moschen, A. R. (2020). Multiple parallel hits hypothesis in nonalcoholic fatty liver disease: Revisited after a decade. *Hepatology, 73*, 833–842. https://doi.org/10.1002/hep.31518 (accessed on 15th June 2025).

53. van der Hee, B., & Wells, J. M. (2021). Microbial regulation of host physiology by short-chain fatty acids. *Trends in Microbiology, 29*, 700–712. https://doi.org/10.1016/j.tim.2021.02.001 (accessed on 15th June 2025).

54. Zheng, D., Liwinski, T., & Elinav, E. (2020). Interaction between microbiota and immunity in health and disease. *Cell Research, 30*, 492–506. https://doi.org/10.1038/s41422-020-0332-7 (accessed on 15th June 2025).

PANCREAS

8

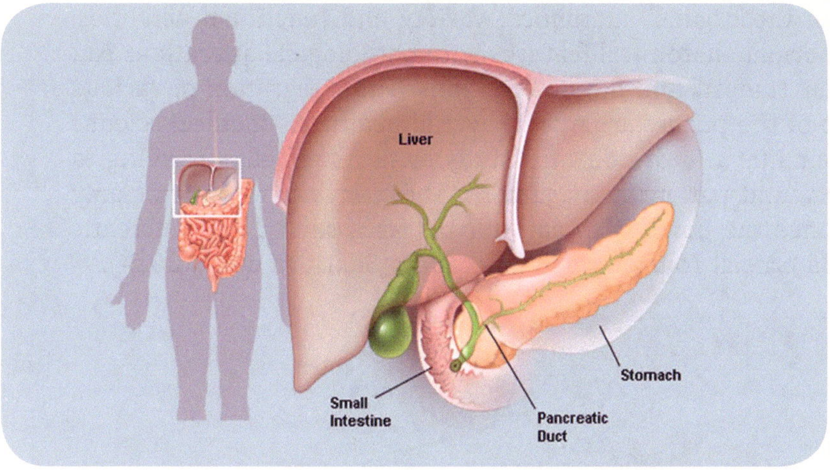

LEARNING OBJECTIVES

After studying this chapter, you will be able to:

1. Understand the anatomy of the pancreas
2. Describe the functions of the pancreas
3. Describe the pancreatic enzymes
4. Understand the hormonal regulation
5. Describe the diseases of the pancreas
6. Learn about diagnostic methods for the pancreas

Introduction

The pancreas is an essential body organ that plays a central role in both the endocrine and digestive systems. It has many functions encompassing the release of digestive enzymes and the regulation of blood glucose levels through hormone secretion. Beyond its physical structure, the significance of understanding the pancreas extends into the physiological processes that propel overall health. With the advent of medical imaging modalities, such as computed tomography, researchers can study the pancreas's complexity in detail. This enhanced capability has enabled researchers to achieve precise diagnoses, including information not only on the organ's structure but also on its disease states, which are increasingly important in clinical assessments. Learning such characteristics, doctors can design more effective treatment strategies for pancreatic pathology, and thus the study of this organ is intrinsic to the essence of medicine (O.V Kuryk et al., 2024). Moreover, the role of the pancreas in perinatal medicine has also become of increasing significance, particularly due to perinatal pathology, which harms newborns. Research into the exocrine function of the pancreas in term neonates has demonstrated that conditions of asphyxia and hypoxia will lead to dramatic alterations in pancreatic enzyme activity. For instance, studies have suggested that neonates experiencing serious perinatal complications exhibit elevated amylase and lipase concentrations, which may be indicative of hyperactivation of pancreatic function in response to injury. With such enzymatic shift analysis, clinicians can better see the role of perinatal trauma to gastrointestinal health and develop more targeted interventions on behalf of at-risk infants. Thus, knowledge of the nuances of pancreatic function during neonatal age not only responds to immediate medical care but also enhances our overall understanding of the organ's role in terms of seminal events in human ontogeny (O.V Kuryk et al., 2024). Finally, ongoing research on the pancreas by newer techniques and clinical findings projects its varied nature. The improvement in imaging technology, added to painstaking clinical research, enables a close inspection of the organs' anatomical variety and functional activities. Thus, for instance, the comparison of normal anatomical features with pathological alterations can elucidate the pan-cancer of pancreatitis, tumors, and other conditions. The integration of various data sources creates a broader picture of the pancreas's role in overall health. As medical science continues to progress, the pancreas remains a focal point for study, with its effects spreading to operative technique, diagnostic criteria, and patient management. These investigations not only increase our knowledge but also enhance the delivery of care for diseases caused by pancreatic dysfunction, acknowledging the organ's crucial role in the human body (Sekisova et al., 2024).

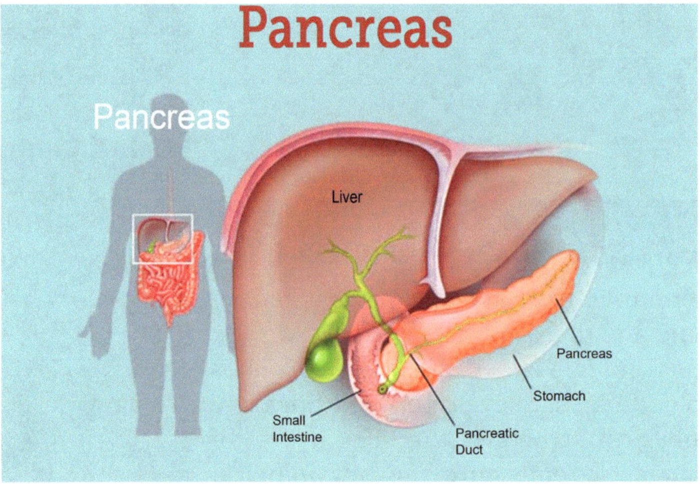

Figure 8.1. Pancreas.

Source: https://assets.lybrate.com/imgs/tic/enadp/image-of-the-pancreas.jpg

Definition and Significance of the Pancreas

The pancreas is an extremely vital organ in the abdominal cavity that has a dual role in the endocrine and exocrine systems. The organ can be structurally classified into four main sites: head, neck, body, and tail. The organ secretes numerous hormones like insulin and glucagon, which are extremely vital in glucose metabolism. Being an exocrine gland, the pancreas releases digestive enzymes—i.e., amylase, lipase, and proteases—into the small intestine to play a central role in digesting carbohydrates, fats, and proteins. The significance of the pancreas is that it possesses multifunctional functions critical to homeostasis, thus having implications on numerous bodily processes, including digestion and metabolic control. The significance of the pancreas extends beyond its physiologic and anatomic characteristics; it is also a focus of interest in various medical disorders. Pancreatitis and diabetes mellitus hint at the pancreas's critical role in disease and health. For instance, in pancreatitis, pancreatic inflammation can lead to intense abdominal pain and gastrointestinal discomfort, along with complications causing damage to its function. Secondly, the understanding of the regenerative ability of the pancreas, demonstrated through experiments in pancreatic-tail duct ligation, suggests a potential for the development of therapeutic interventions for disorders such as diabetes, where insulin-secreting beta cells are impacted. Thus, investigating the pancreas's roles and responses highlights its importance in both clinical use and the development of medical treatments (Chintinne et al., 2012).

Moreover, the intricate relationship between the pancreas and the rest of the organs validates its significance in the digestive and endocrine systems. The pancreas has close interaction with the liver, gallbladder, and small intestine, which provides a collective reaction to most physiological demands. For example, gallbladder atrophy can be linked with pancreatic disorders, thereby indicating that a malfunction in one organ will have an impact on the rest. The interaction among these organs demonstrates the coordinated nature of physiological functions, whereby disturbances in pancreatic health can have systemic impacts. The increasing prevalence of pancreatic diseases demonstrates the need for continued research into the subject area, as understanding these interactions, as well as the regulative roles of the pancreas, is key towards improving health outcomes and deriving effective interventions (Han and Rozengurt, 2023).

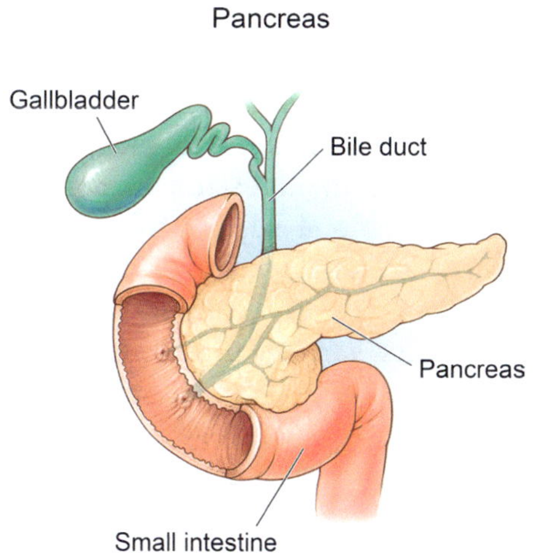

Figure 8.2. Your pancreas is a fish-shaped organ about the length of your hand.

Source: https://my.clevelandclinic.org/-/scassets/Images/org/health/articles/21743-pancreas.jpg

8.1. Anatomy of the Pancreas

Learning Outcome

1. Describe the location and structure of the pancreas
2. Describe the distinct regions of the pancreas
3. Know the blood supply and innervation

The anatomy of the pancreas is characterized by its single structure and multifunctional nature in the human body. Posterior to the peritoneum in location, the pancreas is an exocrine and endocrine glandular organ. Exocrine function is mainly the secretion of digestive enzymes, such as amylase, lipase, and proteases, for carbohydrate, fat, and protein digestion. It is this enzymatic release that is facilitated by the pancreatic ducts, which all come together to form the main pancreatic duct, so that the release of these enzymes into the duodenum is facilitated. The endocrine component, however, is made up of the islets of Langerhans, which release crucial hormones, such as insulin and glucagon, into the circulation to preserve glucose homeostasis. It is significant to recognize the dual function in order to highlight the function of the pancreas in digestion and metabolic processes. The blood supply to the pancreas is a significant anatomical feature because it provides the oxygen and nutrient supply required for its various functions. The blood supply to the pancreas comes primarily from branches of the splenic artery, and secondarily, the superior mesenteric artery. Topographical analysis of the vascular anatomy revealed significant variation in the positioning of the splenic artery relative to the pancreas. It was found in approximately 68.3% of the cases that the splenic artery is suprapancreatic, and in 31.7% of the cases it is retropancreatic. Moreover, moderate to severe tortuosity of the splenic artery was also found, which may influence the risk of surgery in pancreatic surgery. The importance of such differences is of greater than a significant scale, particularly when dealing with pancreatic surgery, because the approach, technique, and general patient outcome of potential complications based on vascular anatomy are influenced (Pronin et al., 2021).

Aside from its vascular and structural aspects, the cellular structure of the pancreas is of interest, particularly how it mimics other glandular structures within the organism. Its lobulated shape is composed of clusters of acini, which are at the center of its exocrine function. The dispositions of these lobules, described by early anatomists, trace the complex pancreatic architecture. Like the liver's lobules, they are composed of small units of glands, or acini, that drain into a ductal system (Kiernan, 1834). But in the course of learning the integrated concept of the pancreas, the particular interconnection of pancreatic cell structure and function remains an area of interest for investigation. Understanding this interconnection will enlighten a variety of pancreatic disease-related pathologies to ultimately result in more refined clinical approaches to treatment and surgery of pancreatic disease.

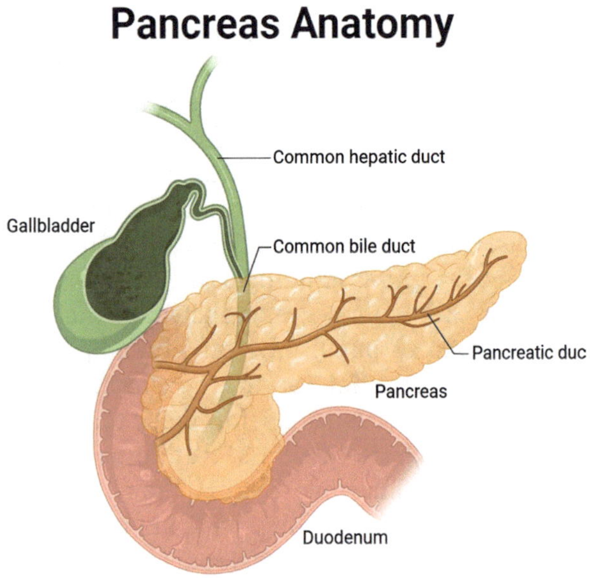

Figure 8.3. Pancreas Anatomy.

Source: https://microbenotes.com/wp-content/uploads/2024/04/Pancreas-Anatomy.jpeg

8.1.1. Location and Structure of the Pancreas

The pancreas is a long, glandular organ in the abdominal cavity, extending horizontally along the posterior abdominal wall. It is located deep back in the peritoneal cavity, between the duodenum on the right and the spleen on the left, and its head is typically found within the curve of the duodenum. Such positioning allows the organ to secrete digestive enzymes and hormones efficiently straight into the gastrointestinal tract so that food can be digested.

The pancreas consists of four different regions: head, neck, body, and tail, of which the head is the most robust segment. It is crucial to know the anatomical location of the pancreas because its proximity to other vital organs, such as the liver and kidneys, influences surgical approaches and the treatment of abdominal pathology (Blagova et al., 2025). The pancreas, functionally, contains endocrine and exocrine components, with each element assuming important roles in body function. Endocrine cells, which primarily occur within the islets of Langerhans, are responsible for the secretion of hormones, including insulin and glucagon, which regulate blood glucose. On the other hand, the exocrine portion, made up of acinar cells, secretes digestive enzymes like amylase, lipase, and proteases that become secreted into the small intestine by the pancreatic duct. This bimodal function emphasizes the role of the pancreas in the regulation of metabolism and digestion. The intricate arrangement of cells and ducts within the pancreas makes this multiplicity of functions possible, and imaging techniques such as MRI and CT scans are able to identify structural pathology that will precede disease (Lucas W Remedios et al., 2025). The pancreas also has a fibrous capsule protecting its structure while allowing blood vessels to penetrate, essential for the transport of nutrients and hormones. This capsule also isolates the pancreas from adjacent structures, making it part of its distinctive location within the abdominal cavity. The organ is highly vascularized, and this is necessary for its metabolic processes; hence, any pathological alterations, like inflammation or tumors, can largely affect its function. Since it is crucial to both endocrine and exocrine systems, maintaining the structure and function of the pancreas is important for the overall health of the individual. Current research on newer imaging modalities and surgery could further elucidate the complexities of pancreatic anatomy and offer enhanced clinical results in the case of pancreatic disease (Lucas W Remedios et al., 2025).

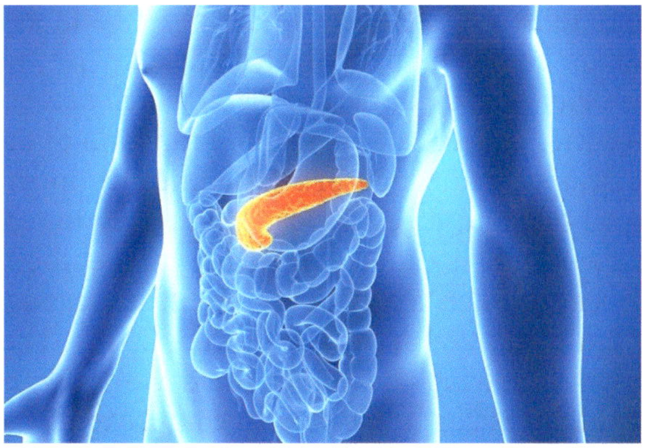

Figure 8.4. The pancreas is located deep inside the abdomen.

Source: https://cdn.mos.cms.futurecdn.net/6nZWaqsX5KvF8AB2QTj7NS.jpg

8.1.2. Distinct Regions: Head, Body, and Tail

The three spatially distinct regions of the pancreas are the head, body, and tail, each with a specialized role in digestive and endocrine processes. The head, due to the hook-shaped position around the duodenum, is centrally located in the gland's exocrine process. It also secretes digestive enzymes from the pancreatic duct into the duodenum, which digest carbohydrates, proteins, and fat in food. Enzymatic digestion is crucial during nutrient absorption, aligning with the head's responsibility of maintaining the body's digestive system intact. Furthermore, head diseases, such as pancreatic adenocarcinoma, can greatly impede digestive functions and lead to severe clinical complications, emphasizing the urgency for an extensive understanding of anatomy and pathology of the area in clinical practice (Arda et al., 2017). Now, going to the body of the pancreas, this region is vital to endocrine as well as exocrine functions. It houses clusters of endocrine cells that are referred to as the islets of Langerhans, secreting hormones such as insulin and glucagon into the blood supply. These hormones lie at the core of glucose metabolism and balancing energy within the human body. The body is also packed with the majority of the pancreatic acini, which secrete digestive enzymes. The two-fold function of the body is an indication of its significance in the metabolic and digestive processes. Any illness of the region is capable of leading to metabolic disorders such as diabetes mellitus because of faulty insulin secretion (Prabu, 2011). This is why knowing the complicated workings of the body makes it possible to comprehend the general implications when it comes to well-being in general terms. Finally, the tail of the pancreas, although smaller, is of importance both anatomically and functionally. Located close to the spleen, the tail is more dense with endocrine cells than the rest of the organ and has a functional aspect in hormonal regulation.

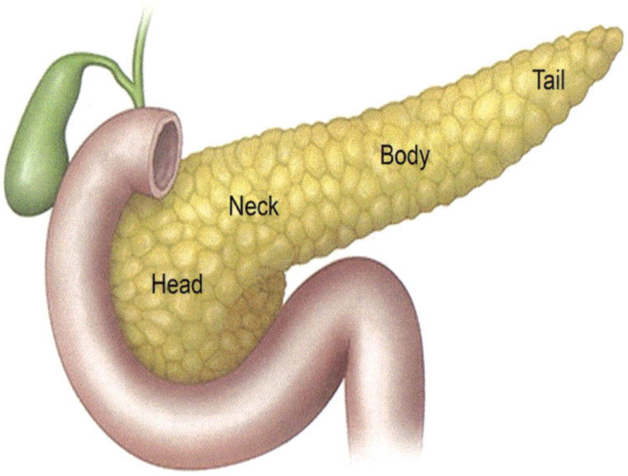

Figure 8.5. Distinct regions of the pancreas.

Source: https://columbiasurgery.org/sites/default/files/styles/large/public/pancreas_anatomy_label.jpg?itok=zvyjdtov

Nearness to the spleen is also suggestive of possible roles in splenic disease or trauma. Tumors and lesions that are derived from within the tail may be latent until advanced, with difficulty in their diagnosis and treatment, thus at early stages. It is essential to understand the pathology of this area because conditions such as pancreatitis may cause inflammation and resultant damage to the surrounding structures, not just the pancreas, but to the organs around it as well (Arda et al., 2017). Hence, it is vital that there is a general understanding of the head, body, and tail by physicians so that they can conceptualize appropriate therapies and treat pancreatic disease.

8.1.3. Blood Supply and Innervation

The pancreas, a vital gland in human physiology, has a complex vascular supply that is a fundamental component of its varied functions, particularly digestive and metabolic activities. The gland's vascular supply is chiefly provided by the pancreaticoduodenal arteries, which originate from the celiac trunk, and the splenic artery. This intricate vascular arrangement is capable of meeting the exocrine and endocrine regions of the pancreas with a sufficient supply of blood, hence facilitating effective delivery of nutrients and hormones to the body. The extensive vascular network not only maintains the metabolic requirement of the pancreatic tissues but also plays an important role in regulatory processes related to digestion and blood glucose homeostasis. Appreciation of this architectural complexity is required to grasp how vascular issues can intrude upon pancreatic function and result in various diseases, enlightening the intricate relationship between blood supply and pancreatic health as discussed in comprehensive anatomical texts (Dolenšek et al., 2017). In addition to its complex blood supply, the pancreas is extensively innervated by the sympathetic and parasympathetic branches of the autonomic nervous system. Whereas the sympathetic fibers primarily regulate blood flow and, in turn, indirectly influence islet cell function, the parasympathetic fibers play a key role in regulating insulin and glucagon secretion. Notably, research revealed that human islets exhibit a unique pattern of innervation compared to other animals, such as mice, and this has great implications for islet function and diabetes mellitus treatment. Specifically, while mouse islets are privileged by rich parasympathetic innervation directly influencing endocrine function, human islets lack this privilege and instead use paracrine mechanisms to regulate hormone secretion (Rodriguez-Diaz, 2012). Such intricate aspects of pancreatic innervation emphasize the importance of a species-specific approach in investigating glucose homeostasis mechanisms and prospects of new therapeutic interventions. The relationship between the neural supply and blood supply to the pancreas is important to facilitate metabolic homeostasis, particularly in diabetes mellitus. The glucagon and insulin hormones secreted by the islets of Langerhans are significantly influenced by the organs' vascular and neural interactions. It has been demonstrated that the sympathetic innervation preferentially targets the smooth muscle cells of the pancreatic vessels, regulating hormone secretion by modulation of blood supply and not by direct effects on endocrine cells (Rodriguez-Diaz, 2012). This highlights the plasticity of human pancreatic function in accordance with physiological demands and, at the same time, signifies the complexity of its regulatory system. Hence, a thorough understanding of vascularization and innervation of the pancreas is required to formulate effective treatments for pancreatic disease, and thus it becomes a priority area for research for upcoming studies aiming to reveal the pathophysiology of diabetes and other metabolic disorders (Dolenšek et al., 2017).

Test Your Knowledge

1. What is the structure of the pancreas?
2. What are the 3 regions of the pancreas?

8.2. Functions of the Pancreas

Learning Outcome

1. Describe the exocrine functions and endocrine functions of the pancreas
2. Understand the role of pancreas in metabolism and nutrient absorption

The pancreas is a dual-functioning organ in human physiology, serving both as exocrine and endocrine gland, essential for the digestion process and the control of metabolism. The exocrine function is basically involved in the secretion and formation of digestive enzymes such as amylase, lipase, and proteases. These enzymes play a significant role in breaking down carbohydrates, fats, and proteins, thus ensuring nutrient absorption from the small intestine. These enzymes are secreted from the pancreas into the duodenum through the pancreatic duct, where they are activated in a neutral pH, which is most favorable to their activity. This function of digestion is indicative of the role played by the pancreas to maintain general metabolic health, enabling efficient nutrient processing and extraction of energy from dietary food. Besides its endocrine role, the pancreas's secretory role also plays a critical role in controlling blood glucose levels. This is primarily due to the secretion of hormones like insulin and glucagon from the islets of Langerhans. Insulin serves to decrease blood sugar content by allowing glucose to enter cells, while glucagon has the opposite effect—triggering the discharge of stored glucose in the liver. There is a need for balance between these two hormones for homeostasis; otherwise, conditions like diabetes mellitus with increased blood sugar levels result. Therefore, the interplay of glucagon and insulin not only reveals the pancreas's function in metabolism but also in long-term health and disease susceptibility. New findings also highlight the pancreas's role in different physiological processes other than digestion and glucose regulation. Recent studies show that the pancreas may exert an influence on energy spending and fat storage, revealing a pivotal role in metabolic syndromes. For instance, the interaction between pancreatic hormones and the remaining body systems, i.e., the gut microbiota, can determine weight regulation and insulin sensitivity. These delicate interactions need to be understood in order to derive overall strategies against metabolic disease, focusing on prevention and treatment that considers the multifunctionality of the pancreas. With further research, our comprehension of these more general functions will improve our understanding of the pancreas's function within the human health dynamics as a whole.

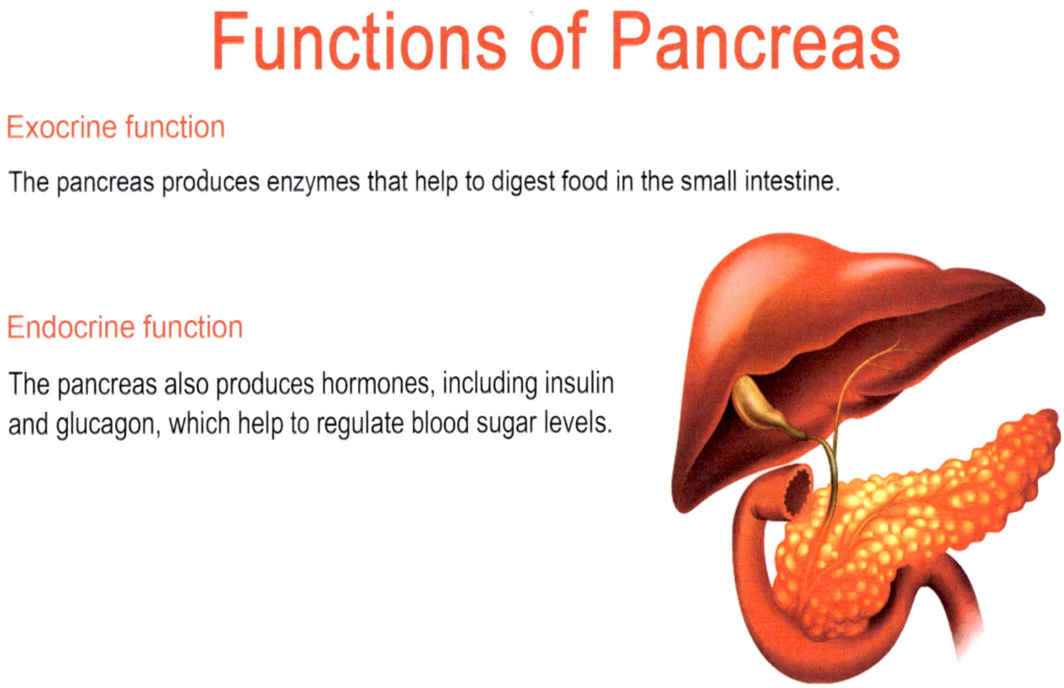

Figure 8.6. Functions of the Pancreas.

Source: https://assets.lybrate.com/imgs/tic/enadp/functions-of-pancreas.webp

8.2.1. Exocrine Functions: Digestive Enzyme Production

The function of the pancreas in the human body is pivotal to the digestive system through its exocrine functions, which are primarily focused on the creation and secretion of digestive enzymes. These enzymes, e.g., amylase, lipase, and proteases, play fundamental roles in the effective digestion of carbohydrates, fats, and proteins, respectively. The pancreas secretes these enzymes in inactive form to prevent autodigestion and releases them into the small intestine, where they become activated by the alkaline pH and other circumstances. This is crucial for nutrient absorption, as digestion efficiency directly affects the body's capacity to extract and utilize essential nutrients from the diet. Inadequate production of these enzymes can lead to malabsorption syndromes, characterized by prominent gastrointestinal disturbances and nutrient deficiencies. Defective exocrine functions can lead to a condition known as pancreatic exocrine insufficiency (PEI) due to a variety of reasons, including surgery such as bariatric surgery. After such procedures, altered GI anatomy renders PEI diagnosis challenging due to the propensity for symptoms to develop together with symptoms of other postoperative complications. For instance, patients may present with steatorrhea, unexplained weight loss, and malabsorption, all of which are indicators of low digestive enzyme activity. Therefore, early diagnosis is important, facilitated by diagnostic tests such as fecal elastase-1 (FE1) to confirm low pancreatic enzyme activity. PEI management is typically by pancreatic enzyme replacement therapy, where required enzymes are replaced to enable digestion and minimize the adverse effect on patient health (Arnelo et al., 2017). The interplay between the pancreas's exocrine functionality and some lifestyle factors, particularly alcohol consumption, has additional intricacies in gastrointestinal health. While most heavy drinkers are not victims of pancreatic diseases, some genetic or environmental susceptibilities may play a crucial role in their occurrence. Specifically, alcohol-induced damage may trigger adaptive responses in the pancreas, e.g., via the unfolded protein response (UPR) of the endoplasmic reticulum. Adaptive responses shield the pancreas against stress, enabling it to maintain enzyme production and thereby preventing acute disease such as pancreatitis in most heavy drinkers. Understanding how to activate such protective UPR responses could be the key to prevention and treatment of most pancreatic diseases, and ultimately in emphasizing the pancreas's pivotal role in digestion and overall health (Lugea et al., 2015).

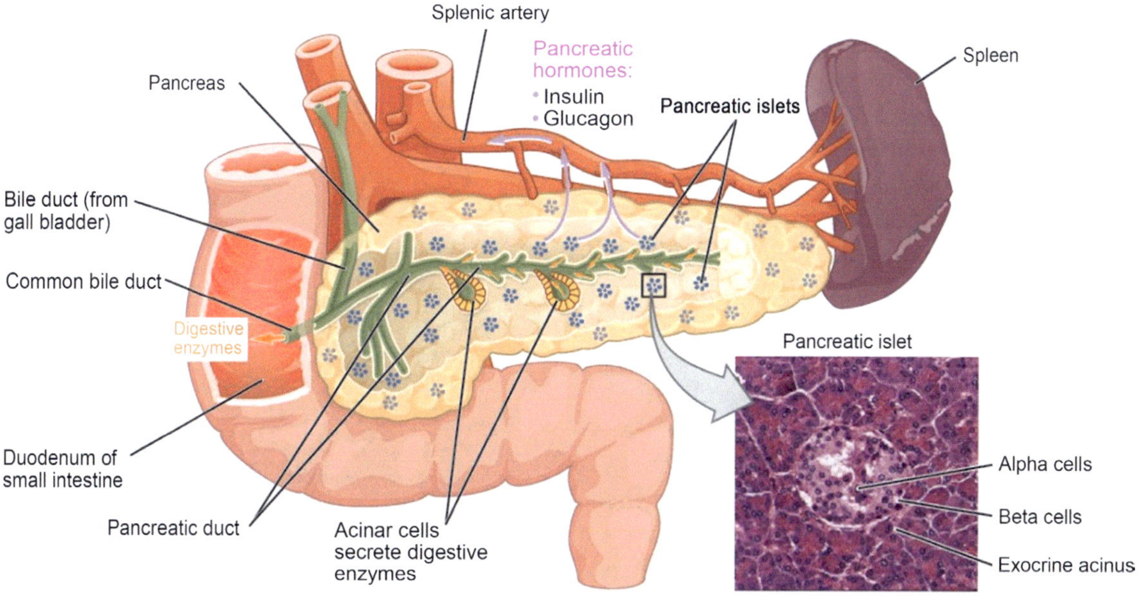

Figure 8.7. The pancreatic exocrine function involves the acinar cells secreting digestive enzymes that are transported into the small intestine by the pancreatic duct. Its endocrine function involves the secretion of insulin (produced by beta cells) and glucagon (produced by alpha cells) within the pancreatic islets. These two hormones regulate the rate of glucose metabolism in the body. The micrograph reveals pancreatic islets.

Source: https://s3-us-west-2.amazonaws.com/courses-images-archive-read-only/wp-content/uploads/sites/403/2015/04/21031221/1820_The_Pancreas.jpg

8.2.2. Endocrine Functions: Hormone Secretion

The pancreas plays a key role in maintaining metabolic homeostasis through its endocrine functions, specifically in regulating the release of hormones. Central to these functions are the islets of Langerhans, which are clusters of endocrine cells that secrete significant hormones such as insulin, glucagon, and somatostatin. Insulin exerts the action of lowering blood glucose via facilitation of cell uptake of glucose, while glucagon has the opposite effect, raising blood sugar levels when the latter is inordinately low. This fine balance is of prime importance for glucose homeostasis, pointing to the function of the pancreas in metabolic regulation. It is essential to appreciate this subtle interaction of hormones, especially under diabetic conditions, where hormone release derangement leads to emergent severe metabolic disturbances. The interaction between such hormones is not only critical to energy metabolism but also suggests a greater systemic effect within the human body (Valente et al., 2024). When considering the pancreas's endocrine roles in more detail, it is clear that hormonal secretion is not a fixed process but one that is dynamic and follows changing physiological conditions. For illustration, insulin release is heavily influenced by changes in blood glucose levels. After ingestion of carbohydrates, elevated glucose levels stimulate the beta cells of the islets to produce insulin rapidly. Conversely, during fasting, low glucose levels stimulate the release of glucagon from alpha cells to activate glucose reserves. In addition, hormones such as somatostatin, produced by delta cells, exert inhibitory effects on insulin and glucagon release, demonstrating an ideally balanced regulatory process. The precise coordination makes it possible for the body to respond in a favorable way to different metabolic demands, indicating the pancreas's significant role in endocrine control and overall well-being (Schl Künder et al., 2024). New research methodologies have enhanced our knowledge of pancreatic hormone secretion and its applicability to diabetes mellitus. New in vitro models, including microphysiological systems, have been developed to simulate the pancreatic endocrine environment so that real-time assessment of hormone secretion and cellular function can be made. These models allow for exploration of pancreatic beta cell response to glucose stimulation and the effects of antidiabetic drugs on insulin kinetics. Such research illuminates the complexities of hormone control and opens doors for therapeutic creativity. By including human pancreatic islet microtissues in these platforms, researchers can preserve endocrine pancreatic tissue's long-term viability, thereby obtaining insights needed for developing effective therapy for metabolic disease caused by pancreatic dysfunction (Valente et al., 2024; Schl Künder et al., 2024).

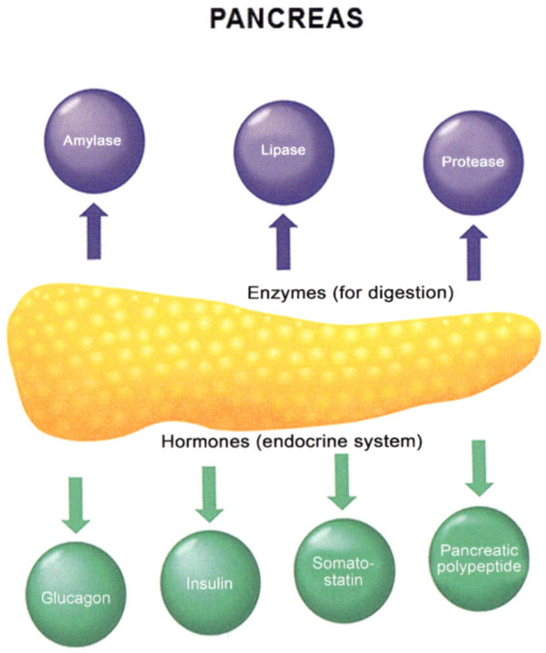

Figure 8.8. Endocrine function of the pancreas.

Source: https://www.bauchspeicheldruese-info.de/files/inhalte-bauchspeicheldruese-info/bilder/fachspezifische-themen/en-funktion_bauchspeicheldruese.jpg

8.2.3. Role in Metabolism and Nutrient Absorption

The pancreas serves a critical role in metabolism and nutrient absorption, primarily through its endocrine and exocrine roles. The exocrine pancreas secretes digestive enzymes such as amylase, lipase, and proteases that are crucial in the digestion of carbohydrates, fats, and proteins in the small intestine. Enzymatic action enables nutrient transport into the circulatory system, which is part of overall metabolic efficiency. In addition, the pancreas secretes bicarbonate to neutralize gastric acid and create a suitable environment for enzymatic action. Disruptions of pancreatic enzyme secretion can cause malabsorption syndromes, emphasizing its significant role in ensuring the body properly absorbs and utilizes nutrients gained through food. Thus, the health of the pancreas is inextricably bound with metabolic process activities, which are important in maintaining homeostasis and energy balance within the human system. The relationship between pancreatic function and dietary fiber further illustrates the pancreas's significant role in metabolism. Research has indicated that a high-fiber diet is able to augment intestinal barrier function as well as potentially inhibit pancreatic enzyme activity within certain populations. In acute pancreatitis, for instance, a prebiotic fiber-rich diet has been associated with low complication rates of infection and systemic inflammation. This protective mechanism emphasizes how fiber preserves stability in the gut and, by extension, pancreatic healing. However, in patients with exocrine pancreatic insufficiency, high fiber intake increases fecal fat excretion, suggesting a complex interaction between dietary components and pancreatic enzyme efficacy. Thus, understanding how fiber influences pancreatic function is critical to developing effective dietary management for pancreatic disease patients (Badiali et al., 2019). With age, the role of the pancreas in nutrient utilization takes on even greater significance. Aging is likely to produce many alterations in the GI tract, including diminished digestive efficacy and lowered rates of nutrient passage, that could ultimately result in nutritional deficiencies. The aged pancreas is also subject to a decrease in insulin secretion, disrupting glucose homeostasis and metabolism. Malnutrition is also high among the aging population, resulting in various health complications that become additive to existing conditions. It is necessary to appreciate the implications of such physiological alterations on pancreatic function to be able to address nutritional needs among the elderly. Tailored dietary interventions considering the aging population's unique physiological impairments can result in improved bioavailability and nutrient uptake, ultimately resulting in improved health outcomes among the population (Bordoni et al., 2015).

Test Your Knowledge

1. What is the exocrine function of the pancreas enzymes?
2. What is the role of pancreas in metabolism and nutrient absorption?

8.3. Pancreatic Enzymes

Learning Outcome

1. Describe the types of digestive enzymes produced
2. Understand the activation and regulation of enzymes
3. Understand the importance of enzymes in digestion

The pancreas significantly assists in digestion by providing pancreatic enzymes, which are very important in degrading macronutrients in the small intestine. They are amylase, lipase, and proteases like trypsin and chymotrypsin. Each of the enzymes serves a specific purpose; for instance, the digestion of carbohydrates starts with amylase, the digestion of fat is performed by lipase, and proteins are digested by proteases. The activation of the enzymes is precise to involve hormonal control in terms of detail and the existence of an alkaline environment sustained by bicarbonate secretions of the pancreas itself. The complex interrelationship guarantees that enzymes are activated within the intestine, where they might best perform their digestive function, underscores the pancreas's vital contribution towards nutritional absorption and overall metabolic health. Disturbances in pancreatic enzyme function may have important clinical outcomes, such as pancreatic exocrine insufficiency (PEI). PEI occurs when the pancreas is unable to secrete a sufficient amount of enzymes for digestion, resulting in malabsorption, steatorrhea, and weight loss. PEI incidence is especially pertinent in patients who have had upper gastrointestinal surgery because changes in anatomy may influence enzyme secretion and activity. Diagnosis also utilizes fecal elastase-1 (FE1) as a biomarker for the level of pancreatic enzymes. Treatment for PEI is most commonly initiated by the administration of pancreatic enzyme replacement therapy, a fundamental feature of patient care that ensures adequate nutrient absorption and metabolic status after such interventions, as reported in recent studies pointing out the influence of surgical operations on the integrity of the pancreas (Arnelo et al., 2017). Diet plays a multifaceted role in the regulation of pancreatic function, particularly in patients with prior pancreatic disease. Dietary fiber has been shown to have a two-faced influence on pancreatic enzyme function. While fiber supplementation is observed to improve the integrity of the intestinal barrier and reduce acute pancreatitis complications, increased fiber may also inhibit enzyme activity in the case of exocrine pancreatic insufficiency, hence accelerating fecal fat excretion and maldigestion. The mechanism by which dietary fiber affects enzyme activity remains to be determined, with some hypothesizing that enzymes become bound to fiber components or trapped by the structure of some fibers. It is necessary to comprehend this dual function of fiber to create nutritional guidelines specific to the patient's requirement so that clinicians can equilibrate the advantage of fiber consumption with its possible drawback of pancreatic enzyme impairment (Badiali et al., 2019).

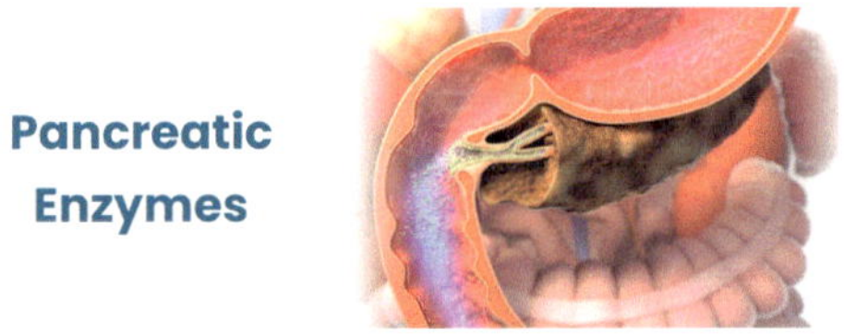

Figure 8.9. Pancreatic Enzymes.

Source: https://www.medicoverhospitals.in/images/articles/pancreatic-enzymes.webp

8.3.1. Types of Digestive Enzymes Produced

The pancreas is indispensable in human digestion through its secretion of digestive enzymes that facilitate the digestion of macromolecules. These enzymes consist of proteases, which cleave proteins to peptides and amino acids.

The most important pancreatic proteases are trypsin, chymotrypsin, and carboxypeptidase. These enzymes are secreted in inactive form as zymogens, which, in the small intestine, are converted to active form in order to prevent self-digestion. Such strict regulation of these enzymes is critical, as they are not only responsible for nutrient uptake but also for maintaining overall gastrointestinal homeostasis. Maintenance of a balance between proteases is what effectively degrades proteins in the diet so that the body may utilize necessary amino acids for various physiological activities. Other than proteases, the pancreas also secretes carbohydrate-digestion enzymes, the most widespread of which is pancreatic amylase. This enzyme breaks down starch and glycogen into simpler sugars, the major ones being maltose and glucose. By breaking down complex carbohydrates, pancreatic amylase enables easier body absorption of energy. Secretion of this enzyme into the duodenum is crucial, especially after a meal rich in carbohydrates. Also, in combination with amylase, α-glucosidase is another enzyme that operates on the intestinal lining brush border to enable glucose absorption. The activity of these enzymes shows the pancreas's pivotal function in controlling glucose homeostasis, which is a pivotal aspect of type 2 diabetes, as shown by studies on other enzyme inhibitors (Daub et al., 2025). Furthermore, the pancreas has a pivotal role to play in the digestion of fats via the release of pancreatic lipase, the major enzyme for the hydrolysis of dietary fats into free fatty acids and glycerol. Lipase cooperates with bile salts to emulsify the fats, making digestion and absorption in the small intestine easy. The enzymic activity is important for energy storage and cell functions, as the fatty acids are key sources of energy. This pancreatic lipase function is supplemented by findings indicating competitive inhibitors with the ability to control activity (Campos F da Silva et al., 2023). Their existence not only enunciates therapeutic possibilities for metabolic diseases and obesity conditions but also elucidates the pancreas's function in regulating nutrient intake and metabolic health overall. Through these intricate enzymatic processes, the pancreas is the foundation of human digestive efficiency and metabolic balance.

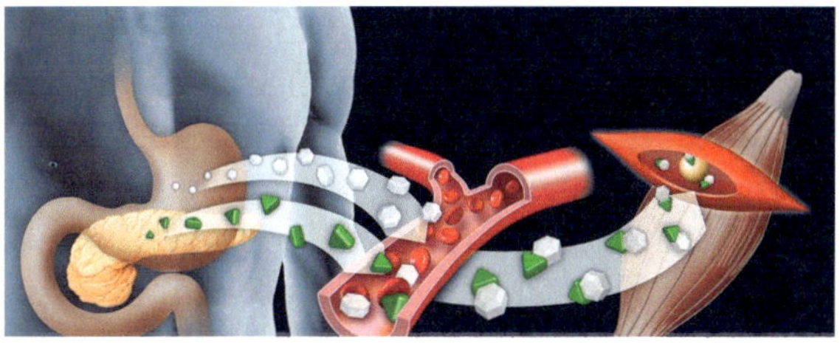

Figure 8.10. Role of Pancreas in Digestion.

Source: https://www.hopkinsmedicine.org/-/media/images/health/1_-conditions/liver-gallbladder-and-pancreas/pancreas-digestion-hero.jpg?h=500&iar=0&mh=500&mw=1300&w=1297&hash=201F001C9F1894CBDF2CBD5830205F0D

8.3.2. Activation and Regulation of Enzymes

Activation and regulation of enzymes are integral components of digestion processes in the human pancreas that impact both metabolic pathways and the overall efficiency of digestion. Digestive enzymes like amylase, lipase, and proteases in the pancreas are synthesized in inactive forms, known as zymogens. Precautions against premature activation safeguard pancreatic tissues against enzyme injury. These zymogens are activated in the duodenum by the action of enteropeptidase, specifically on trypsinogen to generate trypsin. Trypsin proceeds to activate other zymogens, thus generating a cascade that drives enzyme activation and regulates digestion. The highly specific regulation of this activation of the enzyme is essential not only for effective digestion but also for the prevention of pathological conditions such as pancreatitis, which can lead to inappropriate activation in the pancreas itself. Regulation of enzymatic activity in the pancreas is also inextricably linked to hormonal regulation, namely by the action of secretin and cholecystokinin (CCK). Secretin is released when acidic chyme enters the duodenum, stimulating the pancreas to secrete bicarbonate-rich fluid that neutralizes stomach acid. This physiological action forms an ideal pH for enzymatic function and optimizes digestive capacity. Alternatively, CCK is released upon fatty and proteolytic stimuli, stimulating the release of pancreatic enzymes. This interaction between these hormones guarantees proper enzymatic response adaptation to chyme content, proving regulatory dynamic mechanisms of enzyme activity control. With this complex hormonal feedback system, the pancreas maintains a high degree of balance, enabling efficient digestion and preventing digestive system pathologies. Moreover, enzyme activation and regulation dysregulation in the pancreas might lead to severe metabolic disorders or diseases. For instance, in the condition of cystic fibrosis, thick mucus blocks pancreatic ducts, hindering the passage of digestive enzymes and resulting in malabsorption syndromes. Similarly, certain inflammatory conditions have been reported to induce abnormal functioning of enzymes; for example, elevated levels of citrullinated proteins can interfere with enzyme activities, promoting inflammatory responses as observed in rheumatoid arthritis (Martin et al., 2023). Conversely, advances in proteomics research have attributed the dynamic nature of enzyme profiles under various pathological conditions and identified the potential disease progression biomarkers (Li et al., 2022). These processes are significant in that they enhance our knowledge not only of pancreatic functions but also of the broader implications of enzymatic regulation of human health and disease control.

8.3.3. Importance of Enzymes in Digestion

The role of enzymes in digestion is the most important, since they facilitate the breakdown of complex macromolecules to an absorbable state. The pancreas is the epicenter of the activity, secreting an array of digestive enzymes that facilitate effective alimentary processing. These include amylase, lipase, and proteases, which are specific for carbohydrates, fats, and proteins, respectively, thereby making nutrients available for absorption in the small intestine. The efficient functioning of these pancreatic enzymes is critical; deficiencies lead to malabsorption and other gastrointestinal disorders. Furthermore, these enzymes are tightly regulated by hormonal stimuli, which underscores the intricate interaction between the pancreas and the alimentary tract in general. The absence of these enzymes would drastically impair digestion, underscoring their fundamental importance to human physiology and dietetics. In addition to their role in digestion, pancreatic enzymes also play a role in metabolic control and intestinal health. For instance, proteases are not only responsible for protein digestion but also control inflammation and microbiota balance in the gut. The enzymes secreted by the pancreas, such as those being highlighted in current studies, such as studies on bacterial proteases, have potential therapeutic applications in protein digestion disorder treatment and wound care. This emerging understanding indicates that enzymes not only act as facilitators but also as controllers in the digestive system and other systems, enhancing not just digestive efficiency but also healthy gut microbiota. Our understanding of the properties and application of these enzymes is furthered by advanced biotechnological methods, underlining their potential in therapy in the clinical context too. Moreover, the enzyme secretion and action kinetics underline the complex relationship between the pancreas and the rest of the gastrointestinal tract. The pancreatic duct is used as a conduit for pancreatic juice, which is rich in enzymes, to flow into the duodenum and mix with food. This osmosis of digestive material is responsible for proper digestion and illustrates the way the pancreas secretes these enzymes but also regulates their release.

Recent research has even targeted pancreatic ductal organoids, with interest focused on specialized cells in enzyme secretion and gut signaling mechanisms. This new technique sheds light on the subtle homeostasis of balance established in the digestive tract and opens new research directions centering on tuft cells and their potential functions in food constituent perception and regulation of pancreatic enzyme secretion. Overall, the work of enzymes during digestion is more than simple biochemical reactions; they are vital in maintaining homeostasis and health in the human organism.

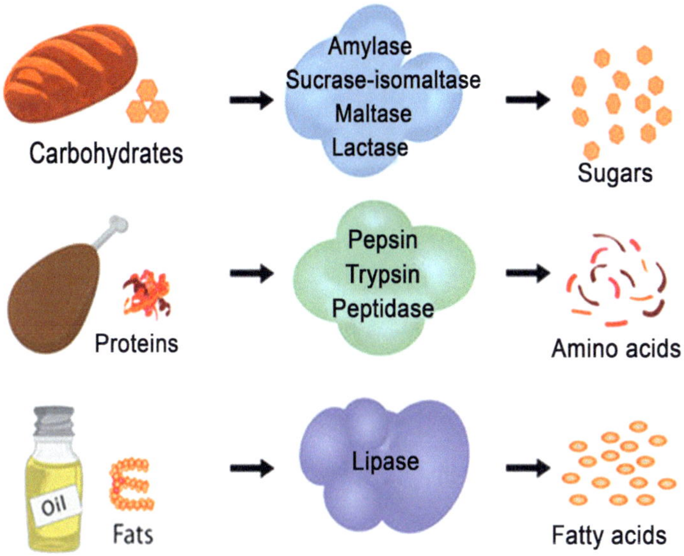

Figure 8.11. Digestive enzymes.

Source: https://classnotes123.com/wp-content/uploads/2021/04/digestive-enzyme.jpg

Test Your Knowledge

1. What are the types of digestive enzymes?
2. What is the role of enzymes in digestion?

8.4. Hormonal Regulation

Learning Outcome

1. Understand insulin and its role in glucose metabolism
2. Know the glucagon and its effects on blood sugar levels
3. Describe the other hormones produced by the pancreas

The pancreas also has the job of ensuring hormonal balance, basically through its endocrine role, and that is releasing hormones such as insulin and glucagon. Insulin and glucagon are key players in glucose homeostasis so that the body can make use of amounts of energy in an effective manner. Insulin, secreted by beta cells of the islets of Langerhans, brings glucose into the cells from the bloodstream after food intake, reducing blood sugar levels. In contrast, glucagon, which is secreted from alpha cells, raises blood glucose through the stimulation of hepatic glycogenolysis and gluconeogenesis during fasting. The fine balance between insulin and glucagon is a demonstration of how sensitive and refined the regulation of hormones is maintained to promote metabolic homeostasis and prevent hypoglycemia or hyperglycemia.

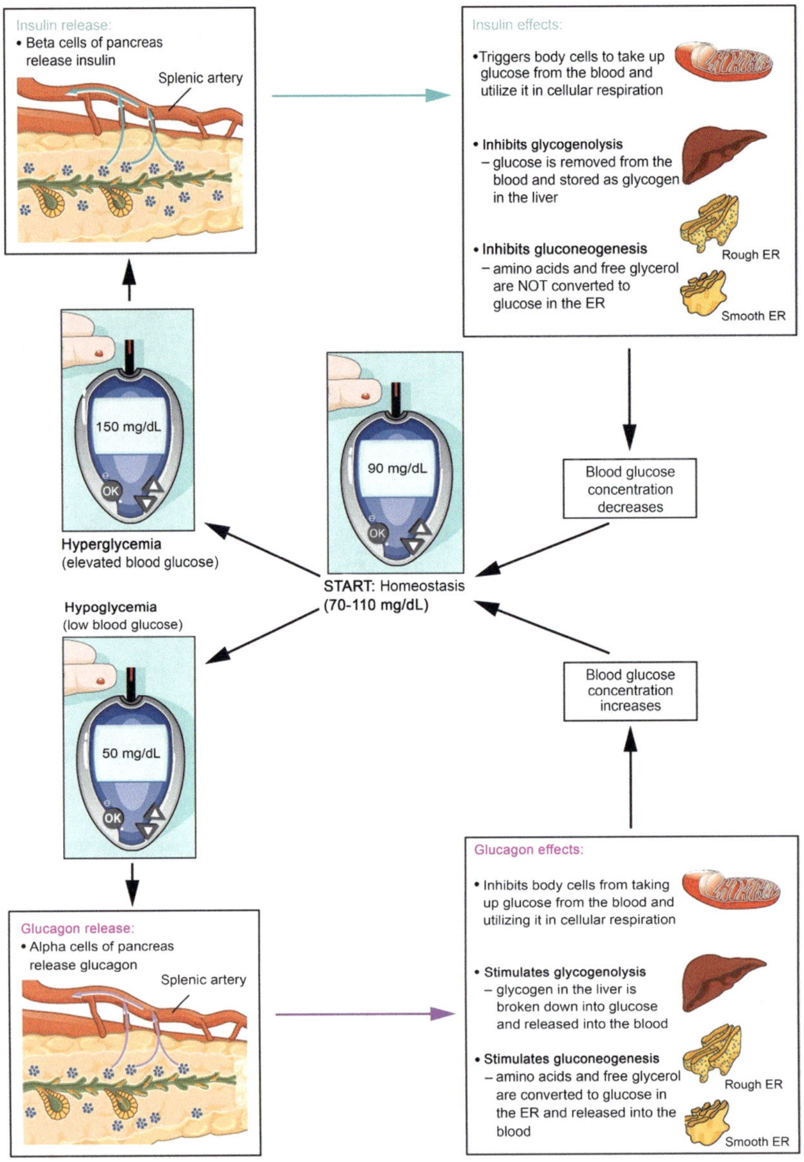

Figure 8.12. Blood glucose concentration is tightly maintained between 70 mg/dL and 110 mg/dL. If blood glucose concentration rises above this range, insulin is released, which stimulates body cells to remove glucose from the blood. If blood glucose concentration drops below this range, glucagon is released, which stimulates body cells to release glucose into the blood.

Source: https://s3-us-west-2.amazonaws.com/courses-images-archive-read-only/wp-content/uploads/sites/403/2015/04/21031225/1822_The_Homostatic_Regulation_of_Blood_Glucose_Levels.jpg

It only serves to illustrate the significant influence of the pancreas on physiological function and metabolic health to enable these mechanisms. Hormonal control is not restricted to insulin and glucagon but encompasses several significant pathways that have relevance in various physiological processes. Pancreatic somatostatin also inhibits the release of insulin and glucagon and therefore functions as a homeostatic mechanism to provide glucose homeostasis despite altered metabolic states. The pancreas also interacts with other endocrine organs, such as the adrenal glands, to respond to stressors by secreting hormones such as cortisol and epinephrine that have the ability to modify insulin sensitivity and glucose metabolism. Disruption of these pathways may lead to such diseases as diabetes mellitus, with significant implications for patient management and treatment outcome. An understanding of these interplaying controls of hormones is essential in moving towards therapeutic interventions towards the restoration of metabolic homeostasis, emphasizing the pancreas's complex function as an integral part of the endocrine apparatus. In addition, hormonal function within the pancreas is inextricably linked with circadian rhythm, emphasizing relative concordance between endogenous biological rhythms and metabolic homeostasis. Recent research has highlighted the crucial role molecular clocks play in controlling rhythms of hormonal secretion in synchrony with feeding and fasting circadian rhythms, both insulin sensitivity and glucose tolerance being influenced. Disruption of these circadian rhythms can potentially lead to metabolic disease and amplify the problem of timing as it comes to hormone discharge and its effect on overall health. In particular, the interaction between pancreatic and circadian regulation suggests that lifestyle factors, such as sleep habits and eating schedules, may affect hormonal control. This observation suggests that therapeutic interventions for harmonizing hormonal activity with internal biological rhythms offer new avenues in the treatment of endocrine and metabolic disorders effectively, placing a new picture on the vision of the role of the pancreas in human well-being (Bruscalupi and Gnocchi, 2017; Arnelo et al., 2017).

8.4.1. Insulin and Its Role in Glucose Metabolism

The connection of insulin to glucose metabolism is central to homeostasis in the human body. Insulin, which is a peptide hormone released from the pancreatic beta cells, is an important regulator of blood glucose concentration. When carbohydrates are consumed, blood glucose levels rise, and the pancreas releases insulin. This hormone allows for glucose entry into various body tissues, predominantly muscle and fat tissues, thereby lowering blood sugar levels. Insulin also stimulates glycogenesis, the conversion of glucose to glycogen to be stored in the liver and muscle tissue, thereby acting as an instant regulator of energy balance. In this, the pancreas is not only an organ of digestion but also a chief control center for the metabolic processes that influence overall human growth and health. The intricate regulation processes involved in insulin release and action are also crucial to understanding glucose metabolism. The endocrine nature of the islets of the pancreas provides for the strict regulation of insulin release in response to variations in blood glucose, although it is also influenced by hormonal stimuli as well as neural input. Consequently, not only is insulin release provoked by an increase in glucose, but other stimuli, such as the presence of certain amino acids or intestinal hormones, can also elicit the release of insulin. This multicompartmental regulatory system is a sophisticated network that governs numerous metabolic needs and emphasizes the pancreas's position as the central point of endocrine control. Insulin's ability to regulate the activity of numerous glucose-sensitive cells is evidence of its significance in maintaining glucose homeostasis and reducing the likelihood of metabolic disease. Despite its crucial role, insulin signaling is susceptible to malfunction, which could lead to diseases such as insulin resistance and diabetes. A classic case is that of type 2 diabetes (T2D), where both environmental and genetic factors perturb insulin secretion and action at the target tissue. As seen in current studies, T2D variants may not only impair insulin release but also the development of the pancreatic islet cells. The Wnt signaling transcription factor Tcf712, linked to susceptibility for T2D, demonstrates the genetic influences that can impact endocrine function as well as vascular health of the pancreas (Argenton et al., 2017). Because islet cells continuously interact with an extensive series of signals, integrated understanding of insulin and its metabolic importance is crucial to create treatment interventions for diabetes therapy to restore the balance of glucose homeostasis (Huising et al., 2019).

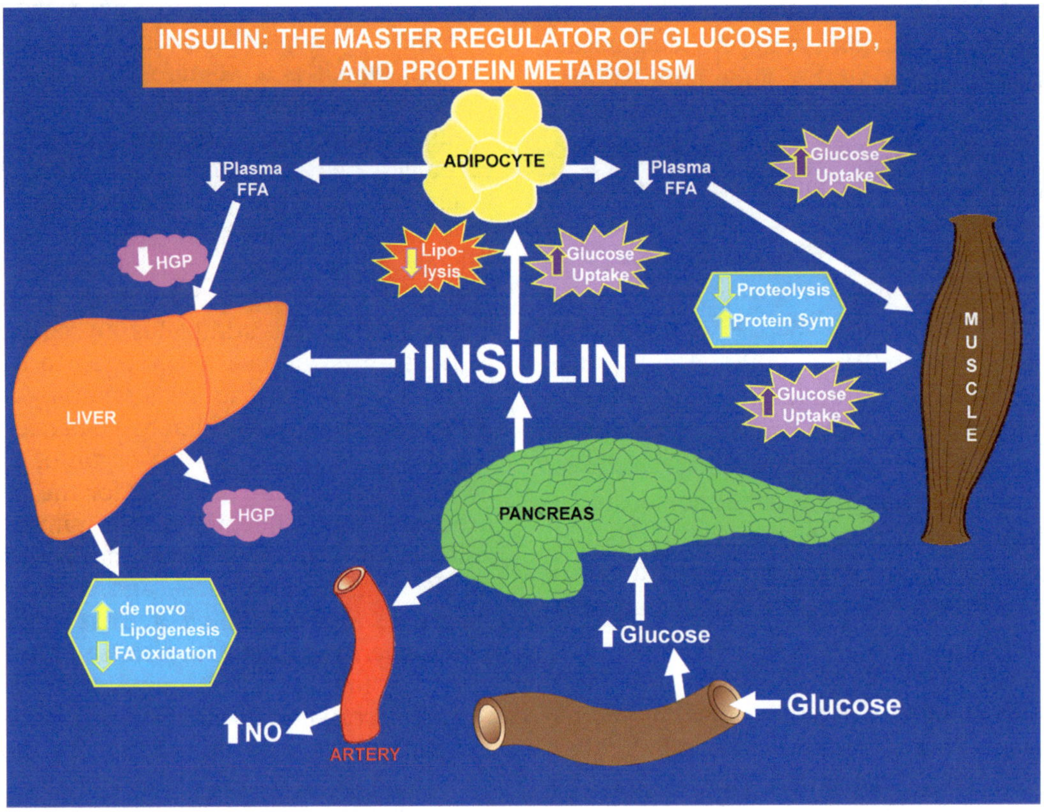

Figure 8.13. Insulin: The master regulator of glucose metabolism.

Source: https://ars.els-cdn.com/content/image/1-s2.0-S0026049522000208-ga1_lrg.jpg

8.4.2. Glucagon and Its Effects on Blood Sugar Levels

Glucagon is a pancreatic alpha-cell-released peptide hormone that plays a crucial role in maintaining blood glucose levels, particularly under fasting or hypoglycemic states. During hypoglycemia, the secretion of glucagon into the circulation occurs, and it only has an effect on the liver, inducing glycogenolysis—glycogen hydrolysis to glucose. This effect increases the available blood glucose, enabling crucial organs, especially the brain, to obtain the energy they need to function optimally. Glucagon also promotes gluconeogenesis, glucose synthesis from non-carbohydrate sources, another way through which it stabilizes blood glucose. The action between insulin and glucagon, a hormone of the pancreas, is mediated by the former to maintain metabolic homeostasis since they interact in the regulation of blood glucose after food intake and during fasting or increased physical activity. The function of glucagon is even more apparent in the case of diabetes mellitus, a chronic disease in which deregulated blood glucose occurs. In type 1 diabetes, with markedly compromised insulin secretion, glucagon secretion can become deregulated and lead to hyperglycemia and disease ease of control problems. In type 2 diabetes, insulin resistance can lead to disrupted glucagon dynamics, with sustained high blood sugars. Studies highlight that dysregulation of glucagon secretion and its impairment of glucose counter-regulation can exacerbate glycemic control problems (Putri MMD et al., 2025). Consequently, understanding glucagon's role is crucial for developing therapeutic strategies aimed at managing diabetes and preventing the associated complications, such as cardiovascular disease and neuropathy. Moreover, recent research suggests that glucagon may also interact with various metabolic pathways, influencing overall energy balance beyond its traditional role in glucose metabolism. This interaction is particularly relevant to the consideration of the evidence for pancreatic function influenced by SARS-CoV-2, as uncovered by Qin et al. (Azoitei et al., 2024). This evidence indicates infection with the virus has the potential to lead to pancreatic dysfunction, shifting insulin and glucagon release, which could eventually lead to dysregulated glucose homeostasis. This action emphasizes the pancreatic organ's pivotal role, not only in regulating blood glucose concentration, but also in maintaining overall metabolic integrity, especially in the face of systemic disease. Recognition of these complex interactions offers valuable insights to gastroenterologists and endocrinologists, as it assures the need for holistic management approaches to disorders of pancreatic function.

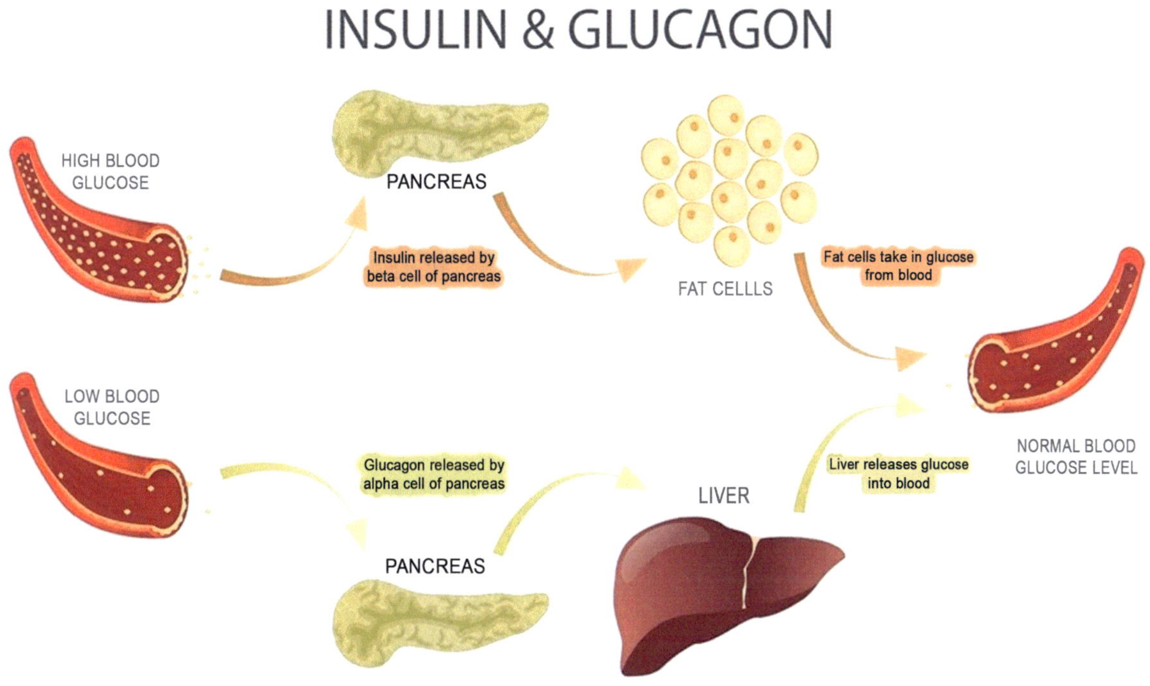

Figure 8.14. Understanding glucagon: The counterpart to insulin.

Source: https://d2jx2rerrg6sh3.cloudfront.net/image-handler/ts/20241122121413/ri/950/src/images/Article_Images/ImageForArticle_25538_17322956522701880.jpg

8.4.3. Other Hormones Produced By the Pancreas

The pancreas is not only at the center of insulin production but also the release of other important hormones that are responsible for regulating a number of physiological body functions. Some of these hormones include glucagon, which is secreted by the alpha cells of the islets of Langerhans. The primary function of glucagon is to increase blood sugar levels, especially during fasting or decreased consumption of carbohydrates. This hormone initiates glycogenolysis—the breakdown of glycogen stored in the liver into glucose — which is released into the bloodstream. Additionally, glucagon triggers gluconeogenesis, a metabolic pathway that generates glucose from non-carbohydrate substrates. By virtue of its opposing activity to insulin, glucagon functions as the master key to the homeostasis of glucose, thus ensuring organs and tissues a constant source of energy, especially under conditions of metabolic stress. Again, another crucial hormone secreted by the pancreas is somatostatin, produced by the delta cells of the islets of Langerhans. Somatostatin is a feedback hormone, and it controls both the release of insulin and glucagon. This negative feedback avoids oscillations between the two hormones and thus is a critical contributor to energy metabolism. Aside from its pancreatic functions, somatostatin has far-reaching effects on the rest of the body, including inhibiting the release of growth hormone from the pituitary and inhibiting gastric emptying. By controlling these systems, somatostatin inhibits blood energy levels from becoming uncontrolled and is involved in the control of metabolic rates in general. This is important in pathologies such as diabetes mellitus, where there is an imbalance in hormone levels, and somatostatin is an important component of endocrine regulation. Klotho, another hormone secreted by the pancreas, is now increasingly implicated in aging and metabolic health. While its primary expression is within the kidneys, Klotho is expressed in other tissues as well, including the pancreas, wherein it serves as an endocrine hormone influencing fibroblast growth factor (FGF) signaling pathways. Klotho's role is brought out by the fact that it plays a role in the prevention of age-related diseases since its levels correlate with chronic illnesses such as diabetes and neurodegenerative diseases. Notably, Klotho inhibits multiple aging pathways like insulin-like growth factor 1 (IGF-1) and transforming growth factor β (TGF-β), which, when not regulated, result in cellular senescence and inflammation. With its multi-faceted strategies, Klotho not only helps in metabolic homeostasis but also presents an optimistic therapeutic target to combat age-related illnesses, further highlighting the diversity of the hormones secreted by the pancreas (Gérald J Prud'homme et al., 2022; Refat MAR et al., 2021).

Test Your Knowledge

1. What is the role of insulin in glucose metabolism?
2. What is glucagon and its effects on blood sugar levels?

8.5. Diseases of the Pancreas

Learning Outcome

1. Describe the types and implications of diabetes mellitus
2. Describe the causes and symptoms of pancreatitis
3. Know the risk factors and prognosis of pancreatic cancer

The pancreas, an abdominal organ, can be affected by a variety of diseases that disrupt its essential roles with respect to digestion and blood sugar control. Of these, pancreatitis is one of the most significant conditions. Pancreatitis, inflammation of the pancreas, can occur as an acute or chronic condition and varies in severity and presentation. Acute pancreatitis will often arise acutely and can be caused by etiologies like gallstones, heavy long-term alcohol use, or some medications. Presentation can include severe abdominal pain, vomiting, and nausea. Proper diagnosis requires that sophisticated imaging techniques such as abdominal ultrasonography, though it is highly dependent on the skill of the operator. In the majority of cases, acute pancreatitis necessitates hospitalization, intensive supportive care, and potentially surgical interventions; thus, the priority is on rapid and accurate diagnosis and management (Daminet et al., 2010). Chronic pancreatitis, in contrast to its acute counterpart, is characterized by prolonged inflammation leading to permanent pancreatic tissue damage. This condition usually occurs after repeated episodes of acute pancreatitis, particularly in individuals with a history of drug use or family history. The patients may experience chronic abdominal pain, weight loss, and malabsorption due to pancreas's diminished ability to secrete digestive enzymes. On progression of the disease, there is a greater likelihood of pancreatic exocrine insufficiency, and dietary adjustments need to be made to address malabsorption issues. In later stages, pancreatitis can lead to diabetes mellitus due to impaired insulin secretion by the damaged pancreas. Understanding the multifactorial nature of chronic pancreatitis is crucial to develop a treatment plan that is holistic with an approach towards symptom control, nutritional management, and lifestyle modification to enhance the quality of life of such patients. Nutritional management of pancreatic disease is a significant aspect that has a great bearing on the outcome of the patient. There is evidence that diet treatment can play an important role in relieving and curing many patients suffering from pancreatic disease. For instance, in acute pancreatitis, the implementation of a prebiotic-enriched diet can lower the incidence of complications such as necrosis infection of the pancreas and hospital stay. The pathophysiology behind this is believed to be due to the fibers' ability to stabilize the intestinal barrier and suppress systemic inflammation. Alternatively, pancreatic exocrine insufficiency patients find it challenging to take high-fiber food since it leads to increased fecal fat excretion by inhibiting the action of pancreatic enzymes (Badiali et al., 2019). Therefore, it is important to personalize nutrition strategies in order to effectively treat such complex diseases, showing the intricate relationship between diet and pancreatic health.

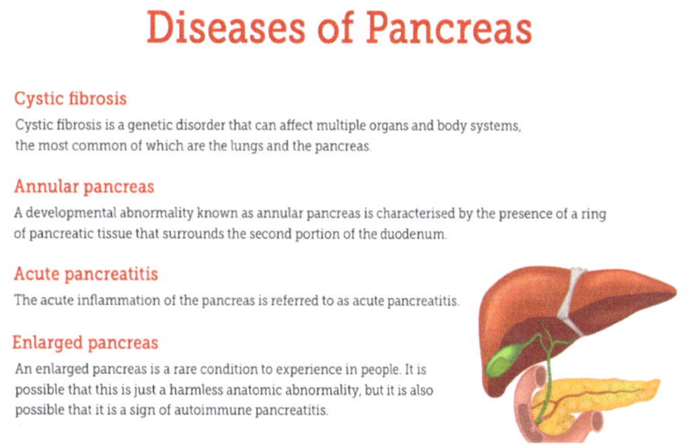

Figure 8.15. Diseases of the pancreas.

Source: https://assets.lybrate.com/imgs/tic/enadp/disease-of-pancreas.webp

8.5.1. Diabetes Mellitus: Types and Implications

Diabetes mellitus is a group of metabolic disorders that are characterized by hyperglycemia resulting from the body's inability to produce or effectively utilize insulin. Diabetes is predominantly categorized into two types: type 1 and type 2. Type 1 diabetes, typically diagnosed at the onset, results from an autoimmune destruction of the pancreatic beta cells and absolute insulin deficiency. This form of diabetes necessitates life-long insulin therapy and strict regulation of blood glucose to prevent acute complications such as diabetic ketoacidosis. Type 2 diabetes, accounting for the majority of the diabetes that exists in the world, is characterized by insulin resistance with relative insulin deficiency. The pathophysiology of these disorders provides a clear indication of how pancreatic dysfunction can significantly impact metabolic homeostasis, reinforcing the importance of pancreatic health to the body as a whole. The burden of diabetes mellitus transcends individual health, as both conditions contribute to significant public health concerns regarding morbidity and mortality. Patients with Type 2 diabetes can often have several comorbidities, including cardiovascular disease, renal impairment, and vision impairment. Type 2 diabetes in children is particularly concerning because, in the last several decades, the rate of development has been increasing. It is in light of this that the role of genetic predisposition and modifiable risk factors, such as lifestyle and obesity, is seen to contribute to the definition of the disease course. Detection and early treatment are the main objectives in the management of such conditions with a view to minimizing long-term complications and enhancing the quality of life in patients. Additionally, understanding the role of diabetes within healthcare systems is essential in long-term planning and the formulation of treatment strategies. Research into the classification of diabetes categories has also resulted in reconsideration of how it should be treated. The contrast between Type 1 and Type 2 diabetes is a model for the need for personalized therapeutic strategies depending on the underlying pathophysiology. For instance, while type 1 diabetes is more commonly defined by the necessity for exogenous insulin replacement, Type 2 diabetes can necessitate a change in lifestyle along with pharmacological therapies to enhance insulin sensitivity. Recent studies have highlighted the importance of diagnosing other forms of diabetes, such as secondary diabetes resulting from pancreatic and other endocrine diseases, so that patients can be cared for in their entirety. (Abdul-Rasoul et al., 2016) takes up the cause of proper classification and diagnosis in humans as well as animals, including how an etiological approach can help in improved treatment. This focus encourages a deeper understanding of diabetes and emphasizes the importance of the pancreas in regulating glucose metabolism and systemic health.

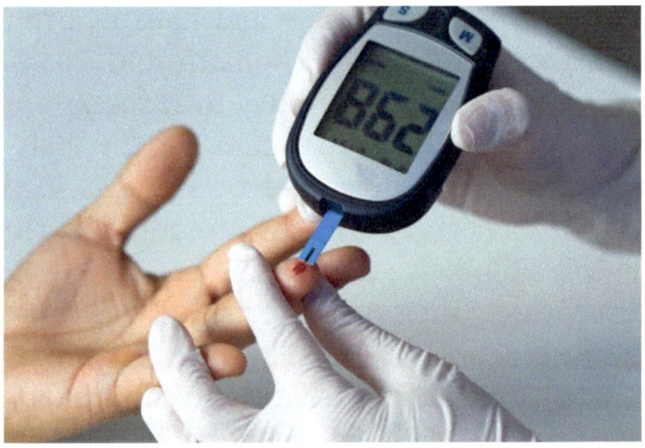

Figure 8.16. Diabetes mellitus.

Source: https://medtour.help/wp-content/uploads/2023/08/diabetes2-1-1.jpg

8.5.2. Pancreatitis: Causes and Symptoms

The pancreas plays a twofold function in the human body, primarily in digestion and glucose regulation, and is therefore prone to a list of diseases, symptoms of which include pancreatitis.

This inflammation can have a number of causes, varying from excessive alcohol consumption and gallstones to metabolic disease and certain drugs. Chronic pancreatitis is usually linked with prolonged exposure to such stressors, leading to massive pancreatic tissue injury and consequent impairment of its enzymatic secretions. The clinical characteristics of the condition include abdominal pain, weight loss, and fatty stools, indicative of derangement in nutrient absorption. Therefore, understanding the cause is very important in a bid to prevent and manage the condition. The symptoms of pancreatitis can present themselves in many different ways, significantly reducing the patient's quality of life. Acute pancreatitis typically starts with an acute presentation of stabbing epigastric pain, often referring to the back, and is associated with nausea and vomiting. Fever and tachycardia can also be seen as evidence of a more marked inflammatory response. Conversely, symptoms of chronic pancreatitis develop more insidiously with recurrent abdominal pain, bloating of the abdomen, and steatorrhea, which is malabsorption secondary to impaired secretion of enzymes. The overlap of these symptoms mandates a discriminating diagnostic evaluation, a mistaken diagnosis can lead to improper management and adverse outcomes for the patient. Complications of pancreatitis can further complicate diagnosis and treatment. For instance, pancreatic exocrine insufficiency (PEI), one of the most common complications of chronic pancreatitis, presents with comparable difficulties to be as challenging to diagnose as in patients undergoing upper gastrointestinal surgeries. As noted, PEI can be responsible for symptoms of maldigestion and malabsorption that are difficult to differentiate from post-bariatric surgery complications, such as steatorrhea and weight loss (Arnelo et al., 2017). Additionally, in some diseases like orthotopic liver transplantation, hyperamylasemia may indicate pancreatitis caused by surgery or surgery complications, which profoundly handicaps postoperative recovery (Gordon et al., 1992). Due to this, the cure of pancreatitis involves teamwork in identifying its myriad causes and symptoms to offer a comprehensive treatment program that reduces the likelihood of developing complications.

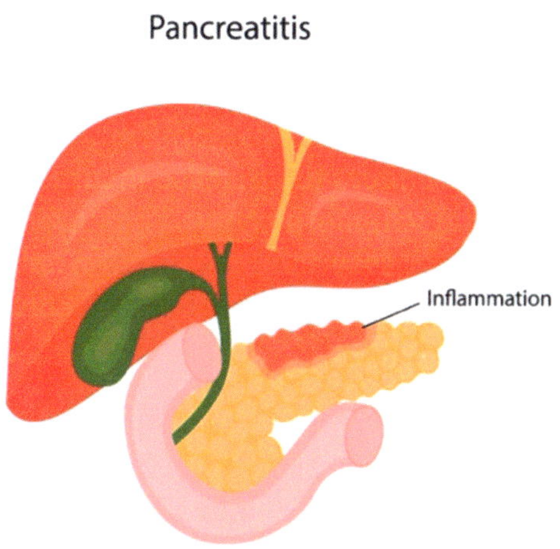

Figure 8.17. Pancreatic disorders.

Source: https://www.centrefordigestivecare.com/images/departments/pancreatic-disorders.jpg

8.5.3. Pancreatic Cancer: Risk Factors and Prognosis

The heterogeneity of pancreatic cancer represents an intricate mix of environmental and genetic factors that profoundly affect its development and prognosis. Of the major genetic elements, KRAS mutations are considered causal events in pancreatic ductal adenocarcinoma (PDAC). The mutations alone are not adequate to promote the invasive nature of the cancer; rather, they need other factors, such as obesity and type-2 diabetes, for the growth of tumors. Evidence shows that the oncogenic KRAS stimulates growth-promoting signaling networks; therefore, it is important to understand related pathways, such as the YAP/TAZ signaling pathway, which underlies PDAC biology. As projections forecast a rising incidence of pancreatic cancer owing in part to obesity, concerted attention towards prevention and interception strategies is more important than ever (Eibl and Rozengurt, 2019). The multimodal risk factors contribute to the pressure to find effective therapeutic approaches to cure this aggressive cancer. The survival rate for pancreatic cancer is poor, highlighting the late diagnosis and the aggressive nature of the disease. The primary reason for this poor survival rate is the extremely fibrotic tumor stroma that renders the disease incurable with conventional chemotherapy. The interaction between cancer cells and their stroma, including inflammatory processes, renders it challenging to treat.

The significance of inflammatory controllers like PPARα has been stressed in recent studies, as they may be a double-edged sword in cancer progression. In PPARα-deficient models, non-neoplastic cells were capable of inhibiting tumor growth, suggesting that the stromal microenvironment plays a critical role in cancer dynamics. These observations hold the promise of therapeutic value, and it implies that inhibition of the PPARα pathway could enhance the effectiveness of treatment and curtail the aggressive nature of pancreatic tumors (Hua et al., 2015). Elucidation of an intricate network of tumor-stroma interactions will be required to further enhance patient outcomes. New therapeutic interventions targeting the key molecular pathways can perhaps bring hope for improved management and results in pancreatic cancer patients. The recognition that conventional therapies are unable to work against the strong tumor microenvironment has generated interest in new therapeutic strategies. One such strategy is the use of PPARα antagonists, which have been potential agents in the growth inhibition of pancreatic tumor cells. By inducing G0/G1 cell cycle arrest, the antagonists cause cellular senescence rather than direct cell death, and this is a potential pathway through which the inefficacies of conventional therapies can be circumvented. Studies have shown that inhibiting the PPARα pathway not only represses tumor cells but also affects non-neoplastic components of the tumor microenvironment. As the biological underpinnings of pancreatic cancer continue to be unraveled, the integration of these new therapies will be central in rewriting prognosis and improving survival among victims. The disease's high mortality rate necessitates a continued exploration of these new therapeutic frontiers.

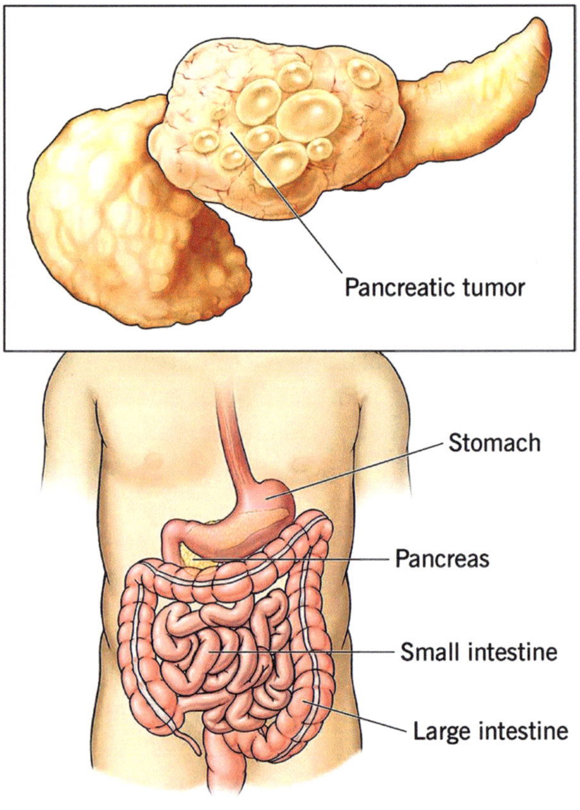

Figure 8.18. Cancer in the pancreas occurs when the cells in the pancreas multiply out of control.

Source: https://my.clevelandclinic.org/-/scassets/images/org/health/articles/21786-pancreatic-cancer-illustration

Test Your Knowledge

1. What are the implications of diabetes mellitus?
2. What are the main causes of pancreatitis?

8.6. Diagnostic Methods

Learning Outcome

1. Know the imaging techniques
2. Understand the blood tests for pancreatic function
3. Describe the biopsy and its role in diagnosis

Technological innovation in pancreatic diagnostic testing is crucial, given its complex role in many physiological processes like digestion and glucose homeostasis. The prevalent conventional histological methods, which are normally employed in studying pancreatic tissues, lack the capability to visualize three-dimensional architectural relationships that play critical functions in tissue pathophysiology. Routine thin-section histology is unable to accurately represent the complexity of pancreatic tissues, and this can lead to inaccurate interpretations of disease states. A novel biphasic hydrogel strategy delivers a substantial leap by enabling high-throughput volumetric quantitative interrogation of irregular and fragile tissue structures. The technique enhances developing and disease pancreatic tissue analysis, thereby making more accurate diagnosis and understanding of pancreatitis and pancreatic cancer possible, a considerable improvement over previous methods in which tissue structure was overlooked (Arda et al., 2017). In addition to histological methods, imaging technologies also play a pivotal role in the diagnosis of the pancreas. Through techniques such as MRI and CT scan, it is possible to have non-invasive methods of observing pancreatic morphology and identifying tumor or other abnormalities. These advanced imaging techniques allow physicians to have thorough information regarding pancreatic well-being without the side effects of invasive methods. For instance, MRI is quite capable of distinguishing normal from diseased tissue, and it offers functional information in terms of structural imaging. Application of such imaging techniques is particularly necessary in the diagnosis of pancreatic cancer, where early diagnosis can be of enormous value in treatment. Additionally, the application of artificial intelligence to interpret imaging data can improve diagnostic accuracy, reducing human error and enhancing the reliability of pancreatic examinations (Arda et al., 2017). Another new technique of diagnosing pancreatic disease is through digital scanning of photographs of the tongue, a technique which entices ancient diagnostic paradigms in some systems of Eastern medicine. This technique surpasses qualitative assessments by using computerized methods to assess color and textural features of the tongue, which may reflect the health of internal organs such as the pancreas. Finally, through complicated modeling, similarities between the condition of the tongue and pancreatic ailments are unveiled after meticulous training from patient data. It is not only a new frontier in diagnosis but also encourages more insight into how systemic disease is manifested in tangible symptoms. As doctors continue exploring the union of technology and traditional diagnostics, the possibility for the creation of an integrative diagnostic paradigm is increasingly obvious, eventually resulting in improved regulation of pancreatic conditions.

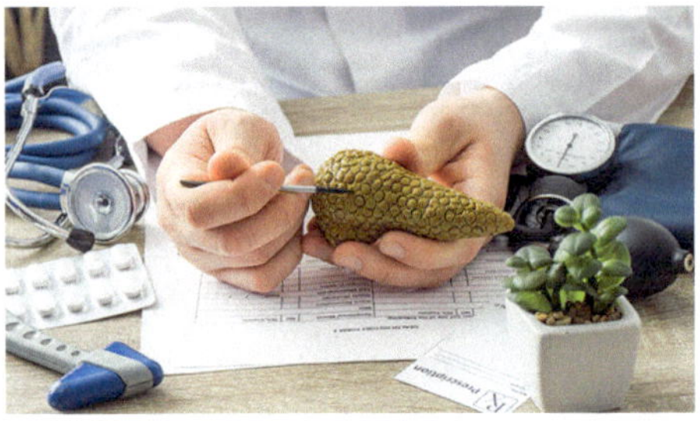

Source: https://www.hopkinsmedicine.org/-/media/images/health/1_-conditions/pancreatic-cancer/pancreatic-cancer-diagnosis-teaser.jpg

8.6.1. Imaging Techniques: Ultrasound and CT Scans

The pancreas is a part of digestion and insulin regulation, and hence the need for a good imaging technique takes center stage in the detection of pancreatic disorders. The two principal modalities employed here are ultrasound and computed tomography (CT) scan. Ultrasound imaging is particularly beneficial because it can be performed without invasive procedures and provides real-time imaging. It uses high-frequency sound waves to create exact images of the pancreas and surrounding structures to help clinicians identify pancreatitis, tumors, or cysts. Moreover, innovation in ultrasound technologies, such as the creation of intraductal and transgastric pathways for thermal treatment, is indicative of its growing role in therapeutic applications. Studies have shown that ultrasound can effectively treat pancreatic tumors with less tissue destruction, thereby enhancing treatment efficacy and patient safety (Adams et al., 2017). CT scans, however, provide a more general picture of the pancreas and are best used for evaluating complex structural anatomy and illness. X-rays are utilized by this technique to create cross-sectional images, detailing close examination of the pancreas and associated organs. One of the key advantages of CT is its ability to distinguish between cystic and solid lesions, which aids in making correct diagnoses. Also, detailed images created by CT scans enable the measurement of a tumor's size and location and its metastasis, which is required for treatment planning. The integration of more advanced techniques, such as the use of attention gates in deep learning frameworks, has been shown to improve the quality of analysis of CT images and, therefore, object localization as well as pancreatic structure segmentation (Glocker et al., 2018).

While both ultrasound scanning and CT scanning have some advantages, the choice of the right imaging technique in the majority of situations depends on the clinical setting as well as the information required. For example, ultrasound will usually be the preferred first-line test due to its ease of use and low cost, and the CT scan will be preferable in cases that require accurate anatomical information in complicated cases. The combination of imaging modalities for the diagnosis of pancreatic disorders will yield a synergy that will enhance patient outcomes. With the continued development of imaging technologies, additional studies must be performed to optimize these techniques and create new applications to help ensure that clinicians can maximize the use of these imaging modalities in the diagnosis and treatment of pancreatitis.

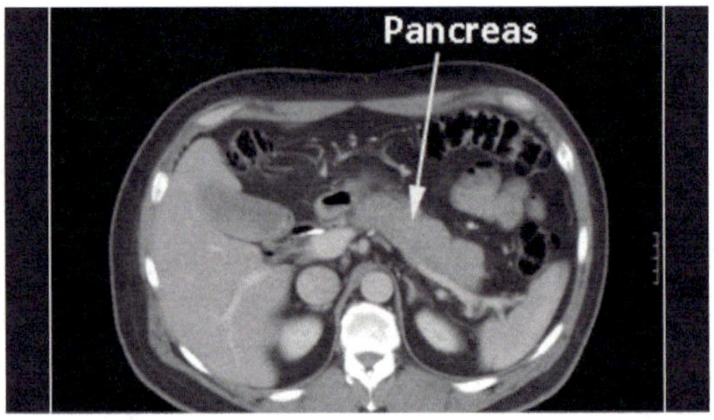

Figure 8.19. Advances in pancreatic CT and MR imaging.

Source: https://cf-images.us-east-1.prod.boltdns.net/v1/static/6168375534001/88ced833-1929-4844-8e12-801a5f450f43/0965017f-6f94-4279-840f-78bda3d97154/1280x720/match/image.jpg

8.6.2. Blood Tests For Pancreatic Function

Blood testing is a vital diagnostic tool that provides information regarding pancreatic function, which proves vital in the understanding of numerous diseases, particularly digestive and metabolic diseases. The pancreas serves both roles as an endocrine gland, where it secretes hormones like insulin, and an exocrine organ, where it secretes digestive enzymes. Blood tests quantify a few biomarkers like amylase and lipase, which are enzymes secreted by the pancreas responsible for carbohydrate and fat digestion, respectively. Elevated activity levels of these enzymes are most typically indicative of pancreatitis or trauma to the pancreas, reflecting the compromised functional state of the pancreas. In addition, blood glucose levels reflect the pancreas's endocrine function, indicating the adequacy of insulin secretion in response to rising blood glucose. Therefore, integrated blood testing is essential for ascertaining the condition of the pancreas and diagnosing related disorders in clinical practice. The addition of genetic analysis in blood tests can also further enrich our understanding of pancreatic diseases. More recent studies emphasize the role of single-nucleotide polymorphisms (SNPs) of the P2X7 receptor, which is linked to pancreatic ductal adenocarcinoma (PDAC) development. Curiously, two SNPs—474G>A and 853G>A—are negatively correlated with PDAC risk, suggesting the role of genetic influences in disease susceptibility. These SNPs have the potential to shape cellular responses in pancreatic stellate and cancer cells to impact variation in calcium signaling and cytokine release. Such findings are a potential step towards individualized medicine, where a blood test would not only determine pancreatic function at any point in time but also determine risk based on genetic predisposition. Such a dual-based strategy has the potential to ultimately enhance diagnostic efficacy and treatment efficacy for pancreatic diseases. In addition, advancements in encapsulation technology mirror the evolving nature of pancreatic function assessment. More recent studies demonstrated that conformal coatings can preserve islet function while providing immunoprotection. For instance, poly(N-vinylpyrrolidone) and tannic acid-mediated islet encapsulation enhanced transplant viability within diabetic models. Such advances can create new blood tests assessing islet function post-transplant, providing better insight into pancreatic health. Because islets encapsulated retain insulin-secretion function, one can monitor their performance through blood glucose levels, giving insight into pancreatic transplant short-term and long-term function. Collectively, these methods constitute a major paradigm shift in the approach whereby we quantify and interpret pancreatic function through blood tests, developing a more integrated model of diagnosis and therapy as outlined in the extensive review of the pancreas in human health.

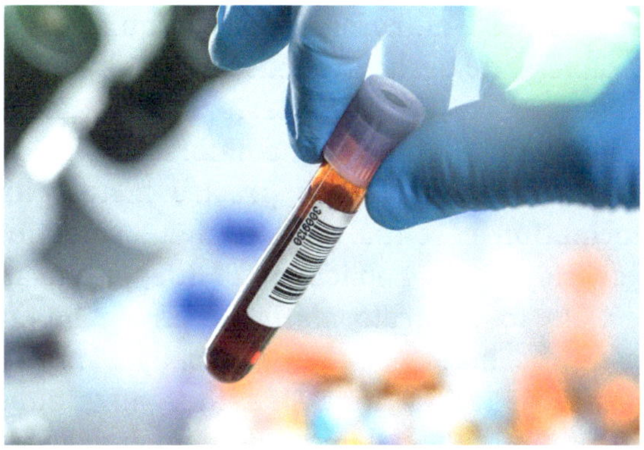

Figure 8.20. Pancreatitis blood tests.

Source: https://www.verywellhealth.com/thmb/g8wDy4eNL77YCQRdVLO4M7aFJtM=/1500x0/filters:no_upscale():max_bytes(150000):strip_icc()/GettyImages-1339206392-2cc6872c9fd64603bbc3e4a27631188d.jpg

8.6.3. Biopsy and Its Role in Diagnosis

In the complex world of pancreatic disease, biopsy stands out as the gold standard of diagnosis. The role of biopsy, particularly in autoimmune pancreatitis (AIP) and other pancreatic diseases, cannot be overstated. In type 1 AIP, for instance, biopsies demonstrate typical histopathological features such as a diffuse infiltrate of lymphocytes and plasmacytoid cells, and an overlying predominance of IgG4-positive plasma cells. All these findings not only confirm the diagnosis but also provide significant information regarding the disease history. The most valuable aspect of the biopsy analysis is the identification of pathognomonic cellular patterns, through which clinicians can differentiate AIP from other neoplasias with high efficiency. Thus, familiarity with such criteria ultimately enhances the validity of clinical assessment by enabling patients to receive appropriate therapeutic interventions tailored to their unique pancreatic states. Endoscopic ultrasound-guided fine-needle aspiration and biopsy is a significant innovation in the diagnostic evaluation of pancreatic diseases. EUS allows real-time acquisition of the pancreatic tissue with ease of tumor staging and detection of cystic lesions. In addition to being safer and more comfortable for the patient, it also provides precise histological information essential in treatment selection. By employing the application of EUS, physicians are able to separate malignant from benign pancreatic masses by cytologically sampling them, an action that provides invaluable information on cell morphology and tumor characteristics. Subsequently, EUS-guided biopsies play an important role in refining diagnosis and contributing to more focused treatment for those patients presenting with pancreatic illnesses, and ultimately improved patient outcomes. Furthermore, the biopsy interpretation test has a solid foundation of both clinical presentation and pathological features. For example, the presence of IgG4-positive plasma cells can be used to diagnose type 1 AIP, suggesting the importance of meticulous observation of the biopsy sample. However, it must be remembered that isolated growth in these cells is not necessarily diagnostic of AIP, since there is always the possibility of overlap with pancreatic ductal adenocarcinoma. Pathologists thus need to recognize the specific histological features and relative proportions that characterize AIP as outlined in existing guidelines. In this way, correlating histologic findings with immunohistochemical markers improves diagnostic specificity and helps overcome the pitfalls of diagnostic imprecision in pancreatic disease, a classic illustration of the role of biopsy in determining diagnosis for pancreatic pathology to resolve hard cases.

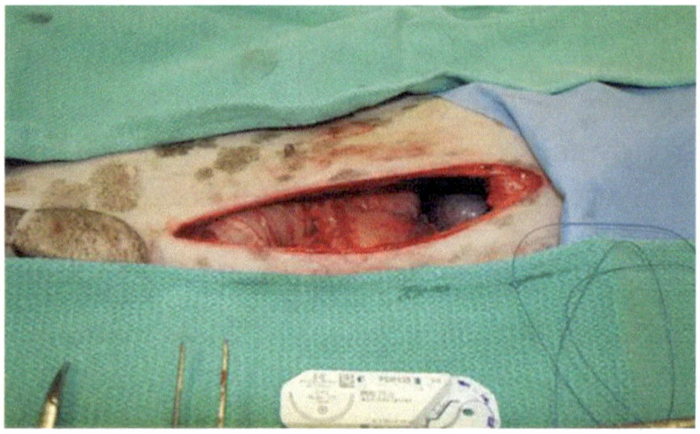

Figure 8.21. Pancreatic biopsy.

Source: https://images.ctfassets.net/4dmg3l1sxd6g/6QqXKGVm5PZtcFn1EPDuPP/ea8e23a3e89c7f69248170009596b746/prop-fig-step-2a_primary-22456-article.png_-_en?fm=webp&q=75

Test Your Knowledge

1. How many imaging techniques are there?
2. What blood test shows pancreas function?

SUMMARY

In summary, the pancreas plays a key role in human physiology because it performs two functions in both endocrine and exocrine systems. The ability of the glands to secrete essential hormones such as insulin and glucagon enables the regulation of blood glucose levels, which is an essential element of metabolic homeostasis. The exocrine component is also essential in digestion because it secretes enzymes such as amylase and lipase, which digest nutrients in the small intestine. Studies have indicated that various factors, including perinatal pathology, affect the function of the pancreas, particularly among newborns who experience physiological stress at birth. The multimodality reflects the need for additional studies on the impact of conditions on the health and disease of the pancreas to guide possible therapeutic targets that can minimize dysfunction of the pancreas and improve clinical outcomes in the affected populations (O.V Kuryk et al., 2024). The findings in relation to the exocrine secretory function of the pancreas, particularly in cases of perinatal pathology in the newborn, demonstrate the significance of separating physiological variations in enzymatic activity. High blood activity of amylase and lipase in full-term neonates with perinatal pathology indicates an adaptation to stress during birth. These variations suggest an association between perinatal severity and pancreatic enzyme activation, providing hints about how the pancreas responds to stress. If doctors can pursue this information, they can more effectively manage newborns with evidence of hypoxic stress, providing proper interventions in due time to meet their metabolic and digestive needs. Another exploration of these events can result in findings that enhance neonate health susceptible to pancreatic dysfunction (Kuryk et al., 2024). Moreover, advances in single-cell RNA sequencing have further enriched understanding of the intricate cellular organization of the pancreas. This cellular diversity meta-analysis of the pancreas not only illuminates the intricacies of transcriptional programs regulating cell-type-specific functions but also highlights the importance of marker genes to future research and therapeutic development. The development of available tools for gene expression study in the pancreas has the potential to drive investigation into connected pancreatic diseases and enables comparison among different biological systems. As our understanding of cellular dynamics in the pancreas grows, there is an unparalleled opportunity to use this knowledge toward therapy and management of diabetes and other pancreatic ailments, thus justifying the need for continued research in this vital gland.

The pancreas, an organ of utmost importance, has dual functions in the human organism as an exocrine and endocrine gland. As an endocrine organ, it regulates blood sugar levels by releasing hormones such as insulin and glucagon. Insulin, produced by beta cells, enables cells to absorb glucose, thereby playing an important role in maintaining energy balance and metabolic stability. In contrast, glucagon secreted by alpha cells initiates the release of glucose into the blood when the concentration drops too low. This intricate interplay of hormones points to the pancreas's essential role in metabolic control and disease when function is deranged, as in diabetes mellitus, which thus underlines its significance in the overall scenario of human pathology and disease. In addition to its endocrine function, the pancreas also has an essential role in digestion as an exocrine gland, producing digestive enzymes. The enzymes, which include amylase, lipase, and proteases, are secreted into the small intestine and are used to digest carbohydrates, fats, and proteins. The process of enzymes is critical for nutrient absorption and use, having direct implications for general health and wellbeing. The enzymes are released in a tightly regulated and meal-coordinated fashion, and this illustrates the role of the pancreas in digestive physiology. Disharmony in the production of enzymes can lead to malabsorption syndromes, which illustrate the essential nature of the pancreas to metabolism as well as the efficiency and functioning of the digestive system. Contributing to the pancreas's complexity of functions, recent research still uncovers its involvement in various pathological conditions, including pancreatic cancer and chronic pancreatitis. Scientists have established that understanding the involvement of biological mechanisms in causing these diseases is essential for developing effective therapies and interventions. The pancreas's double role complicates its pathology, necessitating consideration of pancreatic well-being in a holistic approach. Also, technological and medical advances, such as novel immunosuppression modalities presented at the First International Congress of the Transplantation Society, reflect a widening recognition of the pancreas's function not only in transplantation but in more general biological issues (Cauchi, 1967). Similarly, the intricate involvements of insulin metabolism demonstrate how gains in knowledge acquisition improve our comprehension of pancreatic function and failure (Ensing et al., 1994).

KEY TERMS FROM THIS CHAPTER

- Amylase
- Endocrine cells
- Glucagon
- Hypoxia
- Metabolic regulation
- Pancreatic adenocarcinoma
- Pancreatic dysfunction
- Splenic artery
- Asphyxia
- Exocrine systems
- Hormone secretion
- Lipase
- Pancreas
- Pancreatic duct
- Perinatal trauma

CRITICAL THINKING QUESTIONS

1. **The pancreas is located in which region of the abdomen?**
   a. Right hypochondriac region
   b. Left hypochondriac region
   c. Epigastric region
   d. Umbilical region
2. **The pancreas is classified as which type of gland?**
   a. Exocrine
   b. Endocrine
   c. Mixed (both exocrine and endocrine)
   d. Sebaceous
3. **The exocrine pancreas primarily secretes:**
   a. Hormones such as insulin and glucagon
   b. Digestive enzymes such as amylase and lipase
   c. Bile salts
   d. Glycogen
4. **The endocrine portion of the pancreas is composed of:**
   a. Islets of Langerhans
   b. Hepatocytes
   c. Crypts of Lieberkühn
   d. Acinar cells
5. **Which hormone is produced by beta cells in the pancreas?**
   a. Glucagon
   b. Insulin
   c. Somatostatin
   d. Amylase

Short Answer Questions

1. What is a pancreas?
2. What is the significance of the pancreas?
3. Where is the pancreas located?
4. What are the main functions of the pancreas?
5. What are the pancreatic enzymes?

Answer to Critical Thinking Questions

1. (c) 2. (c) 3. (b) 4. (a) 5. (b)

REFERENCES

1. Abdul-Rasoul, A., Agarwal, A., Ahlgren, A., Alejandro, A., American Diabetes Association, Anderson, A., Appleton, A., et al. (2016). What's in a name? Classification of diabetes mellitus in veterinary medicine and why it matters. https://core.ac.uk/download/76980783.pdf (accessed on 15th June 2025).
2. Adams, M. S., Diederich, C. J., Salgaonkar, V., Scott, S., et al. (2017). Theoretical investigation of transgastric and intraductal approaches for ultrasound-based thermal therapy of the pancreas. https://core.ac.uk/download/323063407.pdf (accessed on 15th June 2025).
3. Arda, H. E., Burns, V. M., Chakravarthy, H., Charville, H., et al. (2017). Pathways to clinical CLARITY: Volumetric analysis of irregular, soft, and heterogeneous tissues in development and disease. https://core.ac.uk/download/129069108.pdf (accessed on 15th June 2025).
4. Argenton, F., Ek, O. F. D., Facchinello, N., Grisan, A., et al. (2017). *Tcf7l2* plays pleiotropic roles in the control of glucose homeostasis, pancreas morphology, vascularization and regeneration. https://core.ac.uk/download/84923362.pdf (accessed on 15th June 2025).
5. Arnelo, U., Haas, S. L., Löhr, J. M., Martin, P., et al. (2017). Pancreatic exocrine insufficiency after bariatric surgery. https://core.ac.uk/download/188827229.pdf (accessed on 15th June 2025).
6. Azoitei, N., Heller, S., & Kleger, A. (2024). Pandemic punch: SARS-CoV-2 hits pancreas. *Signal Transduction and Targeted Therapy, 9*. https://www.semanticscholar.org/paper/eb3cf04e89dcf87c7256e9c23dc5c368a9cf8c88 (accessed on 15th June 2025).
7. Badiali, D., Bruno, G., Ribichini, E., Rossi, M., et al. (2019). Role of fiber in nutritional management of pancreatic diseases. https://core.ac.uk/download/231748461.pdf (accessed on 15th June 2025).
8. Blagova, B., Hristakiev, L., & Malinova, L. (2025). Tubarial organ-like glandular tissue–A comparative histology study in humans and canines. *Journal of IMAB–Annual Proceeding (Scientific Papers)*. https://www.semanticscholar.org/paper/1f21c4de9b226a8a8a9b1afe0ffc184bbcfacec1 (accessed on 15th June 2025).
9. Bordoni, A., Dupont, D., Gille, D., Kachal, J., et al. (2015). Understanding the gastrointestinal tract of the elderly to develop dietary solutions that prevent malnutrition. https://core.ac.uk/download/286575279.pdf (accessed on 15th June 2025).
10. Bruscalupi, G., & Gnocchi, D. (2017). Circadian rhythms and hormonal homeostasis: Pathophysiological implications. https://core.ac.uk/download/98342817.pdf (accessed on 15th June 2025).
11. Campos da Silva, F., Santos, B., Pôssa de Castro, P., Amarante, G., & Sousa, O. (2023). Inhibitory potential of synthetic amino acid derivatives against digestive enzymes as promising hypoglycemic and anti-obesity agents. *Biomolecules, 13*. https://www.semanticscholar.org/paper/e0d7294c4bc9ba6828d13e1a95003123b1b5ec99 (accessed on 15th June 2025).
12. Cauchi, M. N. (1967). Organ and tissue transplantation. https://core.ac.uk/download/46604357.pdf (accessed on 15th June 2025).
13. Chintinne, M., Stangé, G., Denys, B., Ling, Z., in 't Veld, P., & Pipeleers, D. (2012). Beta cell counts instead of beta cell mass to assess and localize growth in beta cell population following pancreatic duct ligation in mice. *PLoS ONE, 7*. https://www.semanticscholar.org/paper/2de0143e5f48392046c58511cb850ee6d39dba1c (accessed on 15th June 2025).

14. Daminet, S., Hesta, M., Paepe, D., Saunders, J., et al. (2010). Acute pancreatitis in dogs and cats: Medical imaging, biopsy, treatment and prognosis. https://core.ac.uk/download/55845908.pdf (accessed on 15th June 2025).

15. Daub, C., Michaels, A. L., Mabate, B., Mkabayi, L., Edkins, A. L., & Pletschke, B. I. (2025). Exploring the inhibitory potential of sodium alginate against digestive enzymes linked to obesity and type 2 diabetes. *Molecules, 30*. https://www.semanticscholar.org/paper/2b2c5b44272aae6c9156f012d6afbfb4a3fdc8cc (accessed on 15th June 2025).

16. Dolenšek, J., Pohorec, V., Rupnik, M. S., Stožer, A., et al. (2017). Pancreas physiology. https://core.ac.uk/download/322428900.pdf (accessed on 15th June 2025).

17. Eibl, G., & Rozengurt, E. (2019). Central role of Yes-associated protein and WW-domain-containing transcriptional co-activator with PDZ-binding motif in pancreatic cancer development. https://core.ac.uk/download/323076522.pdf (accessed on 15th June 2025).

18. Ensing, M., Paton, R., Rada, R., Speel, H., et al. (1994). An object-oriented approach to knowledge representation in a biomedical domain. https://core.ac.uk/download/pdf/11454269.pdf (accessed on 15th June 2025).

19. Euclid Collaboration, Bohringer, H., Chon, G., Cucciati, O., Dannerbauer, H., Bolzonella, M., Lucia, G., Cappi, A., et al. (2024). Euclid preparation. LV. Exploring the properties of proto-clusters in the simulated Euclid wide survey. *Astronomy & Astrophysics*. https://www.semanticscholar.org/paper/6e0bb5a8a1ea66b8fcbf3e8c65bd69d1af81168d (accessed on 15th June 2025).

20. Glocker, B., Heinrich, M., Kainz, B., Oktay, O., et al. (2018). Attention gated networks: Learning to leverage salient regions in medical images. https://core.ac.uk/download/189836581.pdf (accessed on 15th June 2025).

21. Gordon, R. D., Iwatsuki, S., Makowka, L., Marsh, J., et al. (1992). Pancreatic complications following orthotopic liver transplantation. https://core.ac.uk/download/12204775.pdf (accessed on 15th June 2025).

22. H1 Collaboration, Andreev, V., Arratia, M., Baghdasaryan, A., Baty, A., Begzsuren, K., Bolz, A., Boudry, V., et al. (2024). Machine learning-assisted measurement of lepton-jet azimuthal angular asymmetries in deep-inelastic scattering at HERA. https://www.semanticscholar.org/paper/38149e866357c64e1f714d598f393139e53044bc (accessed on 15th June 2025).

23. Han, D., & Jung, D. I. (2023). Gallbladder atrophy associated with pancreatitis: Clinical and advanced imaging diagnosis in a dog. *Veterinární Medicína, 68*, 435–442. https://www.semanticscholar.org/paper/3ee04cef4e447d4a41de826220ee7d2255dbc6d8 (accessed on 15th June 2025).

24. Haris, F., Purnama, K., & Purnomo, M. (2011). Tongue image analysis for diabetes mellitus diagnosis based on SOM Kohonen. https://core.ac.uk/download/12344735.pdf (accessed on 15th June 2025).

25. Hua, A. M. (2015). PPAR-alpha: A novel target in pancreatic cancer. https://core.ac.uk/download/142061797.pdf (accessed on 15th June 2025).

26. Huising, M. O., & Noguchi, G. M. (2019). Integrating the inputs that shape pancreatic islet hormone release. https://core.ac.uk/download/286361735.pdf (accessed on 15th June 2025).

27. Kapke, D. R. (2015). Childhood type II diabetes: The risks and complications. https://core.ac.uk/download/58826199.pdf (accessed on 15th June 2025).

28. Kiernan, F. (1834). The anatomy and physiology of the liver. *The Medical Quarterly Review, 2*, 288–296. https://www.semanticscholar.org/paper/205f1d46234383351f5d1e353ab7bdc76598c0d8 (accessed on 15th June 2025).

29. Li, J., Jiang, X., Wang, Q. H., Wu, X., Qu, Z., Song, T., Wan, W., et al. (2022). Data-independent acquisition proteomics reveals circulating biomarkers of coronary chronic total occlusion in humans. *Frontiers in Cardiovascular Medicine, 9*. https://www.semanticscholar.org/paper/a38b74b3bc96f3bdbc32bc5fcab6738c68f9b60f (accessed on 15th June 2025).

30. Lugea, A., Pandol, S. J., & Waldron, R. T. (2015). Pancreatic adaptive responses in alcohol abuse: Role of the unfolded protein response. https://core.ac.uk/download/323066522.pdf (accessed on 15th June 2025).

31. Magni, L., Yu, H., Christensen, N., Poulsen, M. H., Frueh, A., Deshar, G., Johansen, A., et al. (2024). Human P2X7 receptor variants Gly150Arg and Arg276His polymorphisms have differential effects on risk association and cellular functions in pancreatic cancer. *Cancer Cell International, 24*. https://www.semanticscholar.org/paper/a4d6d40582b231bb81152834a2d3a60f0ad72432 (accessed on 15th June 2025).

32. Martin, M., Nilsson, S. C., Eikrem, D., Fromell, K., Scavenius, C., Vogt, L., Bielecka, E., et al. (2023). Citrullination of C1-inhibitor as a mechanism of impaired complement regulation in rheumatoid arthritis. *Frontiers in Immunology, 14*. https://www.semanticscholar.org/paper/ed4628ea79d7d0ec3e02772d392ec694d98ca3e4 (accessed on 15th June 2025).

33. Muliawan, A., Ananta, Y., & Fitri, S. D. (2025). The role of bacterial protease enzymes and *in silico* prediction on the effectiveness of medical applications. *Dinasti Health and Pharmacy Science*. https://www.semanticscholar.org/paper/1a9d8d9e13bf1783f59cbb3339b33880bebfe605 (accessed on 15th June 2025).

34. Polishevska, K., Kelly, S., Kuppan, P., Seeberger, K., Aggarwal, S., Paramor, J., Unsworth, L., et al. (2023). Nanothin conformal coating with poly(N-vinylpyrrolidone) and tannic acid (PVPON/TA) preserves murine and human pancreatic islet's function. *Pharmaceutics, 15*. https://www.semanticscholar.org/paper/7bd651e0932ee8193a4b730d94fa77f8b8158d0c (accessed on 15th June 2025).

35. Prabu, P. K. (2011). Study of calculus pancreatitis. https://core.ac.uk/download/288215899.pdf (accessed on 15th June 2025).

36. Pronin, N., Pavlov, A., Sekisova, E. V., Lazutina, G. S., Ovchinnikova, N. V., & Ivanov, M. I. (2021). Clinical and variant anatomy of the blood supply to the body and tail of the human pancreas. *Journal of Anatomy and Histopathology*. https://www.semanticscholar.org/paper/22ed2426c0b6e78ccd479c2b63c43055b22539d3 (accessed on 15th June 2025).

37. Prud'homme, G. J., Kurt, M., & Wang, Q. (2022). Pathobiology of the Klotho antiaging protein and therapeutic considerations. *Frontiers in Aging, 3*. https://doi.org/10.3389/fragi.2022.931331 (accessed on 15th June 2025).

38. Putri, M. M. D., Noviza, N., Sari, D. K., Pratiwi, D., Hermalena, Y., Lestari, E. K., Septinawati, S., et al. (2025). Senam tentang diabetes mellitus di Puskesmas Bintuhan Desa Sinar Pagi Kelurahan Bandar Kecamatan Kaur Selatan Kabupaten Kaur. *Jurnal Dehasen Mengabdi*. https://www.semanticscholar.org/paper/e49ea82b30cae00f93b8b954f81037e972f77041 (accessed on 15th June 2025).

39. Refat, M. A. R., Al Amin, M., Kaushal, C., Yeasmin, M. N., & Islam, M. K. (2021). A comparative analysis of early-stage diabetes prediction using machine learning and deep learning approach. https://doi.org/10.1109/ispcc53510.2021.9609364 (accessed on 15th June 2025).

40. Remedios, L. W., Liu, H., Remedios, S. W., Zuo, L., Saunders, A. M., Bao, S., Huo, Y., et al. (2025). Influence of early through late fusion on pancreas segmentation from imperfectly registered multimodal magnetic resonance imaging. *Journal of Medical Imaging, 12*(2), 024008. https://www.semanticscholar.org/paper/51814dc2d59895c34f0be1e0120b2827f055f693 (accessed on 15th June 2025).

41. Rodriguez-Diaz, R. (2012). Regulation of human pancreas hormone secretion by autonomic innervation. https://core.ac.uk/download/70340024.pdf (accessed on 15th June 2025).

42. Rogowska, J., Durko, Ł., & Małecka-Wojciesko, E. (2023). The latest advancements in diagnostic role of endosonographic of pancreatic lesions. *Journal of Clinical Medicine, 12*. https://www.semanticscholar.org/paper/11dcdcafb145446cba288a0be04de001f2b5bee7 (accessed on 15th June 2025).

43. Sakaguchi, K., Kimura-Nakajima, C., Inaba, A., Hatano, Y., Ogawa, H., Koshiishi, Y., Tanaka, K., et al. (2025). Generation and functional characterization of tuft cells in non-human primate pancreatic ducts through organoid culture systems. *Frontiers in Cell and Developmental Biology*. https://www.semanticscholar.org/paper/25c42f0b8b76af14d01f383b97e52ba754327ad7 (accessed on 15th June 2025).

44. Schlünder, K., Cipriano, M., Zbinden, A., Fuchs, S., Mayr, T., Schenke-Layland, K., & Loskill, P. (2024). Micro physiological pancreas-on-chip platform with integrated sensors to model endocrine function and metabolism. *Lab on a Chip*. https://www.semanticscholar.org/paper/755919522be0ee0313fb738e916051f62261ceda (accessed on 15th June 2025).

45. Sekisova, E. V., Pavlov, A., Pronin, N., Zherebyatyeva, S. R., Vvedensky, A. I., Dronova, E. A., & Poludkin, I. A. (2024). Variants of mutual arrangement of parts of human pancreas according to computed tomography data. *I.P. Pavlov Russian Medical Biological Herald*. https://www.semanticscholar.org/paper/0e802e5940c989a21951c800a4540c172d0dcd4a (accessed on 15th June 2025).

46. Sturgill, D., Wang, L., & Arda, H. E. (2024). PancrESS–A meta-analysis resource for understanding cell-type specific expression in the human pancreas. *BMC Genomics, 25*. https://www.semanticscholar.org/paper/9c0c94fb6b739c8793d81eef07ecd0756f0263b5 (accessed on 15th June 2025).

47. Valente, R., Coppola, A., Scandavini, C., Halimi, A., Magnusson, A., Lauro, A., Sotirova, I., et al. (2024). Interactions between the exocrine and the endocrine pancreas. *Journal of Clinical Medicine, 13*. https://www.semanticscholar.org/paper/553f75ccae395169cae9c7e26bf129479ad4fe71 (accessed on 15th June 2025).

48. Zen, Y. (2024). Autoimmune pancreatitis: Biopsy interpretation and differential diagnosis. *Seminars in Diagnostic Pathology*. https://www.semanticscholar.org/paper/55373d19e733c69186195088bc0925a4d1346e61 (accessed on 15th June 2025).

GALLBLADDER

9

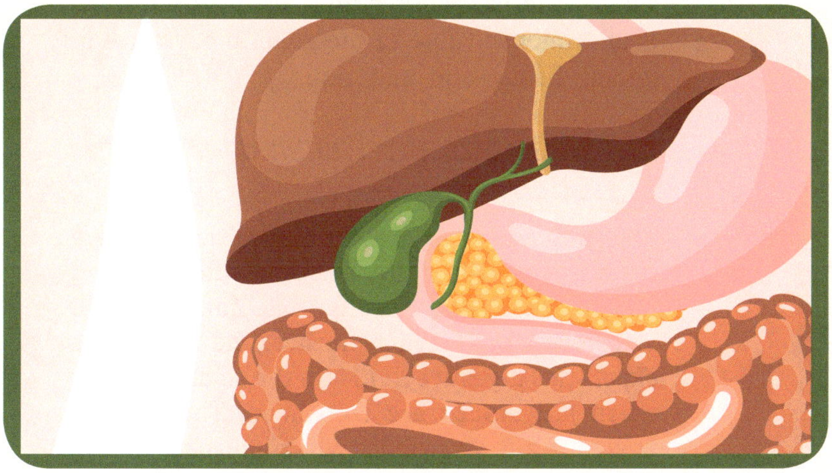

Introduction

The gallbladders, which are small sacs located below the liver, play a critical role in digestion by storing the bile produced by the liver. Bile is utilized to emulsify and digest fat consumed, and therefore, the use of the gallbladders is essential for the digestion process. Bile is released into the small intestine during the digestion of fats, and there it aids digestion. This process is a prime example of the complex interaction among the different organs in the digestive system. Besides retaining bile, the gallbladder also concentrates it, making it more effective when it is required. Knowing its anatomical location and physiological function in digestion is crucial for understanding how gallbladder dysfunction can cause a variety of gastrointestinal problems. Thus, an intense exploration of the gallbladder, its function, and the significance of its malfunction is required for further understanding of human health. Research has indicated that the interaction of the gallbladders with pancreatic juices also plays a significant role. For instance, research has indicated that bile is capable of stimulating pancreatic juice secretion but that

LEARNING OBJECTIVES

After studying this chapter, you will be able to:

1. Understand the anatomy of the gallbladder
- Describe the function of the gallbladder
- Describe the gallbladder disorders
- Learn about the diagnosis of gallbladder conditions
- Know the treatment options for gallbladder issues
- Discuss the prevention of gallbladder diseases

the stimulation does so more intensely under specific conditions. Notably, early experiments by Mellanby demonstrated that the administration of bile into the duodenum elevated pancreatic juice secretion significantly in anesthetized cats. In conscious dogs, though, it was suggested that bile exerted a mild stimulation on pancreatic secretion (Adamczyk et al., 1992).

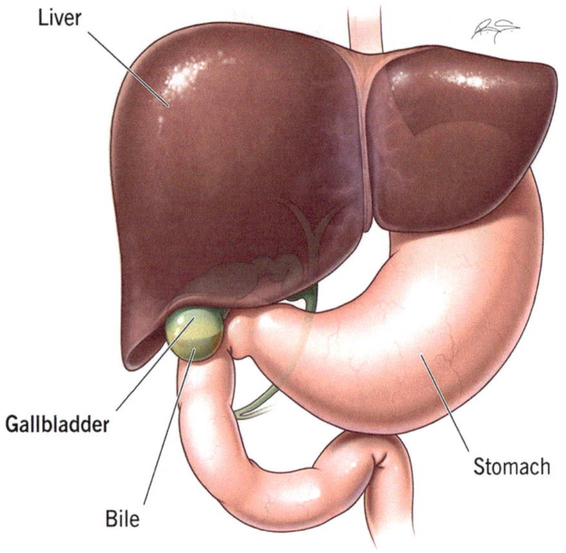

Figure 9.1. Gallbladder.

Source: https://my.clevelandclinic.org/-/scassets/images/org/health/articles/21690-gallbladder

These findings indicate the complexity of digestive mechanisms and demonstrate the way that the actions of adjacent organs can be influenced by modifications in gallbladder function. Such interactions highlight the importance of an adequately functioning gallbladder, since even minimal alterations may have snowballing consequences for health and digestion. Increased investigation into the role of gallbladders further brings about an appreciation of gallbladder pathologies, and these pathologies significantly influence both health and well-being. Gallstones, cholecystitis, and even cancer demand increased attention and research regarding gallbladder health. These pathologies can lead to severe complications if untreated, demonstrating the function of this small organ in overall health. The function of the gallbladder is also demonstrated by its role in nutrient absorption and overall digestion. Gallbladder issues should be treated, either with medicine or diet, to avoid severe digestive illnesses. Therefore, a thorough analysis of the role of the gallbladder and related conditions is of immense value to the general narrative of human health and nutrition.

Importance of the Gallbladder in Digestion

The gallbladder plays a key part in the digestive system, particularly in the emulsification and absorption of fats. Through bile concentration and storage produced by the liver, the gallbladder expels this digestive fluid into the small intestine when fatty foods are consumed. This release is significant since bile, which consists of bile salts, bilirubin, cholesterol, and phospholipids, enables large globules of fats to be degraded into minute micelles and thereby makes fats more vulnerable to enzymatic activity. Bile release affects the effectiveness of digestion directly because coordinated gallbladder contraction during digestion demand ensures proper quantities of bile during digestion. Experiments have also established the function of the gallbladder in the stimulation of the pancreas. For instance, experiments demonstrate that bile infusion into the duodenum tends to stimulate pancreatic juice secretion, a condition significant for protein and carbohydrate digestion. Evidence for the fact that bile is an incomplete stimulant in conscious dogs comes from Mellanby's work, a circumstance that justifies the complex relationship between the gallbladder and pancreas during digestion. Besides this, diversion of bile from the duodenum was also found to be harmful to pancreatic secretions, which indicates that the gallbladder's function does not simply degenerate into storage of bile but has a crucial role in coordinating digestive processes among different organs like the pancreas and intestines (Adamczyk et al., 1992). Interestingly, the bile composition and concentration secreted by the gallbladder are significant in digestive hormone cascades. Bile administration studies revealed that both stimulate pancreatic secretion and elevate secretin and pancreatic polypeptide levels in humans. This implies that the hydrokinetic effect of intraduodenal bile is mediated, at least in part, through such endocrine mechanisms (Scharl et al., 1990). These interactions highlight the gallbladder's vital function not only in the digestion of fat but also in the control of digestive hormone release, thus reaffirming its significance within the overall digestive process. The gallbladder's ability to release bile adaptively based on the intake of diet shows its pivotal role in digestive health.

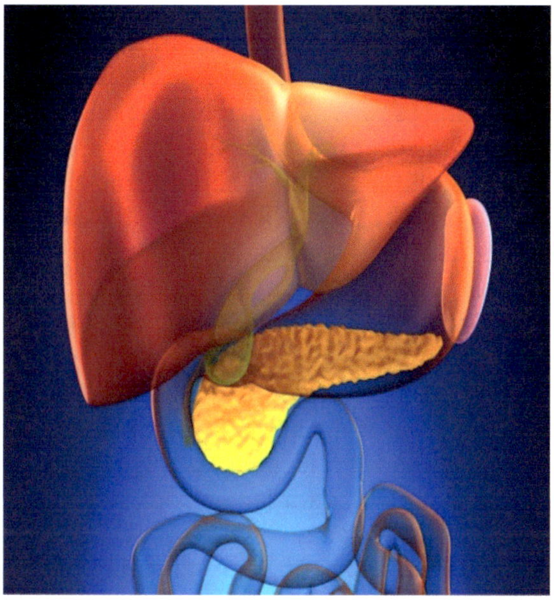

Figure 9.2. The role of gallbladder in digestion.

Source: https://www.drmalladi.com/wp-content/uploads/2016/10/iStock_66621857_MEDIUMtinified.jpg

9.1. Anatomy of the Gallbladder

Learning Outcome

1. Describe the location and physical structure of the gallbladder
2. Know the relationship with the liver and bile ducts
3. Understand the variations in gallbladder anatomy among individuals

The anatomy of the gallbladder is important to understand what role it plays in the human body. Situated below the liver, the gallbladder serves as a reservoir for bile, a digestive juice produced by the liver. The gallbladder is pear-shaped and divided into different segments: the fundus, body, and neck. The gallbladder is joined with the biliary tract by the cystic duct that ends in the common bile duct. This anatomical arrangement is needed for bile storage and release during digestion, particularly after fat intake. The gallbladder has morphological variation in its shape that can influence its functionality and susceptibility to diseases, particularly with increasing age. The literature shows that the length and thickness of the gallbladder vary with age, and thus it is very important to have a clear understanding of its anatomy at different phases of human life (Mansura et al., 2024). Anatomy of the gallbladder is also discussed by learning its histological structure in the form of mucosa, muscularis, and serosa in separate layers. The mucosa is lined by specialized cells facilitating water and electrolyte uptake with the concentration of bile for optimal digestive efficiency. The muscularis is composed of smooth muscle fibers that carry out contraction and release of the bile into the intestinal lumen upon hormonal stimulus, particularly that of cholecystokinin. Besides that, the health of the gallbladder also depends on the integrity of its structure; abnormalities will lead to disease such as cholecystitis and gallstones, which are prevalent clinical conditions. Through comparison of variations in the histological layers and their relation to gallbladder function, medical practitioners can better diagnose and treat gallbladder-related disorders (Ligresti et al., 2019). While pursuing the anatomical variation of the gallbladder, the variations are found to have significant impacts on clinical practice and surgery. For instance, gallbladder size and shape can vary from one population to another, with some populations possessing characteristic gallbladders that could influence risk for gallbladder diseases. Recent studies have shown that, with increasing age, the thickness and length of the gallbladder increase, while the weight and width may not change. Such findings support considering anatomical age-related changes when assessing and managing the health of the gallbladder. The findings are important for healthcare professionals to provide targeted treatment options and improve patient care for common gallbladder diseases (Mansura et al., 2024).

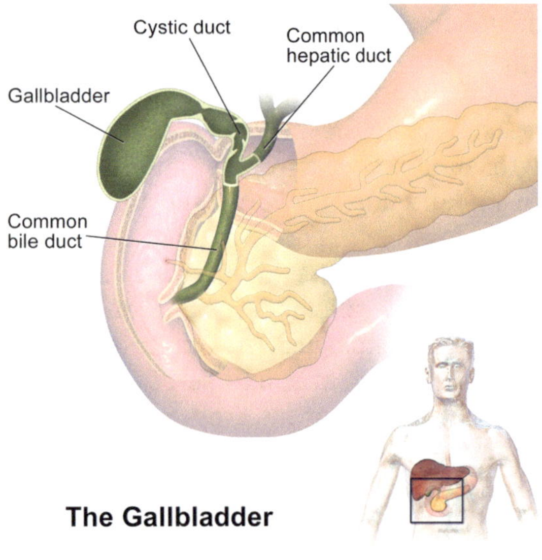

Figure 9.3. Anatomy of the gallbladder.

Source: https://upload.wikimedia.org/wikipedia/commons/e/ed/Gallbladder_%28organ%29.png

9.1.1. Location and Physical Structure

The pear-shaped gallbladder is below the liver, in a fossa on the right lobe of the liver. It has a good position for bile storage and bile secretion, which are required for fat digestion. The gallbladder is connected to the biliary tree via the cystic duct that merges with the common hepatic duct to form the common bile duct. This arrangement offers maximum bile transport—produced by the liver and, in the gallbladder, accumulated to be transported into the duodenum during digestion. The positioning of the gallbladders maximizes digestive efficiency through the regulation of the flow of bile in accordance with food consumption. Physiologically, the gallbladder is composed of a number of discrete layers: mucosa, muscularis, and serosa, each of which is designed to contribute to its functional parameters. Its inner lining, or the mucosa, contains numerous folds in order to spread out when the organ is filled with bile. Over it are columnar epithelial cells that absorb water and electrolytes, thereby concentrating bile. The muscularis contains smooth muscle fibers that contract in response to hormonal stimuli in the form of cholecystokinin, primarily to eject bile into the small intestine. The outermost of the three layers, the serosa, supports and contains the gallbladder to surrounding structures. This complex physical arrangement indicates the organ's primary role in the digestion process, demonstrating the interrelationship between anatomy and physiology. Understanding the anatomic location and physical structure of the gallbladder is particularly critical in the formation of gallstones and subsequent pathologies. Evidence reveals that structural elements, i.e., levels of some proteins such as fibronectin, can influence the susceptibility to form gallstones. Biliary mucin-binding fibronectins suggest mechanisms by which bile composition may be effective in gallstone disease, i.e., in gallstone patients with various levels of fibronectin (Pozo et al., 1994). The involvement of these structural properties with bile emphasizes the importance of the gallbladder's physical features and environment in providing the best possible health. Hence, the thorough understanding of gallbladder anatomy is essential to understand its role in normal physiology as well as disease pathology, i.e., gallstone disease (N/A, 1989).

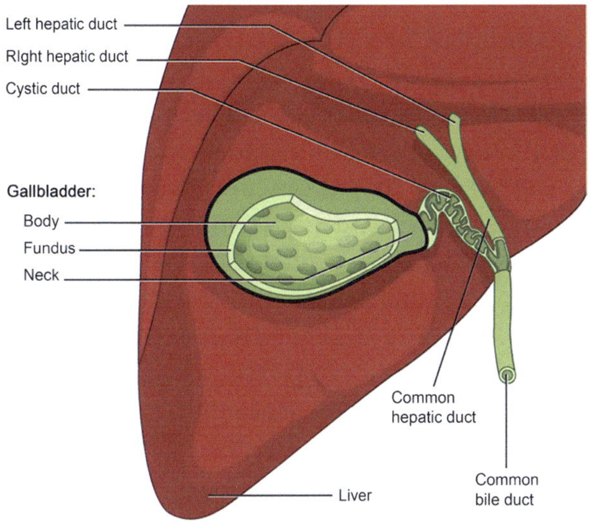

Figure 9.4. Location of the gallbladder.

Source: https://www.researchgate.net/publication/373290407/figure/fig1/AS:11431281183126891@1692723294870/Anatomy-and-location-of-the-gallbladder-5.ppm

9.1.2. Relationship With the Liver and Bile Ducts

The gallbladder plays an essential role in the human digestive system, and it is also responsible for the concentration and storage of bile produced by the liver. The interaction is important because bile is the one that emulsifies and facilitates the absorption of fat by the small intestine. The gallbladder functions as a reservoir, which secretes bile into the biliary tract upon consumption of fatty food. But its function is intimately involved with the bile ducts and liver, and any kind of imbalance in this intricate system can lead to serious health issues. Cholestasis, or a state of diminished bile flow, may be triggered by a variety of causes, including liver disease and gallbladder disease. This exchange between gallbladder function and hepatic function highlights the biliary system's intricacy, in which issues can resonate through the process of digestion (Alpini et al., 2023).

Gallstone development is one of the most frequent complications associated with disruptions in the liver-gallbladder axis. These firm nodules tend to obstruct the bile ducts, with subsequent serious complications such as cholecystitis and pancreatitis. Gallstone formation has a direct relationship with bile composition, such as cholesterol, bilirubin, and bile salt concentration, and the patterns of bile flow. Any changes in these factors can increase crystallization and nucleation, resulting in the formation of gallstones (Jia et al., 2023). Hence, bile flow and content study is crucial in explaining gallstone formation and therapeutic opportunities. Better diagnostic methods, such as microfluidic-based biosensors, are promising prospects for real-time monitoring of bile dynamics, and this allows for more specific measures to address gallbladder disorders and their role in liver health (Jia et al., 2023).

The interaction between the gallbladder, bile ducts, and liver also dominates a number of pathological conditions. Diseases such as cholangiopathies and chronic liver illnesses can lead to widespread abnormalities of the biliary apparatus, both within the liver and gallbladder. The complexity of such interaction suggests that a holistic understanding of the pathology of one organ must take into account the other. For instance, liver disease commonly leads to altered bile production, which can result in acceleration of inflammation within the gallbladder and predisposition to gallstones (Alpini et al., 2023). Moreover, the inflammatory processes of the gallbladders may complicate the management of underlying liver disease, being referred to as a need for simultaneous therapeutic regimes. Investigating these associations can enhance diagnostic accuracy and therapeutic practice and, eventually, patient outcomes within this complicated group of biliary health.

9.1.3. Variations in Gallbladder Anatomy Among Individuals

he gallbladder, one of the key organs of the human gastrointestinal system, exhibits profound anatomical variations among individuals, which may influence both clinical effects and operations. They include size, shape, location, and the morphology of associated structures, for example, the cystic duct. Research indicates that gallbladder thickness and length increase with age, underscoring the importance of examining how these morphological elements change over time.

These time-related changes can complicate the diagnosis of gallbladder disease and require clinicians to be knowledgeable about these changes as they read imaging studies and carry out surgical interventions (Mansura et al., 2024). Also, anatomical variations can influence the success of common procedures like laparoscopic cholecystectomy, validating education that emphasizes the variability that exists in the human anatomy. Variations in anatomy are not solely caused by age but also genetic composition and environmental factors as necessary ingredients in the formation of gallbladder morphology. For instance, studies have recognized that certain populations may have specific anatomical features due to inherited traits or dietary patterns affecting biliary function. Such population-specific characteristics are crucial for clinicians because they can inform preoperative assessment and individualized treatment. Further, these differences can be interspecific; dietary habits and way of life can produce variations in the prevalence of gallbladder disease, which calls for the appreciation of a more nuanced approach to gallbladder health in multicultural populations (Kim I-B et al., 2024). As progress continues in the field of medicine, emphasis on teaching anatomy will be important to preparing practitioners with skills to deal with these differences effectively. In clinical practice, gallbladder anatomical variation is not only valuable for diagnosis and treatment but also useful for gastroenterological research. Research into anatomical variation has the potential to unravel underlying pathophysiological mechanisms, which, in turn, may increase susceptibility to gallbladder diseases, such as cholecystitis and gallstones. For example, one recent study revealed that the absence of gallbladder abnormalities in the target group can be linked to a generally low incidence of gallbladder disease, suggesting the significance of distinguishing these anatomical variations in future studies (Mansura et al., 2024).

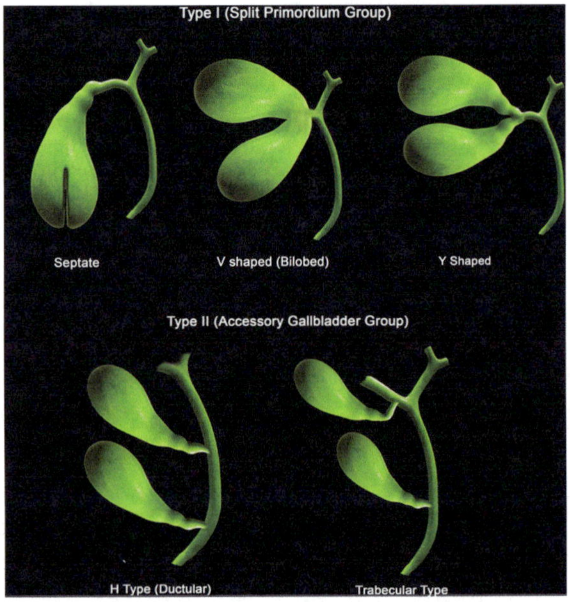

Figure 9.5. Variations of the gallbladder.

Source: https://www.researchgate.net/publication/373290407/figure/fig2/AS:11431281183165299@1692723295390/ariations-of-the-gallbladder.ppm

By fostering a deeper appreciation of interindividual anatomical variation, clinicians and researchers will be able to design more effective preventive measures and therapeutic interventions to optimize gallbladder health and prevent associated complications. Thus, research in gallbladder anatomy remains a vital area of investigation for a complete understanding of human health.

Test Your Knowledge

1. Where is the gallbladder located?
2. What is the relationship between the liver and the bile ducts?

9.2. Function of the Gallbladder

Learning Outcome

1. Describe the storage and concentration of bile
2. Discuss the release of bile into the small intestine

The gallbladder, which is a small pear-shaped organ located beneath the liver, has a key functional role in human digestion primarily through the storage and concentration of bile. Bile, secreted by the liver, is involved in the emulsification of fat, thereby aiding in its digestion and absorption in the intestine. When dietary fats enter the small intestine, they cause the release of cholecystokinin, which is a hormone that causes the gallbladder to contract. This contraction is letting out concentrated bile into the duodenum to facilitate the effective hydrolysis of fats into glycerol and fatty acids, which are absorbed by the intestinal mucosa. Normal gallbladder function is therefore crucial for normal digestive function and nutrient absorption, demonstrating the significance of its function in the digestive process. In addition to its role in helping digest fats, the gallbladder also plays a central position in maintaining general metabolic health. Studies have indicated that individuals with autonomic neuropathy, and particularly those who are diabetic, experience abnormal gallbladder function, which may present as an elevated gallbladder volume and a high incidence of gallstones. Specifically, in a study, it was established that patients with diabetes possess significantly higher fasting and postprandial gallbladder volumes than non-diabetic patients, indicating that gallbladder dysfunction can be a sign of more widespread metabolic disorders (Shekhar and Pradhan, 2023). This association suggests that normal gallbladder function is not only critical to digestive process but also to the prevention of possible complications arising from associated metabolic disorders. Additionally, new research shows the positive impact of dietary supplements such as A-F Betafood® on gallbladder function. When overweight adults underwent supplementation with A-F Betafood®, significant gallbladder values, including volume and ejection fraction emerged, affirming its use in gallbladder wellness maintenance (Evans et al., 2020). This finding further underscores the importance of ongoing research into dietary programs that may enhance gallbladder function, particularly in those individuals at risk for gallbladder failure. Finally, an understanding of the gallbladder's multifaceted roles in digestive competence and metabolic stability is essential to the design of effective prevention against gallbladder disease.

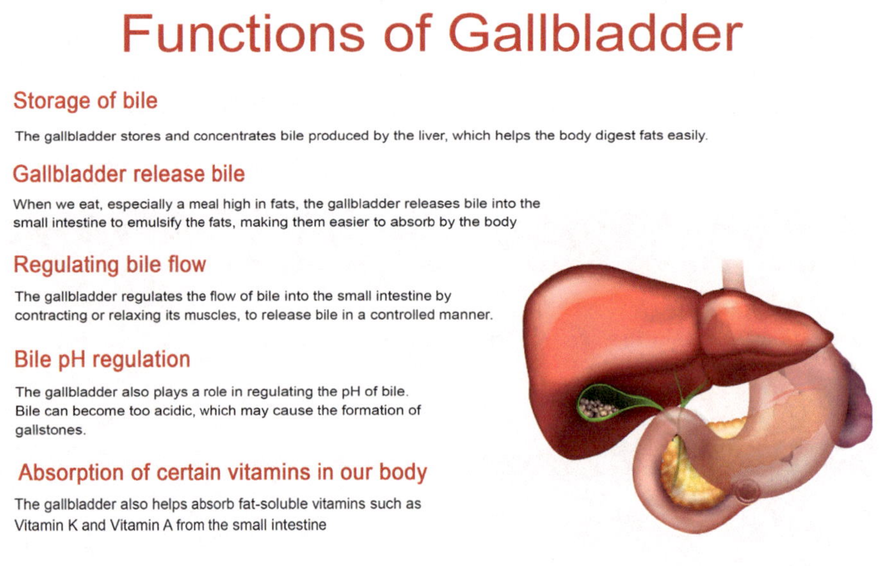

Figure 9.6. Function of the Gallbladder.

Source: https://assets.lybrate.com/imgs/tic/enadp/functions-of-gallbladder.jpg

9.2.1. Storage of Bile

The gallbladder plays a role in the storage of bile, which is used for the digestion and absorption of fats consumed. The gallbladder, a small, pear-shaped organ located below the liver, is a bile reservoir from the liver. Bile, a sophisticated mixture of bile salts, cholesterol, bilirubin, and other substances, is concentrated in the gallbladder, which is used for more efficient mealtime digestion. This dense bile facilitates the emulsification of fats to make them easily susceptible to breakdown by enzymes. Gallbladder storage ensures an adequate supply when food is in the small intestine, in which bile salts facilitate lipid digestion and absorption, and reflect the organ's integral part in digestion. Motility of the gallbladder is vital for efficient storage as well as release of bile and directly influences the efficiency of digestion. On food intake, the hormone cholecystokinin (CCK) is released, causing gallbladder contraction and the discharge of stored bile into the small intestine. Deficits in gallbladder contraction can contribute to a number of gastrointestinal diseases, including gallstone formation. Dysfunctional gallbladder emptying often leads to the existence of an excess of cholesterol and biliary sludge, favoring an enhanced risk of stone formation. Further, studies have demonstrated that genetic expression of receptors like the cholecystokinin A receptor (CCKAR) significantly influences gallbladder motility, where mutations or dysfunctions enhance the likelihood of cholesterol gallstone formation, while stressing the significant interaction between genetic factors and bile storage dynamics (Liu et al., 2020). Apart from their role in the digestion of fat, bile acids are increasingly found to be actively involved in the regulation of metabolism. Evidence from recent studies shows that bile acids play a role in glucose and lipid metabolism, linking them to type 2 diabetes and obesity (Eggink et al., 2018). Storage function of the gallbladders is, therefore, not only affecting results in the gut but also general metabolic health. Abnormal bile acid metabolism, typically marked by abnormal intestinal transit times, might have physiological effects beyond digestion, including metabolic dysfunction. Understanding the complexity of bile storage and its broader implications is paramount to addressing disease in gallbladder dysfunction and metabolic disease, pointing to the gallbladder's centrality in both gastrointestinal and systemic well-being.

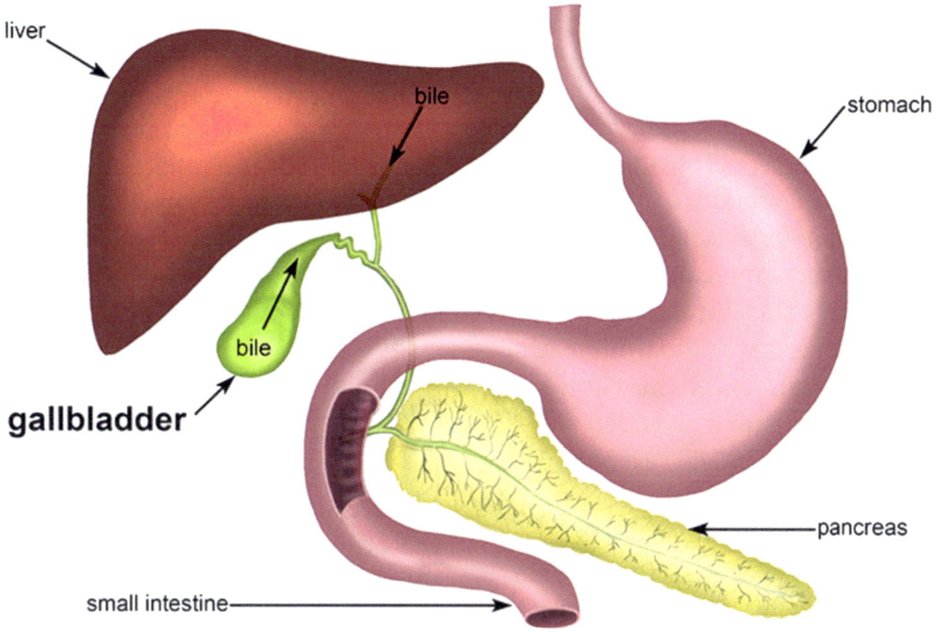

Figure 9.7. The gallbladder stores bile produced in the liver.

Source: https://mammothmemory.net/images/user/base/uncategorised/1.23.4%20Gallbladder%20 position%20image.jpg

9.2.2. Concentration of Bile

The concentration of cholesterol in bile is an important aspect of gallbladder function, influencing the solubility of cholesterol in the bile and, therefore, gallstone formation. Stimulation of the gallbladder results in the secretion of small amounts of bile that contain water, bile salts, phospholipids, and cholesterol. A balance of these components is critical; supersaturation may occur due to a predominance of cholesterol over phospholipids and bile salts. The disease can enhance the crystallization of cholesterol, its precursor in the formation of gallstones. Some recent dietary research has shown that biliary fatty acid composition has the potential to influence the secretion of cholesterol and levels of bile saturation to a high degree, and therefore dietary regulation is a primary issue for those prone to gallstones (Abell et al., 1992). Additionally, biliary proteins, most notably fibronectin, have been identified as pronucleators and may be capable of assisting in crystal formation and development of cholesterol crystals in bile. These proteins attach to other molecular components of bile and may thus influence the process of cholesterol crystal nucleation. While fibronectin is a pronucleator, investigation indicates that its concentration in gallstone patients' bile is low. Interestingly enough, research examining interactions between fibronectin in the biliary and gallbladder mucin has found no notable interaction that impacts cholesterol nucleation time. This indicates that although fibronectin potentially has a place in gallstone disease, it is not strong, and it is likely that other processes contribute more notably to bile concentration dynamics (Pozo et al., 1994).

The importance of bile concentration extends beyond gallstone formation; it influences gallbladder disease treatment approaches as well. Having an understanding of how bile composition and concentration are affected by diet is key to understanding gallstone recurrence prevention. For instance, supplementation of n-3 polyunsaturated fatty acids has been proven to reduce bile cholesterol saturation, indicating dietary changes are an excellent choice in bile concentration management (Abell et al., 1992). Furthermore, continued research into the biochemical interactions of constituents of bile and their relation to gallstone disease can lead to improved clinical advice. This newfound knowledge points to the importance of maintaining maximum bile concentration and composition, for its direct influence on gallbladder health and pathologies associated with improper management of bile.

9.2.3. Release of Bile Into the Small Intestine

The pouring of bile into the small intestine is an essential physiological process that permits fat digestion and absorption. Bile, produced in the liver and secreted into the gallbladder, is made up of bile salts, cholesterol, bilirubin, and proteins. Fatty food intake causes the gallbladder to contract and empty bile into the duodenum. This process is regulated by cholecystokinin, a hormone released by the intestinal walls in response to the presence of protein and fats in the chyme. Bile salts are emulsifying agents that break down fat into large micelles and small globules, increasing the surface area for lipase enzymes to act upon. Thus, normal bile release and subsequent interaction with dietary lipids are crucial for successful nutrient absorption and overall digestive health. The relationship between bile release and bile composition is intricate, with implications for the development of conditions such as gallstones. New evidence has established that dense biliary protein is commonly associated with cholesterol crystals, a significant risk factor for cholesterol gallstones. Cholesterol supersaturation in bile is well documented in gallstone disease, but the interaction between pH, total biliary protein concentration, and cholesterol saturation index has not yet been elucidated. In cholesterol crystal-containing samples, researchers found significantly higher levels of total protein than in samples without crystals, suggesting an interaction warranting further investigation.

This early understanding of the biochemical environment of bile contributes not just to the knowledge of gallstone formation in the gallbladder but also to the role of bile composition at discharge into the small intestine (Abell et al., 1991). Apart from this, bile discharge into the small intestine plays a vital role in regulating pancreatic secretion. Historical studies have shown that bile has an effect of stimulation of pancreatic juice secretion, though the extent differs according to species. Specifically, while it was observed that the duodenal infusion of bile in anesthetized cats results in a high degree of increased pancreatic activity, the response is seen to be diminished in conscious dogs. This finding exemplifies the complexity of digestive processes and the varying physiological responses among animals. Interestingly, diversion of bile from the duodenum does not seem to reduce meal-stimulated volume secretion of the pancreas, implying that bile and pancreatic juices might work by different regulatory pathways, eventually contributing to augmenting overall efficiency of digestion (Adamczyk et al., 1992).

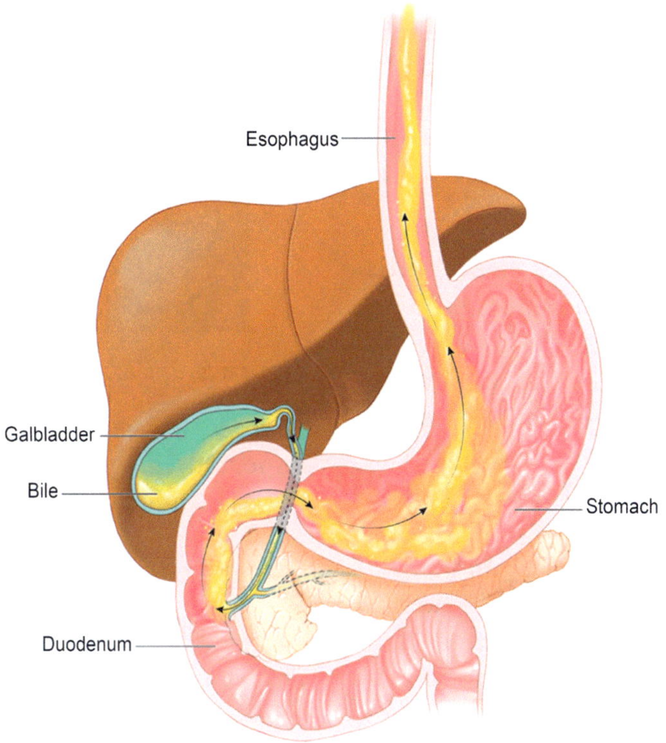

Figure 9.8. Bile refluxes from the small intestine into the stomach and esophagus.

Source: https://my.clevelandclinic.org/-/scassets/images/org/health/articles/22056-bile-reflux-web.ashx

Test Your Knowledge

1. Where is bile mainly stored?
2. What is the concentration of bile?

9.3. Gallbladder Disorders

Learning Outcome

1. Know the causes and symptoms of cholecystitis
2. Describe the formation and types of gallstones
3. Learn about other gallbladder diseases

Diseases of the gallbladder are a collection of conditions that can profoundly impact digestion and overall health. At the very top of the list of these is cholelithiasis, or gallstones, which occur as a result of an imbalance in the ingredients that comprise bile. Gallstones can form due to obesity, diet, and genetic reasons. With the persistence of high levels of obesity globally, incidence levels of gallbladder disease also increase, and the World Health Organization has identified the issue of obesity as a significant public health concern (Kyrou and Weickert, 2010). These hardened deposits can clog the biliary tract, causing acute cholecystitis, or inflammation and severe cramps in the belly. The interplay between gallbladder disease and obesity underscores the preventive function that a healthy life has in reference to gallbladder disease. Gallstones do not occur in isolation; gallbladder disease also includes biliary sludge, along with other inflammatory diseases. Biliary sludge is a mixture of mucus, bilirubin, and cholesterol that, if unattended, could lead to complications.

Moreover, acute and chronic cholecystitis contribute to the medical conditions resulting from gallbladder insufficiency. The etiology of cholecystitis most typically includes gallstones, but sometimes, when the inflammation of the gallbladder is without obstruction, it can result from infections or systemic disease. Latest findings suggest that alterations in gut microbiota are also involved in gallbladder health, as dysbiosis may possibly influence gastrointestinal motility and inflammation (Kyrou and Weickert, 2010). Elucidation of these interconnected pathways is vital in the development of effective treatment modalities and prevention strategies. Surgical treatment, in the form of cholecystectomy, remains the cornerstone therapy for severe gallbladder disease. Laparoscopic surgery is the preferred procedure since it is minimally invasive and has shorter recovery times. Nonetheless, loss of the gallbladder is a risk factor for postoperative complications like bile reflux and alterations in fat digestion. Dietary modifications with an emphasis on adopting a low-fat diet with plenty of fruits and vegetables can reduce some of these consequences and direct patients towards adopting the right diet after surgery. Chronic gallbladder management increasingly recognizes resident intestinal microbiota's role as of critical significance, with the potential to impact not only the digestive system but also homeostasis in general throughout the gastrointestinal tract (Cicala et al., 2016). As such, promoting a healthy diet and understanding the impact of obesity on gallbladder disease are central to the health of both health professionals and patients.

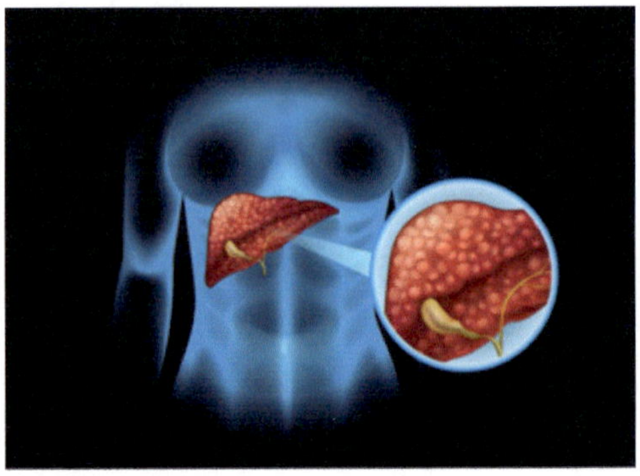

Figure 9.9. Gallbladder disorders.

Source: https://images.onlymyhealth.com/imported/images/2024/April/08_Apr_2024/thumb-gallbladderproblems.jpg

9.3.1. Cholecystitis: Causes and Symptoms

Cholecystitis, or gallbladder inflammation, is most commonly due to the presence of gallstones in the cystic duct to obstruct bile drainage. Obstruction leads to bile stasis and creates optimal conditions for bacterial growth and inflammatory reactions. Acute cholecystitis can develop suddenly and typically has clinical features such as severe pain that is typically localized in the right upper quadrant, nausea, vomiting, and fever. Chronic cholecystitis, on the other hand, may present with intermittent mild abdominal pain and gastrointestinal symptoms. Research suggests that the occurrence of cholecystitis is strongly related to lifestyle factors such as obesity, sudden weight loss, and female gender, highlighting the importance of lifestyle in its pathogenesis. Knowledge of the causative factors is important in effective management plans since it has a substantive influence on patient outcomes and management. The presentation of cholecystitis, though often marked, is extremely variable among patients. Some patients have minimal complaints of pain before sudden evolution to severe pain, while others have difficulty describing the onset of their symptoms. Murphy's sign, in which pain worsens with gallbladder palpation during inspiration of the patient, is the classic presentation. Symptoms in some patients are mimetic of other gastrointestinal diseases and pose a difficulty in diagnosis. Additional symptoms, such as jaundice, when they occur, can be representative of a more complex interaction of gallbladder and liver function. This multi-dimensional symptomatology underscores the relationship between gallbladder integrity and that of the biliary tree, as a dysfunction of one is likely to precipitate the complications of the other, particularly in the instance of cholestatic liver diseases that may arise in association with gallbladder disease (Alpini et al., 2023).

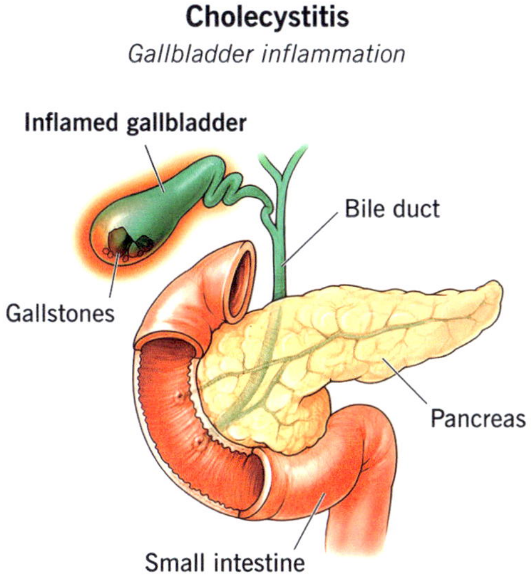

Figure 9.10. Cholecystitis is inflammation in your gallbladder, the small, pear-shaped organ that stores bile.

Source: https://my.clevelandclinic.org/-/scassets/Images/org/health/articles/15265-cholecystitis-gallbladder-inflammation

Diagnosis of cholecystitis primarily relies on imaging tests such as ultrasound and CT scans that are capable of demonstrating the presence of gallstones and inflammation. Laboratory tests in the form of blood tests may be used to estimate disease severity and the potential presence of infectious agents. Cholecystitis must be treated promptly to prevent complications, such as perforation or abscess formation, which can be fatal. The co-existence of gallbladder disease with liver diseases further tightens the association of the health of these vital organs. Research indicates that gallbladder disease may not only arise from, but also progress due to, underlying liver diseases (Kang and Williamson, 1990). It is therefore implied that holistic treatment approaches should involve the proper evaluation of the liver and the gallbladder to enhance diagnostic sensitivity and therapeutic efficacy in cholecystitis patients.

9.3.2. Gallstones: Formation and Types

The process of gallstone formation is a multifactorial one that consists of crystallization of bile components, such as cholesterol, bilirubin, and bile salts. The most frequent type of gallstones are cholesterol gallstones, comprising about 70-80% of all gallstones. They develop when bile is supersaturated with cholesterol, favoring crystal development. Total biliary protein concentrations and bile pH are significant determinants of this process. Studies indicate that higher total protein concentrations of bile are usually associated with cholesterol crystals, suggesting that higher biliary protein may be a risk factor for cholesterol gallstone formation (Abell et al., 1991). It is necessary to understand these mechanisms to develop preventive strategies and effective therapies for gallstone-susceptible individuals. Besides cholesterol stones, the most common second type of gallstones is pigment gallstones that are made up mainly of bilirubin. These will form when there is an excess of bilirubin in the bile, most commonly from hemolysis or liver cirrhosis. Pigment stones are generally brown and may be found in patients with certain conditions, such as sickle cell disease or chronic liver disease, that result in overproduction of bilirubin. The morphogenesis of pigment stones is less clear than that of cholesterol stones, but they may also be susceptible to the influence of some biliary proteins. Despite the reports of the role of certain biliary proteins in cholesterol crystal formation, the subject remains an open area of research concerning the interaction of these proteins and pigment stone formation (Pozo et al., 1994).

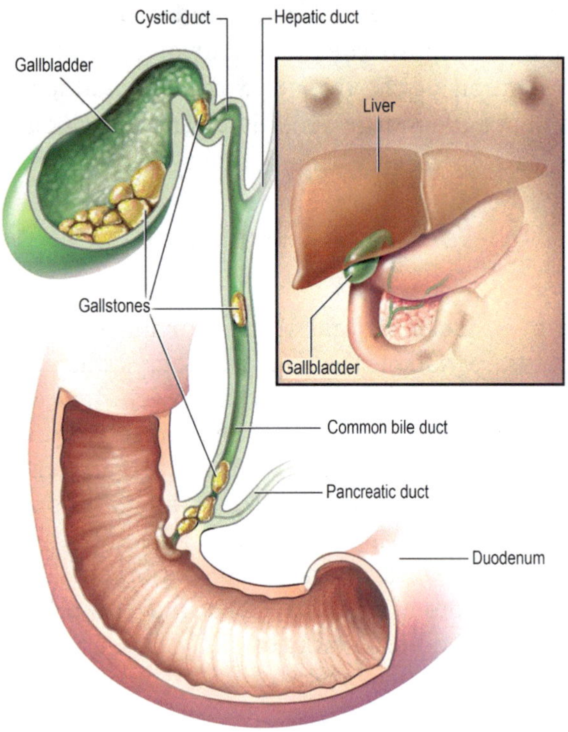

Figure 9.11. Gallstones.

Source: https://assets.mayoclinic.org/content/dam/media/en/images/2023/02/08/gallstones.jpg

These investigations will give us important information on how gallbladder diseases can be prevented and treated. Understanding gallstone type and pathogenesis not only aids in the identification of susceptible patients but also offers a focus on lifestyle and dietary intervention. Specifically, a predisposition to cholesterol gallstones might lead to recommendations to adopt a high-fiber diet with low saturated fats, which could enhance bile fluidity and reducing cholesterol crystallization. Also, a healthy weight will lower the risk of gallstone formation, as obesity is one of the key risk factors. Therefore, ongoing research describing the biochemical pathways and risk factors of gallstone development is important for enhancing clinical practice. With the blend of what is known about cholesterol and pigment stones, physicians can target preventive strategies more precisely and increase the success of patients in all aspects related to gallbladder health.

9.3.3. Other Gallbladder Diseases

Other than gallstones and acute cholecystitis, there exist other gallbladder diseases that require extreme significance, given their effects on human health. One of these is gallbladder dyskinesia, which is characterized by disturbed gallbladder motility that can lead to biliary colic and gastrointestinal discomfort. Patients typically have episodic right upper quadrant pain, which may be reproduced by gallstone attacks but is not due to obstruction. Pathogenesis of gallbladder dyskinesia can be multimodal, perhaps due to inflammation, hormonal influence, or autonomic nervous system disease. Diagnosis typically occurs on imaging studies and functional tests, and treatment may include dietary modification and symptomatic treatment. It is worth learning about such dysfunctions since they highlight the complexities of gallbladder disease beyond the more commonly known entities. Cholecystitis is another severe gallbladder disease and is an inflammation of the gallbladder occurring in an acute or chronic fashion. Initiation of acute cholecystitis is usually caused by gallstones that obstruct the cystic duct, cause bile stasis, bacterial overgrowth, and resultant inflammation. The symptoms typically present with acute abdominal pain, fever, and nausea and require urgent medical care. Chronic cholecystitis is, however, caused by the recurrent inflammatory response to the gallstones, resulting in continuous irritation and follow-up calcification of the gallbladder wall. This long-term condition not only compromises gallbladder function but can also make a person susceptible to gallbladder cancer and other complications. Hence, ongoing study and clinical practice are essential in determining the best management policies, particularly in recurrent cholecystitis and structural change in the gallbladder. Additionally, emerging interest in the function of resident intestinal microbiota in gallbladder disease sheds light on the possible relationship between gut health and gallbladder function. Dysbiosis, a disruption of the balance of gut microbiota, has been recognized as an underlying cause of many gastrointestinal diseases and may also affect biliary health. Alterations in the microbiome have been proposed to affect gastrointestinal motility, including gallbladder contractions and bile flow. The involvement of microbial metabolites and bacterial components in inflammatory processes identifies a complex mechanism in which the gut microbiota may expedite gallbladder diseases either directly or indirectly. Ongoing studies of such complex mechanisms offer novel opportunities for therapeutic approaches that can interfere with gut-microbiota interactions, and it holds promise for novel treatment approaches to gallbladder diseases beyond traditional treatment pathways (Alvaro et al., 2017; Cicala et al., 2016).

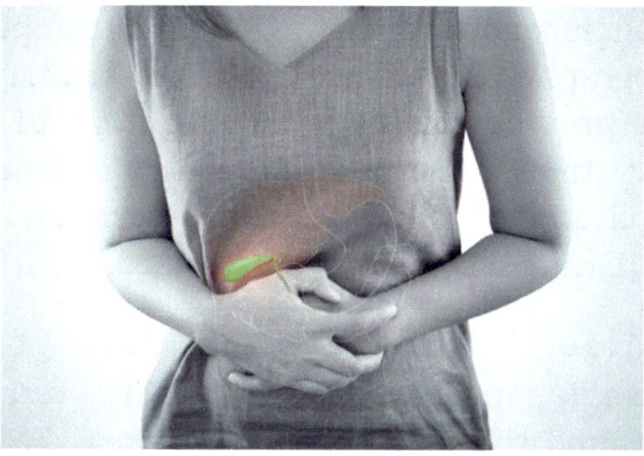

Source: https://www.gastroconsa.com/wp-content/uploads/2024/11/what-does-gallbladder-pain-feel-like-image.jpg

Test Your Knowledge

1. What are the causes of cholecystitis?
2. What are the 3 types of gallstones?

9.4. Diagnosis of Gallbladder Conditions

Learning Outcome

1. Describe the imaging techniques
2. Understand the blood tests and their significance
3. Describe the endoscopic procedures for diagnosing gallbladder diseases

Gallbladder pathology needs a full diagnosis with imaging tests, clinical examination, and laboratory studies. Sufficient medical history is the first requirement because jaundice, abdominal pain, or fever can be the presentation of related gallbladder pathology. During physical examination, right upper quadrant tenderness may be detected and is usually secondary to gallbladder infection or inflammation. Subsequently, laboratory tests, including liver function tests performed under the lab conditions, can identify such anomalies as elevated bilirubin or liver enzymes that can be the indicators of cholestasis or other hepatobiliary diseases. There is added clinical insight that accompanies the incorporation of the results of ultrasound scans, utilized as the primary imaging modality due to its non-invasive nature and ability to detect gallstones, thickening of the gallbladder, and dilatation of bile ducts, and offer a more insightful view of the pathology. Ultrasound is a crucial component in the initial diagnosis of gallbladder disease and in guiding further investigations. If the ultrasound remains unclear, further imaging can be employed, such as magnetic resonance cholangiopancreatography (MRCP) or computed tomography (CT) scans. These newer imaging tests provide excellent visualization of the biliary tree and may be helpful in explaining complications such as gallbladder perforation or pancreatitis secondary to obstructed bile ducts.

Also, endoscopic retrograde cholangiopancreatography (ERCP) can be warranted to remove gallstones from the bile duct or for the treatment of strictures and other gallbladder pathology. All these diagnostic tests combined provide complete insight into gallbladder disease, and the therapeutic measures are considerably determined by the same, and the results of the patient are improved. The clinical manifestations of gallbladder disease may be diverse, and hence the approach to each patient must be individualized. For instance, cholangitis and cholecystitis caused by bacteria, while being infrequently reported in human subjects, are a demonstration of multi-etiology importance in considerations. Clinical presentation may be fever, jaundice, and abdominal pain, accentuated by laboratory testing of leukocytosis and elevated liver enzymes. Ultrasound reports, even though being typically nonspecific, still maintain a central position in gallbladder morphology and function assessment. As evidenced by veterinary reports, equivalent pathology will have specific clinical-pathologic features for differential diagnosis in humans. Monitoring of antimicrobial resistance, resistant cases, and outcome after therapy are important factors for successful therapy. An aggressive diagnostic method will thus result in early intervention and survival of the patient for dogs with gallbladder disease (Allenspach et al., 2016) (Kyrou and Weickert, 2010).

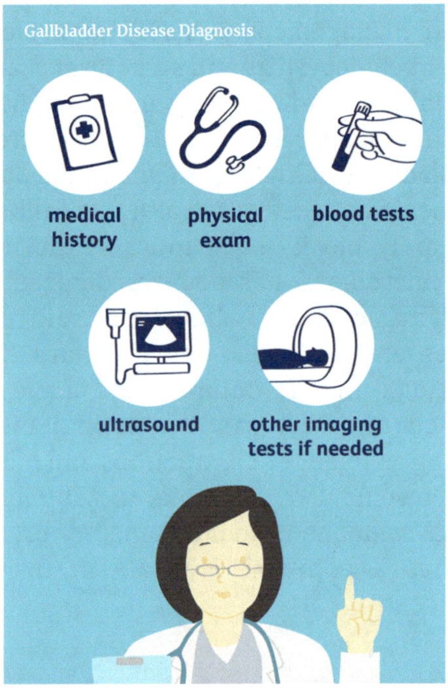

Figure 9.12. Diagnosis of gallbladder disease.

Source: https://www.verywellhealth.com/thmb/A71yTPA4IjTyO-38r4YaCff7OD8=/1500x0/filters:no_upscale():max_bytes(150000):strip_icc()/gallbladder-disease-diagnosis-10-5ae0c0a71f4e130039dc4b27.png

9.4.1. Imaging Techniques (Ultrasound, CT Scan)

Assessment of gallbladder wellness is important since it has a role to play in digestion and may influence some states of disease. Among imaging techniques employed, the primary diagnostic modality is ultrasound due to its non-invasive nature and ease of access. It employs high-frequency ultrasonic waves to produce images of the gallbladder such that clinicians can visualize gallstones, wall thickening, and other pathologies. Ultrasound efficiency stems from its ability to distinguish between solid and fluid-filled structures, making it particularly useful for detecting gallbladder conditions such as cholecystitis. Also, as ultrasound does not expose patients to ionizing radiation, it will generally be the first choice, particularly in populations that are susceptible to the ill effects of exposure to such radiation (N/A, 1989). This basic technique provides important information that guides subsequent management of gallbladder disease. Computed tomography (CT) scan is another way the gallbladder is imaged, particularly when the ultrasound is inconclusive. This new imaging technique employs a series of X-rays from different angles that a computer reformats into accurate cross-sectional images of the body. CT scans are extremely sensitive in identifying complications such as gallbladder perforation or the formation of an abscess, which may be hard to identify using ultrasound. Imaging of surrounding anatomical structures and assessment of potential metastasis is also enormously helpful when malignancies are being evaluated. The drawback of CT is that it uses ionizing radiation, which poses some risk, especially in pregnancy and young patients. Despite these being some limited disadvantages, the high level of detail provided by CT scans makes them an integral component of a comprehensive diagnostic strategy for gallbladder pathology (White et al., 2007). The choice clinically between ultrasound and CT scanning is very much situation and patient-dependent. For instance, ultrasound would be the preferred modality of choice due to convenience, while CT is left in cases of necessity or in suspected complications. Both imaging modalities merged would help enhance diagnostic accuracy and patient outcomes. The combined use can help physicians develop an enhanced knowledge base on gallbladder pathology to inform proper and effective treatment interventions in good time. Furthermore, imaging technology is becoming increasingly advanced, with the potential to refine these modalities' functions. On the basis of evolving research, optimization of imaging protocols, balancing sensitivity, specificity, and safety, will remain a priority in the ongoing search for improved gallbladder health assessment.

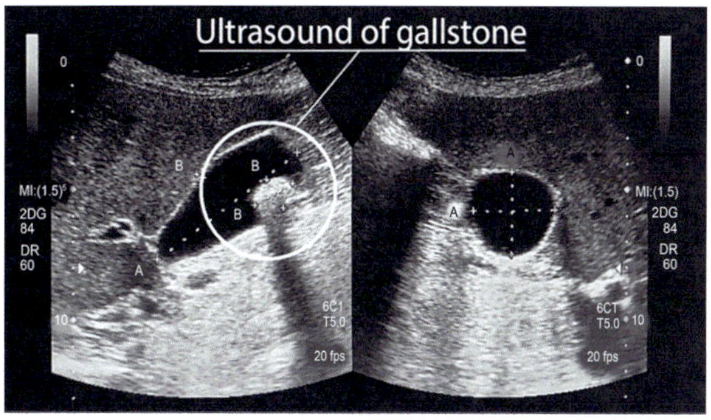

Figure 9.13. An ultrasound showing gallbladder stones.

Source: https://cdn-ilcancn.nitrocdn.com/RimjDkiIALHVXpzCGJAYTPTxgApUQHBS/assets/images/optimized/rev-da34369/www.pockethealth.com/wp-content/uploads/2024/08/gallbladder-stone-1536x864.png

9.4.2. Blood Tests and Their Significance

Blood tests serve a very important role in clinical diagnosis, offering information essential to the evaluation of various organ functions, including the gallbladder. Through the assessment of blood elements, doctors are able to identify alterations associated with gallbladder disease, such as cholecystitis, stones, and other biliary illnesses. Specific biomarkers, such as bilirubin level and liver enzymes, are typically examined to assess gallbladder condition and function. Notably, elevations of alkaline phosphatase and serum bilirubin would point to potential obstructions or inflammation of the biliary tree and render blood tests a valuable component of regular gallbladder disease screening. The combination of history and blood test results allows clinicians to provide an educated diagnosis about the underlying pathophysiology, facilitating earlier intervention and treatment. Further, the relationship between stress, blood pressure, and gallbladder complications highlights the role of blood tests in overall health assessments. Psychological stress has been identified as a causative factor for hypertension, which is a risk factor for gallbladder disease complications (Tanna and Khatri, 2024). The relationship between chronic hypertension and gallbladder function requires follow-up via blood tests. Abnormal blood pressure values and altered markers of stress can reflect the risk of gallbladder dysregulation, where the organ's motility and biochemical homeostasis are compromised. Consequently, blood analyses that include tests of metabolic status, including lipid profile and blood glucose, provide relevant data toward the prediction of gallbladder pathology development. This all-inclusive approach to health screening underscores the significance of blood tests in understanding the interplay among stress, cardiovascular health, and gallbladder function. In the context of cardiometabolic health, the measurement of blood metabolites through tests better illustrates the significance of valuing gallbladder function. Modern studies have also recognized the role of certain metabolites, including acetate and diacylglycerol, in relation to blood pressure regulation and overall metabolic well-being (Parnell et al., 2023). By studying the metabolites involved, healthcare providers can grasp the nutritional and physiological factors of gallbladder well-being. Discovery of genetic markers that relate to cardiometabolic traits also reinforces the importance of personalized medicine in the treatment of gallbladder diseases. Blood tests revealing such metabolic dysregulation may guide lifestyle interventions to decrease gallbladder disease risk. Blood testing thus emerges as a valuable diagnostic tool and a gateway to greater insight into the complex interplay among metabolic health, gallbladder function, and overall body well-being.

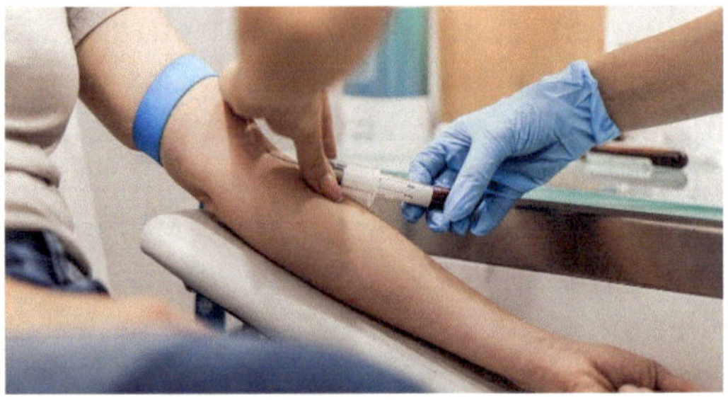

Figure 9.14. Blood test.

Source: https://media-cldnry.s-nbcnews.com/image/upload/t_nbcnews-fp-1200-630,f_auto,q_auto:best/rockcms/2024-08/240829-blood-test-stock-aa-1253p-e88212.jpg

9.4.3. Endoscopic Procedures For Diagnosis

Endoscopic treatment has changed the diagnostic picture of gallbladder disease, especially gallstones and cholecystitis. Through advances in minimally invasive techniques such as endoscopic retrograde cholangiopancreatography (ERCP) and laparoscopic cholecystectomy, medical professionals are now able to precisely assess and treat several gallbladder ailments. ERCP is unique in its dual therapeutic and diagnostic nature, allowing both visualization of biliary obstruction and the ability to extract stones or insert stents as needed. Through these endoscopic techniques, physicians have the ability to offer real-time images and data that significantly enhance gallbladder pathophysiology knowledge, allowing for timely and effective interventions. The role of endoscopy is not only for simple diagnosis but also for biliary composition analysis that can indicate the presence of gallstones. There is recent evidence that highlights the significance of biliary protein content in this context. As an illustration, comparative analysis of samples of gallbladder bile revealed that samples with cholesterol crystals contained significantly higher levels of total protein compared to crystal-free samples. This correlation suggests that higher concentrations of biliary proteins may be a risk factor for cholesterol gallstone formation and hence provide insight into the biochemical conditions under which gallbladder disease exists (Abell et al., 1991). These data serve to underscore the importance of employing endoscopic methods not only for optical inspection but also for the acquisition of information about the biochemical determinants of gallbladder health. In addition to ERCP, other emerging technologies such as transumbilical endoscopic surgery (TUES) have also been promising in enhancing surgical success during gallbladder removal. With this technique, a completely concealed laparoscopic cholecystectomy can be achieved by making incisions less visible and offering better cosmetic results. In clinical trials, TUES had very high rates of patient satisfaction as incisions were largely concealed. With the application of specialized tools through strategically placed trocars, surgeons can navigate the field more efficiently, breaking away from the limitations of conventional methods (Chen et al., 2011). Successful implementation of such endoscopic procedures indicates not only the potential for improved patient outcomes but also the new dynamics of surgical options for gallbladder disease, demonstrating a move towards greater efficacy and patient-focused care.

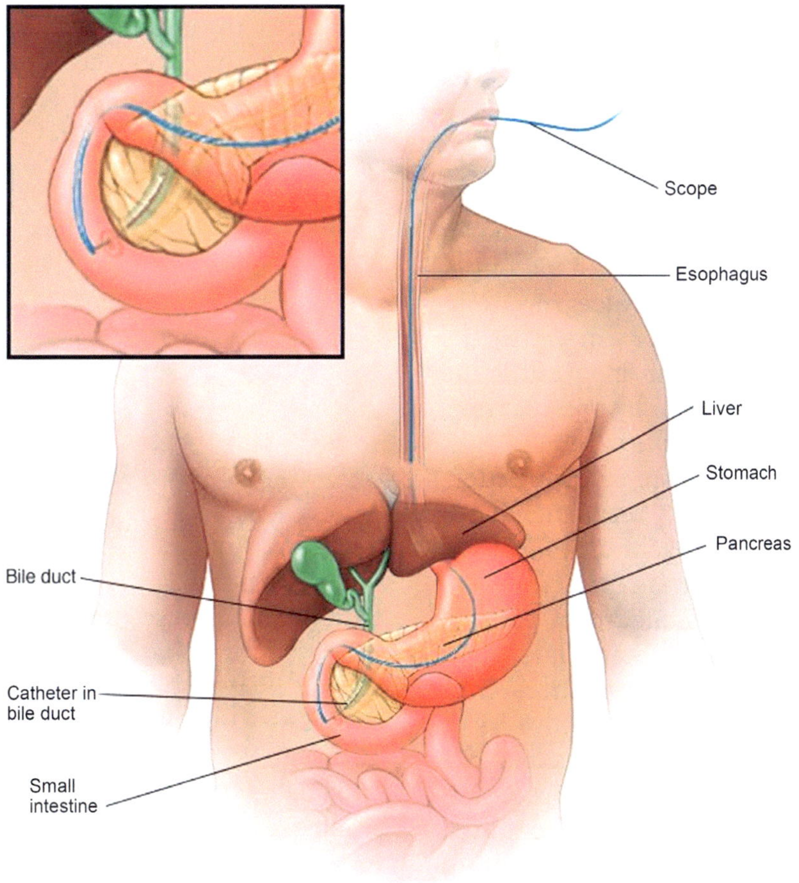

Figure 9.15. Endoscopic retrograde cholangiopancreatography.

Source: https://assets.mayoclinic.org/content/dam/media/en/images/2023/02/09/ercp.jpg

Test Your Knowledge

1. What is the imaging technique for gallstones?
2. What is the significance of a blood test?

9.5. Treatment Options For Gallbladder Issues

Learning Outcome

1. Understand the dietary changes and lifestyle modifications in the management of gallbladder diseases
2. Learn about medications for managing symptoms associated with gallbladder disorders
3. Know the surgical interventions of the gallbladder

Treatment of gallbladder issues is mostly determined by the kind of problem at hand. For instance, cholecystitis, or inflammation of the gallbladder, tends to be treated surgically, particularly by cholecystectomy, in which the gallbladder is removed. This may either be carried out laparoscopically or by open surgery, depending on how bad the issue is and patients' health. If gallstones cause pain or obstruction, this type of surgery is normally recommended to alleviate symptoms and prevent complications in the future. Laparoscopic cholecystectomy has been encouraged as the standard of care by numerous studies due to it being minimally invasive with a shorter recovery time than conventional surgery, and therefore is a treatment option for the majority of gallbladder patients (N/A, 2006). This surgical procedure effectively addresses the underlying condition as well as avoiding future risk. In addition to surgical treatment, non-surgical procedures may also play a role in the treatment of gallbladder conditions, particularly for patients who are unsuitable candidates for surgery. Medication therapy, such as the use of bile acid tablets, may help dissolve cholesterol gallstones but is a therapy that requires a longer course of treatment and is not suitable for all patients. Furthermore, weight management and dietary changes are central to the non-operative therapy of gallbladder disease. By adopting a low-fat, high-fiber diet, patients may significantly reduce the risk of gallstone formation and gallbladder complications. These lifestyle changes have been suggested to, in addition to medication, hold promise for patients who desire to avert surgery in its entirety while still successfully reducing their symptoms (N/A, 2010).

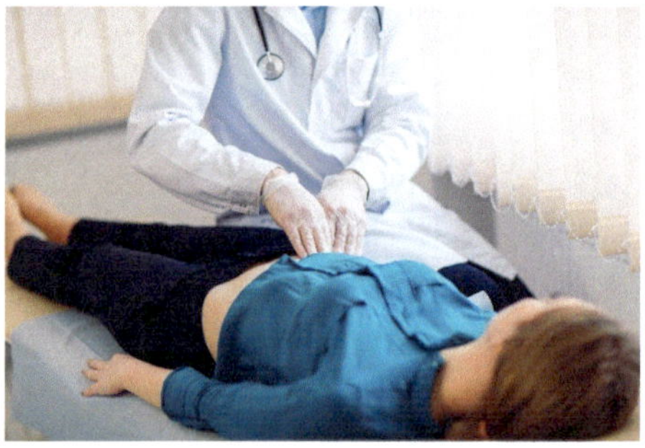

Figure 9.16. Gallbladder treatments.

Source: https://medlineplus.gov/images/GallbladderDiseases_share.jpg

Another progressive consideration in gallbladder treatment includes the use of endoscopic retrograde cholangiopancreatography (ERCP) for patients who have complications such as bile duct stones or stricture. ERCP is a technique that allows direct visualization and intervention of the biliary tract that effectively cures obstructions that otherwise lead to more gallbladder issues. This procedure, while initially non-surgical, can sometimes be employed as a stepping stone to surgery if there are recurrent issues. Utilization of ERCP, or in conjunction with other therapeutic modalities, is selected according to the individual patient's specific clinical scenario and composite health profile. As technology evolves in this field, familiarity with the full scope of therapeutic options is essential for medical professionals and patients who have to deal with gallbladder health (N/A, 2006; N/A, 2010).

9.5.1. Dietary Changes and Lifestyle Modifications

Diet change and lifestyle change are crucial in gallbladder health management, due to the increasing prevalence of gallstones attributed to diet and obesity. Evidence-based facts demonstrate that symptomatic incidence of gallstones can be minimized via application of some diet interventions. Past practice included the prescription of a low-fat diet as a means of gallstone symptom reduction; however, newer evidence refutes the effectiveness of such interventions. Specifically, gallstone disease nutritional fat change literature continues to be scanty, as evidenced by the few top-level randomized clinical trials in the near past. The necessity of adequate research defining dietary patterns, gallstone development, and complications that ensue is crucial in further differentiating such diet interventions and individualizing the nutritional requirements of patients with gallbladder disease (Culkin et al., 2024). Apart from dietary modification, lifestyle modification, such as increased exercise, is also essential in gallbladder maintenance. People who have a sedentary lifestyle are mostly associated with obesity, which is the primary risk factor for developing gallstones. Exercise helps keep one's weight under control and improves digestion, and hence reduces gallstone formation. Also, lifestyle components such as smoking and moderate alcohol use may influence gallbladder function. Because the elderly population suffers from unique gastrointestinal disorders, age alterations of the gastrointestinal tract must be examined. The elderly gastrointestinal tracts suffer from decreased mechanical and chemical function, leading to reduced nutrient absorption and potential malnutrition. This situation emphasizes the significance of lifestyle intervention specifically to ensure gallbladder function and overall health among the elderly (Bordoni et al., 2015). The inclusion of these lifestyle and food interventions is an integrated approach in gallbladder health management. Whole grain, fruit, and vegetable-based foods are advised for consumption with only minimal intake of refined carbohydrates and excessive calories. The same good diet is not only good for the gallbladder but also for overall well-being. In addition, life adjustment before the fact, including stress reduction and hydration, may also improve digestive function. By learning such habits early enough, one can avert gallbladder disease and all its related complications. Lastly, more research is required so that personalized dietetic counseling and life-style therapy could be created, which would counteract the shifting demands of patients with gallstones according to the intricate inter-play between digestion and total body well-being (Culkin et al., 2024).

9.5.2. Medications For Managing Symptoms

Symptom control of gallbladder disease often demands the use of drugs, particularly in the case of cholecystitis or gallstones. The use of the nonsteroidal anti-inflammatory agents (NSAIDs) is typically advocated for in an attempt to reduce pain and inflammation, while the underlying disease is further evaluated in the meantime. Additionally, medications such as ursodeoxycholic acid are held accountable for being vital for the dissolution of cholesterol gallstones. This process is particularly helpful in patients who might not qualify for surgery due to some medical health issues. Therefore, the application of drugs can play an important role in achieving comfort for the patient while simultaneously treating the symptoms, as accepted today (N/A, 2021). This is a proactive solution toward the management of complications and determines overall health and treatment outcomes for individuals suffering from gallbladder disease. In dyspeptic patients with gallbladder disease, which is commonly linked, consideration should be given to some drug regimens aimed at the relief of symptoms. Proton pump inhibitors (PPIs) can successfully reduce gastric acid secretion and thus bring relief of symptoms, as well as treat potential gastric reflux, which may exacerbate gallbladder symptoms. Exploring these options requires a detailed examination of the patient's baseline health and the potential interactions between their gallbladder status and GI health. Notably, the complexity of symptom management presents an appeal for customized treatment plans, as stated by literature in place with greater demands for customized approaches (N/A, 2021). The effectiveness of drugs relies on an intensive assessment process that is critical to attaining the best patient outcomes and satisfaction. Besides, due to the alarming obesity rate, particularly in relation to gallbladder disease, its management requires a multidimensional strategy beyond drugs. The link between the conditions and obesity requires interventional measures that include drugs and lifestyle changes. The use of drugs only may be inadequate in managing such symptoms; hence, doctors recommend dietary modification and exercise as central components of management. This multi-dimensional plan, therefore, not only works towards the treatment of gallbladder symptoms but the public health condition of obesity as well, which in itself is encumbered with dire risks for gallbladder-related complications. As healthcare systems evolve further, integrating therapeutic interventions for obesity alongside gallbladder symptom treatment will continue to be the top priority, justifying the efficacy of the integrated care strategy in improving the health status of those afflicted.

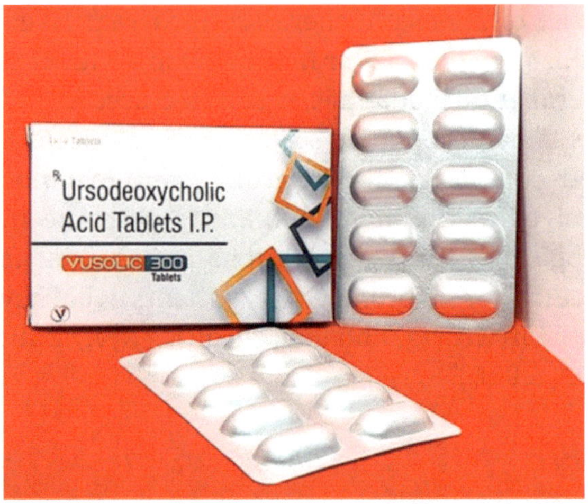

Figure 9.17. Ursodeoxycholic acid for gallstone.

Source: https://tiimg.tistatic.com/fp/1/007/259/ursodeoxycholic-acid-300-mg-gallstone-liver-oral-tablets-878.jpg

9.5.3. Surgical Interventions: Cholecystectomy

The procedure known as cholecystectomy, or gallbladder removal, has become standard treatment for gallbladder disease, particularly symptomatic gallstones. The procedure can either be performed via an open or a laparoscopic technique, but laparoscopic cholecystectomy is usually favored since it is less invasive and therefore results in less pain post-procedure, provides quicker recovery times, and leaves less scarring. With the evolution of laparoscopic techniques, innovations such as TUES have proceeded to further evolve the procedure with even better aesthetic outcomes as well as less trauma. Yet another recent study reported a new concealed laparoscopic technique that had successful outcomes in twelve cases, all of whom had no intraoperative complications and high patient satisfaction with the cosmetic outcome of their wound (Chen et al., 2011). This development of surgical techniques shows the steady advancement in cholecystectomy surgery, both health- and aesthetic-wise. With improvements in surgery, the application of imaging techniques such as near-infrared imaging with indocyanine green (ICG) greatly improved the success rate of laparoscopic cholecystectomy. ICG facilitates better visualization of biliary anatomy, which is crucial to prevent surgical complications. A systematic review cited that utilized at the 2.5-mg dose, ICG significantly improved visualization rates of the cystic duct prior to dissection against traditional methods such as intraoperative cholangiography (IOC). Although results yielded moderate quality evidence only, the promise of ICG in enhancing biliary mapping during cholecystectomy merits optimism (van Dam et al., 2016).

This enhanced visualization allows surgeons to move through complex anatomical settings, reducing the incidence of complications and improving overall surgical results. Postoperative management of patients for cholecystectomy is also highly crucial and has been greatly affected by the minimally invasive nature of laparoscopic surgery techniques. Following surgery, most patients may resume regular activities within a minimal period, most being able to resume a normal diet within hours after the operation. Compared to conventional open surgery, the laparoscopic procedure decreases recovery time and hospital stay, with significant cost-effectiveness to the healthcare system. Furthermore, improvements in analgesia and postoperative care measures ensure that patients experience no significant pain or complications. The potential to perform cholecystectomy through small incisions not only aligns with modern operating techniques but also significantly enhances patient satisfaction. The combined benefits of these postoperative and operative innovations establish the worth of cholecystectomy in the efficient and effective management of gallbladder disease.

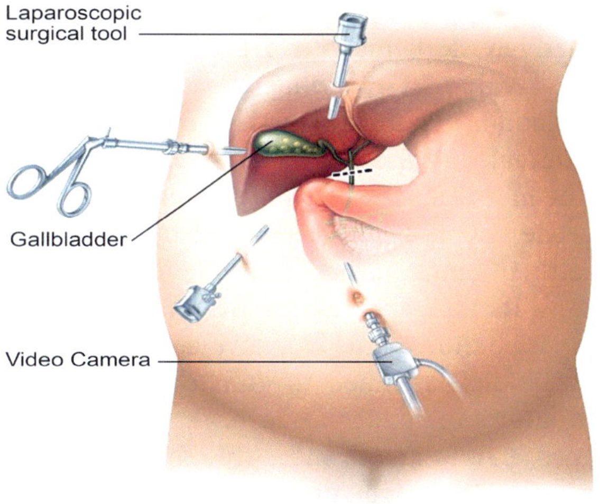

Figure 9.18. Laparoscopic cholecystectomy.

Source: https://assets.mayoclinic.org/content/dam/media/en/images/2023/02/09/laparoscopic-cholecystectomy.jpg

Test Your Knowledge

1. What medication is used to treat gallbladder problems?
2. What is the surgical removal of is called cholecystectomy?

9.6. Prevention of Gallbladder Diseases

Learning Outcome

1. Know the healthy diet and its impact
2. Understand the importance of regular exercise
3. Understand the risk factors associated with gallbladder diseases and how to mitigate them

Effectively implemented preventive measures are of value in reducing the occurrence of gallbladder disease, in particular those related to dietary and lifestyle factors. Obesity is one of the most important etiologies for gallbladder disease and has been classified by the World Health Organization as a worldwide epidemic due to its meteoric rise in incidence, affecting over 1.5 billion adults worldwide. Greater body mass index is linked to gallstone formation and later gallbladder disease. To prevent such issues, public health measures must promote proper weight regulation through the adoption of healthy eating habits and regular exercise. Promotion of the inclusion of a healthy lifestyle can substantially lower gallbladder conditions as well as improve general well-being among the populace. This multi-faceted approach not only encompasses the transition required at the level of an individual but also resources available at the level of a community to enable individuals to make healthier choices and reduce the public expenses of gallbladder disease. Nutritional issues are also a vital part of preventing gallbladder disease. High-refined carbohydrates and saturated fat dietary intake have been linked to an increased risk of gallstones, whereas a diet rich in fiber and healthy fat, such as omega-3 fatty acids, decreases the risk. Supplementing with food sources such as fruits, vegetables, whole grains, and nuts helps in increasing the gallbladder status by promoting a better composition of bile and increased frequency of gallbladder contraction. Moreover, regular normal consumption can prevent bile stasis in the gallbladder, which is one of the primary etiological reasons for the development of stones. Mass public health awareness campaigns to promote healthy eating habits are thus needed. These interventions should include different groups of populations, i.e., children and adolescents, because it could have long-lasting positive impacts on the health of the gallbladder as well as overall well-being if these dietary habits are initiated during early childhood. In addition to diet and lifestyle modification, additional research remains to explain the mechanism of gallbladder disease, and particularly of GBC. Although controversy remains regarding the linking of specific environmental exposures, e.g., arsenic, to GBC, integrated risk evaluation has been initiated in research. As repeated in recent pilot studies, increased levels of arsenic have been observed in patients with GBC compared to non-cancerous gallbladder specimens, pointing to certain areas where prevention measures can be implemented. Creating more awareness regarding these risk factors can make it easier to implement certain measures to minimize GBC incidence. Briefly, an all-round strategy that includes healthy living, nutrition education, and continuous research shall be the key to successful gallbladder disease prevention and control over this important branch of public health (Kyrou and Weickert, 2010; Boffetta et al., 2023).

9.6.1. Healthy Diet and How It Impacts

One important aspect in understanding the role of the gallbladder in human health is to observe the impact of a normal diet on its function. The primary function of the gallbladder is to secrete and concentrate bile, which plays an essential role in the emulsification of fats and later digestion and absorption. With a person on a healthy diet rich in fruits, vegetables, whole grains, and fat, the gallbladder performs at peak level in the emulsification of fats. Conversely, excessive intake of saturated fats and refined sugars may contribute to gallstones and gallbladder dysfunction. The toxic effect may induce cholecystitis, a causative agent of pain and inflammation that causes dysfunction. A healthy diet not only provides support to the gallbladder but also to the overall digestive system, showcasing the connection between food eating habits and gallbladder function. Moreover, the impact of a healthy diet extends beyond the gallbladder to the overall gastrointestinal system. A diet rich in fiber can help regulate digestion and maintain intestinal microbial balance. Normal bowel function is dependent on good fiber intake and can prevent diverticulitis and other inflammatory diseases. There is scientific evidence showing that optimal gallbladder function depends on the optimal functioning of the microbiome, since dysfunction will disrupt bile acid metabolism and drive gallbladder pathologies. For example, patients with an impaired gut microbiota would possess impaired bile composition, which can hasten gallstone disease or other gallbladder conditions. Here, the effects of a healthy dietary lifestyle resonate through a chain of systems of organs to bring out the susceptibility of gallbladders to dietary lifestyle and digestive health. To sum up, the connection between diet and gallbladder health is highlighted by certain medical conditions that are diet-dependent. Celiac disease and non-celiac gluten sensitivity (NCGS) are prototype diseases illustrating how food intake can lead to extensive gastrointestinal distress, along with affecting the gallbladder indirectly. Both diseases are immune-system-related and manifest by symptomatology calling for dietary modification in the form of a gluten-free diet (GFD). In such cases, compliance with a GFD will remit symptoms and return intestinal function to normal, leading to a resultant improvement in gallbladder function too. An explicit understanding of these correlations reiterates the relevance of some nutritional interventions and reiterates the need for patients with some ailments to consider to what extent their diet influences not only their immediate symptoms but also the gallbladder operation and the general digestive system (Bogatyrev et al., 2019; Thomas, 2020).

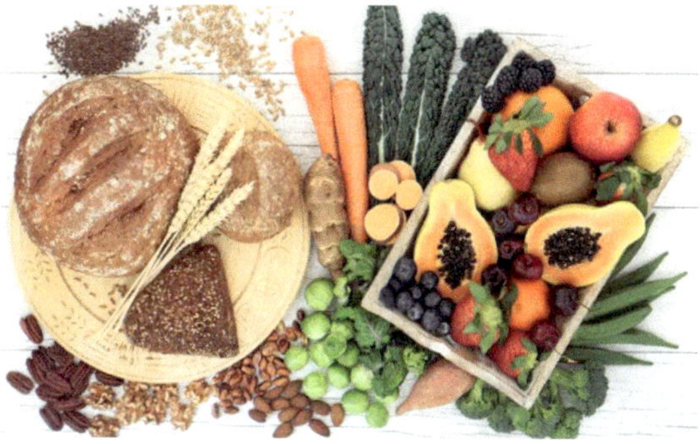

Figure 9.19. Diet for a healthy gallbladder.

Source: https://www.manipalhospitals.com/uploads/blog/healthy-gallbladder-diet.png

9.6.2. Importance of Regular Exercise

In the context of gallbladder health, the importance of regular exercise cannot be overstated. Exercise is a fundamental process whereby individuals are able to regulate their overall metabolic status and minimize the risk of suffering from gallbladder illness. Physical exercise enhances bile acid excretion, which is essential to the digestion and absorption of fat ingested. This mechanism, if supplemented with routine exercise, will hinder the formation of gallstones, which is also, in most cases, associated with intake of high saturated fat diets and physical inactivity. Routine exercise also enhances the metabolism of cholesterol, which, when in excess, leads to the precipitation of cholesterol gallstone formation. By engaging in physical exercise, an individual not only augments metabolic health but also supports gallbladder health, hence optimal functioning in the human body. Secondly, the relationship between exercise and the control of metabolic disorders reveals the preventive aspect of physical exercise towards the functioning of the gallbladder. Conditions such as insulin resistance, diabetes, and obesity have a strong association with gallbladder disease since poor metabolic health is bound to lead to cholesterol deposition in the gallbladder. Physical activity is a protective factor since it manages body weight and increases insulin sensitivity, thus reducing the potential for gallstone formation. The gallbladder functions dynamically since it serves as a reservoir of bile, and lifestyle considerations can play a significant role in maintaining its health. Secondly, physical exercise induces gallbladder contractions so that bile flow occurs and stagnation, which could result in the formation of stones, is minimized. This interaction highlights that exercise is crucial not only for cardiovascular well-being but also for maintaining functional integrity of the hepatobiliary system.

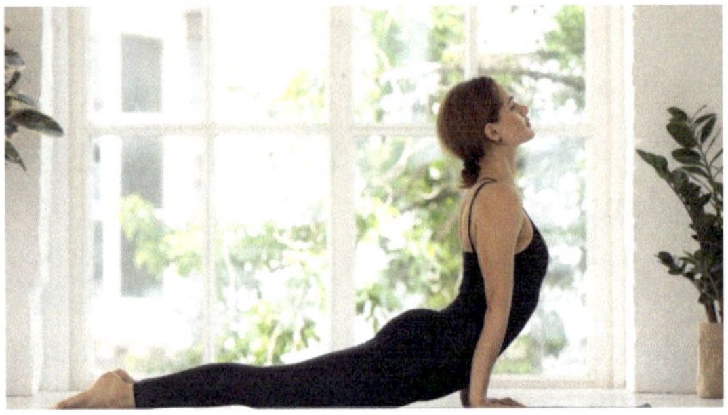

Figure 9.20. A yoga pose.

Source: https://nirva-strapi-soure.s3.us-west-2.amazonaws.com/Yoga_Poses_for_Gallstone_Pain_Relief_d6e40932ac.jpg

Finally, exercise effects on gallbladder disease extend beyond disease prevention; they also encompass optimization of overall digestive health. There is evidence to indicate that exercise facilitates the healthful motility of the gastrointestinal system, integral to bile acid clearance and recycling. With this, exercise can facilitate a more effective process of digestion, resulting in better nutrient uptake and reduced risks of gastrointestinal distress. With lifestyle-related conditions affecting populations more and more, it is then crucial to advocate for the role of exercise to ensure a healthy gallbladder. Scientists should acknowledge that factors such as individual training status, exercise intensity, and general fitness level can affect these results. Hence, encouraging frequent exercise is an essential element not only for overall health but, in particular, to sustain gallbladder performance and avoid associated disorders, thus contributing to overall metabolic health enhancement(David C Goodman et al., 2011; N/A, 2020).

9.6.3. Risk Factors and How to Mitigate Them

Knowledge of the risk factors for gallbladder diseases is crucial for effective prevention and control strategies. The principal risk factors are obesity, physical inactivity, and excessive intake of saturated fats and cholesterol, which are risk factors for gallstones. These risk factors not only predispose a person to cholelithiasis but also compound any conditions that may have followed, such as inflammation and infection of the gallbladder. Furthermore, demographic factors such as age, gender, and ethnicity can influence susceptibility. For instance, studies have revealed that females are more susceptible to gallbladder disease than males, particularly at reproductive ages, with evidence of hormonal influences. Recognition of these risk factors enables medical professionals to target at-risk populations and implement lifestyle modifications and dietary interventions to reduce the risk of gallbladder disease, alongside general health benefits. Prevention of the risks facing gallbladder diseases involves a combination of changes in lifestyle, diet, and periodic health checks. Those at high risk can reduce their likelihood of gallstones and other gallbladder problems by keeping fit, exercising regularly, and having a balanced diet with high fiber and low fat intake. In addition, the inclusion of omega-3 fatty acids and antioxidants can aid in lowering inflammation and improving gallbladder health. Periodic health screening is also important, as it facilitates early observation and treatment of gallbladder disease to prevent it from worsening into major complications. By facilitating the promotion of awareness and education regarding the importance of such lifestyle changes, public health programs can be at the forefront of the reduction in risk and enhancement of the quality of life in those at risk of gallbladder disease. With individual lifestyle change, targeted public health intervention can facilitate greater community involvement in the prevention of gallbladder disease. Initiatives that operate to increase the awareness of the interrelationship between diet, obesity, and gallbladder health are important in reorienting social norms and attitudes regarding nutrition and exercise. For instance, local governments can promote healthy eating campaigns and create recreational spaces for physical activities. At the same time, physicians should encourage active community health programs that familiarize residents with the effects of fatty diets and the benefits of maintaining a healthy weight. Addressing all of these risk factors simultaneously, using both individual responsibility and social support, can reduce the disease burden of gallbladder disease, thereby promoting better health outcomes across different populations and geographic regions.

Test Your Knowledge

1. What is the importance of regular exercise?
2. What are the risk factors for gallbladder disease?

SUMMARY

In general, the gallbladder has a critical role in digestion in efficiently concentrating and storing bile utilized in emulsification and fat absorption. The complex interaction between dietary fats and the gallbladder underscores the importance of understanding dietary influences on gallbladder function. Research indicates that diet exerts a significant influence on modifying the chemical composition of bile, particularly by supplementing n-3 polyunsaturated fatty acids. Studies have shown that the fatty acids can alter biliary phospholipid composition, thus affecting cholesterol saturation and eventually lowering the risk of cholesterol crystal formation among gallstone patients. Modulation of bile composition through diet is a promising way to reduce the incidence of gallstones and improve gallbladder function, thereby enhancing the effectiveness of digestive processes (Abell et al., 1992). Further insight into gallbladder viscoelastic properties can also provide background to gallbladder pathology and physiology. The viscoelastic nature of the gallbladder wall can be an indicator of underlying disease, and examination with progressing technology may have important additional diagnostic potential. Techniques like vibroacoustography, for instance, capitalize on tissue mechanical properties to distinguish disease from health, with the potential for more precise determinations in the clinic. Such a strategy might even bridge the gap between subjective palpatory techniques and objective measurement, with potential applications in gallbladder disease diagnosis and treatment. Apparently, advances in research on the mechanical properties and viscoelasticity of gallbladder tissues have unprecedented implications on future clinical practice and biomedical research (Bajwa et al., 2018). Overall, the gallbladder's multifaceted function in human health extends beyond mere storage and release of bile and involves important interactions with dietary constituents as well as emerging diagnostic methods. As more research is conducted, the study of the role of dietary constituents influencing gallbladder function and the potential of emerging diagnostic technologies will be vital areas of study. The correlations of dietary fatty acids with bile composition not only recapitulate the gallbladder's flexibility but also its susceptibility to dietary choices. Eventually, an enhanced understanding of the gallbladder's highly complex physiology and how it interacts with diet and diagnostic methodologies will provide enhanced health outcomes and prevention strategies against gallbladder disease in the human population. Emphasizing this importance can lead to healthier habits and increased sensitization to the prevention and management of gallbladder pathology.

The gallbladder plays an essential role in human digestion as a bile reservoir and concentrator that is vital for emulsifying and absorbing dietary fats. Its position underneath the liver makes it possible for bile delivery to the small intestine, particularly at the time of fatty food introduction into the duodenum. An understanding of physiological processes underlying gallbladder function is an important key to an appreciation of its contribution to metabolic health. Several causes may influence bile composition and gallbladder motility, for instance, diet, hormonal stimulation, and the overall status of the hepatic system. Furthermore, the alarming rise in obesity rates has significance for gallbladder integrity, as an overweight body condition is a well-documented risk factor for the formation of gallstones and other gastrointestinal diseases, thus underlining the acute nature of the problem for public health due to obesity and metabolic syndromes (Kyrou and Weickert2010). Gallstone formation, which is a widespread disease condition associated with gallbladder dysfunction, is a multicausal process that is influenced by bile composition, gallbladder motility, and diet. It has been postulated that imbalances in bile salts, cholesterol, and bilirubin have a causative role in stone development, and as there is less physical activity, the risk also rises. Clinical presentation of gallstone disease can range from asymptomatic to life-threatening, with the requirement of surgical intervention, demonstrating the heterogeneous nature of gallbladder disorders. Health education campaigns to raise awareness regarding the health of the gallbladder and the impact of lifestyle determinants may decrease the incidence of such conditions. In this context, it is significant to understand the mechanisms of gallbladder function (AR et al., 2002). Furthermore, the implications of gallbladder disease are more extensive than the disease itself, extending into questions of health policy and preventive medicine. With the growing epidemic of obesity and its associated complications, including gallbladder disease, there is a greater need for comprehensive strategies directed toward lifestyle modification, dietary education, and routine health screening. Since obesity has come to be recognized as a global epidemic by the World Health Organization, tackling its effects on the health of the gallbladder holds the highest priority. Promotional programs for physical exercise, healthy diet, and frequent health screenings can serve as a revolutionary force in reducing the prevalence of gallbladder pathology across populations of diverse backgrounds, thereby enhancing public health (Kyrou and Weickert, 2010). The interaction between gallbladder health, obesity, and prevention is a common thread that deserves further study and focus in research and clinical practice.

KEY TERMS FROM THIS CHAPTER

- Bile
- Bilirubin
- Cholecystitis
- Cholecystokinin
- Cholestasis
- Cholesterol
- Cystic duct
- Fibronectin
- Gallbladder
- Gallstone disease
- Gallstones
- Metabolic dysfunction
- Mucosa
- Muscularis
- Phospholipids
- Serosa

CRITICAL THINKING QUESTIONS

1. **The primary function of the gallbladder is to:**
   a. Produce bile
   b. Store and concentrate bile
   c. Digest carbohydrates
   d. Absorb fats
2. **The gallbladder is located beneath which organ?**
   a. Stomach
   b. Liver
   c. Pancreas
   d. Spleen
3. **The bile duct that directly connects the gallbladder to the biliary system is the:**
   a. Cystic duct
   b. Common bile duct
   c. Hepatic duct
   d. Pancreatic duct
4. **Bile is released from the gallbladder in response to which hormone?**
   a. Insulin
   b. Glucagon
   c. Cholecystokinin (CCK)
   d. Gastrin
5. **The gallbladder releases bile into which part of the gastrointestinal tract?**
   a. Stomach
   b. Jejunum
   c. Duodenum
   d. Ileum

Short Answer Questions

1. What is the gallbladder?
2. Why is the gallbladder important in digestion?
3. Name the main parts of the gallbladder.
4. What is the function of the gallbladder?
5. What are common issues that affect the gallbladder?

Answer to Critical Thinking Questions

1. (b) 2. (b) 3. (a) 4. (c) 5. (c)

REFERENCES

1. Adamczyk, W., Andrén-Sandberg, A., Aronchick, C. A., Björnsson, O. G., Björnsson, O. G., Brand, S. J., Burhol, P. G., et al. (1992). The role of bile in the regulation of exocrine pancreatic secretion. https://core.ac.uk/download/12168721.pdf (accessed on 15th June 2025).
2. Allenspach, K., Day, M. J., Hall, E. J., et al. (2016). Bacterial cholangitis, cholecystitis, or both in dogs. https://core.ac.uk/download/36779319.pdf (accessed on 15th June 2025).
3. Alpini, G., Baiocchi, L., Ceci, L., Francis, H., Gaudio, E., Han, Y., Kennedy, L., et al. (2023). Gallstone and gallbladder disease: Biliary tract and cholangiopathies. https://core.ac.uk/download/599513205.pdf (accessed on 15th June 2025).
4. Alvaro, D., Bragazzi, M. C., Cardinale, V., et al. (2017). Cholangiocytes: Cell transplantation. https://core.ac.uk/download/98350472.pdf (accessed on 15th June 2025).
5. AR, A., Babiker, E. M., Becker, W. A., Benos, D. J., Boron, W. F., Brake, J., Cotterill, O. J., et al. (2002). Role of carbon dioxide and ion transport in the formation of sub-embryonic fluid by the blastoderm of the Japanese quail. https://core.ac.uk/download/7486.pdf (accessed on 15th June 2025).
6. Bajwa, N., Grundfest, W., Maccabi, A., et al. (2018). Quantitative characterization of viscoelastic behavior in tissue-mimicking phantoms and *ex vivo* animal tissues. https://core.ac.uk/download/323077188.pdf (accessed on 15th June 2025).
7. Berr, F., Holl, J., Jüngst, D., Fischer, S., Richter, W. O., Seifferth, B., & Paumgartner, G. (1992). Dietary N-3 polyunsaturated fatty acids decrease biliary cholesterol saturation in gallstone disease. *Hepatology, 16*(4), 960–967. https://doi.org/10.1002/hep.1840160418 (accessed on 15th June 2025).
8. Boffetta, P., Cadei, M., Carrasco-Avino, G., De Palma, G., Demartines, N., Gallegos Mendez, I. M., Gilberti, E., et al. (2023). Arsenic may be a carcinogenic determinant of a subset of gallbladder cancer: A pilot study. https://core.ac.uk/download/654535978.pdf (accessed on 15th June 2025).
9. Bogatyrev, S. R., Ismagilov, R. F., & Rolando, J. C. (2019). Self-reinoculation with fecal flora changes microbiota density and composition leading to an altered bile-acid profile in the mouse small intestine. https://core.ac.uk/download/287633428.pdf (accessed on 15th June 2025).
10. Bordoni, A., Dupont, D., Gille, D., et al. (2015). Understanding the gastrointestinal tract of the elderly to develop dietary solutions that prevent malnutrition. https://core.ac.uk/download/286575279.pdf (accessed on 15th June 2025).
11. Chen, B., Hu, H., Huang, A. H., et al. (2011). Covert laparoscopic cholecystectomy: A new minimally invasive technique. https://core.ac.uk/download/12533447.pdf (accessed on 15th June 2025).
12. Cicala, M., Guarino, M. P., Putignani, L., et al. (2016). Gastrointestinal neuromuscular apparatus: An underestimated target of gut microbiota. https://core.ac.uk/download/98336463.pdf (accessed on 15th June 2025).
13. Culkin, A., Madden, A. M., Smeeton, N., et al. (2024). Modified dietary fat intake for treatment of gallstone disease in people of any age. https://core.ac.uk/download/603244426.pdf (accessed on 15th June 2025).

14. Del Pozo, R., Jüngst, D., Lange, V., et al. (1994). Fibronectin in human gallbladder bile: Cholesterol pronucleating and/or mucin "link" protein? https://core.ac.uk/download/12167372.pdf (accessed on 15th June 2025).

15. Eggink, H. M., Groen, A. K., Hilbers, P. A. J., et al. (2018). *In silico* analysis identifies intestinal transit as a key determinant of systemic bile acid metabolism. https://core.ac.uk/download/pdf/159517246.pdf (accessed on 15th June 2025).

16. Evans, M., Guthrie, N., El-Khodor, B., Metzger, B., & Varadharaj, S. (2020). A whole-food-based health product (A-F Betafood®) improves gallbladder function in humans at risk of gallbladder insufficiency: A randomized, placebo-controlled clinical trial. *Nutrients, 12*. https://www.semanticscholar.org/paper/d057f0b35aaff96fbaa4e4dd6bd903ab1cc90f12 (accessed on 15th June 2025).

17. Fernández-Juárez, V., Riedinger, D. J., Gusmao, J. B., Delgado-Zambrano, L. F., Coll-García, G., Papazachariou, V., Herlemann, D. P. R., et al. (2024). Temperature, sediment resuspension, and salinity drive the prevalence of *Vibrio vulnificus* in the coastal Baltic Sea. *mBio, 15*. https://www.semanticscholar.org/paper/716fc3beec55fea4ebf940b976ac9fb99e5344dc (accessed on 15th June 2025).

18. Goodman, D. C., Fisher, E. S., Wennberg, J. E., Bynum, J. P. W., Barry, M. J., & Brownlee, S. (2011). Improving patient decision-making in health care. https://core.ac.uk/download/71358521.pdf (accessed on 15th June 2025).

19. Jia, Y., Lin, X., Liu, Y., et al. (2023). Bile dynamics within the biliary tract and microfluidic-based bile component detection: A review. http://arxiv.org/abs/2311.13117 (accessed on 15th June 2025).

20. Jüngst, D., Lang, T., von Ritter, C., & Paumgartner, G. (1991). Role of high total protein in gallbladder bile in the formation of cholesterol gallstones. *Gastroenterology, 100*(6), 1724–1729. https://doi.org/10.1016/0016-5085(91)90675-b (accessed on 15th June 2025).

21. Kang, J. Y., & Williamson, R. C. N. (1990). Cholecystitis without gallstones. https://core.ac.uk/download/pdf/8088156.pdf (accessed on 15th June 2025).

22. Kim, I. B., Joo, K., Song, C. H., & Rhyu, I. (2024). A brief review of anatomy education in Korea, encompassing its past, present, and future direction. *Journal of Korean Medical Science, 39*. https://www.semanticscholar.org/paper/c12521e1d8446126c21e5fba8cf48569cb5ec7e0 (accessed on 15th June 2025).

23. Kyrou, I., & Weickert, M. O. (2010). Clinical problems caused by obesity. https://core.ac.uk/download/46324.pdf (accessed on 15th June 2025).

24. Ligresti, D., Kuo, Y., Baraldo, S., Chavan, R., Keane, M., Seleem, S., & Seo, D. (2019). EUS anatomy of the pancreatobiliary system in a swine model: The WISE experience. *Endoscopic Ultrasound, 8*, 249–254. https://www.semanticscholar.org/paper/d90cd758c8d257375092c0f1e1362468634f9266 (accessed on 15th June 2025).

25. Liu, M., Portincasa, P., Tso, P., Wang, D. Q. H., & Wang, H. H. (2020). An update on the lithogenic mechanisms of cholecystokinin A receptor (Cckar), an important gallstone gene for lith13. https://core.ac.uk/download/541254019.pdf (accessed on 15th June 2025).

26. Lwande, O., Obanda, V., Lindström, A., Ahlm, C., Evander, M., Näslund, J., & Bucht, G. (2020). Globe-trotting *Aedes aegypti* and *Aedes albopictus*: Risk factors for arbovirus pandemics.

Vector Borne and Zoonotic Diseases, 20, 71–81. https://www.semanticscholar.org/paper/59b470f3f624c3cd9b6cdf97568a32bdb4a2c446 (accessed on 15th June 2025).

27. Mansura, F., Al Mamun, K. A., Al Faisal, A., Khatun, M., & Suchi, H. A. (2024). Morphological parameters of gallbladder are correlated with age. *Medicine Today*. https://www.semanticscholar.org/paper/384bcdaff4eb9b40a54f12fd91751f3d0bdb3ba6 (accessed on 15th June 2025).
28. N/A. (1989). *Focal Spot, Summer 1989*. https://core.ac.uk/download/129069275.pdf (accessed on 15th June 2025).
29. N/A. (2006). *Focal Spot, Spring 2006*. https://core.ac.uk/download/129069350.pdf (accessed on 15th June 2025).
30. N/A. (2007). *Focal Spot, Winter 2006/2007*. https://core.ac.uk/download/129069354.pdf (accessed on 15th June 2025).
31. N/A. (2010). *Focal Spot, Winter 2009/2010*. https://core.ac.uk/download/129069377.pdf (accessed on 15th June 2025).
32. N/A. (2020). *Physical Activity Is Beneficial for Gallbladder Disease*. https://core.ac.uk/download/287852365.pdf (accessed on 15th June 2025).
33. N/A. (2021). *Dyspepsia*. https://core.ac.uk/download/478118073.pdf (accessed on 15th June 2025).
34. Parnell, L., McCaffrey, K. S., Brooks, A. W., Smith, C. E., Lai, C., Christensen, J., Wiley, C. D., et al. (2023). Rate-limiting enzymes in cardiometabolic health and aging in humans. *Lifestyle Genomics, 16*, 124–138. https://www.semanticscholar.org/paper/a394e12611809f449fbacbd199909c25a2d529a7 (accessed on 15th June 2025).
35. Scharl, A., Aronchick, C. A., Bjornsson, O. G., Bondesen, S., Burhol, P. G., Burhol, P. G., Burhol, P. G., et al. (1990). Effect of intraduodenal bile and Na-taurodeoxycholate on exocrine pancreatic secretion and on plasma levels of secretin, pancreatic polypeptide, and gastrin in man. https://core.ac.uk/download/12168700.pdf (accessed on 15th June 2025).
36. Shekhar, H., & Pradhan, V. (2023). Ultrasonographic evaluation of gallbladder volume and its relation with autonomic neuropathy in diabetic patients of Jharkhand. *Indian Journal of Applied Research*. https://www.semanticscholar.org/paper/ad4b28fba6698415e0a93b29961584d555fd01ca (accessed on 15th June 2025).
37. Tanna, K., & Khatri, S. M. (2024). Correlation between perceived stress and blood pressure among adults. *International Journal of Recent Innovations in Medicine and Clinical Research*. https://www.semanticscholar.org/paper/3fd956c0f1c01cb56069ab2e29ec6621ca1df274 (accessed on 15th June 2025).
38. Thomas, V. (2020). Comparisons of celiac disease and non-celiac gluten sensitivity. https://core.ac.uk/download/322851056.pdf (accessed on 15th June 2025).
39. van Dam, D. A., de Lange-de Klerk, E. S. M., Tuynman, J. B., Schoonmade, L. J., Ankersmit, M., Vlek, S. L., Rubinstein, S. M., et al. (2016). Biliary tract visualization using near-infrared imaging with indocyanine green during laparoscopic cholecystectomy: Results of a systematic review. https://core.ac.uk/download/pdf/81728600.pdf (accessed on 15th June 2025).

URINARY SYSTEM

10

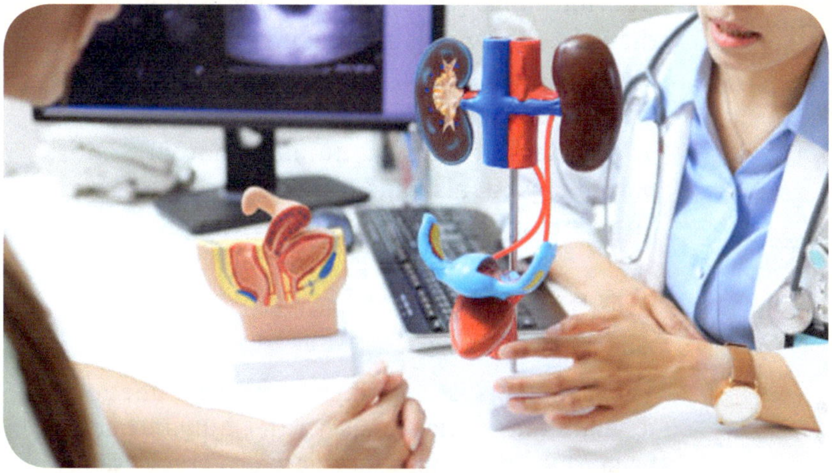

LEARNING OBJECTIVES

After studying this chapter, you will be able to:

1. Understand the anatomy of the urinary system
2. Describe the functions of the urinary system
3. Describe the urine formation process
4. Understand the regulation of urine production
5. Explain the common disorders of the urinary system
6. Describe the diagnostic techniques for the urinary system

Introduction

The urinary system is a vital component of human physiology, charged with maintaining fluid and electrolyte balance, expelling waste products, and supporting homeostasis. The kidneys, ureters, bladder, and urethra comprise this complex system, tasked with the role of filtering blood and generating urine as a means of expelling toxins while maintaining the body's internal equilibrium. The kidneys, traditionally defined as cleansing organs, employ sophisticated mechanisms to dispose of waste while simultaneously reabsorbing essential nutrients and water. This delicate ballet is important not just to the health of the individual but also to the proper functioning of other systems of the body. Thus, an understanding of urinary system anatomy and physiology is critical in making overall body health assessments and diagnosing a variety of clinical conditions that may arise due to its failure (Tyukavin et al., 2025). Historically, examination of the urinary system can be traced back to medical pioneers, among them Hippocrates, who played an essential role in our understanding of renal physiology. His findings made fundamental contributions to the understanding of the anatomy of the kidneys and the urinary flow ways, opening the way for later nephrology research. Principles outlined in his teaching are valid today in medical texts and practice too, and demonstrate the significance of studying anatomy in comprehending urinary tract diseases. Moreover, Hippocrates' discrimination of various urinary pathologies and the corresponding treatments, such as the diagnosis of bladder stone and kidney pathology, illustrates the early recognition of complex urinary pathologies (Hashim et al., 2024).

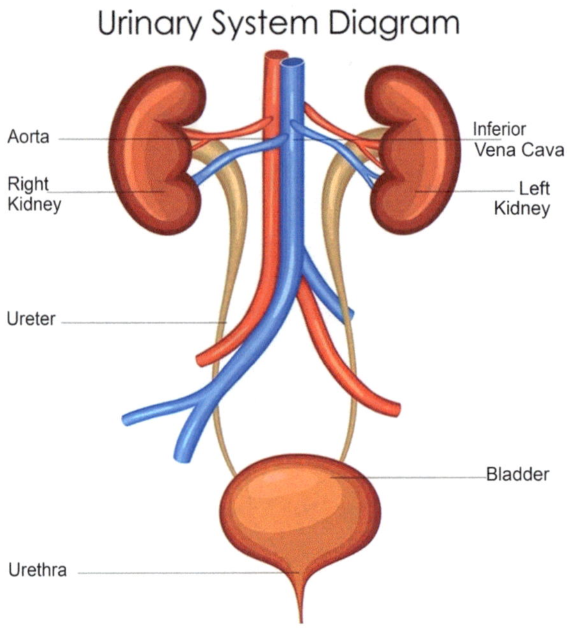

Figure 10.1. Urinary system diagram.

Source: https://d2jx2rerrg6sh3.cloudfront.net/image-handler/ts/20180902092316/ri/673/picture/2018/9/shutterstock_638539345.jpg

With this background, it is easy to see how beneficial an examination of today's developments in urinary health can be. In contemporary times, the urinary system has a multifunctional role going beyond simple waste elimination, influencing many body functions and overall well-being. Advances in medical technology and research have established new fields of knowledge in the complexity of renal functioning and its interfacing with other body systems. Nephrology as a subspecialty has grown significantly, with advances in diagnosis and treatment that are compatible with a wide range of renal diseases and disorders. Critical awareness of the urinary system's significance stimulates a more in-depth examination of diseases such as chronic kidney disease, urinary tract infections (UTIs), and bladder dysfunctions that are becoming increasingly common in modern populations. A careful analysis of the urinary system, therefore, not only enriches our understanding of human anatomy and physiology but also underscores its pivotal role in maintaining health and preventing illness.

Importance of the Urinary System in Human Health

The urinary system plays a crucial function to maintain homeostasis in the human body, primarily through fluid and electrolyte regulation. By blood filtration and urine excretion, the kidneys remove excessive electrolytes, urea, and other undesirable products from the blood and, thus, avoid the buildup of harmful materials. This position is particularly vital in the context of antimicrobial resistance (AMR), with the kidneys being involved in the systemic distribution and clearance of antibiotics, dysregulation of which would very likely lead to increased rates of resistance. In light of recent evidence suggesting that disturbances in kidney function would likely exacerbate the effects of AMR, research into the ways in which variations in renal function might affect infection susceptibility and overall health outcomes is therefore crucial. Therefore, the effectiveness of the urinary system has a direct bearing not only on a person's health but also on global public health initiatives against AMR (Murray et al., 2022). In addition to waste removal, the urinary system is important in regulating blood pressure and acid-base balance. The kidneys respond to changes in blood pressure by adjusting the rate of excretion or reabsorption of fluid and thus keeping an ideal internal environment. This process is sustained by the renin-angiotensin-aldosterone system and has a marked effect on systemic blood pressure. Kidney dysfunction, as in chronic kidney disease or acute renal failure, can have a marked cardiovascular impact, including hypertension and increased risk of heart disease. Moreover, renal handling of acids and bases is essential to maintaining blood pH within a narrow range. Its disturbance causes metabolic acidosis or alkalosis with repercussions on patient outcomes for other clinical syndromes. Renal physiology offers insights into the clinical practices that avoid their occurrence (Biggins et al., 2021).

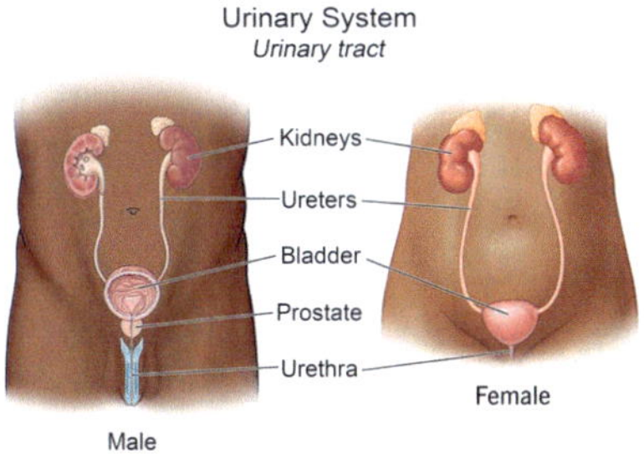

Figure 10.2. Your urinary system is your body's filtering system and produces your pee. The organs of the urinary system include kidneys, ureters, bladder and urethra.

Source: https://my.clevelandclinic.org/-/scassets/images/org/health/articles/21197-urinary-systems

The urinary system also plays a dominant role in the body's adaptation to metabolic needs and environmental stimuli. Beyond the excretion of wastes and fluid homeostasis, kidneys also participate in the secretion of required hormones, such as erythropoietin, which stimulates red blood cell formation in response to insufficient oxygen. This function calls attention to the urinary system's participation in hematopoiesis and overall oxygen delivery to tissues, critical to the upkeep of body functions. Moreover, the kidneys contribute to calcium homeostasis via their activation of vitamin D, impacting bone metabolism and health. When renal function is lost, cascading effects will extend through several body systems as the interdependence of physiological processes is illustrated. Thus, advances in understanding the significance of the urinary system not only enhance patient care but also emphasize preventive health steps to ensure renal function (Biggins et al., 2021).

10.1. Anatomy of the Urinary System

Learning Outcome

1. Describe the major organs of the urinary system
2. Understand the location and structure of the kidneys
3. Understand the role of the urinary system in excretion

The anatomy of the urinary system is elegantly described to provide the essential functions of waste elimination, fluid balance, and electrolyte regulation. The kidneys are the key organs involved in the process of filtration. Each kidney contains approximately one million nephrons, the functional units that filter blood, eliminate waste products, and regulate water and electrolyte balance. This filtration process begins when blood is transported through the renal arteries into the kidneys and through the nephrons glomerulus where water and solutes are filtered to exit, and larger molecules like proteins and blood cells are left behind. The intricately designed anatomy of the kidneys provides support for the efficiency of the urinary system, ensuring homeostasis through the creation and constitution of urine, which matches the body's metabolic state and hydration level. The urinary system further includes a network of tubular structures: the ureters, bladder, and urethra. Once formed, urine travels through the ureters, hollow tubes connecting the kidneys to the bladder, where it is temporarily stored. The bladder's muscular walls allow it to expand as it fills and contract during urination, facilitating the expulsion of urine through the urethra. This expulsion process is facilitated by an advanced coordination of sphincter muscles that provide continence and control the passage of urine. Notably, pathological conditions such as bladder-ureteral reflux have the ability to disrupt this function and result in complications that underscore the importance of the anti-reflux mechanism of the vesicoureteral segment.

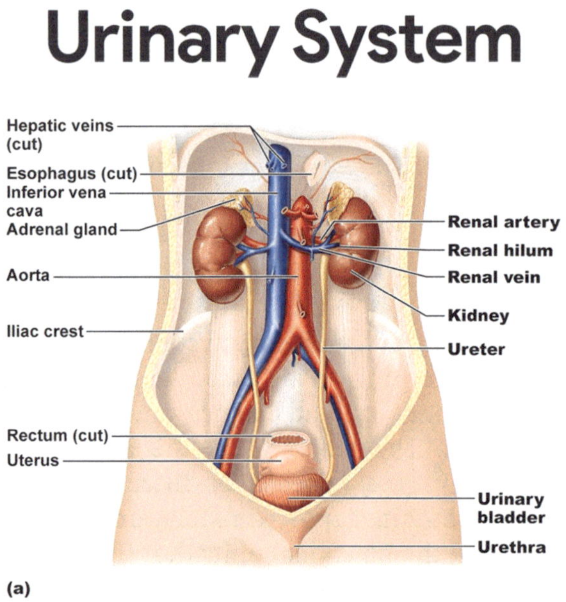

Figure 10.3. Anatomy of the urinary system.

Source: https://nurseslabs.com/wp-content/uploads/2017/04/Urinary-System-Urinary-System-Anatomy-and-Physiology.png

Understanding of such anatomical relationships is critical when treating and diagnosing conditions of the urinary tract, and therefore interventions are effective and appropriate for the maintenance of urinary health. Developments in imaging technology during the last decade or so, such as magnetic resonance imaging (MRI) and computed tomography angiography (CTA), have enriched our understanding regarding the anatomy of the urinary tracts. Three-dimensional model reconstruction from such imaging data sets provides precise anatomical visualization for understanding the spatial relationships of the urinary organs. MRI data studies, for instance, have revealed significant geometric parameters of the bladder and urethra that contribute to our knowledge of functional variation across populations. These meticulous anatomical aspects not only dictate clinical practice but also enhance surgical planning, especially in pediatric urology, where congenital malformations may present unique challenges. Overall, the thorough understanding of urinary anatomy forms the basis of refining diagnostic, therapeutic, and surgical techniques in urological medicine, and thereby enhancing patient care and results.

10.1.1. Major Organs Involved: Kidneys, Ureters, Bladder, Urethra

The kidneys are the important filtration organs of the urinary apparatus, carrying out the essential duty of attaining homeostasis within the human organism. Anatomically, each kidney is a bean-shaped organ and retroperitoneal in location, with the primary function of filtering the blood to remove waste products and excess substances. It is not merely an excretion of toxins but also electrolyte balance, blood volume, and pH level in the organism. The intricate structure of the nephron, the body's functional unit in the kidneys, facilitates this filtering process through glomerular filtration, tubular reabsorption, and secretion. Any dysfunction of the kidneys can lead to serious metabolic derangement, demonstrating the dominant role these organs play in overall well-being. Understanding the complexity of kidney function is an important introduction to effective handling of kidney diseases, underscoring their vital position in the urogenital system that encompasses the key organs of the ureters, bladder, and the urethra, underscoring the interlinkage of these factors (Wang et al., 2025). Urine is drained through the ureters from filtration by the kidneys, a pair of muscular tubes that connect each of the kidneys to the urinary bladder. The ureters play a crucial role in moving urine along peristaltic waves, a wavelike constriction that propels urine downward, preventing reverse flow. This is significant in the provision of a one-way system so waste products are not transported back to the kidney. The transitional epithelium covers the ureters so they may stretch with changing quantities of urine. Infection or obstruction in the ureters can lead to serious complications, looking at the bigger picture of kidney and urinary tract function. As conduits for the conduction of urine, the ureters emphasize the interactive process between the kidneys and the bladder and reinforce the necessity of thinking about these organs as part of the greater scheme of the urinary system (Kutia et al., 2023). The urinary bladder is a temporary reservoir for urine before it is eliminated from the body. It is a muscular, saccular organ with unparalleled elastic properties, accepting varying volumes of urine while serving as an essential structure for preserving urinary continence. Micturition is a coordinated function between the bladder and urethra that is controlled by voluntary and involuntary mechanisms. The wall of the bladder is composed of smooth muscle fibers referred to as detrusor muscles, which contract when urinating in order to push the urine out of the body through the urethra. The internal and external sphincters also regulate the flow of urine, such that the act of urination can be regulated consciously. Bladder failure can cause incontinence or retention of urine, which can significantly impact the quality of a person's life. Its proper functioning is necessary because it works harmoniously with the kidneys, ureters, and urethra, thus reflecting the urinary system's overall complexity (Wang et al., 2025).

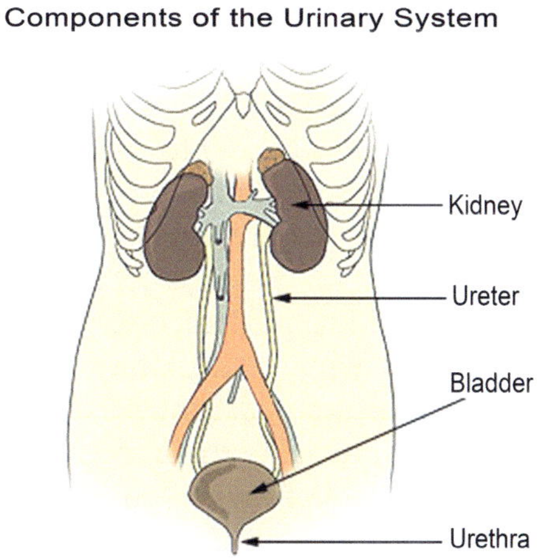

Figure 10.4. Components of the Urinary system: Here are the major organs of the renal system.

Source: https://s3-us-west-2.amazonaws.com/courses-images/wp-content/uploads/sites/1940/2017/05/31172635/illu-urinary-system.jpeg

10.1.2. Location and Structure of the Kidneys

The kidneys, key organs of the human urinary system, are located retroperitoneally, pressed against the dorsal body wall. This allows them to carry out their filtering functions under protection provided by layers of fat and connective tissue. Each kidney is approximately fist-sized, elliptical in shape, and possesses a discernible structural plan enveloped by a fibrous capsule. The renal cortex, beneath the capsule, is composed of nephrons, the functional units that process blood. The medulla, the inner structure, is made up of renal pyramids, which have collecting ducts that transport urine. The renal pelvis, a widening of the ureter, transports urine to the bladder. The intricate organization of such structures underscores the kidneys' role in fluid and waste elimination, which demonstrates their critical roles in the homeostasis of the human body. At the structural level, the kidneys consist of a unique combination of cortical and medullary areas that support their filtering processes. The renal cortex consists of nephron structures, including glomeruli, where blood filtration begins. This area is critical to the regulation of electrolytes and blood pressure by the renin-angiotensin-aldosterone system. The renal medulla also includes the Loop of Henle and collecting ducts that concentrate urine by reabsorbing water and sodium. The kidney also has a complex vascular organization with afferent and efferent arterioles that tightly regulate blood flow. The presence of glomerular capillaries confirms the mechanism of filtration, demonstrating the complexity of the kidneys in the management of wastes and volumes of fluid in the blood. Each part's individual structure plays a unique function, ensuring proper renal operation essential to wellness as a whole. The kidneys also possess noteworthy anatomical variation, particularly regarding blood supply and innervation. Supplied predominantly by the renal arteries and arising from the aorta in the abdominal region, each kidney receives a robust blood supply to facilitate its filtration function. Moreover, venous blood is evacuated by the renal veins into the inferior vena cava. A tight relationship between the vascular and nephron structures is crucial for the proper functioning of the kidneys. Further, the kidneys are innervated by sympathetic fibers of the renal plexus, which modulate renal blood flow and excretion rate accordingly. Because of the kidneys' central roles in many physiological phenomena, knowledge of these positional and structural factors is significant in realizing their fundamental roles in the urinary system as well as general human health. Significance is highlighted in clinical cases where structural alterations—like material migration—can cause complications, highlighting the requirement of constant research and knowledge (Baulina et al., 2025; Tsyhykalo and Vladychenko, 2024).

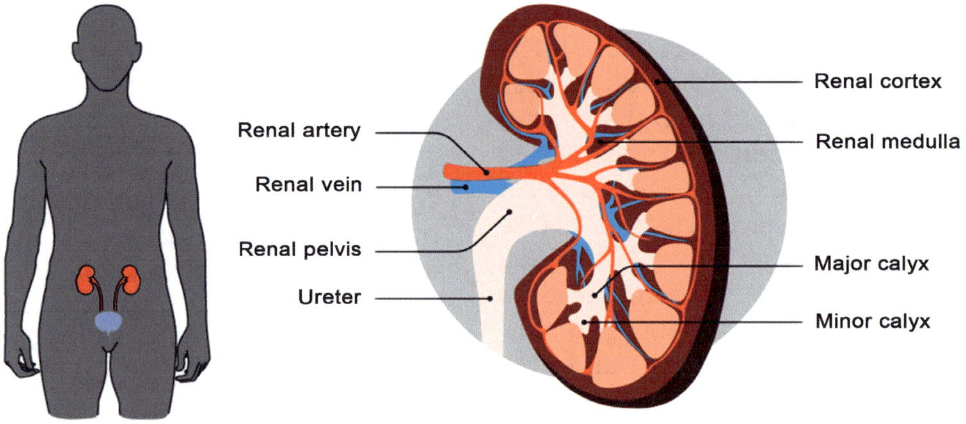

Figure 10.5. Location and anatomy of the kidneys.

Source: https://i0.wp.com/post.medicalnewstoday.com/wp-content/uploads/sites/3/2021/11/1450092-Where-Are-the-Kidneys-Located-What-Do-They-Do-What-Do-They-Look-Like_Header_1296x728-1024x575.png?w=1155&h=1528

10.1.3. Role of the Urinary System in Excretion

Excretion is mainly carried out by the urinary system, which is a regulatory system as well as a major system for removing waste and excess material from the body. Made up of the kidneys, the ureters, the bladder, and the urethra, the urinary system, with exact precision, filters blood to produce urine to maintain homeostasis. The kidneys, as the primary organs of filtration, utilize nephrons to eliminate toxins, metabolic waste products, and excess ions while conserving essential nutrients and water. The dual roles of excretion and conservation are essential to fluid balance, electrolyte, and blood pressure control. The urinary system also maintains acid-base balance, again highlighting the function of the urinary system in metabolism. The general knowledge of the physiology of the urinary system describes how it functions, not just as an organ of excretion but also as part of the whole physiology of humans (Sharma et al., 2025). Central to effective excretion of waste is the mechanism of urine production by way of three primary processes: filtration, reabsorption, and secretion. At the filtration phase, blood passes through the nephron glomeruli, where water, ions, and small molecules are removed from larger proteins and cells. Afterwards, in reabsorption, essential nutrients and water are taken up from the filtrate into the bloodstream. This is precisely regulated so that the body remains in balance and does not become dehydrated or experience electrolyte imbalances. Finally, secretion involves active transport of wastes other than urea from the blood into renal tubules for excretion. The combined action of these mechanisms enables the urinary system to excrete toxic substances efficiently while maintaining vital homeostatic values (Wang et al., 2025). Besides the mere elimination of wastes, the urinary system carries significant meaning for overall well-being. Functional abnormalities in urinary function can significantly impact body systems, with the possibility of leading to pathological processes. For instance, disturbances in urine production can result in the accumulation of toxic products and cause problems within the body. Ayurveda emphasizes the overall understanding of the urinary system as a whole, highlighting its anatomical and physiological significance in maintaining human health. According to Ayurveda principles, the Mutravaha Samsthana, or the excretory system, is part of grasping excretion-related illness and emphasizes the interdependence of various body systems. Thus, not only does the urinary system facilitate the elimination of waste, which is a necessity, but it also reflects on the health condition of an individual through variations in the composition and amount of urine (Sharma et al., 2025).

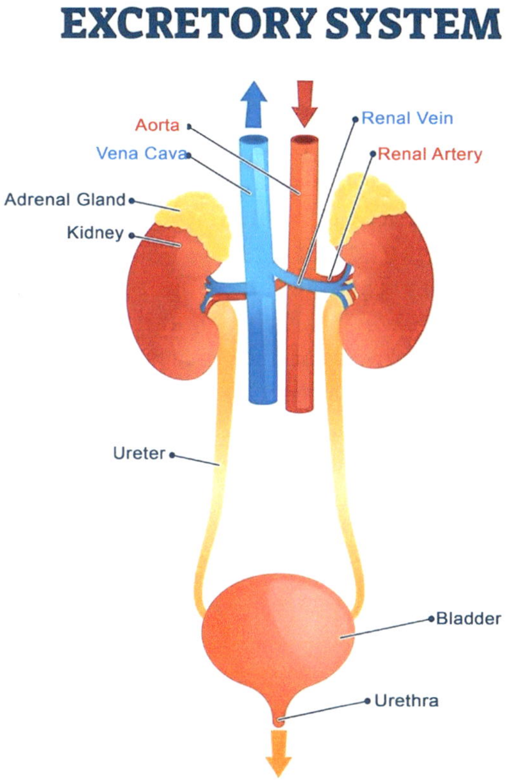

Figure 10.6. Excretory system.

Source: https://images.myacare.com/uploads/CKEditorImages/31903530c8e749568b43d0a7ca70feb7.webp

Test Your Knowledge

1. What are the 4 organs of the urinary system?
2. What is the role of the urinary system in excretion?

10.2. Functions of the Urinary System

Learning Outcome

1. Describe the filtration of blood and waste removal
2. Understand the regulation of electrolyte balance
3. Discuss the maintenance of fluid balance and blood pressure

The urinary system carries out several significant functions crucial to the maintenance of homeostasis and general human health. Essentially, it is responsible for the filtration and elimination of waste products from the blood. This is a primary function aimed at preventing the accumulation of harmful substances. The principal organs of the urinary system are the kidneys. They purify blood in an effort to rid the body of excess salts, urea, and creatinine, which are the end products of metabolism and the breakdown of proteins. In the regulation of blood volume and fluid composition, the urinary system plays a vital role in maintaining electrolyte balance. It also assists in acid-base homeostasis by way of the excretion of hydrogen ions and bicarbonate production, maintaining appropriate pH levels of the blood and metabolic functions smoothly. Regulation of blood pressure and fluid balance is another fundamental function of the urinary system. The kidneys regulate these parameters through the renin-angiotensin-aldosterone system (RAAS), which is responsive to alterations in blood volume and sodium. When renin is released during a drop in blood pressure, a cascade is initiated that ultimately raises blood pressure by maintaining sodium and water in the body. This not only makes urine more concentrated but also provides sufficient blood flow to the vital organs. In addition, the urinary system assists in maintaining fluid balance through altering urine output in accordance with hydration levels, and this is particularly crucial during dehydration or excessive fluid intake. Therefore, the different roles of the urinary system in managing blood pressure and fluid flow underscore the pivotal role of the system within human physiology. Barring waste elimination and fluid equilibrium, the urinary tract also supports overall well-being through its interaction with the human microbiome. It has been proven in recent research that the urinary tract harbors an extraordinarily rich microbiota community whose role is pivotal regarding urinary conditions and disease susceptibility. Disruption of this microbiome can lead to a number of urological diseases, including UTIs (Aggarwal et al., 2022). Here, the urinary system not only performs its classic excretory functions but also plays a role in immunological responses and protective mechanisms against infection. Moreover, the materials filtered by the kidneys can influence systemic health, e.g., the impact of materials like caffeine on urinary function, which can lead to a change in diuresis patterns and influence total hydration status (Rodak et al., 2021). Therefore, the urinary system maintains a complex interplay of functions that cumulatively safeguard systemic well-being as well as biological homeostasis.

10.2.1. Filtration of Blood and Waste Removal

Excretion of waste and purification of blood are vital functions of the urinary system, primarily performed by the kidneys. The retroperitoneal cavity is filled by the kidneys, which always work to gain homeostasis by purifying the blood and regulating the fluid, electrolytes, and waste products. The renal arteries bring blood to the kidneys, where it is purified within the nephrons, the functional units of the kidneys. Within the nephron, that is, within the glomerulus, blood plasma is filtered to allow small molecules to pass through, but the larger proteins and cells are left behind. The sophisticated process of filtration ensures that metabolic waste products such as urea, creatinine, and uric acid are efficiently removed from circulation in order to prevent toxicity as well as maintain overall health. Besides, regulation of blood volume and pressure through fluid balance is intimately connected with this process of filtration, illustrating the kidneys' pivotal role in physiological homeostasis. Once the process of filtration is over, the kidneys reabsorb essential materials back into circulation and concentrate waste materials to form urine, which is subsequently excreted from the body. In the renal tubules, there are distinctive segments to reabsorb nutrients such as glucose, amino acids, and certain ions, indicating a selective process that preserves useful substances. The excretion of hydrogen ions and other metabolites in the tubular fluid also acts to enhance the renal system's function in acid-base balance. The final product, waste and excess material, is transported through the ureters to the bladder for storage before it is excreted. Such complex interaction between filtration, reabsorption, and secretion brings out the complexity of the urinary system, demonstrating its critical function in waste elimination and fluid homeostasis in the organism. The discovery of the molecular mechanisms of renal physiology has significant implications in diagnostics and therapeutics. Abundant evidence indicates that exosomes, nanoscale vesicles containing a heterogeneous cargo of molecules, are involved in intercellular communication and can affect kidney function and disease. Exosomes can be used as informative biomarkers for a wide range of kidney diseases that give insight into the state and development of the disease. Their ability to deliver molecular messages between cells can also affect renal responses to injury and inflammation. Specifically, as researchers venture deeper into exosomal activity processes in renal physiology, efficient illumination of these processes could lead to new treatment approaches and improved control of kidney conditions. Through the integration of exosome research with traditional renal physiology, the future of kidney disease control may be brighter, with therapeutic options for improved patient outcomes (Zhang et al., 2019; Manyi-Loh et al., 2018).

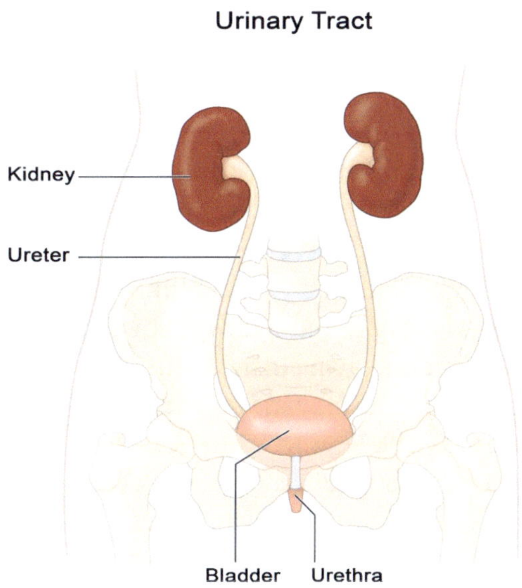

Figure 10.7. You have two kidneys that filter your blood, removing wastes and extra water to make urine.

Source: https://www.niddk.nih.gov/-/media/Images/Health-Information/Kidney/B1Image-01A--Urinary-TrackMainFINALLabels.jpg

10.2.2. Regulation of Electrolyte Balance

Regulation of electrolyte balance is a vital function of the urinary system, largely mediated through the kidneys. The kidneys cleanse blood and allow for selective excretion and reabsorption of electrolytes such as sodium, potassium, calcium, and chloride. This active process not only maintains physiological homeostasis but also contributes importantly to blood pressure and fluid balance regulation. Kidneys adapt to changes in physical and dietary requirements by adjusting electrolyte levels accordingly to maintain the internal body environment as stable. Deviation from normal electrolyte balance will lead to severe body complications, including arrhythmias, muscle weakness, and neurological malfunction, so it is crucial that renal function intervenes in this adjustment (Sarma et al., 2021).

Urinary prokallikrein is a critical component in the regulation of water and electrolyte homeostasis in the human body. The protein controls blood pressure and volume by regulating the renin-angiotensin-aldosterone system, which, in turn, regulates sodium reabsorption and potassium excretion. The biochemical properties of urinary prokallikrein, such as molecular weight and hydrophobicity, are vital to the function, giving insights into how kidney-secreted proteins influence electrolyte regulation (Gun et al., 2017). Having gained knowledge of the properties of urinary prokallikrein and its action under varying physiological conditions, researchers are in a better position to understand the mechanism of electrolyte balance and its relationship with the overall condition of the kidneys, leading to more efficient therapeutic strategies in their pathologies. In addition, the kidneys are highly versatile, employing various regulatory mechanisms to maintain electrolyte homeostasis.

Hormonal signals, such as aldosterone from the adrenal cortex, stimulate sodium reabsorption but increase potassium secretion in the distal nephron. Antidiuretic hormone (ADH) also controls water reabsorption and, in turn, influences electrolyte composition. Such hormonal interactions illustrate the intricate feedback regulation responsible for maintaining electrolyte homeostasis under varying needs. Anomalies in these processes may lead to pathologies such as hyponatremia or hyperkalemia, underscoring the need for normal kidney function to maintain electrolyte balance. Hence, understanding control of electrolyte balance is crucial for preventive treatment and regulation of renal disease (Sarma et al., 2021).

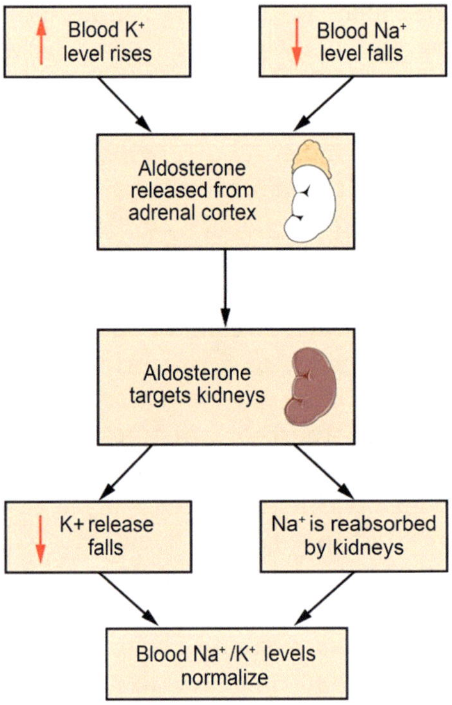

Figure 10.8. Aldosterone, which is released by the adrenal gland, facilitates the reabsorption of Na+ and thus the reabsorption of water.

Source: https://s3-us-west-2.amazonaws.com/courses-images/wp-content/uploads/sites/3148/2018/03/29184557/2711_Aldosterone_Feedback_Loop-01.jpg

10.2.3. Maintenance of Fluid Balance and Blood Pressure

Fluid balance and blood pressure are vital aspects of the function of the urinary system; hence, they directly contribute to homeostasis in the body. The kidneys are a key part of filtering the blood and regulating the level of fluids in the body via various processes like glomerular filtration and tubular reabsorption. By controlling the amount lost in urine, the kidneys help to maintain blood pressure within an optimal level. Importantly, with decreasing blood volume or dehydration, the kidneys move to conserve water, a function of gigantic importance in maintaining blood pressure and perfusion of vital organs. This regulatory function is not only essential for fluid balance but also for overall health, since disturbance leads to complications such as hypertension and renal disease, and emphasizes the significant interrelationship between these physiological mechanisms. Fluid balance is in close association with the body's electrolytes, which are responsible for maintaining osmotic pressure and thus blood pressure. The kidneys regulate the concentration of sodium, potassium, and other electrolytes that play a significant role in hydrostatic and osmotic pressures to affect fluid movement through cell membranes. For instance, sodium retention leads to water retention, increases blood volume, and ultimately increases blood pressure. Conversely, excess sodium loss decreases blood volume and thus reduces blood pressure. This dynamic interaction between fluid regulation and electrolyte control underscores the urinary system's importance to cardiovascular health. Moreover, any impairment of renal function, whether by disease or injury, can greatly destabilize this system. These processes are thus of critical importance in the development of successful treatments for fluid imbalance disorders and hypertension, according to recent studies (Hou et al., 2022). Aside from renal function, the general impact of fluid dynamics extends to broader physiological functions and microbial interactions. The Starling principle model of fluid exchange across capillary membranes has been expanded to incorporate the intricate roles of the endothelial surface layer and its influences on vascular permeability and blood pressure (Ding et al., 2017). Moreover, alterations in the gut microbiome can also affect fluid balance and blood pressure through mechanisms such as inflammation and immune modulation. Dysbiosis or disruption in the gut microbiota has been linked with myriad diseases, including those that affect cardiovascular health. This exchange illustrates how the process of maintaining fluid balance is not a simple renal function but one that is part of a holistic system interacting with other bodily processes and external sources, reflecting the intricacy of homeostasis in the human body.

Test Your Knowledge

1. What filters the blood and removes waste?
2. What is the regulation of electrolyte balance?

10.3. Urine Formation Process

Learning Outcome

1. Understand the process of glomerular filtration
2. Describe the process of tubular reabsorption
3. Know the process of tubular secretion

The mechanism of urine generation in human beings is a complex physiological process that occurs primarily in the nephron, the functional and structural unit of the kidney. The mechanism involves three extremely crucial phases: filtration, reabsorption, and secretion. Blood enters the glomerulus first, where filtration by the glomerular membrane occurs, allowing water, ions, and a few molecules to pass into the Bowman's capsule. This filtrate development is important because it sets the stage for subsequent processes of reabsorption and secretion that further alter the original urine. Through the renal tubules, the substances required to maintain homeostasis, such as glucose and some ions, are reabsorbed from the filtrate into the blood and have a significant impact on the composition and volume of the final urine. Following initial filtration, reabsorption occurs primarily in the proximal convoluted tubule and extends to the loop of Henle, the distal convoluted tubule, and the collecting duct. Reabsorption is meant to keep essential nutrients and electrolytes while also regulating water balance. It's interesting to mention that the hormone aldosterone plays a vital role at this point by telling the nephron to reabsorb sodium, therefore setting water retention and blood pressure control. Changes in reabsorption can cause a myriad of health conditions, highlighting the fine balance the urinary system must achieve. Moreover, as noted in recent research, aspects like the extent of ureteral obstruction may influence the composition of urine. For instance, significant differences in urine parameters, including citrate and pH, have been observed in obstructive condition research, pointing out the complexity of urine formation and susceptibility to physiological changes (Demirhan et al., 2025). Secretion, which helps actively remove substances from blood into the renal tubules, is the final phase of urine formation. This function allows the body to eliminate many of its waste products, including urea, creatinine, and certain drugs, thus playing a crucial part in detoxification. Furthermore, the secretory process is selectively regulated to permit the body's homeostasis to be maintained. For example, potassium ions are secreted in relation to diet and blood levels, a change that is extremely significant for cardiac and neurological function. As illustrated by recent research, dysregulation of these processes can lead to excess toxin buildup, potentially leading to the creation of antibiotic-resistant infections, such as those caused by Klebsiella pneumoniae in UTIs (Farag et al., 2025). Together, the intricate interplay of filtration, reabsorption, and secretion characterizes a highly sophisticated urine formation process essential to overall health and well-being.

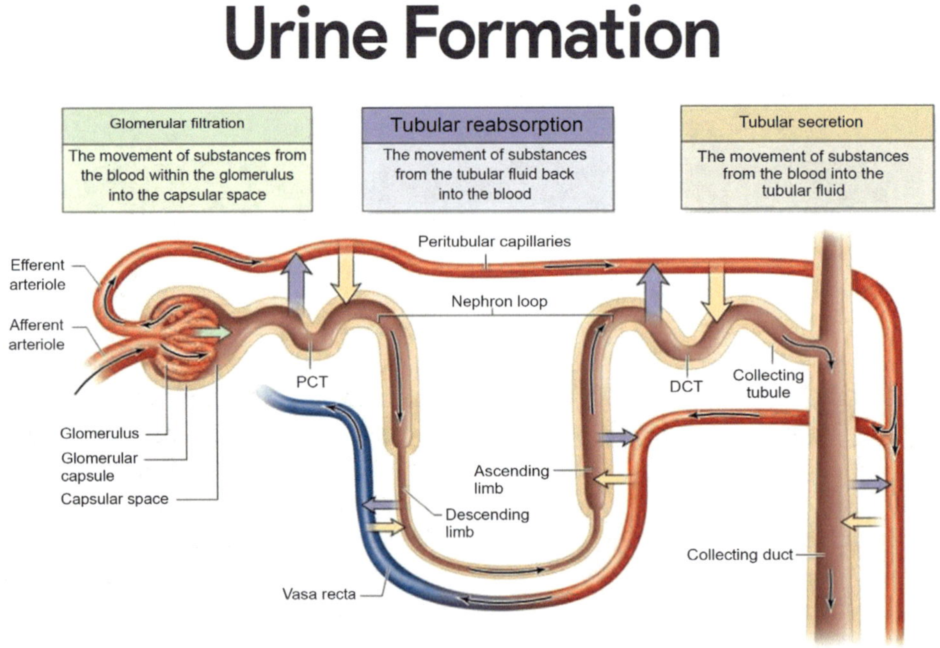

Figure 10.9. Urine formation.

Source: https://nurseslabs.com/wp-content/uploads/2017/04/Urine-Formation-Urinary-System-Anatomy-and-Physiology.png

10.3.1. Glomerular Filtration

The glomerular filtration mechanism is crucial to the normal functioning of the urinary apparatus and begins in the nephron, the workhorse of the kidney. It is controlled by the glomerulus, a group of capillaries that is found inside a capsule known as Bowman's capsule. By filtration, the blood is pumped into the glomerulus under pressure so that water, electrolytes, and small molecules are filtered off from bigger proteins and circulating blood cells. This selectivity is necessary for homeostasis and to prevent loss of vital components from circulation. Disturbance of filtration can lead to renal pathologies, and diabetic kidney disease directly corresponds with impaired glomerular function. The interdependency of glomerular filtration rate (GFR) with renal health is indicative of the importance of such a complex and vital physiological process. The integrity of the glomerular filtration barrier is fundamental in regulating substance entry into urine. The barrier consists of three layers: the capillary endothelium, glomerular basement membrane, and podocytes that envelop the glomerular capillaries. These layers complement each other in providing selective permeability. For instance, podocytes possess foot processes that form slit diaphragms, essential in controlling the molecular size that can pass through them. Interference with this architecture—through inflammation or disease—can lead to disease such as albuminuria, where proteins leak into the urine. Proteins like endomucin have been found to play a pivotal role in the structural and functional integrity of the glomerular filtration barrier and, therefore, imply that endothelial health and podocyte function are inseparable (Hu et al., 2024). Exposure of these associations further our insights into disease mechanisms and probable therapeutic options for renal dysfunction. Glomerular filtration rate (GFR) measurement remains a clinical mainstay in the evaluation of renal function. A decrease in GFR indicates deteriorating kidney function, typically with an array of pathological processes, e.g., diabetic kidney disease (DKD). In DKD itself, the urinary albumin presence and decrease in estimated GFR are mandatory diagnostic signs (Zou and Sun, 2024). GFR biomarkers may indicate the degree of disease severity and progression. Evidence has lately indicated that high urinary levels of proteins such as osteopontin correlate with the onset and progression of renal disease among diabetic patients. The correlation emphasizes the potential in the integration of biochemical markers into practice to enhance earlier detection and treatment results. Therefore, glomerular filtration is perhaps the most significant factor to understand in efforts to control and minimize kidney disease in human populations.

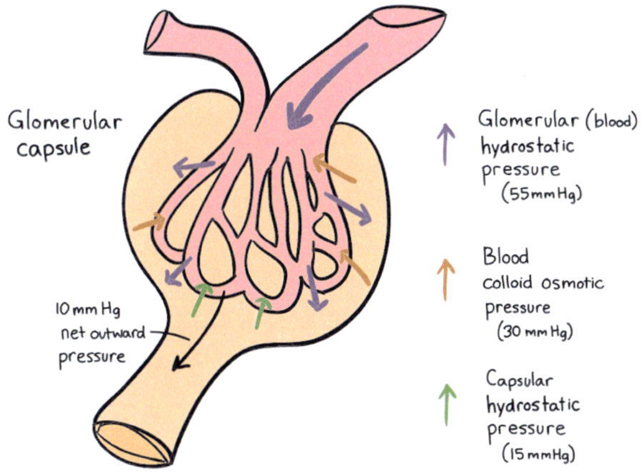

Figure 10.10. The glomerular filtration rate.

Source: https://cdn.kastatic.org/ka-perseus-images/0e7bfc98302c3e45dc7ec73ab142566a57513ec3.svg

10.3.2. Tubular Reabsorption

Tubular reabsorption is a critical function in the nephron, where it becomes possible to conserve essential substances and body fluids. With the flow of fluid through renal tubules, several processes are engaged to retrieve valuable solutes such as glucose, amino acids, and ions from the filtrate. This is mainly done in the proximal convoluted tubule, where approximately 65-70% of filtered water, sodium, and chloride are reabsorbed. Bicarbonate is also reabsorbed here and has a vital role to play in acid-base balance. These transport functions are essential not just to keep electrolytes in balance but to prevent dehydration and maintain blood pressure. The efficacy of tubular reabsorption is further exemplified by the nephron's remarkable capacity to adapt to varying degrees of diet consumption and hydration status, and also to preserve homeostasis within the urinary system in man. Furthermore, the intricate mechanism of tubular reabsorption involves both passive and active transport mechanisms acting in concert with one another. For instance, sodium-potassium ATPase on the basolateral membrane utilizes ATP to pump sodium out of the cell and leaves it with a concentration gradient such that sodium can passively move from the tubular lumen through the dedicated co-transporters. Active sodium transport allows other molecules like glucose and amino acids to be passively reabsorbed through co-transport. Furthermore, within the collecting duct and distal convoluted tubule, rates of reabsorption are controlled even further by aldosterone and antidiuretic hormone (ADH). Their activity demonstrates the nephron's ability to control reabsorption in response to bodily needs, thereby highlighting the complex nature of the urinary system's controls on tubular reabsorption in the human organism. In pathologic states, tubular reabsorption can produce dramatic clinical presentations, such as in distal renal tubular acidosis (dRTA). Research indicates that patients with dRTA possess impaired bicarbonate reabsorption and therefore retain metabolic acidosis, emblematic of the importance of tubular reabsorption in maintaining body pH levels within normal parameters. Later research into the genetic mutations in intercalated cells and their role in regulating proton and bicarbonate transport has added further detail to the underlying pathophysiology of the disease. These studies indicate the way in which disruption of tubular reabsorption affects not only ion homeostasis but also nephron function and fluid balance in general.

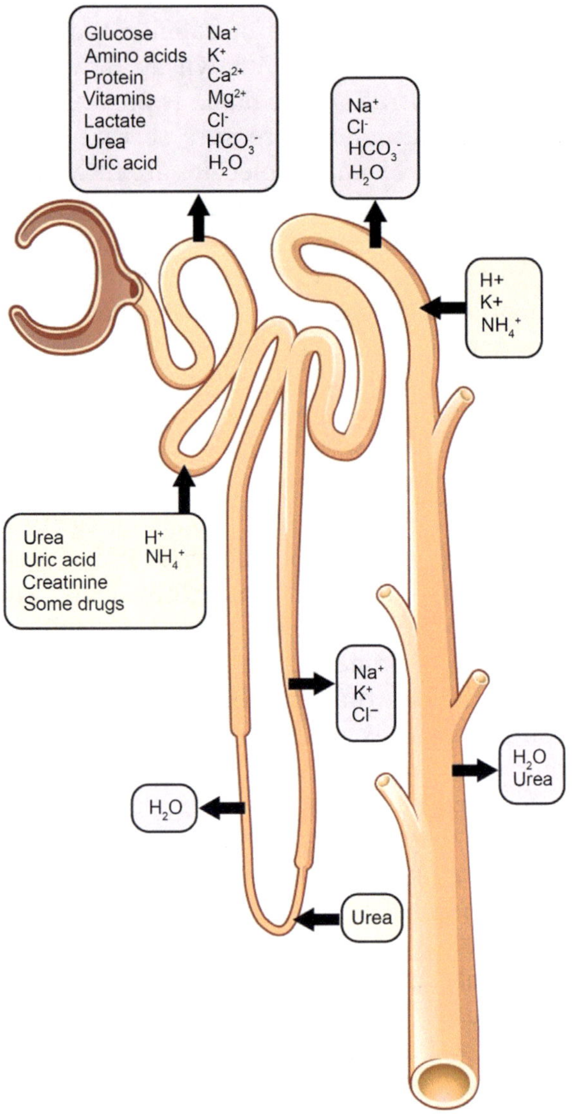

Figure 10.11. Substances filtered and reabsorbed by the nephron.

Source: https://textimgs.s3.amazonaws.com/osanp/m46443/2618_Nephron_Secretion_Reabsorption.jpg

These findings inform potential interventions, illustrating the value of understanding tubular reabsorption within the broader context of the urinary system in humans, as illustrated by research into urinary ion loss and compensatory mechanisms under various conditions (Mungara et al., 2024; Zapf et al., 2023).

10.3.3. Tubular Secretion

The tubular secretory process is essential for the urinary system to facilitate the excretion of unwanted substances from the blood to the renal tubules. The primary function occurs in the proximal convoluted tubule, in which the active transport of drugs, toxins, and metabolic waste products is facilitated. The ions and small molecules are secreted from the peritubular capillaries into the tubular lumen by specialized transport proteins. This process not only contributes to the elimination of xenobiotics—substances alien to the body—but also the regulation of essential body fluids and electrolytes, thereby maintaining homeostasis. The efficacy and discrimination of tubular secretion are crucial in renal clearance rates, which are essential in the practice of pharmacokinetics and organismal health in general, emphasizing its value in the field of renal physiology and therapeutic interventions (Olivia C Klatt et al., 2025). In addition, different regions of the nephron are involved in different ways with tubular secretion, and the distal nephron has specific roles. In particular, collecting duct intercalated cells participate in acid-base balance by secreting protons and reabsorbing bicarbonate, which is vital for maintaining the body's pH. Abnormalities in this secreting mechanism could lead to a variety of pathological conditions, such as distal renal tubular acidosis (dRTA), in which there is impaired acid secretion that results in metabolic acidosis that is accompanied by alkaline urine (Mungara et al., 2024). Understanding the mechanisms of proton and bicarbonate transport allows researchers to explore the potential therapeutic avenues for the restoration of normal renal function in such patients, thereby bridging tubular secretion directly to clinical advantages. Cellular modeling advances over the past decade have also contributed to a better understanding of mechanisms of tubular secretion, particularly in xenobiotic metabolism.

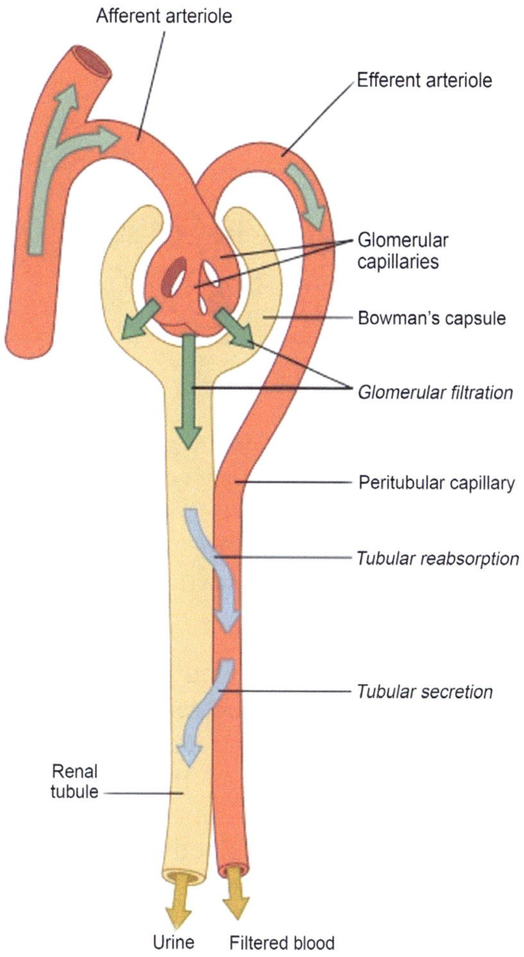

Figure 10.12. Tubular secretion.

Source: https://www.pharmacy180.com/media/imgph04/J6LEhMv.jpg

Proximal tubule models have been developed in vitro to study the expression and function of renal transporters employed in secretory mechanisms. Gene editing and organoid cultures have provided entry into the complex nature and efficiencies of these transport systems.

Moreover, renal clearance and transport functions research can elucidate variations observed in humans, that is, in response to drugs, by accurately simulating kidney responses in a human-like manner under controlled situations (Klatt et al., 2025). This integration of advanced study techniques into the investigation of tubular secretion holds promise for improved therapy and understanding of renal function, pointing to the dynamic nature of the urinary system.

Test Your Knowledge

1. What is the process of glomerular filtration?
2. What is the process of tubular reabsorption?

10.4. Regulation of Urine Production

Learning Outcome

1. Understand the role of hormonal control in regulating the human urinary system
2. Describe the neural regulation and the role of the autonomic nervous system
3. Know the impact of hydration levels on urine concentration

Urine formation is controlled to serve a vital function of fluid and electrolyte balance in the body. This complex process is primarily performed in the kidneys in the nephron, which is the functional unit of the kidney responsible for filtering blood and producing urine. Through filtration in the glomerulus in the nephron, filtrate is formed and is then altered by reabsorption and secretion processes. Hormones such as antidiuretic hormone (ADH) and aldosterone play a significant role in these processes. ADH increases collecting duct permeability, resulting in greater water reabsorption, urine concentration, and reduced urine volume. Aldosterone, meanwhile, increases sodium reabsorption, resulting in the retention of water and also maintaining blood pressure and blood volume, both essential to homeostasis. The nuances of the regulation of urine formation are thus essential to optimal body function. The coordination of neural and endocrine messages is at the very foundation of the regulation of urine production. ADH release is regulated by the posterior pituitary gland and hypothalamus in response to changes in blood osmolality and volume. With a reduction in body water, osmoreceptors within the hypothalamus detect increased serum osmolality, which triggers the release of ADH. This effect causes water retention, thus concentrating the urine but causing the kidneys to retain fluid. Moreover, cardiovascular baroreceptors monitor blood volume. A decrease in blood volume, for instance, during hemorrhage, triggers a cascade that enhances fluid retention and stimulates thirst. These sophisticated feedback controls guarantee that the production of urine is dynamically controlled to balance the body's hydration needs, reflecting the delicate equilibrium in which the urinary system functions among other bodily systems (Faisal, 2025). Moreover, regulation of urine production also encompasses pathological issues, particularly with kidney function. Diabetes insipidus and chronic kidney disease are two examples of how disruption of normal regulatory mechanisms can lead to significant clinical consequences. In diabetes insipidus, the deficiency of ADH leads to inappropriate hypersecretion of urine and excessive thirst, the hormone's critical role in water conservation. Similarly, chronic kidney disease may impair the kidneys' function of effectively filtering blood, resulting in altered urine production and fluid imbalance. The impact of these diseases transcends the urinary system, affecting overall fluid homeostasis and potentially resulting in complications, such as electrolyte imbalance or UTI. Hence, it is crucial to understand the regulatory mechanisms of urine production not just for the sake of normal physiology but also in order to comprehend various pathological conditions that affect the urinary system's function (Assimos, 2020).

10.4.1. Hormonal Control (e.g., ADH, Aldosterone)

Hormonal control plays a significant role in the regulation of the human urinary system, the secreted antidiuretic hormone (ADH) and aldosterone, which are the principal active hormones of the posterior pituitary gland. ADH has direct control over water reabsorption in the kidney. It acts to encourage the collecting tubules' permeability to water, thus increasing reabsorption of water into the body.

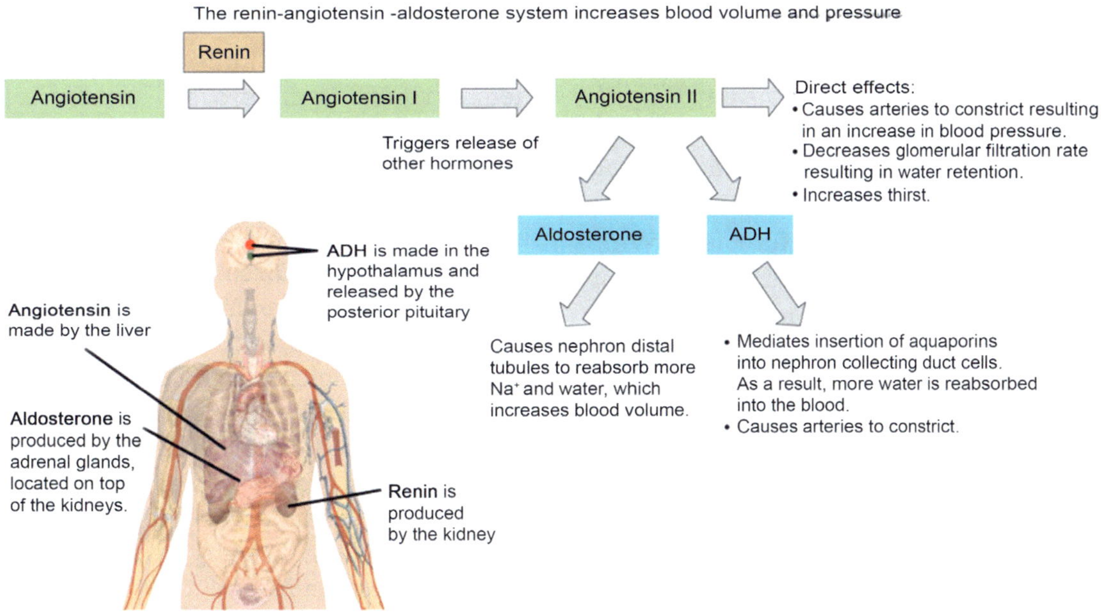

Figure 10.13. ADH and aldosterone increase blood pressure and volume. Angiotensin II stimulates the release of these hormones. Angiotensin II, in turn, is formed when renin cleaves angiotensin.

Source: https://s3-us-west-2.amazonaws.com/courses-images/wp-content/uploads/sites/1223/2017/02/07230054/Figure_37_03_01-1024x554.jpeg

This is important to maintain fluid balance and prevent dehydration, particularly during times of reduced water intake or extreme fluid loss. As body osmolarity rises, ADH secretion is stimulated to conserve water in the kidneys. ADH is thus important in regulating the volume and osmolality of urine and effectively managing hydration status and electrolyte balance in the body. Aldosterone, another significant hormone of the urinary system, is secreted from the adrenal cortex and principally regulates sodium and potassium balance. Its effect is mediated largely through its effect on the collecting ducts and distal convoluted tubule, where it is responsible for enhancing sodium reabsorption and potassium secretion. Sodium reabsorption induces the secondary retention of water, which increases blood volume and consequently blood pressure. Moreover, aldosterone secretion is also linked closely to the renin-angiotensin-aldosterone system (RAAS), which is activated by reduced blood pressure or diminished sodium chloride delivery to the kidneys. Dysregulation of this endocrine control mechanism might lead to conditions such as hypertension and heart failure, further emphasizing the need for balance in aldosterone levels for the overall maintenance of general renal function and cardiovascular well-being. New work has begun to explore other hormone impacts on renal function, contributing to our understanding of the regulation of the urinary system. Recent evidence suggests that hormones like glucagon-like peptide-1 (GLP-1) also potentially play an important role in renal physiology, namely, sodium handling and global kidney function. GLP-1, for instance, has been shown to enhance natriuresis, driving sodium excretion without altering glomerular filtration rate (GFR) or renal plasma flow (RPF) to a large degree. This implies that other hormonal mechanisms might then interact with dominant mechanisms such as those for ADH and aldosterone and thereby determine renal actions to other physiological needs. While the complexity of endocrine regulation of the urinary system becomes apparent, the more their interdependence will be necessary in developing targeted therapies for renal and cardiovascular disease, which are prone to endocrine disturbances (Santoro et al., 2015; Skov et al., 2013).

10.4.2. Neural Regulation and the Role of the Autonomic Nervous System

The autonomic nervous system (ANS) regulates the urinary system in a way that homeostasis of the body is maintained. A combination of sympathetic and parasympathetic components, the ANS regulates activities such as bladder relaxation and contraction, ureteral peristalsis, and urine production overall. The sympathetic nervous system inhibits the contraction of the bladder when the body is stressed or physically moving, thereby preserving energy and resources. Conversely, the parasympathetic division, with the vagus nerve playing a leading role, governs bladder contraction during relaxation and rest, enabling efficient urine expulsion. This neural control is not only important for the mechanical process of micturition, but also for coordinating the urinary system's function with other processes in the body, an expression of the intricate interplay in the ANS that is vital to the regulation of fluid balance and disposal within the human body. Central to neural control is the process of interoception, by which the nervous system interprets signals from within the body, such as urinary-related signals. Interoceptive consciousness allows individuals to develop an awareness of a full bladder and the requirement to urinate. It forms the core function of planning when and why to urinate, resonating with the brain's ability to synthesize physiological messages into conscious perception. Interoceptive signaling dysfunction can cause urinary disorders, underscoring the importance of proper neural feedback within the ANS. By looking into the role played by interoception in the urinary system, researchers are able to learn more about how disruption can cause a range of conditions affecting bladder control, hence gaining insight into potential therapeutic methods for those suffering because interoception impacts both the psychological condition and physiological condition relating to the urinary system (Sahib S Khalsa et al., 2017). Secondly, the modulation of the ANS by varied stimuli may produce marked consequences on urinary function and health. Exercise, nutrition, and stress may each influence the balance between parasympathetic and sympathetic stimulation and thereby both urinary output and urinary tract health in general. For instance, activation of the sympathetic nervous system through stress can lead to increased urine retention, potentially causing UTIs or other difficulties if continued. Yet, activities that promote vagal tone, such as meditation and slow breathing, can enhance parasympathetic function, resulting in improved bladder function as well as overall well-being. An understanding of these dynamics highlights the importance of an integrated model of urinary health, considering both neural control and lifestyle factors that can optimize the function of the autonomic nervous system for maintaining a healthy urinary system (Breit et al., 2018).

10.4.3. Effect of Water Levels On Urine Concentration

The fluid level is an important determinant of urine concentration and, as a result, of urine volume and composition. When well-hydrated, the kidneys can efficiently remove excess water, and they also secrete dilute urine with decreased specific gravity.

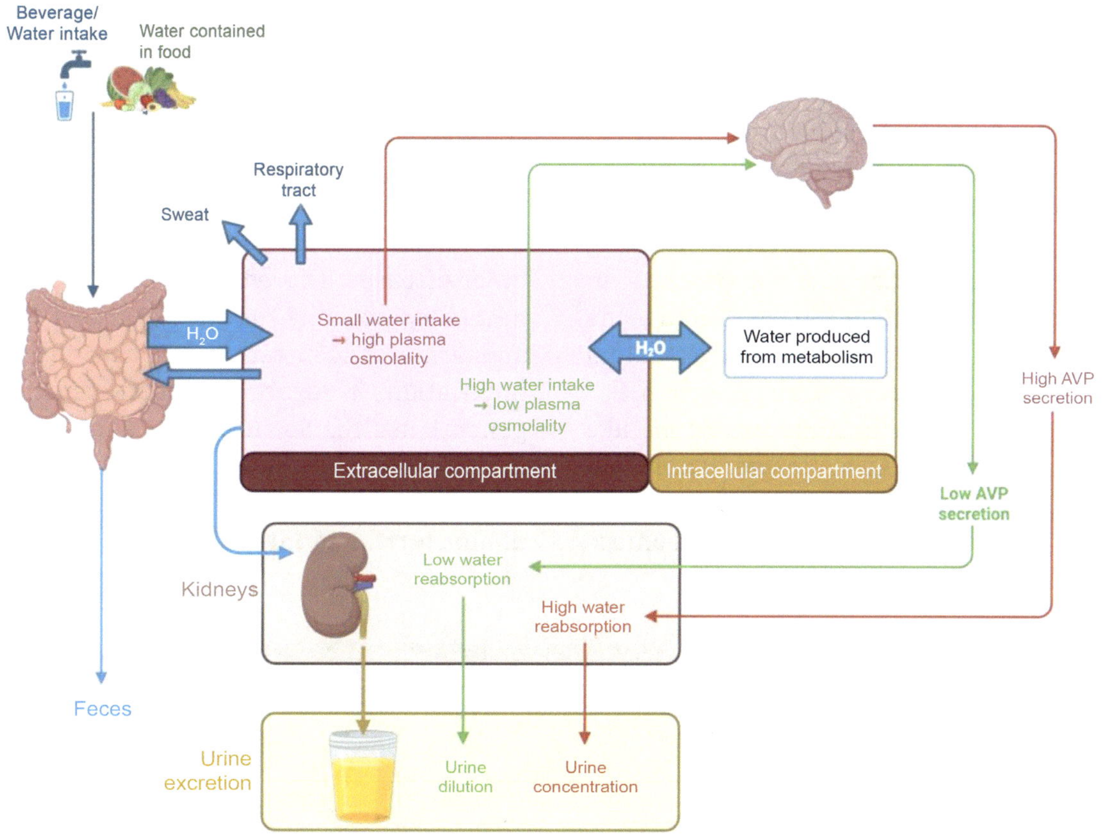

Figure 10.14. Physiological regulation of water balance. Fluid intake is mostly excreted by kidneys in response to water balance and AVP release. In the case of limited water intake (red arrows), intracellular volume decreased, leading to high AVP release and thus maximum water reabsorption by the kidney. Finally, a small amount of concentrated urine is excreted. On the other hand, high fluid intake (green arrows) leads to increased intracellular volume and thus to suppression of AVP release, and finally to an increased amount of diluted urine.

Source: https://www.mdpi.com/nutrients/nutrients-15-01642/article_deploy/html/images/nutrients-15-01642-g001.png

This is due to the activity of the antidiuretic hormone (ADH), which controls the water reabsorption in the collecting ducts of the nephron. Conversely, dehydration triggers ADH secretion, resulting in the kidneys conserving water as they concentrate the urine. The action of hydration on urine concentration demonstrates the body's sophisticated equilibrium between water intake and elimination, which is essential to maintain homeostasis in the urinary system. The alterations in urine concentration can be important diagnostic indicators of overall health as well as hydration. Insufficient hydration is associated with more concentrated urine, typically leading to such conditions as oliguria, which is marked by decreased urine output. These alterations in physiological condition can increase UTI risk since concentrated urine contains greater amounts of solutes, including urea and creatinine, that have the potential to irritate the bladder's lining. Concentrated urine also has the potential to act as a culture medium for bacterial growth, complicating infection. For instance, the presence of some pathogens like Carbapenem-resistant Acinetobacter baumannii has been correlated with changes in urines chemical environment that may promote infection. The interplay between hydration and urine concentration is thus not merely crucial in the formation of urine but also pivotal in understanding recurring infection risk factors, as seen in a number of clinical findings in UTI patients. Stringent monitoring of hydration levels is crucial in preventing the adverse effects of concentrated urine on the urinary tract. Healthy hydration behaviors can lead to better urine concentration patterns, reducing the risk of diseases such as kidney stones and UTIs. Proper fluid intake has been scientifically demonstrated to have a profound impact on serum levels of essential nutrients such as vitamin D3 and zinc, which are already shown to be significant players in urinary health (Faisal and Hasan, 2024). Conversely, chronic dehydration may exacerbate such deficiencies and further increase the risk of infection and other diseases. Therefore, optimal hydration is necessary, not only for effective renal function and urine concentration but also for overall implications in regard to immune function and general health. So, knowing and promoting hydration can be utilized as a preventative measure to maintain urinary tract health and diminish risks of infection.

Test Your Knowledge

1. What role do hormones play in the urinary system?
2. What is the impact of hydration levels on urine concentration?

10.5. Common Disorders of the Urinary System

Learning Outcome

1. Understand the urinary tract infections
2. Describe the kidney stones and their formation
3. Know the chronic kidney disease and its implications

The urinary system is susceptible to a number of common disorders that influence human health greatly. One of the commonly known conditions is UTI, which is caused by the infection of any urinary system structure, such as the kidneys, ureters, bladder, or urethra. UTIs are much more prevalent in females, typically due to anatomy facilitating easier bacterial colonization. Symptoms range from slight dysuria to more disabling symptoms, such as fever and flank pain, indicative of a possible upper UTI. Prompt diagnosis is critical, with antibiotic therapy the usual treatment. However, frequent UTIs pose a challenge, for which ongoing monitoring and preventive interventions are necessary in order to minimize complications. This highlights the importance of ongoing research into the risk factors and pathogen dynamics within the urinary system, as evidenced in present research into the function of urinary biomarkers to enhance sensitivity for diagnosis (Weldon et al., 2025). Another critical disorder of the urinary system is chronic kidney disease (CKD), which is characterized by a gradual, insidious loss of kidney function. Some of the etiologic factors, including diabetes mellitus and hypertension, make a person susceptible to CKD. The patient is mostly asymptomatic in the initial stages, leading to late diagnosis and treatment. While the disease is progressing, the patient shows symptoms such as weakness, edema, and incontinence or a change in urine output. Furthermore, CKD has also been associated with a variety of complications like cardiovascular disease and electrolyte imbalance, which further complicate the management and quality of life for the patient. Therefore, early detection and intervention are necessary in order to slow disease progression and optimize patient outcomes. Secondly, the use of multimodal therapy in the management of CKD has been found effective in promoting holistic care, suggestive of the benefits of health professionals' collaboration (Shajari et al., 2024). Lastly, kidney stones represent a frequent disorder of the urinary tract with significant implications for patient health and healthcare utilization. Made up of crystallization of a number of substances, such as calcium, oxalate, and uric acid, kidney stones can lead to severe pain, hematuria, and urinary tract obstruction. Risk factors for kidney stone development include diet, dehydration, and heredity. Treatment is primarily symptomatic and involves pain relief, fluids, and, in complicated cases, surgery or lithotripsy for stone passage. Furthermore, lifestyle modification is also necessary in the prevention of recurrence, as underscored by patient education regarding dietary patterns and water intake behavior. Understanding of the metabolic processes predisposing one to developing stones would similarly enhance prevention strategies, underlining the need for further research into effective management strategies for kidney stone disease in susceptible populations (Weldon et al., 2025).

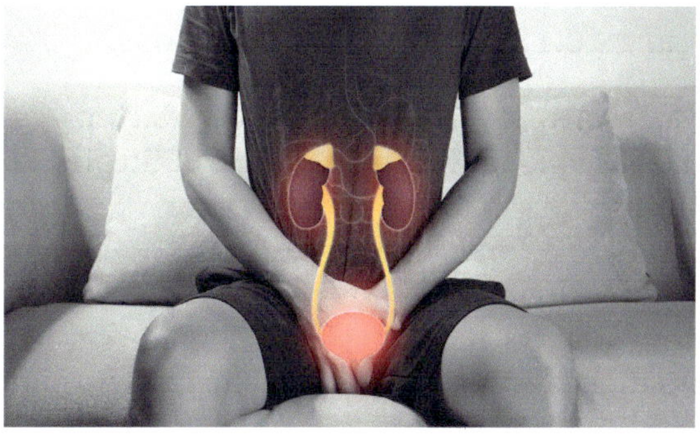

Source: https://www.drpiyushpatawari.com/blog/images/post/04-08-2023-Dr-Piyush-Kumar-Patawari-Web-blog-1-img-1.jpg

10.5.1. Urinary Tract Infections (UTIS)

UTI is a prevalent health issue that affects all demographics of individuals, particularly women. *Escherichia coli* is the leading causative agent for most UTIs, which are particular strains known as uropathogenic *E. coli* (UPEC). These pathogens employ an array of virulence factors in order to bind to the uroepithelial cells, facilitating colonization and eventual infection of the urinary tract. The high rate of UTI recurrence, especially in women, is indicative of the bacterium's ability to evade the host's immune system and necessitates a thorough understanding of UPEC's pathogenic processes to lead to successful treatment and prevention. In addition, identification of the phylogroups of *E. coli* strains that cause UTIs helps in marking risk factors differently attributed to different strains, from research evidence where phylogroups B2 and C were most commonly implicated in UPEC infections (Ketkhao et al., 2024). UTIs are not merely the identification of causative organisms; they are a dynamic interplay of interaction between uropathogens and host defense mechanisms. Explanation of these interactions is vital in developing effective treatment regimens. It has been seen in research that toxin-antitoxin (TA) systems in UPEC are key players in the pathogenesis of rUTIs. The systems enable bacteria to survive in the host, maintain stress response, and form biofilms, which are famously resistant both to the immune system and antibiotics.

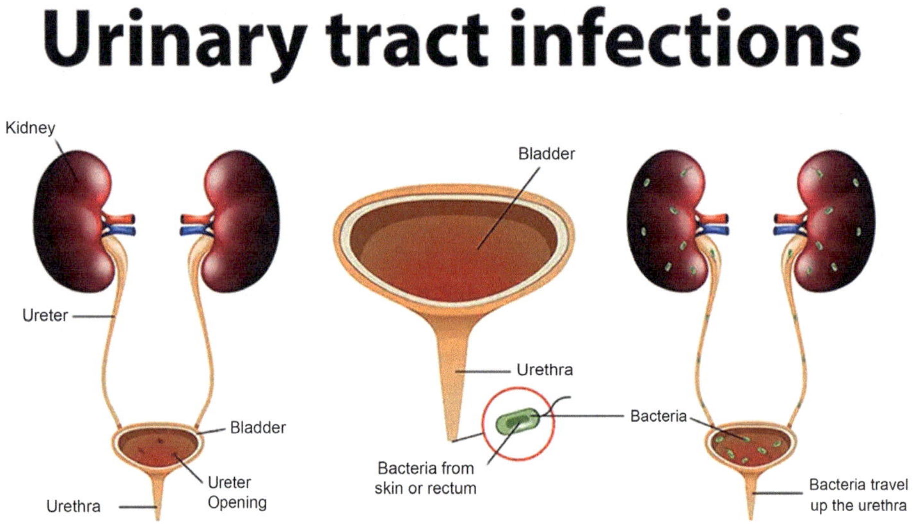

Figure 10.15. Urinary tract infections.

Source: https://www.apexhospitals.com/_next/image?url=https%3A%2F%2Fbed.apexhospitals.com%2Fuploads%2FUTI_3d1a698556.png&w=1920&q=75

The prevalence of certain TA systems, e.g., ccdAB, has been linked with bacterial persistence in the urinary tract, indicating their role as possible targets for new therapeutic strategies to avoid UTI recurrence (Zhang et al., 2024). The implications of UPEC-driven UTIs go beyond personal health and affect public health issues as well. The speeding trend of antibiotic resistance complicates the treatment process, and therefore, preventive care and other types of therapy need more focus. UPEC strains that occur due to urinary infections as well as through food sources such as pork indicate the possibility of interaction among such strains, and therefore, stringent food safety protocols must be followed to minimize the risk of cross-contamination (Ketkhao et al., 2024). As ongoing research continues to refine mechanisms of UTI pathogenesis, healthcare professionals are increasingly well placed to implement preventive strategies, such as customized treatment protocols and enhanced patient education. Lastly, a thorough understanding of UTIs is essential within the larger framework of urinary system health in order to address the escalating issues related to these diseases.

10.5.2. Kidney Stones and Their Formation

Kidney stone development, a critical element of urinary tract pathology, is a complex interplay of etiologies that lead to crystallization of the renal tract. Nephrolithiasis, or kidney stones, develops due to an imbalance of the concentration of calcium, oxalate, and uric acid in urine. This imbalance may be due to dehydration, diet, or metabolic derangements, leading to urinary saturation with these stone constituents. These solutes come together to form tiny crystals, which coalesce into larger stones with the passage of time. The process can lead to severe complications, including acute pain, urinary tract obstruction, infection, and even potential kidney failure, underlining the importance of understanding stone-forming mechanisms in the overall scheme of urinary health (Ahmed et al., 2024). In evaluating potential preventative strategies, historical practices and modern medicine are both of some use in understanding kidney stone care. Traditional Persian Medicine (TPM), as discussed in various literary works, suggests dietetic treatments founded on centuries of clinical practice in stone development and treatment. A review of such classical practices shows that some dietary changes and plant medicines can be highly successful in preventing stone formation. For example, the infusion of fluids with adequate minerals, along with an appropriate dietetic intake of components, may influence urinary chemical content and thereby reduce the risk of stone formation. In addition, ongoing searches of such ancient modalities in conjunction with current medical technology may offer a broad arena for the prevention and treatment of urolithiasis (Rameshk, 2024). The integration of technological advancements in the treatment and diagnosis of kidney stones is making our knowledge and treatment capabilities better. Advances in artificial intelligence, in utilizing the application of machine learning algorithms like VGG16, have been encouraging in accurately diagnosing kidney stones from KUB X-ray images. This method, besides speeding up the process of diagnosis, also enhances the predictive power, achieving testing accuracy levels of 97.41% (Ahmed et al., 2024). This is crucial in guiding treatment interventions and improving the patients' outcomes. Through the blending of traditional knowledge systems with modern diagnostic practices, there is a unique possibility to develop a more unified and more powerful approach for those at risk of or suffering from kidney stones, thereby fostering a balanced understanding of the complexity of the urinary system.

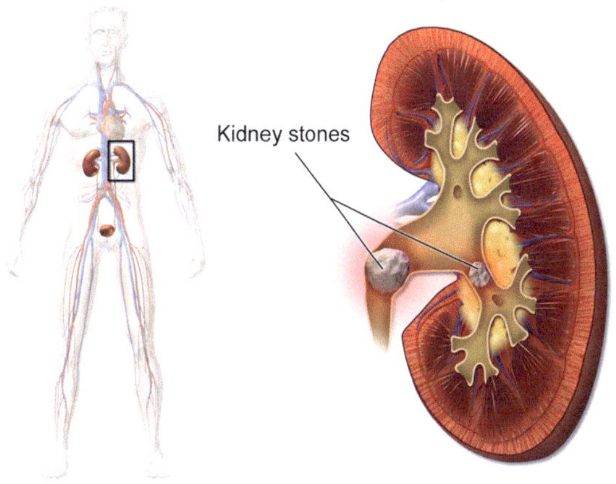

Figure 10.16. Kidney stones form in the kidney and may grow large enough to block the major calyx or ureter.

Source: https://upload.wikimedia.org/wikipedia/commons/d/d8/Blausen_0595_KidneyStones.png

10.5.3. Chronic Kidney Disease and Its Implications

Chronic kidney disease (CKD) refers to irreversible loss of renal function, and if left untreated, it can progress to severe conditions that mostly affect an individual's life. Reduction in filtering capacity of the kidneys leads to accumulation of waste products in the blood, triggering a cascade of ill health throughout the body. One of the implications of CKD is its association with cardiovascular disease, as the patients exhibit a predisposition to developing hypertension and deranged lipid metabolism, thereby aggravating cardiac conditions. Secondly, the renal injury that comes with CKD has a severe effect on the bones via deranged mineral and bone metabolism, thereby putting it at risk of fracture and osteoporosis. This intricate interaction between renal impairment and global health necessitates integrated management strategies to prevent such risks and realize optimal patient outcomes while stressing the unique interaction of the urinary system's anatomy and physiology in managing chronic disease. The implications of chronic kidney disease are not merely physical, with relevant correlation to psychological status and functional level in patients. CKD patients tend to have a chronic pattern of physician consultations, dietary limitations, and drug therapy, all resulting in cumulative stress and depression. Psychiatric burden further complicates disease management and makes more integrated care absolutely indispensable. Psychological support therapies, i.e., social support groups and counseling, can enable better adherence to treatment and coping in CKD patients, based on research. Some of the symptoms are alleviated as well as overall kidney function by lifestyle change—e.g., increased hydration, dietary adjustment. With an awareness of the emotional and psychological aspects of CKD, clinicians are now better positioned to shape more sensitive and comprehensive interventions for each patient's overall experience. There has been renewed interest in investigating the potential role of environmental agents in chronic kidney disease, particularly in the setting of microplastics in renal tissue. Microplastics and nanoplastics have been found in the urinary tract and linked to kidney injury and urinary system disease, including bladder cancer and chronic UTI. The indicated cytotoxicity of microplastics, which would enhance inflammation and disrupt normal cellular signaling mechanisms, has a significant implication in public health. As plastic contamination keeps expanding in everyday life, public health agencies such as the World Health Organization should reconsider their position regarding environmental poisons and their impacts on health. Identification of such environmental etiologies of CKD is key to developing forward-thinking strategies that fix kidney function and kidney sustainability in the environment, thereby forming part of our urinary system care strategy.

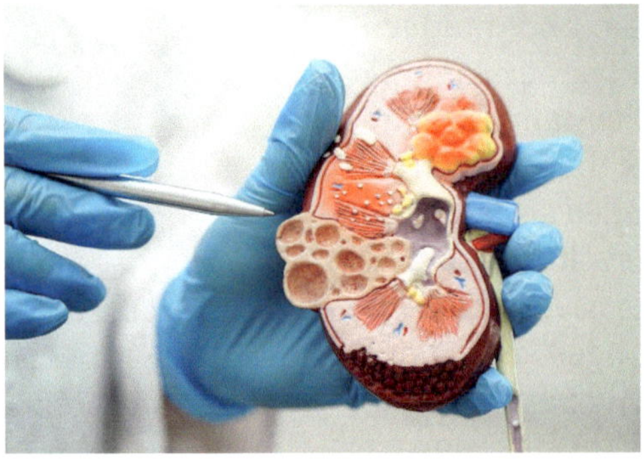

Figure 10.17. Chronic kidney disease.

Source: https://dam.northwell.edu/m/1a4d1b4b068a12c6/Drupal-TheWell_kidney-disease_AS_598468387.jpg

Test Your Knowledge

1. What is a urinary tract infection (UTI)?
2. What is the chronic kidney disease?

10.6. Diagnostic Techniques

Learning Outcome

1. Understand the urinalysis and its significance
2. Describe the role of imaging techniques in the evaluation and diagnosis of the urinary system
3. Understand the importance of blood tests in assessing kidney function

The urinary system has an important role in homeostasis, and diagnostic techniques are important in assessing its functioning and integrity. Older techniques such as urinalysis provide initial information about many pathological disorders, identifying abnormalities of constituents such as glucose, protein, and blood, which can indicate diseases such as diabetes or pyelonephritis. Also, imaging techniques such as X-rays and ultrasound are critical in the visualization of the urinary tract, allowing clinicians to detect structural issues such as obstructions or stones. Such diagnostic tools play a key role in creating a thorough understanding of an inpatient's urinary condition, essentially guiding the process of treatment and disease monitoring. Advancements in diagnostic equipment have greatly enhanced the examination of the urinary system. For instance, the incorporation of robotic-assisted techniques into ultrasound has improved accuracy in imaging and reduced the role of operators. In addition, the application of machine learning algorithms in data analysis allows for real-time, automated interpretation of diagnosis results, which means faster and more accurate assessments. As discussed in recent summaries, including summaries of the applications of ultrasonic technology, these developments avoid difficulties with traditional diagnostic practices while simultaneously compensating for sample variability and environmental factors that can skew measurement precision (Yan et al., 2024). Not only are these developments making the diagnostic process easier, but they ultimately lead to better patient outcomes as a result of timely treatments. In addition, the potential of automated processes in lab diagnosis has also transformed the way renal pathologies are being evaluated.

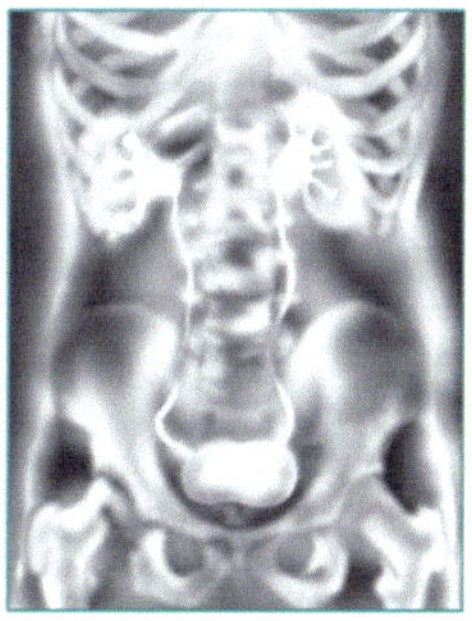

Figure 10.18. IVP image showing the kidneys, ureters, and bladder.

Source: https://www.niddk.nih.gov/-/media/Images/Health-Information/Diagnostic-Tests/IVPimage.jpg

Laboratory automation can efficiently handle the increasing number of tests required for urinary tract analysis, from pre-test sample preparation to end analysis (Dakhilallah et al., 2024). This advancement eliminates the risk of human error and significantly speeds up turnaround time, thus facilitating timely clinical decision-making. Furthermore, by combining automation with advanced imaging techniques, clinicians better understand a patient's urinary condition. As advances in such fusion keep expanding, their impact on urinary diagnosis is likely to create new lines of research, ultimately altering standards of care and patient management in nephrology and urology.

10.6.1. Urinalysis and Its Significance

Urinalysis is a key function in renal and systemic disease assessment, being a non-invasive diagnostic screen that assists in communicating the urinary systems' status in an effective manner. Through observation of the physical, chemical, and microscopic properties of the urine, clinical staff can identify a range of medical conditions from UTIs to renal dysfunction. The value of this analysis is brought out by its ability to detect abnormalities early on, potentially guiding early interventions that can maximize patient outcomes. For instance, in one of the studies, detection of white blood cells (WBCs) in urinalysis yielded the best diagnostic accuracy to predict uropathogens from urine cultures, thus enabling diagnostic stewardship to prevent unnecessary treatment (Kupferwasser et al., 2025). This function highlights urinalysis not only as a diagnostic tool but also as a cornerstone in the management of many urinary pathologies with possible more systemic significance. Moreover, the use of urinalysis is beyond the detection of urinary pathology. Recent research has given credence to its role in the context of new diseases, such as COVID-19, where urinary pathology has been linked with acute kidney injury in affected patients. These findings indicate that urinalysis is capable of disclosing significant immune reactions and renal features of systemic infections (Axmedjanova, 2025). The analysis of cytokines and other markers in the urine can deliver crucial data about renal function and inflammation and therefore disclose latent kidney issues, particularly in individuals who are inclined towards long-term conditions. Thus, the intersection of urinalysis with more recent health concerns underscores its dynamic utility and underscores the need for continuous improvement in diagnostic standards and methods. In the context of public health, too, a relatively low-cost screening tool with the ability to identify high-risk populations and facilitate preventive healthcare interventions is no less essential. The overall approach to this evaluation assists in the identification of conditions that might otherwise go unnoticed, thereby assisting in the promotion of preemptive health intervention. As an example, urinalysis as a routine screening is frequently conducted during community health assessments since it can readily identify early markers of diabetes, hypertension, and other systemic diseases. The integration of urinalysis in routine medical tests not just makes diagnosis easier but also facilitates overall healthcare efficiency through ease of timely interventions. The significance of urinalysis in practice is thus undoubtedly substantial, ensuring its ongoing reliance as a central aspect of urinary tract examination and general medical checkups.

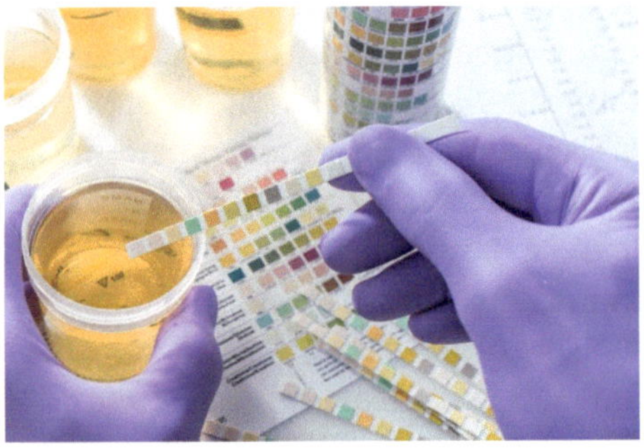

Figure 10.19. Urinalysis.

Source: https://aareurology.sg/wp-content/uploads/2022/04/shutterstock_1245033115-1024x683.jpg

10.6.2. Imaging Techniques (e.g., Ultrasound, CT Scans)

Imaging modalities play a critical function in the assessment and diagnosis of the urinary system and provide distinct information about its anatomical and physiological condition. Among them, ultrasound stands out as non-invasive and capable of dynamic imaging. It utilizes high-frequency sound waves to produce images and, hence, allows clinicians to visualize structures such as the kidneys, ureters, and bladder. Of particular mention, ultrasound is particularly valuable in assessing conditions such as hydronephrosis, kidney stones, and tumors. Abnormality detection without exposing patients to the application of ionizing radiation makes it more appealing, particularly in sensitive groups of individuals such as pregnant women and children. With the continuous advancement of ultrasound technology, i.e., the application of Doppler imaging for monitoring blood flow, it serves as a more vital tool in clinical practice for urinary system diagnosis and will remain so in the future. CT scanning combined with ultrasound is another cornerstone of urinary system imaging that provides high-resolution cross-sectional images enabling more precise diagnoses. CT scans are able to identify a broad array of urinary tract pathology, including tumors, cysts, and trauma-related injuries. Enhanced visualization using contrast media enhances the imaging of structures with better definition of pathology. In addition, CT urograms are specifically focused on renal and urinary tract disease and provide superior information on urinary tract morphology. Significantly, while the benefits of CT are substantial, most notably in emergency practice with the imperative of expeditious diagnosis, risk of exposure to radiation is a vital consideration. Thus, the appropriate use of CT imaging is paramount, balancing the need for the best diagnosis against the dangers of ionizing radiation exposure, especially among younger or more vulnerable patient groups. Whereas both CT scans and ultrasound are useful, each procedure has its own limitations inherent within it, which are also to be considered in the practice setting. For instance, whereas ultrasound is highly effective in certain disease states, it will not always provide sufficient information in others, such as when dealing with small renal cancers or with certain pathologies obscured by bowel gas. In contrast, while CT scans provide better resolution, their application is constrained by radiation exposure, which requires cautious planning in instances of repetitive imaging. Furthermore, imaging modalities may have varying availability across institutions and thereby influence the scope of availability of these diagnostic tools. Finally, it involves a full understanding of the relative advantages and limitations of each imaging modality so that health practitioners can best make informed decisions in the diagnosis and treatment of urinary tract ailments. By strategic integration of multiple imaging modalities, clinicians can optimize diagnostic efficacy and ensure improved patient outcomes in managing urinary well-being.

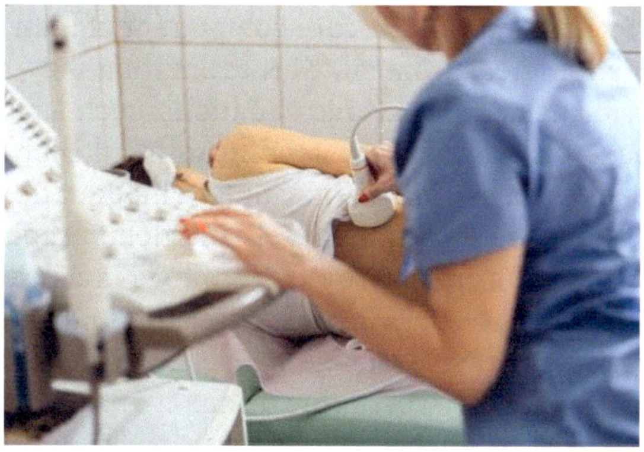

Figure 10.20. Ultrasound transducers bounce safe, painless sound waves off different organs to create an image of their structure.

Source: https://www.niddk.nih.gov/-/media/Images/Health-Information/Diagnostic-Tests/Woman-doctor-doing-ultrasound-patient.jpg

10.6.3. Blood Tests Related to Kidney Function

The role of blood tests in assessing kidney function should not be exaggerated, as they provide essential information about the health of the urinary system. Two markers that are most essential are blood urea nitrogen (BUN) and serum creatinine. The concentration of creatinine reflects how well the kidneys function; an elevated creatinine concentration suggests kidney dysfunction because the kidneys excrete this substance from the circulation. Similarly, BUN levels are used to gauge the ability of the kidneys to remove nitrogenous waste. Anything that's outside normal values could be a sign of chronic kidney disease or acute renal failure. Ongoing monitoring of these blood work-ups enables physicians to diagnose kidney failure early, enabling timely treatment that is crucial in patient outcomes. These markers combined are key to understanding not only kidney function but also its broader influence on overall health, with the interconnectedness present in the urinary system as well as in other bodily systems. In addition to serum creatinine and BUN, glomerular filtration rate (GFR) estimation is a core component of kidney function measurement. GFR estimation may be performed using various equations, such as the Cockcroft-Gault or the Modification of Diet in Renal Disease (MDRD) formula. The equations consider the creatinine levels and demographic information and provide a more accurate representation of kidney function. GFR indicates how efficiently the kidneys handle blood; a falling GFR indicates worsening renal insufficiency, such as in diabetes and hypertension. As CKD can occur without evident symptoms, it is necessary that blood tests should be applied to track kidney function in clinical settings. By quantifying the kidneys' filtration capacity, GFR facilitates informing treatment decisions and improving patient management practice, demonstrating the crucial role of blood tests to maintain urinary tract health. New research has unveiled other kidney function biomarkers, further enhancing our knowledge of renal health. A good example is the urotensin II (UII) system, whose involvement in cardiovascular disease as well as kidney pathologies has been suggested. Urotensin levels are elevated in conditions of hypertension and diabetic kidney disease (DKD), suggesting the UII system could be a therapeutic target (Olugbenga S Michael et al., 2024). UII levels in blood or urine can not only serve as markers of kidney disease but also as a starting point for developing new therapeutic strategies. Moreover, as the function of UII in the kidneys is further characterized, future blood tests could incorporate these newer biomarkers to have a complete view of renal function. These advances indicate an active development in the field of nephrology, expressing the consistent effort toward enhancing diagnostic accuracy and treatment strategies in understanding the urinary system in humans.

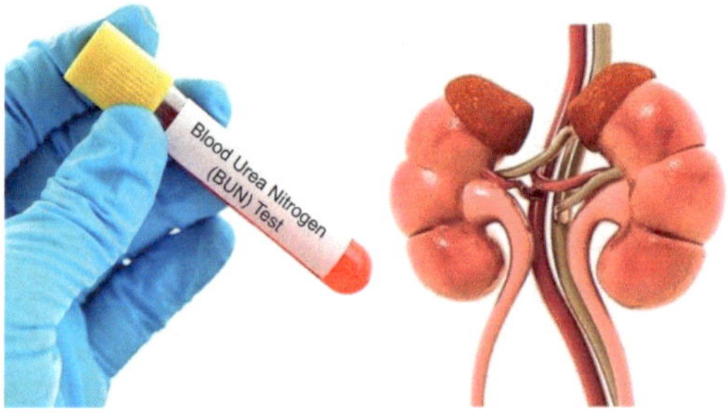

Figure 10.21. Blood urea nitrogen test.

Source: https://requestatest.com/includes/uploads/blog/BUN.jpg

Test Your Knowledge

1. What is urinalysis and its significance?
2. What blood tests detect kidney function?

SUMMARY

The dynamic and intricate nature of the human urinary system highlights its critical role in maintaining homeostasis in the body. In addition to facilitating the elimination of waste products, it plays a critical role in fluid balance, electrolyte composition, and blood pressure regulation. As a crucial component of the renal system, the kidneys cleanse blood, allowing the body to keep essential substances and eliminate excess and toxic elements. Further, the interrelation of the kidneys, ureters, bladder, and urethra is a highly integrated physiological process that eventually results in overall well-being. Understanding the role of this system is vital in determining possible effects of urinary pathology, which can arise as a result of derangement at any point along this process. Thus, there is an urgent need for medical practitioners to be well aware of the urinary system in order to diagnose and treat various renal pathologies. Besides, emerging technologies such as hyperspectral imaging (HSI) allow medical technologists to pursue new avenues in understanding and diagnosing urinary system pathologies. This new imaging technique offers a non-invasive method of comprehending tissue composition, structure, and function, possibly significantly enhancing the monitoring and detection of urinary diseases. Through providing precise measurements of body tissues in a way other imaging technologies are incapable of, HSI has the potential to alter the direction of diagnostic methods and patient treatment. Additionally, ongoing research into the application of HSI in clinical settings has the potential to reveal further knowledge about the urinary system and its pathology, and thus to innovative standards of treatment. Thus, persistent integration of technology into knowledge about human physiology, including that of the urinary system, is an important step towards sophisticated medicine. As a whole, the intricacy of the urinary system and its vital roles solidify the significance of ongoing research and education in this field. An understanding of urinary system processes deepens our knowledge of human health and the potential complications that arise from its dysfunction. As demonstrated, application of advanced imaging modalities such as HSI presents an exhilarating new frontier for the study of the urinary system, with the promise of greater diagnostic capability and patient care. Therefore, with further discoveries and learning of the urinary system, it becomes increasingly imperative to share all this information with the medical community and educate the future generation of healthcare professionals. Through this way, we can ensure that individuals who are afflicted with urinary disorders are given the best care possible and benefit from the ongoing advancements in medical science, keeping our vow to advance the welfare of humans and their health.

The urinary system serves to regulate homeostasis in the human body. Its primary functions include fluid balance, balance of electrolytes, and removal of waste, which are required for proper physiological functioning. By removing waste products of metabolism, excess ions, and poisons from the blood through the filtration of blood by the kidneys, the urinary system subsequently excretes them as urine. In addition, the kidneys are also at the hub of blood pressure regulation through the renin-angiotensin-aldosterone system. Through this active process, it is shown how urinary function defects can lead to systemic illnesses and, in the process, emphasize the system's importance in the general body regulation and health upkeep. Apart from the elimination of waste, the urinary system has a key function in acid-base balance. The kidneys also help in regulating the pH of the body by secreting hydrogen ions and recovering bicarbonate from the urine. This becomes critical in keeping the extracellular fluid within the pH range that allows enzymatic activity and metabolic processes. The ability of the urinary system to adapt to dietary consumption, dehydration, and other physiological demands similarly accentuates its adaptive potential and function in metabolic equilibrium. Any failure of the regulations in these mechanisms can lead to serious conditions such as metabolic alkalosis or acidosis, thus the need for the proper functioning of the urinary system for health and prevention of complications (Biggins et al., 2021). The urinary system is also crucial in endocrine function as it releases hormones required in regulating a variety of processes in the body. For instance, the kidneys secrete erythropoietin that stimulates the bone marrow to produce red blood cells in response to a lack of oxygen in the blood. The kidneys also stimulate vitamin D as calcitriol, an agent crucial in calcium absorption from the intestines as well as in bone health. These endocrine functions illustrate that the urinary system does not just excrete waste but is also critically involved in systemic biological regulation. This complex function underscores the need for ongoing research and clinical interest in the urinary system, particularly with respect to chronic diseases that can impair its function (Liguori et al., 2018).

KEY TERMS FROM THIS CHAPTER

Ayurveda	Bladder dysfunctions
Blood cells	Blood volume
Chronic kidney disease	Detrusor muscles
Electrolyte balance	Hypertension
Kidneys	Nephrology
Proteins	Renal cortex
Renal diseases	Ureters
Urethra	Urinary tract infections

CRITICAL THINKING QUESTIONS

1. The functional unit of the kidney is:

a. Nephron

b. Alveolus

c. Lobule

d. Glomerulus

2. Which organ is responsible for filtering blood and producing urine?

a. Bladder

b. Kidney

c. Ureter

d. Urethra

3. The tube that carries urine from the kidneys to the bladder is called:

a. Urethra

b. Collecting duct

c. Ureter

d. Renal vein

4. The urinary bladder stores urine and is located in the:

a. Thoracic cavity

b. Pelvic cavity

c. Abdominal cavity

d. Cranial cavity

5. The region of the kidney where blood vessels, nerves, and the ureter enter is called the:

a. Cortex

b. Medulla

c. Renal pelvis

d. Hilum

Short Answer Questions

1. What is the urinary system?
2. Why is urinary system important in human health?
3. Name the 4 organs of the urinary system.
4. What is the main function of the urinary system?
5. What is the most common disorder of the urinary system?

Answer to Critical Thinking Questions

1. (a) 2. (b) 3. (c) 4. (b) 5. (d)

REFERENCES

1. Aggarwal, N., Kitano, S., Puah, G. R. Y., Kittelmann, S., Hwang, I. Y., & Chang, M. W. (2022). Microbiome and human health: Current understanding, engineering, and enabling technologies. *Chemical Reviews, 123*, 31–72. https://doi.org/10.1021/acs.chemrev.2c00431 (accessed on 15th June 2025).
2. Ahmed, F., Abbas, S., Athar, A., Shahzad, T., Khan, W., Alharbi, M., Khan, M. A., et al. (2024). Identification of kidney stones in KUB X-ray images using VGG16 empowered with explainable artificial intelligence. *Scientific Reports, 14*. https://www.semanticscholar.org/paper/3a34a49cebc3df9725f281ad8887d023f89aba0f (accessed on 15th June 2025).
3. Andronico, L. A., Jiang, Y., Carannante, V., Iskrak, S., Sandoz, P. A., Mikeš, J., Klymchenko, A. S., et al. (2024). High-throughput analysis of membrane fluidity unveils a hidden dimension in immune cell states. *bioRxiv*. https://www.semanticscholar.org/paper/ef9297058d1491810e8565d5e1dc07376d021680 (accessed on 15th June 2025).
4. Assimos, D. (2020). Re: Safety of high-dose vitamin D supplementation: Secondary analysis of a randomized controlled trial. *The Journal of Urology*. https://www.semanticscholar.org/paper/e6dc6fb7e402eda21457f6ad18f2473d942f18cb (accessed on 15th June 2025).
5. Axmedjanova, N. I. (2025). Significance of cytokine profile in renal complications in children during the COVID-19 pandemic: An observational cohort retrospective clinical study. *Kuban Scientific Medical Bulletin*. https://www.semanticscholar.org/paper/29ae1be7399fa60e39cd08c2caa633134c0ac27f (accessed on 15th June 2025).
6. Baulina, O., Baulin, A., Baulin, V. A., & Aver'yanova, L. A. (2025). Migration of foreign bodies through the urinary system (clinical cases). *Bulletin of the Medical Institute "REAVIZ" (Rehabilitation, Doctor and Health)*. https://www.semanticscholar.org/paper/d3abf95052698b0e909fd9021f64534b1e0b8228 (accessed on 15th June 2025).
7. Biggins, S. W., Angeli, P., García-Tsao, G., Ginés, P., Ling, S. C., Nadim, M. K., Wong, F., et al. (2021). Diagnosis, evaluation, and management of ascites, spontaneous bacterial peritonitis and hepatorenal syndrome: 2021 practice guidance by the American Association for the Study of Liver Diseases. *Hepatology, 74*, 1014–1048. https://doi.org/10.1002/hep.31884 (accessed on 15th June 2025).
8. Bordeianou, L., Paquette, I. M., Johnson, E. K., Holubar, S. D., Gaertner, W. B., Feingold, D. L., & Steele, S. R. (2017). Clinical practice guidelines for the treatment of rectal prolapse. *Diseases of the Colon & Rectum, 60*, 1121–1131. https://doi.org/10.1097/dcr.0000000000000889 (accessed on 15th June 2025).
9. Breit, S., Kupferberg, A., Rogler, G., & Hasler, G. (2018). Vagas nerve as modulator of the brain–gut axis in psychiatric and inflammatory disorders. *Frontiers in Psychiatry, 9*. https://doi.org/10.3389/fpsyt.2018.00044 (accessed on 15th June 2025).
10. Chen, L., Chen, C., Liu, P., Chen, R., Li, C., Tang, L., Liao, K., et al. (2020). [Three-dimensional modeling of female urinary system based on MRI and CT data]. *Nan fang yi ke da xue xue bao. Journal of Southern Medical University, 40*(7), 1056–1061. https://www.semanticscholar.org/paper/a3fc820fa2bbdc461daa54f696ee8ef0c0ea4d34 (accessed on 15th June 2025).
11. Dakhilallah, S., Almalki, S., Nasser, M., Al Inkis, A., Alrashdan, S., Ateeq, A. A., et al. (2024). Automation in laboratories: How it's changing diagnostic techniques. *Power System Technology*.

https://www.semanticscholar.org/paper/c189ef6f85976209371f187144896d41380e3845 (accessed on 15th June 2025).

12. Demirhan, K., Saglam, H., Cimen, H., Elcin, B., & Çokluk, E. (2025). Effect of the location and severity of partial ureteral obstruction on urinary system stone disease formation. *Scientific Reports, 15*. https://www.semanticscholar.org/paper/deaa27da02bc834cff099ea6d7149644d7f159ba (accessed on 15th June 2025).

13. Ding, X., Cheng, Z., & Qian, Q. (2017). Intravenous fluids and acute kidney injury. *Blood Purification, 43*, 163–172. https://doi.org/10.1159/000452702 (accessed on 15th June 2025).

14. Escalante, J., Hamza, M., Nishimura, B., Melecio, M., Davies-Sala, C., Tuttobene, M., Subils, T., et al. (2024). Carbapenem-resistant *Acinetobacter baumannii* (CRAB): Metabolic adaptation and transcriptional response to human urine (HU). *Scientific Reports, 14*. https://www.semanticscholar.org/paper/3d5d0bad08a9d95d6be58c009bed09449c1b5c1d (accessed on 15th June 2025).

15. Faisal, A., & Hasan, S. F. (2024). Evaluation of Vit. D3 and Zn levels in patients with urinary tract infections. *Kufa Journal for Nursing Sciences*. https://www.semanticscholar.org/paper/739a5b5577f6782857af779dab24eb52be2c6533 (accessed on 15th June 2025).

16. Faisal, M. S. (2025). The healing power of nature: Herbal medications in treating urinary tract infections. *International Journal of Pathology*. https://www.semanticscholar.org/paper/9174f78cfe9e254877f29ad5d616b72b96685353 (accessed on 15th June 2025).

17. Farag, M., Elghazaly, E., & Khaliel, S. (2025). The relation between antibiotic resistance and biofilm formation in *Klebsiella* species isolated from human, sheep and goats at Matrouh Governorate, Egypt. *Alexandria Journal of Veterinary Sciences*. https://www.semanticscholar.org/paper/580774a68d31bc5174b6f73a3927eb0b231c3961 (accessed on 15th June 2025).

18. Gun, L., Ru, Y., Han, T., & Lu, J. (2017). Bioinformatics tools study on the sequence and structure characteristics of urinary prokallikrein. *(2)*, 9–11. https://www.semanticscholar.org/paper/6ec9baf04f62e0f109b6e285f01e4ef053db9d68 (accessed on 15th June 2025).

19. Hashim, R., Qadri, M. A. B., Malik, A., Ansari, N. A., & Khan, M. I. (2024). Hippocrates's contribution exploring the Tashrih-Al-Nizam-E-Baul (anatomy of urinary system): A comprehensive review. *SAR Journal of Anatomy and Physiology*. https://www.semanticscholar.org/paper/0d0e6b04ce0016ee465b47d8af1074dbc6b57d21 (accessed on 15th June 2025).

20. Hou, K., Wu, Z. X., Chen, X. Y., Wang, J. Q., Zhang, D., Xiao, C., Zhu, D., et al. (2022). Microbiota in health and diseases. *Signal Transduction and Targeted Therapy, 7*. https://doi.org/10.1038/s41392-022-00974-4 (accessed on 15th June 2025).

21. Hu, Z., Cano, I., Lei, F., Liu, J., Ramos, R. B., Gordon, H., Paschalis, E. I., et al. (2024). Loss of the endothelial glycocalyx component EMCN leads to glomerular impairment. *Circulation Research, 136*, 59–74. https://www.semanticscholar.org/paper/addd21020c879dd5300e612aa6d449c43c8e1086 (accessed on 15th June 2025).

22. Ketkhao, P., Utrarachkij, F., Parikumsil, N., Poonchareon, K., Kerdsin, A., Ekchariyawat, P., Narongpun, P., et al. (2024). Phylogenetic diversity and virulence gene characteristics of *Escherichia coli* from pork and patients with urinary tract infections in Thailand. *PLOS ONE, 19*. https://www.semanticscholar.org/paper/4860c7a251f59d0a15da9e808c58a2e29be4f1d0 (accessed on 15th June 2025).

23. Khalsa, S. S., Adolphs, R., Cameron, O. G., Critchley, H., Davenport, P. W., Feinstein, J. S., Feusner, J. D., et al. (2017). Interoception and mental health: A roadmap. *Biological Psychiatry: Cognitive Neuroscience and Neuroimaging, 3*, 501–513. https://doi.org/10.1016/j.bpsc.2017.12.004 (accessed on 15th June 2025).

24. Khan, A., Jamil, M., Ullah, M., Ullah, I., Zubair, M., & Saheem, S. (2023). Causes, precautions and management of risk factors associated with dehydration among athletes. *The Therapist (Journal of Therapies & Rehabilitation Sciences)*. https://www.semanticscholar.org/paper/e092c31ed2ac9404d3e66e1e8a408b6d039b0d16 (accessed on 15th June 2025).

25. Klatt, O. C., de Brouwer, L., Hendriks, F., Dehne, E., Ataç Wagegg, B., Jennings, P., & Wilmes, A. (2025). Human and rat renal proximal tubule *in vitro* models for ADME applications. *Archives of Toxicology*. https://www.semanticscholar.org/paper/e14d3814f27ffbfae1421b623b88884e16da20ab (accessed on 15th June 2025).

26. Kupferwasser, D., Kang, A. Y., Chen, L., Huse, H. K., & Miller, L. G. (2025). P-1592. Diagnostic stewardship cutoffs for urinalysis results prior to performing a urine culture: Analysis of data from a healthcare system. *Open Forum Infectious Diseases, 12*. https://www.semanticscholar.org/paper/24824a20f2dc8e9e05756631eec14836a1f0347c (accessed on 15th June 2025).

27. Kutia, S., Eremin, A. V., & Alekseev, M. A. (2023). [Etymology of Russian terms in the anatomy of the urinary system]. *Urologic, 3*, 114–116. https://www.semanticscholar.org/paper/b79f79a4d091cefee7d0263d64c69eaf7625d469 (accessed on 15th June 2025).

28. Labayen, M., Ochoa de Eribe, D., Aramburu, A., Nieto, M., & Aginako, N. (2024). European common data management platform definition for railway AI function development. *Transportation Development Research*. https://www.semanticscholar.org/paper/8cf4fd0285463ee8458d6d1168e3263ceef82d41 (accessed on 15th June 2025).

29. LeBoff, M. S., Greenspan, S. L., Insogna, K., Lewiecki, E. M., Saag, K. G., Singer, A., & Siris, E. S. (2022). The clinician's guide to prevention and treatment of osteoporosis. *Osteoporosis International, 33*, 2049–2102. https://doi.org/10.1007/s00198-021-05900-y (accessed on 15th June 2025).

30. Liguori, I., Russo, G., Curcio, F., Bulli, G., Aran, L., Della-Morte, D., Gargiulo, G., et al. (2018). Oxidative stress, aging, and diseases. *Clinical Interventions in Aging, 13*, 757–772. https://doi.org/10.2147/cia.s158513 (accessed on 15th June 2025).

31. Lu, G., & Fei, B. (2014). Medical hyperspectral imaging: A review. *Journal of Biomedical Optics, 19*, 010901. https://doi.org/10.1117/1.jbo.19.1.010901 (accessed on 15th June 2025).

32. Mahajan, T., Sarma, K., & Devi, J. (2021). Prenatal histological development of the nephron in goat fetus (*Capra hircus*). *International Journal of Current Microbiology and Applied Sciences, 10*, 1493–1499. https://www.semanticscholar.org/paper/3ca5457b5581226813b7ebd284f98e7df568bbac (accessed on 15th June 2025).

33. Manyi-Loh, C. E., Mamphweli, S., Meyer, E. L., & Okoh, A. I. (2018). Antibiotic use in agriculture and its consequential resistance in environmental sources: Potential public health implications. *Molecules, 23*, 795. https://doi.org/10.3390/molecules23040795 (accessed on 15th June 2025).

34. Michael, O. S., Kanthakumar, P., Soni, H. M., Lenin, R., Jha, K. A., Gangaraju, R., & Adebiyi, A. (2024). Upregulation of the urotensin II system in diabetic kidney disease includes urotensin II-related peptide. *Physiology*. https://www.semanticscholar.org/paper/fd7e54203f7b0aecdba4f8b56bc6c70de7a921fd (accessed on 15th June 2025).

35. Mungara, P., MacNaughton, K., & Cordat, E. (2024). Investigating the urinary salt losing phenotype in R607H and L919X mutant mice with distal renal tubular acidosis. *Physiology*. https://www.semanticscholar.org/paper/05f829c6c1be8d85ce89eb154b95da123063abc2 (accessed on 15th June 2025).

36. Murray, C. J. L., Ikuta, K. S., Sharara, F., Swetschinski, L. R., Robles Aguilar, G., Gray, A. P., Han, C., et al. (2022). Global burden of bacterial antimicrobial resistance in 2019: A systematic analysis. *The Lancet, 399*, 629–655. https://doi.org/10.1016/s0140-6736(21)02724-0 (accessed on 15th June 2025).

37. O'Callaghan, L. A., Olsen, M., Tajouri, L., Beaver, D., Hudson, C., Alghafri, R., McKirdy, S. J., et al. (2024). Plastic induced urinary tract disease and dysfunction: A scoping review. *Journal of Exposure Science & Environmental Epidemiology*. https://www.semanticscholar.org/paper/7709ada00c1cee64153f035b54d4c4c1c7179d18 (accessed on 15th June 2025).

38. Rameshk, M. (2024). The cause of kidney stone formation and treatment from the perspective of conventional and traditional Persian medicine. *Traditional and Integrative Medicine*. https://www.semanticscholar.org/paper/cd5c8138584da974be4d44246dfae67b97b23902 (accessed on 15th June 2025).

39. Rodak, K., Kokot, I., & Kratz, E. M. (2021). Caffeine as a factor influencing the functioning of the human body—Friend or foe? *Nutrients, 13*, 3088–3088. https://doi.org/10.3390/nu13093088 (accessed on 15th June 2025).

40. Santoro, D., Šebeková, K., Teta, D., & De Nicola, L. (2015). Extra skeletal functions of vitamin D. *BioMed Research International, 2015*. https://www.semanticscholar.org/paper/5889f705a0e93d22643964aae5756f9a3338e6de (accessed on 15th June 2025).

41. Savitska, A. A., Konoplitskyi, V. S., & Korobko, Y. (2024). Evolution of views on the functional anatomy of the vesicoureteral segment and etiopathogenetic features of vesicoureteral reflux in children. *Pediatric Surgery. Ukraine*. https://www.semanticscholar.org/paper/f1b709168f39e33c36567d879d54c4a3cd0b708b (accessed on 15th June 2025).

42. Shajari, A., Ahmadabadi, A. Z., Ashrafi, M. M., Mahdavi, T., Mirzaee, M., Mohkam, M., Sharafian, S., et al. (2024). Inborn errors of immunity with kidney and urinary tract disorders: A review. *International Urology and Nephrology, 56*, 1965–1972. https://www.semanticscholar.org/paper/913b6f50ab9af2c7e18d51ad0794e8488f416232 (accessed on 15th June 2025).

43. Sharma, N., Sharma, A. K., & Meena, R. R. (2025). A critical study of the physiological concept of "Mutra Utpatt"–Ayurveda and modern science perspective. *International Journal of Pharmaceutical Research and Applications*. https://www.semanticscholar.org/paper/95b473333975bd0028d0e84b042b1a8877dabd0a (accessed on 15th June 2025).

44. Skov, J., Dejgaard, A., Frøkiær, J., Holst, J., Jonassen, T., Rittig, S., & Christiansen, J. (2013). Glucagon-like peptide-1 (GLP-1): Effect on kidney hemodynamics and renin-angiotensin-aldosterone system in healthy men. *The Journal of Clinical Endocrinology and Metabolism, 98*(4), E664–E671. https://www.semanticscholar.org/paper/dc87f52d3e40047fc05ffa7f6303b5458118a70e (accessed on 15th June 2025).

45. Spahn, D. R., Bouillon, B., Černý, V., Duranteau, J., Filipescu, D., Hunt, B. J., Komadina, R., et al. (2019). The European guideline on management of major bleeding and coagulopathy following trauma: Fifth edition. *Critical Care, 23*. https://doi.org/10.1186/s13054-019-2347-3 (accessed on 15th June 2025).

46. Tsyhykalo, O., & Vladychenko, K. (2024). Comparative morphology of prenatal angiogenesis of the urinary system of humans and domestic pig (*Sus domestica*). *Bukovina Medical Herald*. https://www.semanticscholar.org/paper/88fb986b7a2c2f31f180ee42649d28a43fc514a9 (accessed on 15th June 2025).

47. Tyukavin, A., Gayvoronskiy, I., Maystrenko, V., & Nichiporuk, G. (2025). *Human Anatomy and Physiology*. https://www.semanticscholar.org/paper/bafe8bd3c43be23121274e95625ac68ac05c3581 (accessed on 15th June 2025).

48. Wang, J., Yu, Z., Chen, Z., Ye, F., & Sun, Z. (2025). The potential role of Zika and dengue virus infection in the urogenital system disorders: An overview. *Reviews in Medical Virology, 35*. https://www.semanticscholar.org/paper/8f1cec100464715009be02a8728bb7940176d89e (accessed on 15th June 2025).

49. Weldon, K. C., Panitchpakdi, M., Caraballo-Rodríguez, A., Wolfe, A. J., Dorrestein, P. C., Brubaker, L., & Burnett, L. A. (2025). Urinary metabolomic profile is minimally impacted by common storage conditions and additives. *International Urogynecology Journal, 36*, 839–847. https://www.semanticscholar.org/paper/e288f5aec81f66164b0ecee29d67863564cf54d3 (accessed on 15th June 2025).

50. Yan, J., Zhang, Y., Jiao, Z., Song, L., Wang, Z., Zhang, Q., Liu, Y., et al. (2024). Opportunities and challenges of ultrasonic diagnostic techniques for plant-based food monitoring: Principle, machine system, and application strategies. *Critical Reviews in Food Science and Nutrition*. https://www.semanticscholar.org/paper/807d341443dacded407ada8a1745052a84801cab (accessed on 15th June 2025).

51. Zapf, A. M., Halperin Kuhns, V. L., & Woodward, O. (2023). Renal tubular uric acid influences water reabsorption, urine concentration, and K+ homeostasis. *Physiology*. https://www.semanticscholar.org/paper/3e09b86131181f9e1305b376a5a84dd828ffef93 (accessed on 15th June 2025).

52. Zhang, H., Tao, S., Chen, H., Fang, Y., Xu, Y., Chen, L., Ma, F., et al. (2024). The biological function of the type II toxin-antitoxin system ccdAB in recurrent urinary tract infections. *Frontiers in Microbiology, 15*, 1379625. https://www.semanticscholar.org/paper/770c7466c4b1d5ccf201ef28d5453f5a175d695b (accessed on 15th June 2025).

53. Zhang, Y., Liu, Y., Liu, H., & Tang, W. H. (2019). Exosomes: Biogenesis, biologic function and clinical potential. *Cell & Bioscience, 9*. https://doi.org/10.1186/s13578-019-0282-2 (accessed on 15th June 2025).

54. Zou, L., & Sun, L. (2024). #635 Effect of multi-biomarker panels based on urinary N-terminal osteopenia on prediction of diabetic kidney disease in patients with diabetes mellitus. *Nephrology Dialysis Transplantation*. https://www.semanticscholar.org/paper/8e448afb6b0b8d5fe6d6078809c91f2388b17179 (accessed on 15th June 2025).

MALE REPRODUCTIVE SYSTEM

11

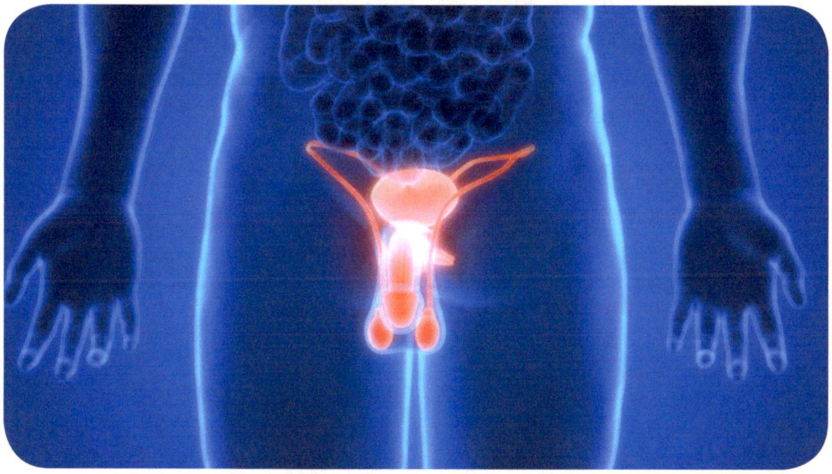

LEARNING OBJECTIVES

After studying this chapter, you will be able to:

1. Understand the anatomy of the male reproductive system
2. Describe the function of the male reproductive system
3. Learn about common disorders of the male reproductive system
4. Understand the male reproductive health and wellness
5 Describe the male reproductive system and sexual health
6. Understand the advances in male reproductive medicine

Introduction

The male reproductive system is an essential biological system utilized in an attempt to produce, develop, and deliver sperm, as well as to secrete masculine hormones. A thorough investigation of the system not only explains its physiological complexity but also its critical role in human reproduction. The system is created by a series of anatomical structures like the testes, seminal vesicles, prostate gland, and ductal systems, all of which are functionally controlled to facilitate reproduction. A critical analysis of the male reproductive system allows us to develop an appreciation of its functions from gamete production to hormonal regulation, and it is a vital part of maintaining male reproductive health. In addition, research into interactions among environmental, genetic, and lifestyle factors affecting male reproductive function provides an overview of contemporary health problems, underscoring the need for highly focused research into male reproductive physiology (Souza et al., 2019). It is shown that there are female and male reproductive health issues in common. In recent times, it has been proposed to examine a Male Athlete Triad similar to the highly reported Female Athlete Triad. Such research further contributes to a broader spectrum of thought on energy availability and its consequences on reproductive function and fueling controversy in male reproductive health (Laing et al., 2017). Disruptions in energy balance, usually caused by a bad diet or excessive exercise, could have quantifiable effects on the male reproductive axis and affect testosterone and sperm production levels. Such correlations are used to estimate lifestyle's contribution to effects on reproductive health and point out pathways through which prevention and therapies can reverse the on-rising problems with male fertility and health.

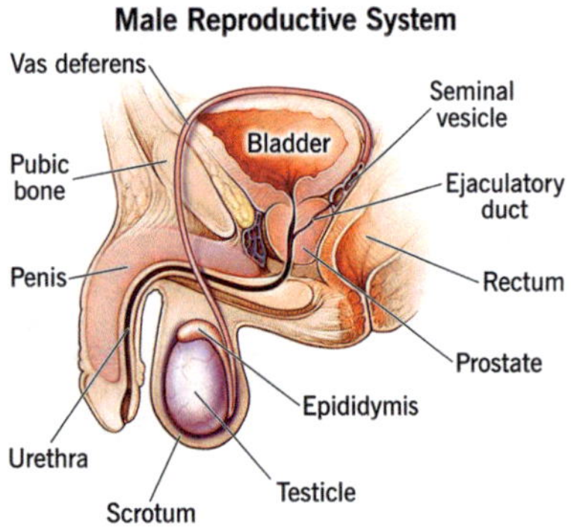

Figure 11.1. The male reproductive system consists of internal and external organs. These organs help you have sexual intercourse and pee.

Source: https://my.clevelandclinic.org/-/scassets/images/org/health/articles/9117-male-reproductive-system

This model is a first point of thought for future research in the academic field of male reproductive physiology. Since the male reproductive system is increasingly threatened by determinants of lifestyle in today's world and disease states, there is a pressing requirement to examine such dynamics under critical scrutiny. Endocrine imbalance, lifestyle determinants, and environmental determinants are causing issues like declining fertility and diseases related to reproduction among men. With signs tending to suggest poor sperm quality as linked to a variety of ailments, once more, the necessity for general health care is impressed upon us. Understanding of biological and environmental mechanisms in the male reproductive tract can be applied to make public health policy and personal health behavior more effective in optimizing reproductive function. With greater awareness of such factors, the stakeholders can come up with revolutionary strategies to favor male reproductive health and counter prevalent issues within this field, towards healthier future generations (Souza et al., 2019).

11.1. Anatomy of the Male Reproductive System

Learning Outcome

1. Describe the external and internal structures of the male reproductive system
2. Learn about the accessory glands of the male reproductive system

The anatomy of the male reproductive system is a sensitive relationship between the organs and structures that support reproduction. Central to the system is the testes, which perform several functions like spermatozoa formation and testosterone secretion. The testes are located in the scrotum, whose external environment not only favors spermatogenesis but also functions in regulating temperature, a factor that is extremely important for sperm viability. Located alongside the testes is the epididymis, where sperm mature and are stored. The vas deferens passes from the epididymis, transporting sperm on ejaculation. As they travel through the male reproductive tract, sperm become mixed with seminal fluid that is secreted by accessory glands such as the seminal vesicles and prostate gland to create semen, the fluid used in internal fertilization (Kelly and Moore, 2016). Morphological variation in the male reproductive system is used to highlight evolutionary adaptations that enhance reproductive fitness. Intromittent organs, like the penis, exhibit a highly varied array of morphological adaptations across species, aimed at maximizing sperm delivery into the female reproductive system.

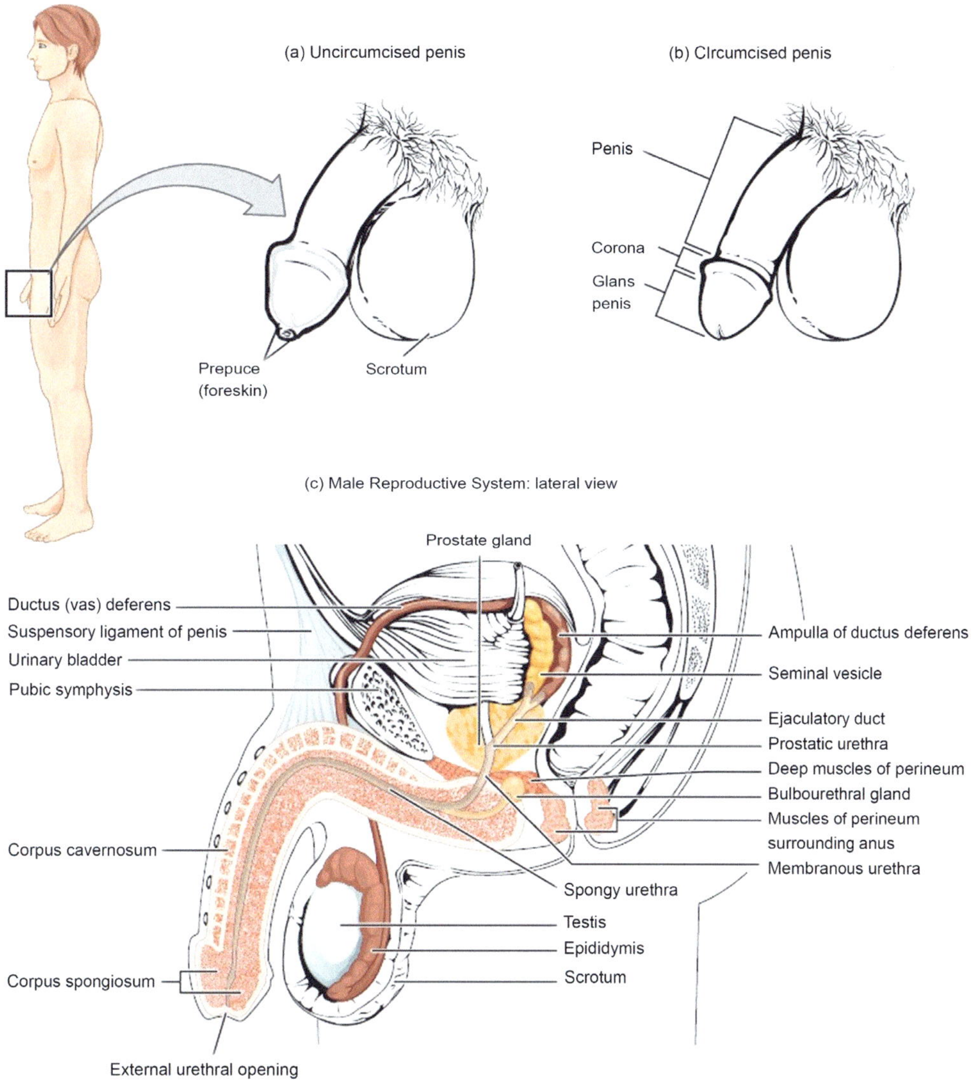

Figure 11.2. The structures of the male reproductive system include the testes, the epididymides, the penis, and the ducts and glands that produce and carry semen. Sperm exit the scrotum through the ductus deferens, which is bundled in the spermatic cord. The seminal vesicles and prostate gland add fluids to the sperm to create semen.

Source: https://s3-us-west-2.amazonaws.com/courses-images-archive-read-only/wp-content/uploads/sites/403/2015/04/21031908/Figure_28_01_01.jpg

Sexual selection forces and coevolutionary processes between male and female reproductive morphologies are illustrated as mechanisms that produce such variation. For instance, anatomical structure variations enable various species to cope with challenges posed by female anatomy and reproductive strategies. Additionally, copulation biomechanics can inform the evolutionary path of these structures, illustrating to us the complex interplay between anatomy, functionality, and sexual dynamics (Kelly and Moore, 2016). This points out how essential it is to understand the anatomy of the male reproductive system because it is part of not only individual species reproductive strategy but also general ecological and evolutionary processes. Moreover, the functioning and health of the male reproductive system can be negatively affected by environmental factors, particularly endocrine-disrupting chemicals (EDCs). These compounds disrupt hormone synthesis and signaling pathways and lead to a variety of reproductive health issues. Research has documented the harmful effects of EDCs on sperm development, virility, and male reproductive general health. The clinical and epidemiological findings substantiate mounting alarm regarding EDCs and their potential to disrupt normal reproductive mechanisms, therefore threatening public health. Resolution of these problems requires a multidisciplinary approach, necessitating increased research into the mechanism of action of EDCs on male reproductive anatomy and function, and public education on minimizing exposure to such harmful chemicals. Knowledge of these interactions between anatomy, environmental health, and reproductive outcome is vital for ensuring long-term male reproductive health.

11.1.1. External Structures: Penis and Scrotum

The external reproductive organs in males are primarily the penis and scrotum, which both play significant roles in sexual and reproductive life. The penis is the organ employed for copulation and the ejaculation of sperm into the female reproductive system. Its anatomy includes the shaft, glans, and the urethra, from which semen is pushed out at ejaculation. The penis contains erectile tissues like corpora cavernosa and corpus spongiosum, which enable its enlargement and stiffening upon sexual arousal. The distal end of the penis also contains the urethral opening through which urine and semen are expelled from the body. This functional arrangement highlights the penis's double purpose during urination and reproduction, with reference to its significance in the male reproductive system as described in research on other anatomical arrangements. The scrotum is a sack-like structure containing and supporting the testes, responsible for testosterone and sperm production. Sitting behind the penis, the scrotum is typically composed of a layer of cremaster muscle and skin, allowing it to regulate the testes' temperature in the optimal manner. Being slightly below the body's core temperature is necessary for the health of sperm production, a role facilitated by the capacity of the scrotum to constrict or relax with assistance from the dartos and cremaster muscles. The anatomical location of the scrotum and its mobility are essential in ensuring the ideal environment for spermatogenesis. The thermoregulatory role ensures testicular function, thereby enhancing reproductive success (Yllera et al., 2024). The penis and scrotum are not fixed structures; they are dynamic components of the male reproductive system, adapting to the influence of hormones as well as other physiological processes. For example, the presence of testosterone significantly impacts both organs, stimulating libido and facilitating growth and maintenance of reproductive tissue. Furthermore, the penis's capacity to become engorged when stimulated not only displays anatomical sophistication but also demonstrates the coordination of the circulatory and nervous systems. The coordination identifies the importance of extrinsic organs within the grand design of male fertility and reproductive health. As with other alternative species, such as the sugar glider, variation in these structures is used to emphasize evolutionary adaptations related to reproductive success across a range of settings, while requiring comprehensive knowledge of anatomy for clinical practice (Yllera et al., 2024).

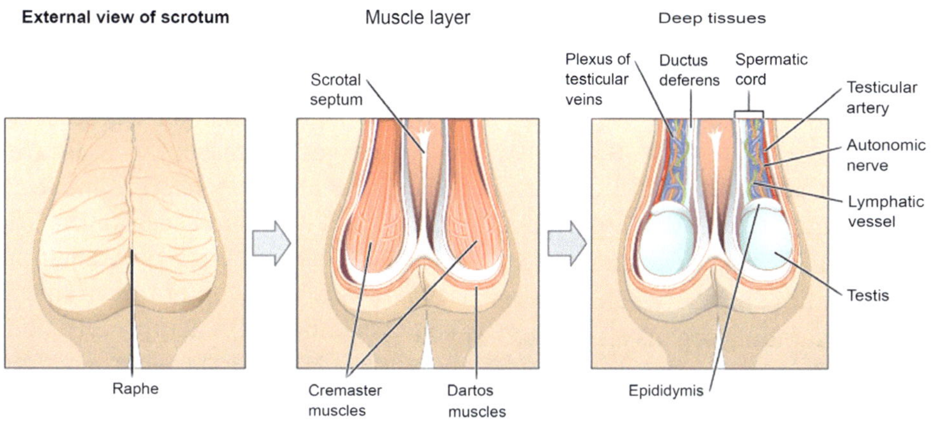

Figure 11.3. This anterior view shows the structures of the scrotum and testes.

Source: https://s3-us-west-2.amazonaws.com/courses-images-archive-read-only/wp-content/uploads/sites/403/2015/04/21031909/Figure_28_01_02.jpg

11.1.2. Internal Structures: Testes, Epididymis, and Vas Deferens

Testes belonging to the male reproductive system play numerous functions essential for reproduction, in addition to endocrine homeostasis. The testes that lie in the scrotum not only manufacture the sperm cells and the testosterone hormone required for secondary sexual characteristics of the male, but also the spermatogenesis of the seminiferous tubules of the testes occurs to produce immature spermatozoa. These tubules are controlled by Leydig cells, which secrete testosterone upon stimulation by luteinizing hormone. In this way, not only do the testes function to manufacture sperm but they also have a tremendous role in controlling the regulation of male reproductive wellness through hormonal control, thereby showing their double importance in the reproductive process. There needs to be an understanding of the anatomical and functional properties of the testes since the failure of the testes will cause infertility, along with disturbance in hormones and overall debilitation. Following spermatogenesis in the testes, immature spermatozoa are transported to the epididymis, a very specialized organ that is also attributed with the responsibility of assuming the central role in taking part during maturation of the spermatozoa. The epididymis is composed of four functionally different segments: the initial segment, caput, corpus, and cauda, each playing a unique role in the maturation process. Through the passage through all of them, sperm acquire motility and fertilizing capability, the critical attributes to ensure reproduction. The luminal environment of the epididymis is unique and facilitates extensive biochemical interaction required to maintain sperm function. Not surprisingly, the epididymis is also a defensive one, holding sperm until ejaculation and occasionally concentrating and filtering them. The function names the epididymis as a necessary reproductive organ, one that is integrated into the activity of the entire male reproductive system, as emphasized by the recent controversy surrounding sperm competence and how exosomes secreted by the epididymis influence them (James et al., 2020). Vas deferens, as a muscular tube, is a critical structure serving to carry mature sperm from the epididymis into the ejaculatory duct, hence leading to semen expulsion upon ejaculation. The vas deferens has functionally thick muscular walls that enable peristaltic contractions for efficient expulsion of sperm during male reproduction. In addition, it is noteworthy that the male genital tract is susceptible to certain viral infections that can significantly impact health and fertility (Tortorec et al., 2020).

The infections would lead to infertility, disease transmission, and more, and hence it is important to take into account the importance of the vas deferens in addition to its anatomical significance. The relationship between the vas deferens and the surrounding organs also places it in the male reproductive system and in the limelight for research on reproductive disease and possible therapies for the treatment of males.

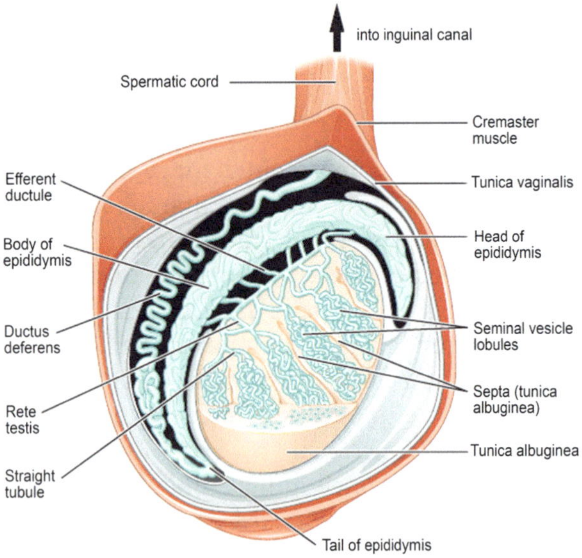

Figure 11.4. This sagittal view shows the seminiferous tubules, the site of sperm production. Formed sperm are transferred to the epididymis, where they mature. They leave the epididymis during an ejaculation via the ductus deferens.

Source: https://s3-us-west-2.amazonaws.com/courses-images-archive-read-only/wp-content/uploads/sites/403/2015/04/21031910/Figure_28_01_03.jpg

11.1.3. Accessory Glands: Seminal Vesicles, Prostate Gland, and Bulbourethral Glands

The male accessory glands play a crucial role in the production and secretion of seminal fluid, which is essential for successful fertilization. The largest accessory glands are the seminal vesicles, and they secrete most of the seminal plasma. The glands secrete the sticky fructose-rich fluid along with prostaglandins and other chemicals that contain nutrients and maintain sperm motility. A supply of such nutrients is needed because the sperm would have to be fueled and supplied once they are outside the male's body. The seminal vesicles also influence sperm motility and viability, thereby increasing the likelihood of successful fertilization. The complexity of the operations suggests that semen is not a passive transport fluid but a bioactive form, actively contributing to reproductive success and fertility. Following the seminal vesicles comes the second major accessory male reproductive system gland, which is the prostate gland. Its secretion contains enzymes, citric acid, and prostate-specific antigen (PSA), which aid in liquefying the semen following ejaculation and increase the sperm motility in the female reproductive system. The prostate is also involved in pH regulation to facilitate the sperm's viability within the vaginal canal's acidic environment. Prostate dysfunction because of inflammation, benign prostatic enlargement, or carcinoma may have a direct effect on male reproductive health and fertility. Issues in this area bring to the center consideration of research on the function of the prostate gland and its role in male reproductive illness, such as its function in elements of infertility included in research on the male microbiome and its role in reproductive health (Jendraszak et al., 2024; Das et al., 2023). BESIDES the prostate and seminal vesicles, the bulbourethral glands, also known as Cowper's glands, contribute yet another dimension of sophistication to male reproductive physiology. These little glands discharge a watery alkaline secretion prior to ejaculation that rinses away urethral acidity, thus paving the way for a more spermopoietic-friendly environment to proceed through. The secretion also lubricates the canal of the urethra so that semen may flow smoothly. Although the bulbourethral glands are smaller than the seminal vesicles and prostate, they play an essential pre-ejaculatory support that speaks volumes regarding the fine collaboration of these accessory glands. Understanding the functional mechanisms of the glands further complicates male fertility and highlights the necessity of further research into the degree to which their activity could be affected by various physiological and pathological factors (Jendraszak et al., 2024; Das et al., 2023).

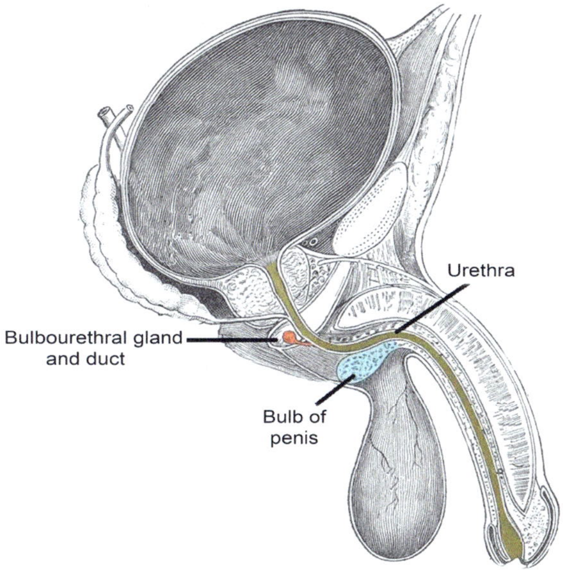

Figure 11.5. Anatomical position of the bulbourethral gland.

Source: https://teachmeanatomy.info/wp-content/uploads/Anatomical-Position-of-the-Bulbourethral-Glands.jpg.webp

Test Your Knowledge

1. What is the external structure of the scrotum?
2. What is the internal structure of the testes?

11.2. Function of the Male Reproductive System

Learning Outcome

1. Describe the sperm production and maturation
2. Understand the role of hormonal regulation in the functionality and health of the male reproductive system
3. Understand the role of the male reproductive system in sexual reproduction

The male reproductive system has several vital functions required for sexual reproduction, primarily sperm production, maturation, and ejaculation. The process initiates in the testes, where spermatogenesis is finalized and results in sperm cells through a series of complicated cell divisions. The sperm cells are then matured and stored in the epididymis to gain motility and capacity for fertilization. The systemic control of androgen hormones, primarily testosterone, performs a key function in the execution of these roles. The hormone is involved not just in sperm formation but also in secondary sexual characteristics and reproductive health overall. An impeccable mix of these factors again suggests the key role adopted by the male reproductive system in the fulfillment of reproduction and species existence. Apart from spermatogenesis, the male reproductive system also possesses specialized intromittent structures supporting intromission of sperm into the female reproductive system during coition. The intromittent organ is the penis, which is an important instrument in internal fertilization. This is an evolved anatomical device designed to place the sperm directly inside the female reproductive system in order to offer a higher chance of successful fertilization. Morphology of the penis differs greatly between species, as it has been influenced by sexual selection and compatibility with the female reproductive organs. These differences highlight the way in which morphological specializations contribute to reproductive efficiency optimization and, as such, seemingly the male reproductive system evolved not only functionally but also based on ecological and evolutionary constraints, as described in more recent literature regarding the intricacies of intromittent organ evolution and function, as detailed in Kelly and Moore (2016). Apart from this, recent endocrine-disrupting chemicals (EDCs) issues refer to the potential harm or damage inflicted on the male reproductive system function. EDCs are widespread within the environment and consumer products, which compromise hormonal biosynthesis as well as action and thus attack reproductive health. These chemicals have been linked to cause pathological effects on the generation, quality, and overall reproductive health of both humans and animals. Exposure to EDCs bears consequences beyond personal health, and population dynamics and genetic diversity may be impaired. Consequences of EDCs are analyzed through a multi-disciplinary approach, including toxicology, endocrinology, and epidemiology, as has been confirmed in recent research studies (Diamanti E-Kandarakis et al., 2009). As individuals become more sensitized to the risk induced by such substances, interventions aimed at preventing them from inhibiting exposure and maintaining the integrity of male reproductive functions need to be sought.

11.2.1. Spermatogenesis and Sperm Maturation

Spermatogenesis, or spermogenesis, is a developmentally and regulatively complex process that occurs in the testes. Spermatogenesis begins with mitosis of spermatogonial stem cells, which are located in the seminiferous tubules. Spermatogonial cells undergo successive processes of differentiation culminating in the formation of mature spermatozoa. The tubular microenvironment of the seminiferous tubules is crucial to spermatogenesis and is under the regulation of Sertoli cells, which provide the necessary support and nourishment. The process culminates in round spermatids, which, through a series of morphological changes, are transformed into elongated spermatozoa. As spermatogenesis is very susceptible to hormonal fluctuations, particularly testosterone, any disruption in the hormones will harm the sperm development and lead to male infertility, which illustrates how carefully the balance needs to be struck in order to attain optimal reproductive fitness. Once the process of spermatogenesis is complete, the sperm must mature in the epididymis, a coiled tubular organ near the testes. Recently expelled sperm are immature and do not have the ability to fertilize. During their journey through the epididymis, sperm gain motility and acquire fertilizing capacity by undergoing chemical changes under the direction of epididymal secretions. A strange mention is due to epididymosomes, extracellular vesicles released by epididymal epithelial cells, which have a significant contribution in sperm maturation by sharing proteins, lipids, and RNAs with sperm. All these factors contribute to remodeling the sperm proteome, function, and viability potential. Also, the epididymis contributes towards the establishment of protective mechanisms of the sperm to safeguard them against the female reproductive tract immune system to enable the sperm to successfully fertilize when they reach their destination. The role of defensins, identified as antimicrobial peptides, once more highlights the importance of an intact epididymis in sperm maturation. Defensins have also been found to be expressed in the male reproductive tract, i.e., the epididymis, where they contribute to sperm viability by providing protection from bacterial infection. This antimicrobial function is essential for infection causes male infertility through impaired immune motility of sperm and reproductive overall fitness. Not only protect the sperm but also enable them to mature by maintaining the local immune microenvironment and enabling maximally effective interaction between sperm and the encompassing fluid environment. As there is greater knowledge gained in terms of such molecular mechanisms, one such possible therapy that can enhance the fertility of men is targeted therapy, with the new avenues in treating infertility conditions of men with a focus on the production and development of sperm in male reproductive health (Zhai et al., 2022; Barrachina et al., 2022).

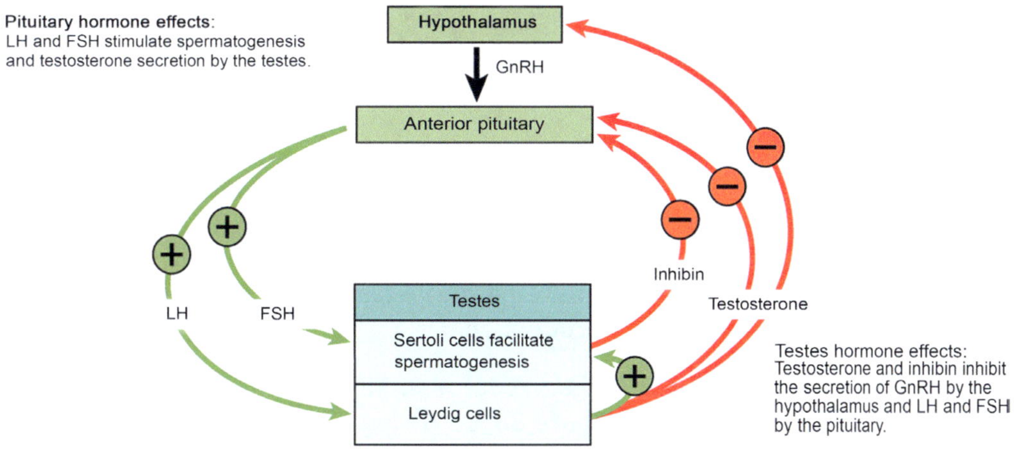

Figure 11.6. Hormones control sperm production in a negative feedback system.

Source: https://s3-us-west-2.amazonaws.com/courses-images/wp-content/uploads/sites/3206/2018/05/04134322/Figure_43_04_01.jpg

11.2.2. Hormonal Regulation: Testosterone and Other Hormones

Hormonal control is essential to the function and health of the male reproductive system, primarily through the action of testosterone and other hormones of equivalent significance. Testosterone, which is produced in the testes, plays a critical role in spermatogenesis, or sperm cell formation. It is synthesized under tightly regulated control by the hypothalamic-pituitary-gonadal (HPG) axis, which activates the testes by the action of luteinizing hormone (LH). The secretory patterns of these hormones have the capacity to significantly influence male fertility; thus, any disruption of the axis will lead to reproductive disorders. As has been observed in Li et al. (2024), coordination of androgens like testosterone with follicle-stimulating hormone (FSH) facilitates Sertoli and germ cell development, which are vital determinants of healthy production of spermatozoa. Without such coordination of hormones, male fertility can be influenced, and this creates reproductive health issues.

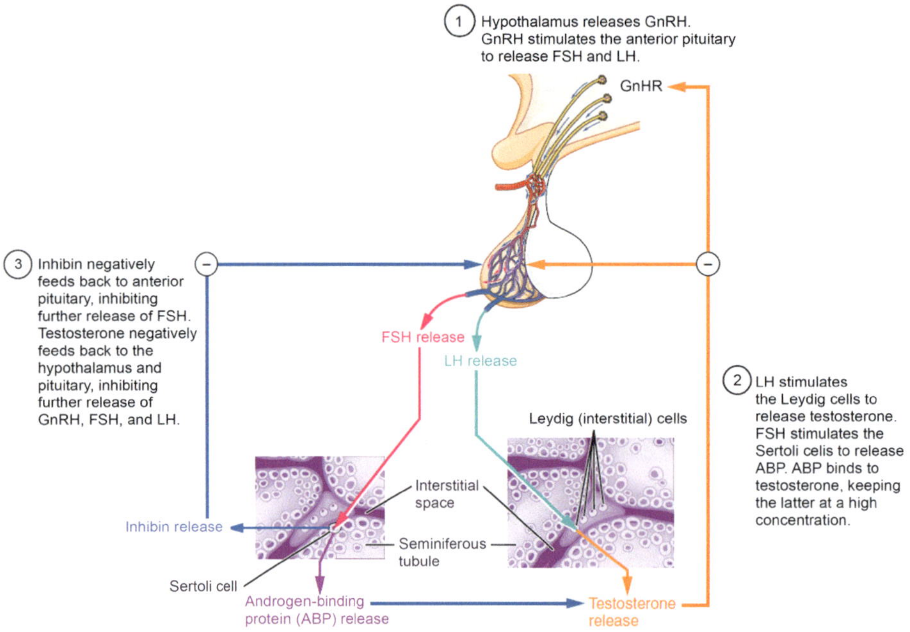

Figure 11.7. The hypothalamus and pituitary gland regulate the production of testosterone and the cells that assist in spermatogenesis. GnRH activates the anterior pituitary to produce LH and FSH, which in turn stimulate Leydig cells and Sertoli cells, respectively. The system is a negative feedback loop because the end products of the pathway, testosterone and inhibin, interact with the activity of GnRH to inhibit their own production.

Source: https://s3-us-west-2.amazonaws.com/courses-images-archive-read-only/wp-content/uploads/sites/403/2015/04/21031919/Figure_28_01_07.jpg

Furthermore, the impact of external factors on hormonal regulation cannot be overstated. The GnRH pulsatile secretion by the hypothalamus is regulated by numerous external and internal variables, including nutritional status, stress levels, and photoperiodic changes. These factors dictate the HPG axis dynamics and, consequently, testosterone release. As has been noted in Zhao et al. (2023), dialogue between nutrition and reproductive physiology is critical; hormonal communication will be modulated based on energy availability, therefore directly impacting sperm development and overall reproductive quality. Such biological responsiveness is the evolutionary significance of hormonal regulation for allowing male organisms to optimize reproductive primacy under varying environmental conditions. A good understanding of such interactions can facilitate the driving of improvements in fertility drugs and contraceptives. Lastly, the intricate balance between testosterone and other hormones underscores the combined effect on broader-ranging physiological and behavioral aspects of male reproduction. Changes in levels of testosterone are well known to affect aggression, libido, and physiological metabolic rate, all toward reproductive success. The regulation of these hormones is not only limited to reproductive processes but also encompasses the regulation of social behaviors and interactions critical to mating and reproductive behavior. The study of neuropeptides and their role in GnRH release, as opened up by current research, is a promising area of reproductive endocrinology. In particular, findings on the kisspeptin-neurokinin-dynorphin neuronal network significantly enhance our understanding of mechanisms of hormonal regulation in male reproductive efficiency (Zhao et al., 2023). Proper management and enhancement of male reproductive health in farm animals and humans alike are contingent on this comprehensive understanding of hormonal regulation.

11.2.3. Role in Sexual Reproduction

The male system of reproduction is a vital aspect of sexual reproduction and is responsible primarily for the production of sperm and fertilization. At the center of the functioning of the system lies the process of spermatogenesis, which occurs in the seminiferous tubules of the testes. The process is a multifaceted one and is regulated by a cascade of hormonal signals, including luteinizing hormone (LH) and follicle-stimulating hormone (FSH), that stimulate the testes to produce spermatozoa. After sperm cells reach maturity, they undergo a series of modifications needed for successful fertilization, including the development of motility and the formation of an acrosome. An acrosomal reaction is crucial as it allows the sperm to penetrate the protective sheath of the ovum, creating the coming together of genetic material. Furthermore, fertility and quality of sperm have a direct correlation with reproductive success, emphasizing the critical role that male reproductive health contributes to the sexual reproduction continuum. In addition to sperm production, the male reproductive system also plays a significant role in regulating hormones, which is achieved through the action of kisspeptin, a neuropeptide with wide-ranging effects on reproductive function. Kisspeptin controls the secretion and synthesis of gonadotropin-releasing hormone (GnRH), which in turn activates the release of other key hormones—LH and FSH. They not only contribute decisively to spermatogenesis but also control sexual urge and arousal in males. The action of kisspeptin on the hypothalamic-pituitary-gonadal (HPG) axis is, therefore, a way of underlining the importance of hormonal equilibrium in male reproductive function. Dysregulation of kisspeptin signaling could lead to a number of reproductive disorders, ultimately depicting its inherent role in guaranteeing fertility as well as the regulation of reproductive behavior in males, as evident from research linking its dysregulation with disorders such as infertility and other hormonal disorders (Korkmaz, 2024). Moreover, the evolutionary significance of male reproductive strategies also cannot be overlooked when considering their function in sexual reproduction. The reproductive value theory (RV), conceived by Grafen and expanded by Gardner, proposes that males' reproductive efforts are intimately intertwined with genetic machinery and life history strategies. The implication is that male reproductive tactics influence individual fitness, population-level processes, and within-population genetic variation. Males typically exhibit alternative strategies ranging from monogamous pair bonding to competitive polygyny, which can lead to varying reproductive fortunes in reaction to different environmental and social contexts. Understanding these strategies puts into context how the male adapts and optimizes his reproductive yield, solidifying the assertion that the male reproductive system plays a pivotal role in propagating genetic lines and contributing to the broader sexual reproduction canvas (Rautiala and Lehtonen., 2024).

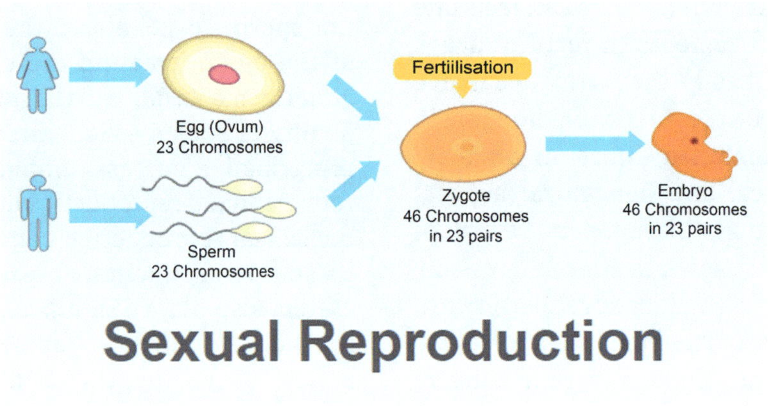

Figure 11.8. Sexual Reproduction.

Source: https://www.careerpower.in/blog/wp-content/uploads/sites/2/2023/08/31135454/sexual-reproduction..png

Test Your Knowledge

1. What is the production and maturation of sperm?
2. What are the roles of hormones in the male reproductive system?

11.3. Common Disorders of the Male Reproductive System

Learning Outcome

1. Know the erectile dysfunction and its causes
2. Describe the prostate disorders
3. Describe the testicular conditions

The male reproductive system is susceptible to numerous disorders that can create a meaningful impact on overall reproductive health. Among the most common fertility conditions of males is varicocele, characterized by the enlargement of scrotal veins. Varicocele can lead to impaired sperm production and endocrine status, predisposing to infertility. Evidence demonstrates that the condition exists in approximately 15% of the total male population and 40% of men who are infertile. The pathophysiological mechanisms are believed to involve increased testicular temperature and altered blood flow, which could inhibit spermatogenesis. Diagnosis also typically involves physica examination, an ultrasound scan, and sometimes semen analysis to identify the level of fertility impairment.

Surgical therapy of varicocele has been documented to yield promising results in restoring fertility among some men with the condition, a sign of the necessity of early diagnosis and intervention to preserve reproductive capabilities. Another common disorder of the male reproductive apparatus is benign prostatic hyperplasia (BPH), a non-malignant hypertrophy of the prostate gland. This disease increases with advancing age and occurs in nearly 50% of men aged over 60 years. Enlargement of the prostate can lead to blockage of the urethra and cause urinary symptoms of frequency, urgency, and nocturia, which can impair quality of life. The etiology of BPH is not clearly established, but hormonal changes with aging have been thought to have a central etiologic role. Pharmacological management with alpha-blockers and 5-alpha-reductase inhibitors is common for control of symptoms as well as improvement in urinary flow. In complex and severe conditions, surgical treatments like transurethral resection of the prostate (TURP) are indicated, considering various treatment modalities for control of BPH and complications. Diseases of the testes, like testicular torsion and hypogonadism, are critical concerns of male reproductive health. Testicular torsion is an emergent condition where the spermatic cord twists, potentially causing testicular compromise of blood supply and necrosis if not immediately addressed. It classically presents with acute-onset scrotal pain and demands urgent surgical exploration to save the involved testicle. Hypogonadism, however, refers to low levels of testosterone production that can be caused by genetic conditions, trauma, or overall body disease. Hypogonadism is often characterized by lowered libido, lethargy, and infertility. Their treatment would include replacement with testosterone or treating the underlying medical condition, highlighting the necessity for detection and treatment of these disorders in order to preserve male reproductive health. In conclusion, knowledge of these prevalent disorders facilitates awareness, early detection, and proper management measures in the preservation of male reproductive function.

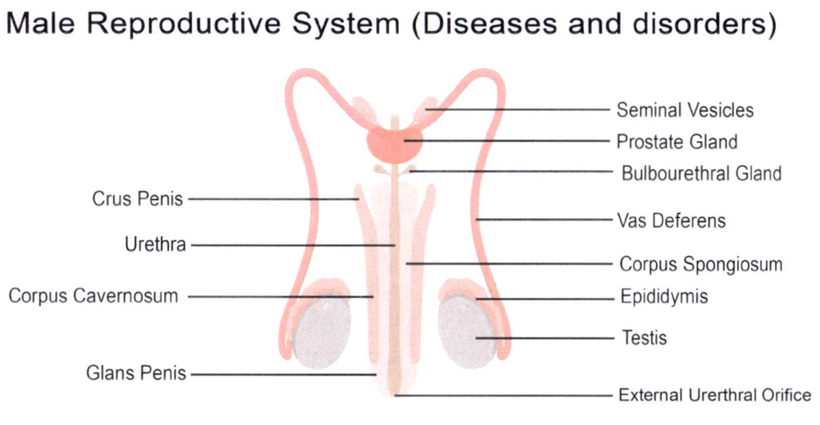

Figure 11.9. Diseases and disorders of the male reproductive system.

Source: https://microbenotes.com/wp-content/uploads/2020/11/Diseases-and-disorders-of-the-male-reproductive-system.jpeg

11.3.1. Erectile Dysfunction and Its Causes

Erectile dysfunction (ED) is a polyetiologic condition more prone to result from an aggregation of physiological and psychological etiologies. Physiological etiologies can be vascular, neurological, hormonal, or structural malfunctions of the male genital organs. Vascular status is particularly critical since it relates to blood inflow into the penis that is needed in order to produce and sustain an erection. Hypertension and atherosclerotic diseases encroach on blood circulation, consequently, erectile dysfunction. And hormonal imbalance, testosterone levels in particular, cause impaired libido and erectile function. The culmination of all this serves to emphasize the intricacy of both the diagnosis and treatment of erectile dysfunction within the overall framework of healthcare of the male reproductive system. Apart from physiological causes, psychological causes play a significant role in erectile dysfunction. Stress, depression, and anxiety are likely to have a suppressive effect on the libido and sexual responsiveness overall. Performance anxiety, especially, is likely to put a patient into a negative feedback loop where fear of failing to perform worsens the situation.

Psychological testing is usually part of treatment plans since treating the mental status of the patients will most likely result in better outcomes. Surprisingly, as other research shows, a large proportion of men with ED also have co-morbid mental illness, something that suggests that proper management of erectile dysfunction should be done from both the physical and mental health perspectives. The exploration of recent scientific advances also touches on the link between erectile dysfunction and underlying medical conditions. New data show that H2S is also involved in the modulation of vascular functions and penile smooth muscle relaxation, which are new therapeutic targets for treating ED (Song et al., 2024). Moreover, leprosy was shown to influence hormonal and testicular parameters and therefore to contribute to erectile dysfunction in infected individuals (Hegde et al., 2024). These findings underscore the importance of delineating the general significance of systemic health to sexual function in men. By establishing the pathophysiology of erectile dysfunction, clinicians are able to create more specific and effective treatment plans that maximize the sexual health and quality of life of men who suffer from this troublesome condition.

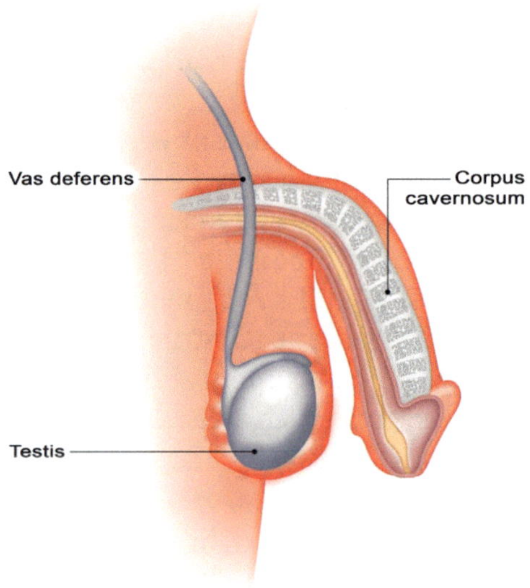

Figure 11.10. Erectile dysfunction.

Source: https://mindbodysoulmentalhealth.com/wp-content/uploads/2023/08/Erectile-Dysfunction-and-Vasectomy-768x863.jpg.webp

11.3.2. Prostate Disorders: Benign Prostatic Hyperplasia and Prostate Cancer

Prostate disorders like benign prostatic hyperplasia (BPH) and prostate cancer (PCa) are medical conditions prevalent in a significant proportion of the male population, especially with advancing age. BPH is a prostate enlargement causing urinary dysfunction and lower urinary tract symptoms. BPH frequently manifests as a hurried need to urinate, straining to void, and an incomplete emptying sensation of the bladder. Even though BPH is not cancerous, it has a substantial impact on quality of life. On the other hand, prostate cancer is a malignancy of prostate tissue that can be distinguished from normal by abnormal cellular growth with metastatic capability. Epidemiological studies have proved that early detection and treatment of BPH may well lower risks for subsequent development of prostate cancer and thereby highlight the interactive nature of these diseases in the field of male reproductive medicine. Investigation of the molecular and inflammatory processes underlying these prostate pathologies holds the secrets to their pathogenesis. Chronic inflammation, in fact, has become an impeller in BPH and PCa, with markers IL-8 and IL-6 being significantly increased in BPH tissues, proportionally to the degree of high-grade inflammation. Contrary to expectation, studies have shown that prostate cancer tissues contain greater levels of fibroblast growth factor-2 (FGF2), suggesting divergence of the mechanisms underlying these two conditions. Understanding the function of these inflammatory biomarkers could potentially uncover targeted therapies to reverse symptoms of BPH or to inhibit the onset of PCa. Further, the role of some microRNAs, such as members of the miR-29 family, has been highlighted for their ability to regulate DNA methyltransferases, making them therapeutic targets in prostate disease treatment (Foenna et al., 2025).

Implications of such research extend beyond symptomatology, and the potential exists to reshape treatment paradigms for prostate diseases. In particular, the convergence of inflammation, growth factors, and microRNA regulation allows a multi-aspect therapeutic strategy. For instance, research into miRNA-driven means of targeting DNMT3A and DNMT3B expression levels may open a new avenue for targeted therapy in opposition to cancer therapies targeting the inhibition of PCa progression while preserving prostatic function in BPH patients (Foenna et al., 2025). In addition, addressing the inflammatory component of BPH progression through interventions targeting IL-8 and IL-6 levels may be effective, underscoring the need for an integrated treatment approach. As research evolves, knowledge of these interactions will be crucial in developing comprehensive care plans within the context of male reproductive disorders with the objective of enhancing outcomes and quality of life.

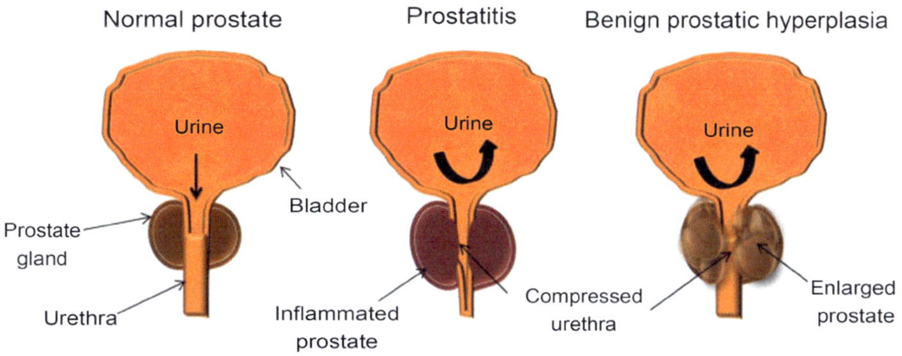

Figure 11.11. Representation of normal prostate gland, prostatitis and benign prostatic hyperplasia.

Source: https://ars.els-cdn.com/content/image/1-s2.0-S0009898119319916-gr1.jpg

11.3.3. Testicular Conditions: Torsion and Cancer

Testicular torsion refers to an urgent urological condition where the spermatic cord twists, thereby reducing blood supply to the testis. It typically affects adolescent males with the highest prevalence, but can affect any age group. It usually involves severe and acute pain, swelling of the affected testicle, and, in some cases, nausea, which may require immediate medical examination. Early treatment and diagnosis are crucial, as delayed treatment—usually surgical detorsion—is likely to lead to permanent loss of the testicle or damage to the testicle. In addition, within the broader context of the male reproductive system as a whole, consideration should also be given to the possibility of environmental exposures, for instance, to endocrine-disrupting chemicals (EDCs), playing a role in increased vulnerability to the conditions of torsion. Awareness of these associations enables more efficient preventive interventions and emphasizes reproductive health and potential risk factors for testicular torsion among young men (Pan et al., 2024). In contrast to torsion, testicular cancer is also a significant concern in male reproductive health and the most common solid tumor in young men. The pathogenesis of the condition is multi-factorial, with complex interactions among environmental factors, genetic susceptibility, and lifestyle. While the exact etiology is unknown, a few of the risk factors are cryptorchidism, family history of testicular malignancy, and EDC exposure.

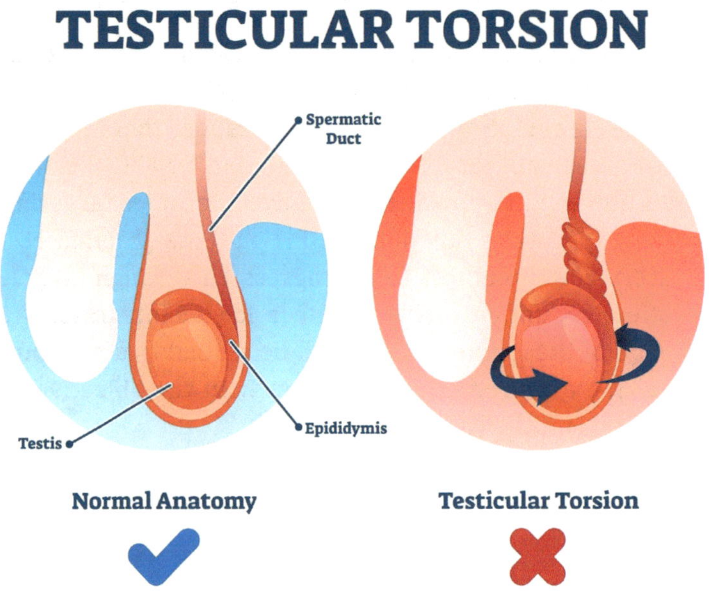

Figure 11.12. Testicular torsion.

Source: https://d2jx2rerrg6sh3.cloudfront.net/images/Article_Images/ImageForArticle_23682_16796634576666689.jpg

These risk factors have been implicated in conferring the higher risk of testicular tumors. Prompt detection by self-examination and surveillance for peculiar symptoms significantly increases cure rates. Besides, oncologic therapies like chemotherapy and radiotherapy have been shown to impact fertility significantly, and hence the necessity of pre-treatment counseling for sperm banking. Effective communication among care providers and patients is essential in making well-informed decisions regarding reproductive functions post-cancer treatment (Santaballa et al., 2021). Furthermore, enhanced awareness of testicular ailments such as torsion and cancer has necessitated the inclusion of multidisciplinary approaches in male reproductive health. The collaborative practice of urologists, oncologists, and reproductive health professionals underscores the importance of an integrated strategy that considers prevention, diagnosis, and treatment. Dealing with the substances that may trigger testicular torsion, for instance, EDC exposure, requires a unified approach in public health policy as well as in awareness campaigns at the individual level. Similarly, testicular cancer treatment should include discussions about fertility preservation and sperm banking avenues before initiating therapy. By adopting this integrated view of the male reproductive organ, medical practitioners can more effectively empower patients with the knowledge and tools to challenge the testicular pathology challenge (Pan et al., 2024; Santaballa et al., 2021).

Test Your Knowledge

1. What is the main cause of erectile dysfunction?
2. What are testicular conditions?

11.4. Male Reproductive Health and Wellness

Learning Outcome

1. Understand the importance of regular check-ups and screenings
2. Describe the lifestyle factors affecting reproductive health
3. Describe the role of nutrition in promoting optimal reproductive function

The male reproductive health and well-being encompasses a range of environmental and biological elements that play a role in overall fertility and reproductive success. Glue to the concept is the male reproductive microbiome, which has been highlighted in its contribution to reproductive health. From research, it has been established that healthy microbiota within the male reproductive tract is important for the normal functioning of sperm and reproductive health. Interference in this delicate equilibrium is said to result in dysbiosis, and this has caused a variety of reproductive challenges, among them infertility. The seminal microbiota not only affects male fertility but also has implications for potential offspring well-being, and thus the inter-dependence of male reproductive well-being with overall health outcomes. Furthermore, probiotics and their relation to the well-being of men is a relatively new research frontier. Probiotics refer to live bacteria that offer health benefits to the host and have been promising in enhancing fertility. By modulating the male microbiota, probiotics may improve sperm quality and function, thereby influencing reproductive outcomes. The studies have proved that the health-enhancing bacteria strengthen the immune function of the reproductive tract and enhance homeostasis, thereby lessening the risk of reproductive illness. Furthermore, the bidirectional effects of male and female microbiota suggest that probiotic treatment not only has the potential to promote male reproductive health but can, by extension, also benefit female partners and offspring (Adnane and Chapwanya, 2022).

Tackling male reproductive health calls for an appreciation of the need for multidisciplinary therapeutic approaches in consideration of microbiological, immunological, and life parameter factors. Integrated health approaches with adequate nutrition, stress, and reduced environmental toxin exposure can be a potent reinforcement of male reproductive health. That of the male microbiome should not be discounted, as it provides structural integrity and immunomodulation within the reproductive tract, as evidenced by endometrial flora in women (Adnane and Chapwanya, 2022). Hence, an effective framework for enhancing male reproductive health must be comprised of a grasp of these microbial communities and their interactions, part of the overarching public health effort of One World, One Health. By recognizing and responding to these intricate interdependencies, we can advance reproductive outcomes and overall health in males.

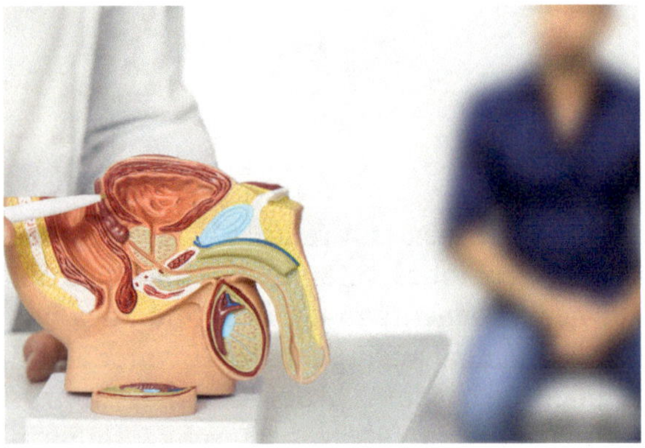

Figure 11.13. Male Reproductive Health.

Source: https://www.center4reproduction.com/wp-content/themes/yootheme/cache/e1/male-reproductive-health-1-e146cb12.png

11.4.1. Importance of Regular Check-Ups and Screenings

Regular check-ups and screening are also vital components of maintaining mens' health, particularly that of the male reproductive system. Routine preventive care enables any potential health issues to be identified early on, thus improving health a lot. For instance, regular checks can identify such diseases as prostate cancer, testicular conditions, and sexually transmitted diseases (STIs) at a stage that is more manageable when their impact is reduced. Furthermore, regular screenings allow for discussion between patients and healthcare professionals on reproductive health in order to give men the chance to address matters that would go unheard otherwise. Being proactive can lead to greater awareness of personal health risks and healthier lifestyle choices that can lower such risks. The rise of telemedicine during the COVID-19 pandemic has shifted how men engage with their healthcare providers, affecting regular check-ups and screenings. As governments reacted to the pandemic difficulties, most embraced remote care services in a move to preserve continuity of care. While telemedicine has enhanced access to healthcare, it has also identified potential inadequacies in the quality of some remote consultations, raising concerns about the effectiveness of such screenings. Therefore, while telemedicine offers an alternative, men are supposed to know the importance of check-ups and screenings conducted in person for complete assessment and accurate diagnosis of conditions involving the male reproductive system (N/A, 2023).

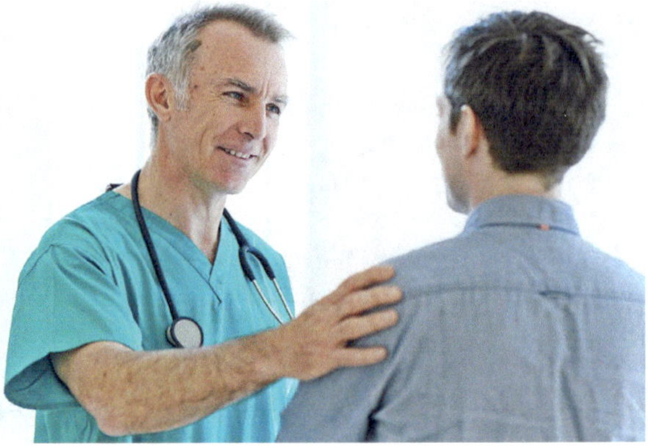

Figure 11.14. The Importance of regular sexual and reproductive health screenings.

Source: https://news.uams.edu/wp-content/uploads/2024/08/6.jpg

Moreover, discussing the importance of mental health in respect to physical health through regular screenings with men will lead to better care for men. The COVID-19 pandemic showed how physical and mental health are related to each other because most individuals experienced greater depression and anxiety as a result of public health-related stressors. Periodic medical check-ups offer an opportunity for healthcare providers to tackle not only reproductive well-being but also mental well-being, since stress and psychological disorders may directly affect the outcomes of reproductive health (Clemente VJ-Suárez et al., 2021). By incorporating both physical and mental health conversations during screening, medical practitioners can ensure that men receive comprehensive care that addresses all their needs. This will, in the long term, result in better health outcomes and quality of life.

11.4.2. Lifestyle Factors Affecting Reproductive Health

Lifestyle factors play a significant part in contributing to their impact on male reproductive well-being, particularly sperm quality and fertility. The most important lifestyle factor is tobacco use or, indeed, tobacco smoking. It has been demonstrated to have detrimental effects on semen volume and absolute sperm count, which are extremely important parameters in assessing male fertility. Although some parameters, for instance, morphology and motility, fail to produce statistically significant changes, the trend suggests that smoking can compromise reproductive integrity. The study identified that a high concentration of heat shock protein 27 (HSP27) in semen is able to demarcate tobacco-induced stress, once again correlating lifestyle to potential infertility. Identification of such adverse effects of tobacco cigarette smoking on reproductive health has also brought into focus the importance of public health policy interventions for raising awareness among men regarding the contribution of life changes towards enhancing their fertility potential as well as overall reproductive health (Henriques et al., 2023). Drinking alcohol is one more significant lifestyle factor that influences male reproductive health. Heavy drinking is always linked to semen quality diminishment as alcohol drinking may undermine hormonal equilibrium, leading to an imbalance of testosterone levels and thus upending the sperm creation process. Long-term drinking also may induce oxidative stress, which impacts sperm vitality and function. Reviews suggest that heavy drinkers may experience reduced libido, erectile dysfunction, and risk of infertility. Because contemporary life typically involves social alcohol consumption, information on the impact of alcohol on reproductive health is highly relevant. When more awareness exists, individuals will be able to make decisions on alcohol consumption, and moderation can be used as a strategy to minimize the risk to fertility and promote healthier reproduction in the long term (Medenica et al., 2022). Lifestyle and diet and exercise, too, have a tremendous amount to do with male reproductive health. Regular exercise has been associated with improved hormone levels and reproductive function, which serves not only cardiovascular health but also fertility. A lifestyle of being inactive will result in obesity, which will only add more risk to hormonal balance and sperm production. At the dietary level, equilibrious intake of required nutrients like antioxidants, vitamins, and minerals protects the sperm from oxidative stress and maximizes reproductive success. Male reproductive health strategy is based on habits of lifestyle, such as physical exercise and diet. Encouraging men to exercise regularly and eat well can trigger healthier production of sperm and overall reproductive activity as a whole, hence boosting fertility and minimizing the risk of infertility (Medenica et al., 2022).

11.4.3. Nutritional Requirements For Optimum Reproductive Ability

Nutrition has the greatest contribution to enhancing maximal reproductive function, especially in relation to male reproductive well-being. Sperm integrity and testosterone status are constructed and maintained by a harmonious diet intake. Micronutrients zinc, selenium, and vitamins C and E have been recognized as optimal modulators of avoiding oxidative stress that negatively impacts sperm motility and viability. Besides, polyunsaturated fatty acids, being the omega-3s, also contribute to structural integrity in sperm membranes and have been linked to improved reproductive performance. Malnutrition has been shown to lead to increased infertility and reduced reproductive performance, and men therefore embrace nutrient-dense food in their diets to improve general health as well as reproductive competence. Revealing the influence of specific diets may expose how they impact male fertility. For instance, traditional Mediterranean diets rich in fruits, vegetables, whole grains, and healthy fats have been associated with improved reproductive health. Not only does the diet deliver the body with all the required nutrients, but it also encourages a more desirable body weight and hormone balance, both of which are crucial for reproductive success. Of special interest is that obesity negatively affects testosterone status and sperm quality, offering a further stimulus towards optimal nutrition application. Apart from isolated nutrient focus, the interplay between overall diet and lifestyle with moderate exercise and stress control also implies multi-factor causation of male reproductive health. Promotion of nutritional intake on a more generic basis may thus improve fertility potential in men. Furthermore, the role of sustainability in choosing food cannot be overemphasized when considering its greater role for best reproductive functioning. The solution to favoring plant foods, which tend to be lower in calories and higher in antioxidants, is that men not only optimize their own reproductive health but also do their part for environmental sustainability. Evidence highlights the link among diet, health, and the environment, such that diets rich in processed foods and saturated fat may have adverse effects both on individual health and population trends in reproduction. Increasingly, clinicians and researchers recognize nutrition's key function to fertility, enabling dietary change that includes a focus on whole foods as aligning with evidence-based interventions to enhance health outcomes. This general strategy can further guide the following practices of reproductive health, with more emphasis placed on nutrition factor awareness for optimal reproductive performance among men, based on available guidelines (Mauvais F-Jarvis et al., 2020) and (Teede et al., 2018).

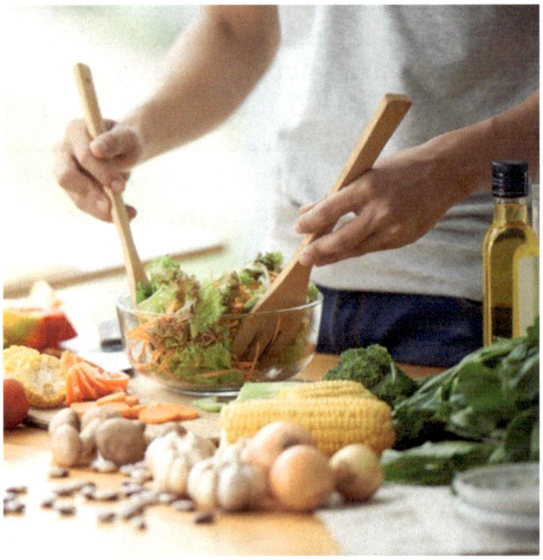

Figure 11.15. The Role of Nutrition in Male Fertility.

Source: https://www.drrajeshdhakeurologist.com/wp-content/uploads/2023/06/nutrition-brunswick.jpg

Test Your Knowledge

1. How do lifestyle factors affect reproductive health?
2. What is the role of nutrition in reproductive health?

11.5. Male Reproductive System and Sexual Health

Learning Outcome

1. Understand the sexual function and libido
2. Describe the impact of mental health on reproductive health
3. Learn about safe sex practices and sexually transmitted infections

The male reproductive system plays a central role in sexual health and consists of anatomical structures and physiological processes. Testes, epididymis, vas deferens, seminal vesicles, and prostate are the primary components, all of which work together to facilitate sperm production, maturation, and transport. This complicated system can be threatened by disease conditions that can significantly impair reproductive function. For instance, hormonal imbalance can lead to low levels of testosterone, which eventually cause a decrease in libido and sperm count. Besides that, age, lifestyle, and environment can be responsible for considerable variation in male reproductive health, which would necessitate general methods of well-being and preventive medicine. With the increasing prevalence of infertility complications, the need to understand the intricate function of such systems in general male sexual well-being and the significance of targeted interventions in reversing such complications is more crucial now than ever before. It is only recently that studies have turned their attention towards understanding how outside factors influence the reproductive well-being of men, particularly in the case of contagious illnesses like COVID-19. Research has found the SARS-CoV-2 virus to be harmful to male reproductive function by exerting effects on spermatogenesis and endocrine homeostasis. Changes in semen quality among infected male patients have shown the promising role of viral infection on fertility outcome. Virus entry mechanisms into reproductive cells, as mediated through male reproductive system receptors, show evident overlap between infectious disease and sexual health. As a result of ongoing research in this matter, fertility levels and health statuses for men whose lives are influenced by these latest health crises need to be monitored so that care plans can be better established to mitigate long-term impacts. Aside from this, aging is a cause of affecting the overall health of the male reproductive system as well. With advancing age, a man loses testosterone and declining testicular function, which leads to various reproductive changes. Such changes can include compromised motility of sperm, altered morphology, and even probabilities of sterility. There is growing evidence of some biomarkers of reproductive aging that may serve as markers of potential fertility issues. Notably, immune responses to aging have been related to systemic and reproductive modification, which suggests that interfaces between reproductive health and immune function need to be explored. Modulation of such factors by preventive and therapeutic interventions may maximize male reproductive health and fertility, yielding valuable information on how aging affects the male reproductive process and sex in general.

11.5.1. Understanding Sexual Function and Libido

Sexual function and libido can best be explained by an interdisciplinary approach to understanding involving physiological, psychological, and endocrine factors of the male reproductive system. Sexual function is primarily regulated by the complex interaction of hormones, namely testosterone, whose role is central to the modulation of libido. Adequate levels of testosterone are required to evoke sexual desire and promote healthy erectile function. In addition, libidinous growth is also affected by psychological conditions such as stress, worry, and relationship issues. The data indicate that psychologically disturbed men receive low sexual interest and function ratings, highlighting the importance of mental health in sexual health. As such, any full conceptualization of sexual function has to account for these various influences, illustrating that libido is more a convergence of several domains than a biological process. The engagement of the CNS and hormonal processes in the regulation of libido is not something of the volume of hormone. The CNS also functions to synthesize sexual stimuli and respond with appropriate physiology through neuroendocrine processes. As recently reviewed, the performance of certain natural supplements, such as Tribulus terrestris, has been said to enhance sexual desire and sexual performance. The plant's compounds were said to trigger significant physiological events, including pituitary and gonadal hormone regulation and enhancement of gamete quality. All of these effects are significant since they show the therapeutic action potential under conditions of reduced libido or sexual dysfunction. The collaboration of evidence from traditional and modern medicine provides data on male sexual health promotion on an integrated level. Furthermore, the importance of improving sexual function extends beyond individual health to societal considerations. Infertility and sexual performance dissatisfaction can lead to extreme emotional distress in addition to affecting interpersonal relationships. Plant substances such as Tribulus terrestris that have been said to enhance male reproductive activities are of significant therapeutic potential. Such treatments have the ability to enhance factors pertaining to libido and fertility, treat diseases like polycystic ovarian syndrome, and promote the reproductive health of both genders. With greater awareness of the intricacy of libido and sexuality, the problem is evident in that both the physiological and psychological factors need to be addressed. Not only does this integrated strategy support better sexual health outcomes, but it also maximizes relational and emotional fulfillment in the male reproduction process.

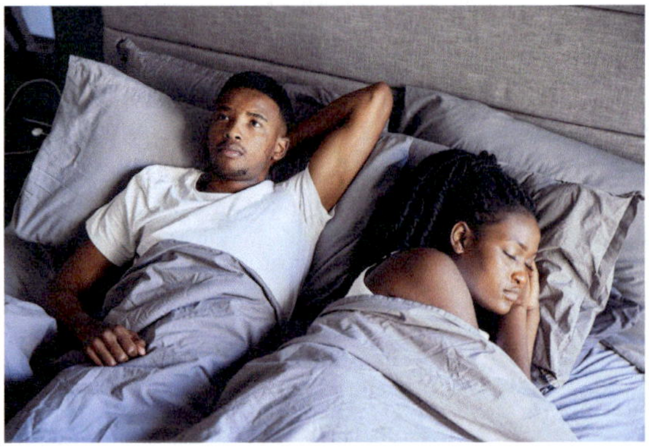

Source: https://www.health.com/thmb/xeTbFidMYbPof6NzD7_QkC_Vxv4=/1500x0/filters:no_upscale():max_bytes(150000):strip_icc()/Health-GettyImages-1407486910-776c38694b2845d784abb9c42300fe3e.jpg

11.5.2. Impact of Mental Health on Reproductive Health

The interplay between mental health and reproductive health is increasingly valued as a priority area, most notably when focusing on the reproductive health of men. Findings have revealed that mental disorders, especially depression and anxiety, negatively affect hormonal balance and fertility. Such mental disorders can lead to hormonal imbalances that disrupt normal testicular functioning and therefore influence sperm development and quality. Further, the stress that is associated with mental illness can lead to behavioral changes that complicate reproductive health issues further, such as decreased libido and sexual dysfunction. These complexities speak to the necessity of holistic approaches in mental health treatment, which reach far beyond end outcomes of reproductive function, making it imperative for medical practitioners to consider mental and reproductive health in their evaluations and treatment plans. Pharmacological treatments of mental illness, particularly the use of selective serotonin reuptake inhibitors (SSRIs), have proven helpful in male reproductive health. Despite the drugs' action against depressive disorders, they are also found to have adverse impacts on reproductive processes. SSRIs have been associated with reproductive toxicity, which affects the development of germ cells and even results in adverse effects such as congenital malformations in children. These mechanisms are complex and involve everything from sperm motility to endocrine control. An imperative need, therefore, exists for further research to shed light on the magnitude of the impact of SSRIs on male reproductive health, particularly as their use becomes increasingly prevalent in populations suffering from mental illnesses (Feng et al., 2025). In addition, studies on other pharmacological agents, such as hydroxyurea, recognize the delicate balance between treatments of mental illness and fertility.

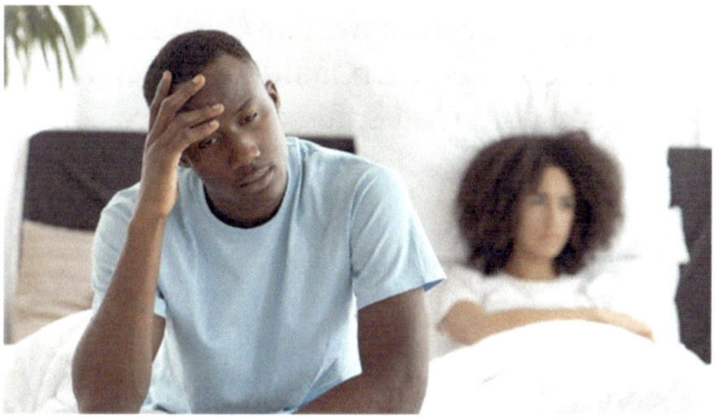

Source: https://static.wixstatic.com/media/cae34d_f095ad820fb24c97894c1e48001858ff~mv2.jpg/v1/fill/w_568,h_320,al_c,q_80,usm_0.66_1.00_0.01,enc_avif,quality_auto/cae34d_f095ad820fb24c97894c1e48001858ff~mv2.jpg

Hydroxyurea has become a promising medication in the treatment of various diseases, but is linked to side effects on spermatogenesis. Hydroxyurea was found to reduce testicular weight and disrupt hormone levels in male fertility in treated animal model experiments. However, interventions that included antioxidants like Vitamin C were found to be protective against hydroxyurea-induced testicular injury, pointing towards the potential of mitigation therapies. That is, while mental health treatments presently ongoing could be harmful to reproductive health, appropriate adjunctive treatments might offer a way to safeguard male fertility and overall well-being in patients undergoing mental health treatment (Abdulhadi et al., 2024).

11.5.3. Safe Sex Practices and Sexually Transmitted Infections

In men's reproductive health, safe sex is essential in the prevention of sexually transmitted diseases (STIs) and maintenance of sexual health. Practice and application of standard and consistent use of condoms have been recognized as one of the most effective HIV/AIDS and STIs prevention practices. Despite this, pregnancy prevention is the choice of the majority of people, including young people, over the risk of infection. It was found through a survey of students in the tertiary level of The Gambia that even though a considerable percentage of the respondents had indicated that they knew HIV/AIDS, condom use among them was very low. In particular, 62.2% of sexually active respondents indicated condom use unanimously, while only a paltry 24.4% used condoms on a regular basis, recording a glaring deficit between knowledge and practice that calls for additional educational interventions to promote safer sexual practice(Anaetor ISC et al., 2025). Additionally, the sexual health sector's complexity is exacerbated by other extraneous factors, such as the degree of societal attitude and misinformation on STIs. Findings of a survey of youths in The Gambia show that although there was a good level of HIV knowledge, a vast majority of the respondents held misconceptions regarding its spread. For instance, some respondents believed on a false basis that HIV can be contracted through casual contact like being bitten by mosquitoes or sharing a plate. This behavior-information gap is one of the reasons for the longstanding STI epidemic, like chlamydia and gonorrhea, among vulnerable groups like left-behind rural women. Women like these have unique issues in which restricted sexual health care access and unwanted sexual experiences leave them more susceptible to infection, and thus, education-centered and accessibility-centered interventions become more important(Li et al., 2025). There is a call for instituting quality sexual health education and intervention in targeted populations to avoid STIs and ensure safe sex behavior. Sexual education, for instance, should involve breaking down the stigma of HIV testing and myths of modes of transmission with a view to enhancing individuals' preparedness to adopt prevention strategies. Through lessons obtained from learning with youth and vulnerable populations, there can be evidence-based public health interventions that put emphasis on putting reproductive health complications out of reach through condoms. In addition, simplifying the process of HIV testing and offering healthcare services can empower the citizenry to assume control over their sexual life, which can contribute to a sharp reduction of STI cases in urban as well as rural areas. A shared approach to de-mystifying the problems of STIs is the basis of healthier sex practices that improve the health of the male reproductive system and indirectly benefit broader public health.

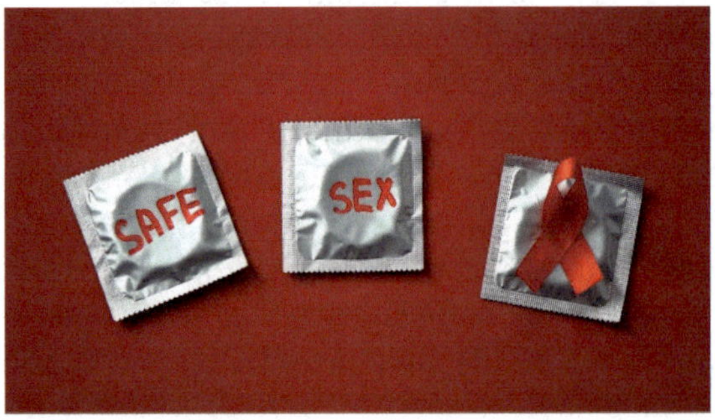

Figure 11.16. Safe Sex Practices Recommended by Expert to Avoid Infections.

Source: https://www.newmi.in/s/6123687a0e3882eabaee1e6e/64e70b29af0bd73bbcb470a4/expert-recommended-safe-sex-practices.jpg

Test Your Knowledge

1. What is meant by sexual function?
2. what are the impact of mental health on reproductive health?

11.6. Advances in Male Reproductive Medicine

Learning Outcome

1. Understand the innovations in fertility treatments
2. Describe the research of male contraceptives
3. Learn about emerging technologies in reproductive health

Recent advances in male reproductive medicine represent a revolutionary age in the understanding of male fertility and its complexities. Traditional approaches to examining reproductive biology relied on animal models or descriptive clinical studies, which provided limited data on human-specific reproductive mechanisms. However, novel approaches, particularly the generation of three-dimensional (3D) epithelial stem cell-derived organoid cultures, have provided new avenues of research. These organoids are closer models of human reproductive organ development and function, allowing for closer examination of cellular behavior, differentiation, and even preclinical pharmacological screening. With the application of these in vitro systems, researchers expect to have a better understanding of normal and disease states affecting male reproduction, with the hope for more efficient therapeutic strategies tailored to each patient's requirements (Haider and Beristain, 2023). Furthermore, the genetic underpinning of male infertility has, for the first time, ever gained unparalleled interest, highlighting the intricate interface between genetics and reproductive health. The establishment of exhaustive lists of male subfertility syndromes has become paramount in elucidating such intersections. This endeavor recognized several underlying genetic defects producing several infertility syndromes, creating a genome–phenome network that showed the intricate interface between genes and clinical features.

The studies in this aspect have not only upgraded the diagnostic methods but also led to the introduction of personalized medicine protocols in male reproductive well-being. By identifying the genetic processes affected, practitioners can offer targeted interventions to address specific reasons for infertility, beyond generic interventions (Špela Mikec et al., 2022). The addition of regenerative medicine techniques is also a significant advancement in this field. Techniques such as organoid use and stem cell therapy for modeling reproductive processes have proved promising in reproductive medicine, and they have generated new avenues for treatment. The ability to manipulate and in vitro cultivate human gametes and reproductive tissues guarantees not only improved knowledge of development but also prospects for the treatment of infertility. This new approach has the potential to restore damaged reproductive tissue or fertility in men who are experiencing difficult circumstances, like cancer treatments or genetic disorders. As these new methods evolve, they have promising potential for improving male reproductive health results, paving the way to more effective treatments that are tailored to each patient's individual requirements (Haider and Beristain, 2023).

11.6.1. Innovations in Fertility Treatments

The field of fertility treatment has also seen tremendous leaps in recent times, mainly driven by developments in medical science and reproductive technologies. Among these, procedures such as in vitro fertilization (IVF) have seen tremendous improvement in success rates due to improved methods of selecting embryos and genetic screening facilities. The incorporation of preimplantation genetic diagnosis (PGD) allows physicians to identify genetic flaws before implanting, hence guaranteeing a normal pregnancy. These advancements have transformed the landscape of assisted reproductive technology, transgressing previously untransgressed male infertility issues. Besides, such progress has assisted in the development of enhanced awareness of the effect of environmental conditions on male fertility, which is the area of focus exemplified by the growing concern at the levels of chemical pollutants that affect reproductive health (Naidu et al., 2021). Yet another area of fertility care is hormone therapy and its mechanism in relation to addressing hormonal imbalances that affect male fertility. Recent studies underscore the importance of testosterone replacement therapy among men afflicted with low testosterone levels, causing decreased sperm counts and, ultimately, sterility. Further, the advances in cryopreservation techniques in use today make it feasible to successfully bank sperm with preservation of fertility potential before submitting to medical treatments for various conditions. This increase in options is a shift in the view of men's reproductive health, with new avenues of approach for those who are affected by disease or age. Other possible hormone treatments are also being researched that would further augment libido and sperm performance, which would have a drastically altered effect on male fertility (Kyle J Foreman et al., 2018). Lastly, lifestyle interventions in conjunction with modern fertility care have come to be placed more in the forefront. Recent studies have highlighted the interplay among factors such as diet, exercise, and environmental exposures and male reproductive success. Developments in the area of personalized medicine address these factors by presenting treatment protocols that are tailored to an individual based on their lifestyle characteristics. The integrative model provides new hope for both patients and practitioners in that they can work together in creating fertility a reality through medical and lifestyle changes. The incorporation of technology within monitoring these variables, along with medical interventions, provides an overall model for advancing male fertility treatments. Hence, the ongoing innovation of fertility treatment holds the promise not only of addressing current reproductive needs but also of enhancing overall male reproductive health in the future (Naidu et al., 2021).

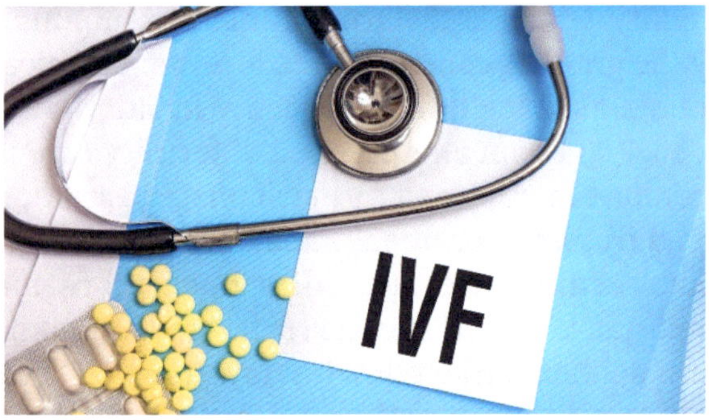

Figure 11.17. IVF Treatment.

Source: https://images.squarespace-cdn.com/content/v1/5bac99efb2cf79a76d80781d/bb35dc92-9045-4867-a7cb-9fb153c4988e/HE+image+%285%29.jpg

11.6.2. Research on Male Contraceptives

Male contraceptive studies have been extremely trendy in the last decade or so, particularly as cultural attitudes toward family planning and reproductive rights keep evolving. Women have long carried the responsibility of contraception, a reality that has fueled attempts at equitable responsibility between genders. Current studies examine an array of male contraceptive methods, ranging from hormonal to non-hormonal. Hormonal methods typically involve alterations in testosterone and other hormones critical to spermatogenesis. These findings highlight the complex interaction between the male reproductive tract and endocrine regulation, underscoring the central role of hormones such as follicle-stimulating hormone (FSH) in supporting sperm production. As researchers move in new directions, it is important to consider these effects of hormones so that effective male contraceptive methods can be developed according to the needs of both partners within the framework of mutual control over fertility (Li et al., 2024). The development of non-hormonal male contraceptives also holds promise as they offer unique alternatives that can bypass the unwanted side effects of hormonal treatments. All these methods focus primarily on inhibiting sperm motility or function chemically or inhibiting differentiation processes during sperm development. Breakthroughs in this area can lead to methods not only reversible in their mode of contraception but also respecting the natural hormonal balance of the male reproductive system. These advances have the capability to diminish such global phobias against hormonal contraceptive usage, such as weight gain or mood changes. Also, alongside shifting expectations from society towards mutual reproductive responsibilities, there is an increased need for thorough education on male contraceptive methods to ensure men are properly educated and empowered to take an active part in family planning and reproductive health decisions (Morgen A Chalmiers et al., 2021). Despite ongoing research and development into male contraceptives, several barriers remain that could hamper mass adoption. These are masculine attitudes, male contraceptive stigma, and a general lack of knowledge about what exists. In addition, clinical trials and research are faced with the challenge of enrolling men as trial participants, typically due to skepticism concerning the efficacy or safety of new methods and what such use will do to their bodies. Also worth examining is the broader impact on sexual relationships and sexual health of male contraception, as shared responsibility in contraception can facilitate increased partnership. As the field moves forward, overcoming such barriers through collaborative public health efforts and focused research will be needed to make male contraceptive use mainstream culture and, ultimately, promote shared reproductive responsibility (Li et al., 2024).

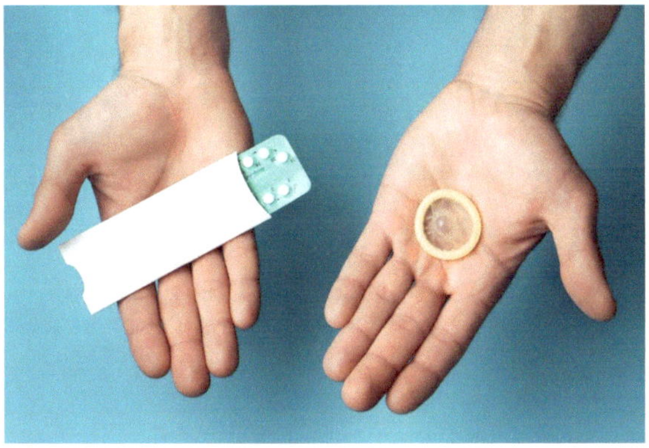

Figure 11.18. Methods of contraception for men.

Source: https://dreminozbek.com/wp-content/uploads/2024/10/Erkekler-icin-Dogum-Kontrol-Yontemleri.jpg

11.6.3. Emerging Technologies in Reproductive Health

The advent of novel technologies for reproductive health has generated a lot of interest, particularly in the male reproductive system. The advancements in molecular diagnosis and newer imaging technologies have revolutionized the capacity to assess male reproductive potential effectively. The technologies allow for the identification of genetic, epigenetic, and morphological determinants of reproduction. For instance, artificial intelligence and machine learning-based technology assess sperm motility and morphology to predict fertilization probability more precisely. With their implementation in clinical practice, healthcare providers are able to offer personalized treatment regimens for individual patients, improving the overall quality of male infertility management. The advent of such technology not only enhances the precision of diagnosis but also educates couples and individuals with reproductive problems, bridging the gap to successful conception and healthier outcomes. In combination with diagnostic advancement, pioneering treatments with regenerative medicine are transforming the care of male reproductive health. Stem cell treatment and tissue engineering have attracted significant attention with the potential of their restoration of function in states of compromised reproductive ability owing to congenital disease or trauma. Research indicates that stem cells derived from various sources may differentiate into spermatogenic cells, thereby correcting infertility-related issues. Furthermore, new techniques, such as organoids, allow researchers to replicate male reproductive tissues in a lab dish, furthering our understanding of development and pathology. As these regenerative medicines become more advanced, they can potentially restore fertility and provide options for those who suffer because of environmental factors or genetic predisposition, significantly enhancing the field of reproductive medicine. The intersection of emerging technologies and issues of environmental health is rapidly becoming pivotal in shaping contemporary discourse regarding male reproductive systems. Studies have indicated that exposure to toxic chemicals in the environment, such as bisphenol A (BPA), poses serious threats to reproductive health, possibly disrupting endocrine functions. The merging of biosensors and wearable technologies has enabled users to monitor their exposure levels to such poisonous substances. In addition, the application of traditional medicinal plants, like Eruca sativa, showcases the importance of applying holistic approaches in combination with modern technological advancements. Research showcases the phytochemical compounds in these types of plants with antioxidant activity, which can reverse the adverse effects of environmental contaminants on male fertility performance. As the discipline delves further into these complex interactions, it is imperative to integrate both technological advancements and conventional practices into a progressive framework to optimize overall reproductive health measures intended to protect male fertility.

Test Your Knowledge

1. What is the most advanced fertility treatment?
2. What are the new technologies in reproductive health?

SUMMARY

The physiology of the male reproductive system illustrates a delicate interdependence between anatomical structures and physiological processes, and places in foreground position emphasis on environmental factors and hormone regulation. Elaborate regulation of spermatogenesis, hormone discharge, and sexuality is under the control of a vast number of external agents, including chemicals and illness. Current studies have established the fearsome impact of endocrine disruptors such as bisphenol A (BPA) on reproductive function, as exposure has been established to lead to significant dysfunction and apoptosis in the reproductive tissues. This interaction is pertinent as cumulative evidence has recognized the risk that environmental agents present to male fertility and reproductive health. For this purpose, increasingly evident is the need to preserve the integrity of the male reproductive system through further studies and public health education regarding environmental exposures and their lasting consequences on reproductive function (Kadry M Sadek et al., 2024). Clinical presentation of disease of the male reproductive system also underscores the interplay of environmental and biological processes. Diseases such as leprosy have been reported to adversely affect testicular function and hormone levels, leading to significant issues in the quality of life of the patients. Addition of clinical examination with hormonal and radiological studies has re-established dismal prevalence of reproductive dysfunction in the infected patients. For instance, the prevalence of 'nepler' of the testicles and endocrine level fluctuations, including elevated follicle-stimulating hormone (FSH) and luteinizing hormone (LH), reflects the intricate interaction between the endogenous diseases and the effect on reproductive wellness. The study highlights the employment of early diagnosis methods and intervention strategies according to individual needs, such as hormone replacement therapy, in an attempt to shorten the adverse effects on fertility and overall health (Hegde et al., 2024). Finally, the study of the male reproductive system provides a case for interdisciplinary research and public policy to preserve reproductive health. Knowledge of determinants of male reproductive function in clear terms enables researchers and medical practitioners to strategize intervention and inform the public of potential hazards. This is achieved by creating awareness of the effects of environmental contaminants, optimizing lifestyle choices, and avoiding delayed intervention for reproductive diseases. By promoting prevention, early intervention, and sound management, society can make an effort to improve male reproductive health outcomes as well as safeguard the fertility of future generations. Finally, an evidence-based strategy can reduce environmental and clinical impacts on male reproductive health, maximizing well-being and quality of life (Kadry M Sadek et al., 2024; Hegde et al., 2024).

As one learns about the male reproductive system, there are a few important points that greatly increase our knowledge regarding its function and components. Simple structures, such as the testes, are responsible for important functions in spermatogenesis and the secretion of hormones, primarily testosterone. Spermatogenesis in the seminiferous tubules is the complex process by which the germ cells form spermatozoa. This is regulated by hormonal stimulation by luteinizing hormone (LH) and follicle-stimulating hormone (FSH), highlighting the central role of the endocrine system in regulating male reproduction. Neurobiology also highlights the coordination between the nervous and reproductive systems by starting to show the mechanisms behind not only spermogenesis but also mating behaviors. The research into neurobiological mechanisms, particularly on the male reproductive system, has revealed complex correlates that go beyond physical and biological understanding. Contemporary research emphasizes the central key function of neurons in the control of reproductive behaviors, such as mating and copulation. Notably, one study using the fruit fly species Drosophila melanogaster has found major neural circuits that have been shown to have effects on reproductive behaviors through sensory feedback systems. Sensory neurons in the reproductive tract transmit information about partner availability and sperm maturity, eliciting subsequent behavioral responses. Such integration of reproductive biology with neurobiology research does not merely account for simple reproductive processes but also opens up novel avenues to study evolutionary adaptations of mating behavior across species, as seen through sensory signal observation and neuronal control mechanisms (Afkhami, 2024). Moreover, an understanding of how environmental inputs drive the male reproductive system sheds light on our broad understanding of its biology. Research, including a variety of external inputs such as diet and social structure, outlines how they can impact reproductive success. For example, evidence shows that neurotrophic factors, such as nerve growth factor (NGF), are involved in testicular development and hormone regulation in males and represent a new target for controlling reproductive health in invasive species such as the grey squirrel (Mercati et al., 2024). This reality highlights the importance of considering ecological environments while researching reproductive mechanisms. As science endeavors to unravel the intricacies of the male reproductive system, the intersection of neurobiology, hormones, and environmental stress is a fascinating topic of research that holds broad implications for basic science and applied conservation.

KEY TERMS FROM THIS CHAPTER

- Autophagy
- Bulbourethral glands
- Epididymis
- Erectile dysfunction
- Hormone regulation
- Luteinizing hormone
- Male hormones
- Prostate disorders
- Prostate-specific antigen
- Scrotum
- Seminal vesicles
- Sertoli cells
- Sperm cell
- Spermatogenesis
- Testicular torsion
- Testosterone

CRITICAL THINKING QUESTIONS

1. **The primary male reproductive organ responsible for sperm production is the:**
   a. Prostate gland
   b. Testes
   c. Seminal vesicle
   d. Epididymis
2. **Sperm mature and are stored in the:**
   a. Vas deferens
   b. Epididymis
   c. Seminal vesicle
   d. Urethra
3. **The tube that transports sperm from the epididymis to the urethra is called the:**
   a. Vas deferens
   b. Ejaculatory duct
   c. Seminal duct
   d. Ureter
4. **The structure that produces seminal fluid to nourish sperm is the:**
   a. Prostate gland
   b. Bulbourethral gland
   c. Seminal vesicle
   d. Testes
5. **The muscular tube that conveys both urine and semen out of the body is the:**
   a. Vas deferens
   b. Ureter
   c. Urethra
   d. Ejaculatory duct

Short Answer Questions

1. What is the male reproductive system?
2. What are the 7 organs of the male reproductive system?
3. Where are the testes located?
4. What are the main functions of the male reproductive system?
5. What are the most common disorders of the male reproductive system?

Answer to Critical Thinking Questions

1. (b) 2. (b) 3. (a) 4. (c) 5. (c)

REFERENCES

1. Abdulhadi, E., Aqeelah, G., & Milad, F. (2024). Impact of vitamin C and hydroxyurea on the reproductive system health in male rats. *AlQalam Journal of Medical and Applied Sciences*. https://www.semanticscholar.org/paper/64b9f54322ff72ac07b728328a7e5790abded53d (accessed on 15th June 2025).
2. Adnane, M., & Chapwanya, A. (2022). A review of the diversity of the genital tract microbiome and implications for fertility of cattle. *Animals, 12*, 460. https://doi.org/10.3390/ani12040460 (accessed on 15th June 2025).
3. Afkhami, M. (2024). Neurobiology of egg-laying behavior in *Drosophila*: Neural control of the female reproductive system. *Journal of Neurogenetics, 38*, 47–61. https://www.semanticscholar.org/paper/d84ee733df95c53ec723310f739d30b595cfc89e (accessed on 15th June 2025).
4. Anaetor, I. S. C., Ikwuka, A. O., & Udeh, F. C. (2025). HIV/AIDS: Safe sex practices, condom use and knowledge among students attending selected tertiary institutions in the Gambia. *World Journal of Advanced Research and Reviews*. https://www.semanticscholar.org/paper/6355ca8b2e5d247c5e12356261b2f0c9d69595ef (accessed on 15th June 2025).
5. Azhar, M. M., Chandar, K., Salam, K. A., Khan, V. M., Shahzeb, A., Ali, P. S., Rahman, I. U., et al. (2024). Potential role of autophagy in the male reproductive system. *International Journal of Sexual and Reproductive Health Care*. https://www.semanticscholar.org/paper/b20ef7ff95940b95002044a1b219d62e67260c5e (accessed on 15th June 2025).
6. Bahreiny, S. S., Ahangarpour, A., & Aghaei, M. (2024). Assessment of the effects of subclinical hypothyroidism on male reproductive parameters: A meta-analysis approach. *Reproductive and Developmental Medicine, 9*, 57–65. https://www.semanticscholar.org/paper/9090bb71 9b0f608d337819238f4d40d726da1dd0 (accessed on 15th June 2025).
7. Barrachina, F., Battistone, M. A., Castillo, J., Mallofré, C., Jodar, M., Breton, S., & Oliva, R. (2022). Sperm acquire epididymis-derived proteins through epididymosomes. *Human Reproduction, 37*, 651–668. https://doi.org/10.1093/humrep/deac015 (accessed on 15th June 2025).
8. Bhavsar, U. G., Tamboli, F., Chaudhari, A. J., Bahalkar, N. S., Chaudhari, B. S., & Mali, U. S. (2024). Male reproductive health at risk: Examining the impact of coronaviruses on fertility and potential sexual transmission of SARS-CoV-2. *International Journal of Pharmaceutical Chemistry and Analysis*. https://www.semanticscholar.org/paper/c5e104d23085d1b8cea72d634c641aa14a8c8c15 (accessed on 15th June 2025).
9. Chalmiers, M. A., Karaki, F., Muriki, M., Mody, S. K., Chen, A., & Thiel de Bocanegra, H. (2021). Refugee women's experiences with contraceptive care after resettlement in high-income countries: A critical interpretive synthesis. *Contraception, 108*, 7–18. https://doi.org/10.1016/j.contraception.2021.11.004 (accessed on 15th June 2025).
10. Clemente-Suárez, V. J., Martínez–González, M. B., Benítez-Agudelo, J. C., Navarro-Jiménez, E., Beltrán-Velasco, A. I., Ruisoto, P., Diaz Arroyo, E., et al. (2021). The impact of the COVID-19 pandemic on mental disorders: A critical review. *International Journal of Environmental Research and Public Health, 18*, 10041. https://doi.org/10.3390/ijerph181910041 (accessed on 15th June 2025).
11. Das, P. K., Mukherjee, J., & Banerjee, D. (2023). Functional morphology of the male reproductive system. https://doi.org/10.1007/978-981-19-9410-4_19 (accessed on 15th June 2025).

12. De Souza, M. J., Koltun, K. J., & Williams, N. I. (2019). The role of energy availability in reproductive function in the female athlete triad and extension of its effects to men: An initial working model of a similar syndrome in male athletes. *Sports Medicine, 49*, 125–137. https://doi.org/10.1007/s40279-019-01217-3 (accessed on 15th June 2025).

13. Diamanti-Kandarakis, E., Bourguignon, J. P., Giudice, L. C., Hauser, R., Prins, G. S., Soto, A. M., Zoeller, R. T., et al. (2009). Endocrine-disrupting chemicals: An Endocrine Society scientific statement. *Endocrine Reviews, 30*, 293–342. https://doi.org/10.1210/er.2009-0002 (accessed on 15th June 2025).

14. Feng, T., & Liu, Y. (2022). Microorganisms in the reproductive system and probiotic's regulatory effects on reproductive health. *Computational and Structural Biotechnology Journal, 20*, 1541–1553. https://doi.org/10.1016/j.csbj.2022.03.017 (accessed on 15th June 2025).

15. Feng, Y., Qu, X., & Hao, H. (2025). Progress in the study of the effects of selective serotonin reuptake inhibitors (SSRIs) on the reproductive system. *Frontiers in Pharmacology*. https://www.semanticscholar.org/paper/6aa6a798bb696dae829b2b028cf31b8ea25028c2 (accessed on 15th June 2025).

16. Foenna, Y. G., Calapoglu, N. S., Sancer, O., Tepebaşı, M. Y., & Calapoğlu, M. (2025). miR-29 family as epigenetic regulators of DNMTs in prostate cancer and benign prostatic hyperplasia. *The Indonesian Biomedical Journal*. https://www.semanticscholar.org/paper/fdb3110d014af1ead13ce5f84355003b178de769 (accessed on 15th June 2025).

17. Foreman, K. J., Marquez, N., Dolgert, A. J., Fukutaki, K., Fullman, N., McGaughey, M., Pletcher, M. A., et al. (2018). Forecasting life expectancy, years of life lost, and all-cause and cause-specific mortality for 250 causes of death: Reference and alternative scenarios for 2016–40 for 195 countries and territories. *The Lancet, 392*, 2052–2090. https://doi.org/10.1016/s0140-6736(18)31694-5 (accessed on 15th June 2025).

18. Gautam, R., Priyadarshini, E., Patel, A. K., & Arora, T. (2024). Assessing the impact and mechanisms of environmental pollutants (heavy metals and pesticides) on the male reproductive system: A comprehensive review. *Journal of Environmental Science and Health, Part C, 42*, 126–153. https://www.semanticscholar.org/paper/e97a9e7f54bc4710e151230ed75732fb55e3267a (accessed on 15th June 2025).

19. Grami, D., Selmi, S., Rtibi, K., Sebai, H., & De Toni, L. (2024). Emerging role of *Eruca sativa* Mill. in male reproductive health. *Nutrients, 16*. https://www.semanticscholar.org/paper/6d1b8691eca5340a7a9d7ee38168c5e3513ab136 (accessed on 15th June 2025).

20. Haider, S., & Beristain, A. G. (2023). Human organoid systems in modeling reproductive tissue development, function, and disease. *Human Reproduction, 38*, 1449–1463. https://doi.org/10.1093/humrep/dead085 (accessed on 15th June 2025).

21. Hegde, M., Kanathur, S., Shanmukhappa, A., & Srinivas, M. R. (2024). Evaluation of clinical, hormonal and ultrasound parameters of male reproductive system in leprosy: A cross-sectional study. *Indian Journal of Dermatology, 68*, 723. https://www.semanticscholar.org/paper/83a5a98a1d656e486845407d0f0bd8680ac8a283 (accessed on 15th June 2025).

22. Henriques, M. C., Santiago, J., Patrício, A., Herdeiro, M. T., Loureiro, S., & Fardilha, M. (2023). Smoking induces a decline in semen quality and the activation of stress response pathways in sperm. *Antioxidants, 12*, 1828. https://doi.org/10.3390/antiox12101828 (accessed on 15th June 2025).

23. Huang, Y., Li, X., Yao, J., Liu, W., Lu, M., & Xie, Y. (2024). (221) Anatomical transcriptome atlas of the male mouse reproductive system during aging. *The Journal of Sexual Medicine.* https://www.semanticscholar.org/paper/5968dc235fddb8901365477a702d276d7753f124 (accessed on 15th June 2025).

24. James, E., Carrell, D. T., Aston, K. I., Jenkins, T. G., Yeste, M., & Salas-Huetos, A. (2020). The role of the epididymis and the contribution of epididymosomes to mammalian reproduction. *International Journal of Molecular Sciences, 21*, 5377. https://doi.org/10.3390/ijms21155377 (accessed on 15th June 2025).

25. Jendraszak, M., Skibińska, I., Kotwicka, M., & Andrusiewicz, M. (2024). The elusive male microbiome: Revealing the link between the genital microbiota and fertility. Critical review and future perspectives. *Critical Reviews in Clinical Laboratory Sciences.* https://doi.org/10.1080/10408363.2024.2331489 (accessed on 15th June 2025).

26. Kelly, D. A., & Moore, B. C. (2016). The morphological diversity of intromittent organs: An introduction to the symposium. *Integrative and Comparative Biology, 56*, 630–634. https://doi.org/10.1093/icb/icw103 (accessed on 15th June 2025).

27. Korkmaz, O. (2024). Role of kisspeptin in female and male reproduction. *Journal of Medical Topics and Updates.* https://www.semanticscholar.org/paper/0ce7dfb8f9168497aa8f4220ba027dcf99c1d3d2 (accessed on 15th June 2025).

28. Laing, R., Gillan, V., & Devaney, E. (2017). Ivermectin–Old drug, new tricks? *Trends in Parasitology, 33*, 463–472. https://doi.org/10.1016/j.pt.2017.02.004 (accessed on 15th June 2025).

29. Le Tortorec, A., Matusali, G., Mahé, D., Aubry, F., Mazaud-Guittot, S., Houzet, L., & Dejucq-Rainsford, N. (2020). From ancient to emerging infections: The odyssey of viruses in the male genital tract. *Physiological Reviews, 100*, 1349–1414. https://doi.org/10.1152/physrev.00021.2019 (accessed on 15th June 2025).

30. Li, L., Lin, W., Wang, Z., Huang, R., Xia, H., Li, Z., Deng, J., et al. (2024). Hormone regulation in testicular development and function. *International Journal of Molecular Sciences, 25*, 5805. https://doi.org/10.3390/ijms25115805 (accessed on 15th June 2025).

31. Li, Q., Ye, Y., & An, L. (2025). Reduced sexual activity and increased sexually transmitted infections risk among left-behind women in rural China. *African Journal of Reproductive Health, 29*(2), 78–85. https://www.semanticscholar.org/paper/e2981631dc2d3340afef8adbd8337c3781cfe6b3 (accessed on 15th June 2025).

32. Mauvais-Jarvis, F., Bairey Merz, C. N., Barnes, P. J., Díaz Brinton, R., Carrero, J. J., DeMeo, D. L., De Vries, G. J., et al. (2020). Sex and gender: Modifiers of health, disease, and medicine. *The Lancet, 396*, 565–582. https://doi.org/10.1016/s0140-6736(20)31561-0 (accessed on 15th June 2025).

33. Medenica, S., Zivanovic, D., Batkoska, L., Marinelli, S., Basile, G., Perino, A., Cucinella, G., et al. (2022). The future is coming: Artificial intelligence in the treatment of infertility could improve assisted reproduction outcomes—The value of regulatory frameworks. *Diagnostics, 12*, 2979. https://doi.org/10.3390/diagnostics12122979 (accessed on 15th June 2025).

34. Mercati, F., Guelfi, G., Bufalari, A., Dall'Aglio, C., Suvieri, C., Cocci, P., Palermo, F., et al. (2024). From gene to protein: Unraveling the reproductive blueprint of male grey squirrels via nerve growth factor (NGF) and cognate receptors. *Animals, 14.* https://www.semanticscholar.org/

paper/45b65223ff16a91059ff9f9c95f00c877fbde45e (accessed on 15th June 2025).

35. Mikec, Š., Kolenc, Ž., Peterlin, B., Horvat, S., Pogorevc, N., & Kunej, T. (2022). Syndromic male subfertility: A network view of genome–phenome associations. *Andrology, 10*, 720–732. https://doi.org/10.1111/andr.13167 (accessed on 15th June 2025).

36. Naidu, R., Biswas, B., Willett, I. R., Cribb, J., Singh, B. K., Nathanail, C. P., Coulon, F., et al. (2021). Chemical pollution: A growing peril and potential catastrophic risk to humanity. *Environment International, 156*, 106616. https://doi.org/10.1016/j.envint.2021.106616 (accessed on 15th June 2025).

37. Obukohwo, O. M., Kingsley, N. E., Rume, R. A. R., & Victor, E. (2021). The concept of male reproductive anatomy. *Male Reproductive Anatomy*. https://www.semanticscholar.org/paper/eb746e080b047e8c90861d34c8ddce5beaa50dc4 (accessed on 15th June 2025).

38. Pan, J., Liu, P., Yu, X., Zhang, Z., & Liu, J. (2024). The adverse role of endocrine disrupting chemicals in the reproductive system. *Frontiers in Endocrinology, 14*. https://doi.org/10.3389/fendo.2023.1324993 (accessed on 15th June 2025).

39. Rautiala, P., & Lehtonen, J. (2024). Juvenile and total reproductive values for sexual reproduction under any genetic system. *Evolution: International Journal of Organic Evolution*. https://www.semanticscholar.org/paper/ed0afb1f170cff8564e9667faf1551290acb2c15 (accessed on 15th June 2025).

40. Sadek, K. M., Khalifa, N. E., Alshial, E. E., Abdelnour, S. A., Mohamed, A. R., & Noreldin, A. E. (2024). Potential hazards of bisphenol A on the male reproductive system: Induction of programmed cell death in testicular cells. *Journal of Biochemical and Molecular Toxicology, 38*. https://www.semanticscholar.org/paper/1ced330c63d32ffe7409cc93ebe77f8153881167 (accessed on 15th June 2025).

41. Santaballa, A., Márquez-Vega, C., Rodríguez-Lescure, Á., Rovirosa, Á., Vázquez, L., Zeberio-Etxetxipia, I., Andrés, M. M., et al. (2021). Multidisciplinary consensus on the criteria for fertility preservation in cancer patients. *Clinical & Translational Oncology, 24*, 227–243. https://doi.org/10.1007/s12094-021-02699-2 (accessed on 15th June 2025).

42. Sirotkin, A. V., & Kolesárová, A. (2021). Puncture vine (*Tribulus terrestris* L.) in control of health and reproduction. *Physiological Research*. https://doi.org/10.33549/physiolres.934711 (accessed on 15th June 2025).

43. Song, Y., Mao, C., Zhong, Q., Zhang, R., Jiang, D., & Sun, X. (2024). Role of hydrogen sulfide in the male reproductive system. *Frontiers in Endocrinology, 15*. https://www.semanticscholar.org/paper/e5a067bcc1d165ef2cb15823e873726905ca6def (accessed on 15th June 2025).

44. Syahrir, S., Palinrungi, M., Hatta, M., Kholis, K., Syarif, S., Azis, A., & Faruk, M. (2025). The impact of inflammation on prostate tumor dynamics: A pathological perspective on prostate cancer and benign prostatic hyperplasia. *Archive Italiano di Urologic, Andrologies: Organo Ufficiale [di] Societa Italian di Ecografia Urological e Nephrological*. https://www.semanticscholar.org/paper/1c8adaf55309d167d3892c2ec9e2afdffd1dbd24 (accessed on 15th June 2025).

45. Teede, H., Misso, M., Costello, M., Dokras, A., Laven, J. S. E., Moran, L., Piltonen, T., et al. (2018). Recommendations from the international evidence-based guideline for the assessment and management of polycystic ovary syndrome. *Clinical Endocrinology, 89*, 251–268. https://doi.org/10.1111/cen.13795 (accessed on 15th June 2025).

46. Yllera, M., Alonso-Peñarando, D., & Lombardero, M. (2024). Anatomy of the male reproductive system of sugar gliders (*Petaurus breviceps*). *Animals, 14.* https://www.semanticscholar.org/paper/81b98cc9bdd1552557d72a438b6c61d7b4ded065 (accessed on 15th June 2025).

47. Zaks, N., Batuure, A., Lin, E., Rommel, A. S., Reichenberg, A., Grice, D., Bergink, V., et al. (2023). Association between mental health and reproductive system disorders in women: A systematic review and meta-analysis. *JAMA Network Open, 6*(4), e238685. https://www.semanticscholar.org/paper/49a3b63d8c6d1631d77335867811d1856f2ae46e (accessed on 15th June 2025).

48. Zhai, Y., Feng, Y., Ma, X., & Ma, F. (2022). Defensins: Defenders of human reproductive health. *Human Reproduction Update, 29*, 126–154. https://doi.org/10.1093/humupd/dmac032 (accessed on 15th June 2025).

49. Zhao, W., Adjei, M., Zhang, Z., Yuan, Z., Cisang, Z., & Song, T. (2023). The role of GnRH in Tibetan male sheep and goat reproduction. *Reproduction in Domestic Animals, 58*, 1179–1187. https://doi.org/10.1111/rda.14432 (accessed on 15th June 2025).

FEMALE REPRODUCTIVE SYSTEM

12

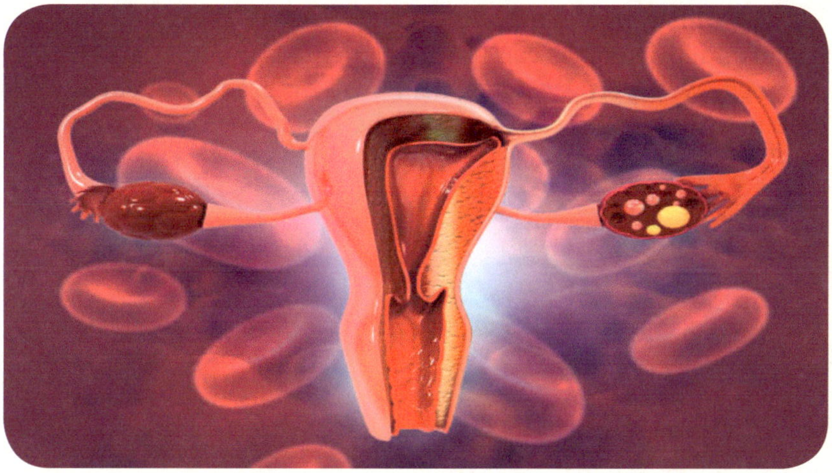

Introduction

The female reproductive system is not only important to the biological processes of reproduction but also to women's general health and wellness. Describing this intricate system is in urgent need in the medical field and in health education. The female reproductive system comprises structures such as the ovaries, fallopian tubes, uterus, and vagina, each contributing to specific functions related to fertility, hormonal balance, and sexual health. Physiological and psychological factors also play a role in terms of their impact on reproduction, which results in diverse experiences among women. By comprehension of the female reproductive tract, medical practitioners are able to enhance diagnosis, treatment, and prevention of reproductive health conditions, indicating a fundamental aspect of women's care. Beyond the anatomy basics, however, are complex issues with regard to the female reproductive tract, such as varied social and cultural determinants. Cultural factors, education, and availability of health services affect attitudes towards female reproductive health. In managing women's health, it

LEARNING OBJECTIVES

After studying this chapter, you will be able to:

1. Understand the anatomy of the female reproductive system
2. Describe the ovarian function
3. Explain the fertilization and early development
4 Understand the pregnancy and fetal development
5 Discuss the menopause and aging
6. Describe the common disorders of the female reproductive system

is essential to incorporate understanding of sex and gender differences that can be articulated in treatment and diagnostic interventions. Evidence supports that the differences can affect many areas of health, including disease causation and treatment responses. Managing the differences, identification, and elimination of differences are crucial for clinicians to construct holistic care plans that are equitable and inclusive. As recommended in recent proposals, clinicians should do their best to translate these concerns into practice to deliver higher-quality care to women (Baumgartner et al., 2020). In the process of providing the optimum healthcare practices, there is an urgent necessity for critical analysis of both biological and social determinants that influence the female reproductive tract. With advanced research, it seems more and more that precision medicine must include sex and gender as the underlying diagnostic, preventive, and treatment variables. This requires an interprofessional model of women's health that closes knowledge gaps and responds to the unique health needs of women. Bypassing the consideration of these factors can lead to overlooked health complications and low-quality care protocols. Therefore, it is crucial that clinicians and researchers adopt an inclusive approach recognizing the different influences that impact the female reproductive system and arguing for improved health in women across populations (Mauvais F-Jarvis et al., 2020).

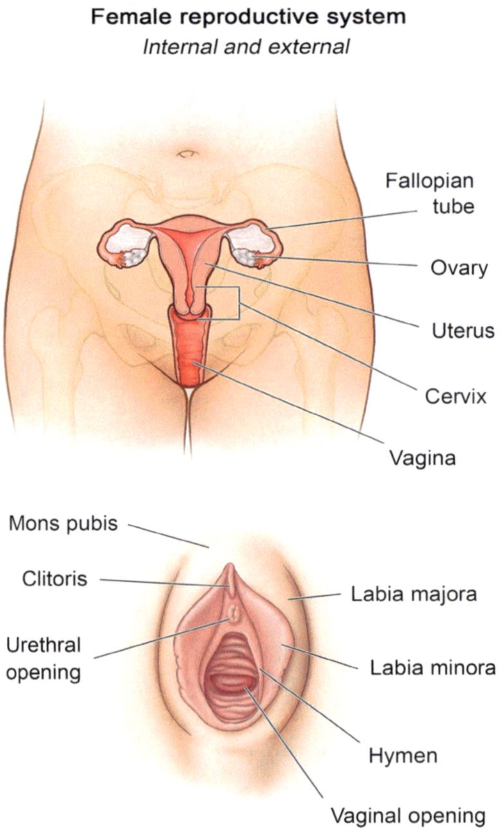

Figure 12.1. Internal and external organs of the female reproductive system.

Source: https://my.clevelandclinic.org/-/scassets/images/org/health/articles/9118-female-reproductive-system

12.1. Anatomy of the Female Reproductive System

Learning Outcome

1. Describe the external and internal structures of the female reproductive system
2. Understand the role of ligaments and supporting tissues

The female reproductive system is typical of a series of organs essential to reproduction, hormonal regulation, and overall well-being. The primary organs include the ovaries, the fallopian tubes, the uterus, and the vagina. The ovaries, usually two pairs, supply ova and release hormones such as estrogen and progesterone, crucial in controlling the menstrual cycle and supporting pregnancy. The fallopian tubes serve as the conduit for ova to travel from the ovaries to the uterus, where fertilization would typically occur. The muscular uterus is where a fertilized egg implants and develops. Familiarity with these structures interconnected functions is fundamental to comprehending the physiological mechanisms that regulate female reproductive health. Hormonal regulation is crucial for the function of the female reproductive apparatus, where estrogen and progesterone are key in the cycle of reproduction. Estrogen, primarily produced by the ovaries, triggers the development of the uterine lining to prepare it for potential implantation of a fertilized ovum. Estrogen also triggers vaginal epithelium changes, which are extremely important in ensuring reproductive tissue health. For instance, studies indicate estradiol, an estrogen, induces widespread proliferation within the vaginal epithelium, a response that is readily ascertainable under experimental conditions, such as in ovariectomized mice (Pai et al., 2006). The interactions between these hormones not only play vital roles in reproduction but also in women's health in general and influence many physiological processes throughout a woman's life. Due to the subtleties in visualizing human reproductive anatomy, researchers resort to using animal models, primarily mice, in order to better understand development and hormones.

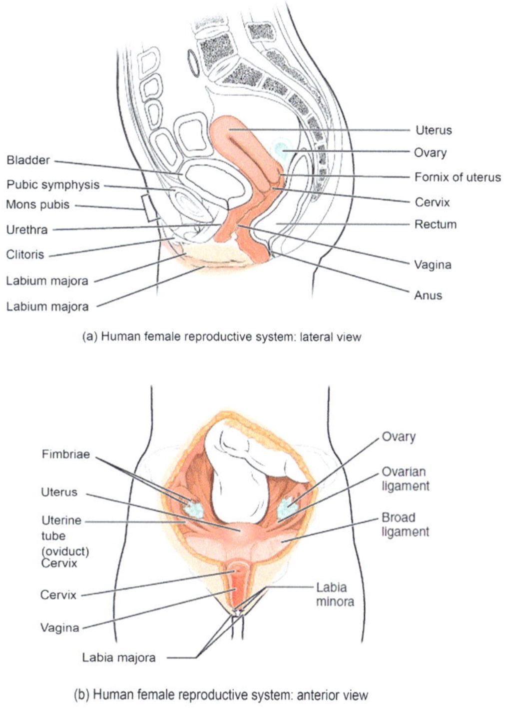

Figure 12.2. The major organs of the female reproductive system are located inside the pelvic cavity.

Source: https://s3-us-west-2.amazonaws.com/courses-images-archive-read-only/wp-content/uploads/sites/403/2015/04/21031921/Figure_28_02_01.jpg

The process employed in such studies presents both similarities and inherent differences between the mouse and human reproductive systems. While mouse models prove to be advantageous due to similarities between developmental biology and endocrine functions, their limitations should also be considered. Species-specific anatomical, developmental, and endocrine differences mandate caution during extrapolation. Careful knowledge of these differences enables researchers to select elements of the mouse model that have clear-cut relevance for human reproductive tract development and disease (Baskin et al., 2019). For this reason, sensitivity exists in both understanding women's health issues and providing better therapeutic responses.

12.1.1. External Structures: Vulva and Clitoris

The female reproductive system's external organs, the vulva and especially the clitoris, play a crucial role in reproduction but also sexual health and enjoyment. The vulva has various structures, including the labia majora, labia minora, clitoris, and vaginal opening. All structures are defined by certain anatomical features and functions that contribute to overall female sexual health. Periodic hormonal changes at different phases of life, such as puberty, menstruation, and menopause, influence the physiological properties of such organs, which can also be assessed with the aid of advanced imaging techniques. To illustrate, high-frequency ultrasonography has facilitated the presentation of the layered vulvar anatomy in a differential pattern, allowing for accurate assessment of its structural integrity and status, as indicated by research on this topic (Deng et al., 2024).

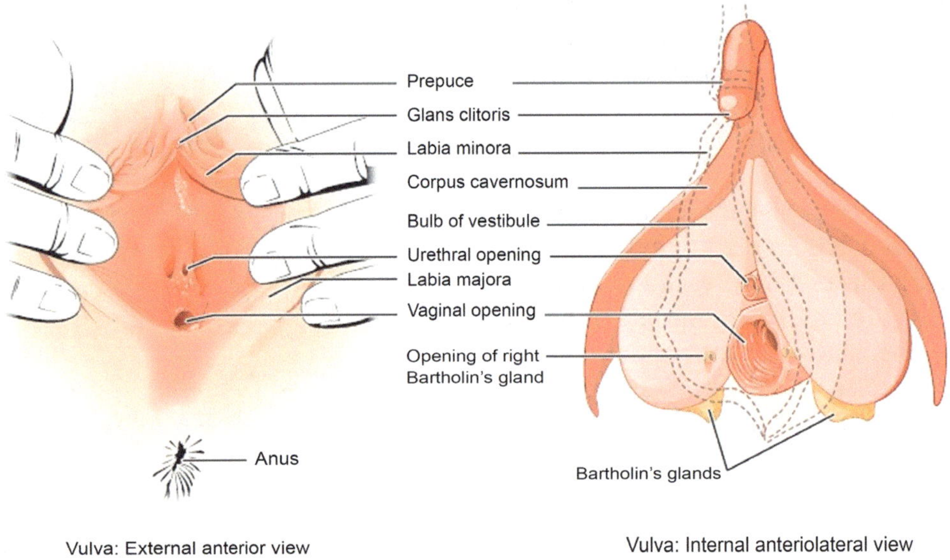

Figure 12.3. The external female genitalia are referred to collectively as the vulva.

Source: https://s3-us-west-2.amazonaws.com/courses-images-archive-read-only/wp-content/uploads/sites/403/2015/04/21031923/Figure_28_02_02.jpg

This advance leaves the door open for further research into female reproductive anatomy and disease. The clitoris, specifically, is among the most sensitive areas of the vulva, with a dense plexus of nerve endings involved in sexual pleasure and arousal. The clitoris's anatomical complexity is often overlooked in light of the fact that the visible external portion is only a small fraction of an enormous internal structure. Research affirms that the clitoral network spreads outside of the glans, branching into a network of erectile tissue that engorges with blood during sexual arousal. Such a conceptualization resists dominant knowledge about female anatomy and sexual function. As noted in various studies on women's sexual arousal, a thorough knowledge of the clitoris not only adds to women's sexual health knowledge but also directs to sexual pleasure as a fundamental part of general health (Deng et al., 2024). Such knowledge supports fuller and correct representation of the female body in medical education and popular thought. The importance of being aware of the vulva and clitoris has implications in the healthcare and social environments, where having knowledge of the importance of such an organ can inform healthcare interventions for women. Healthcare professionals must ensure that they provide adequate education regarding the anatomy and functions of such reproductive exterior organs to facilitate informed discussions on reproductive choices and sexual health. In addition, improvements in imaging technology, such as the application of high-frequency ultrasonography as in certain recent studies, underscore the value of visual understanding of the layering of the vulva (Migda et al., 2019). This can lead to improved diagnostic tools and specially designed treatments for various conditions that affect the female reproductive tract and ultimately contribute to better health outcomes for women. By putting the door open to a better understanding of the outer anatomy of the female reproductive system, society can start dismantling stigmas around female sexual health and work towards more acceptance of diversity within women's bodies.

12.1.2. Internal Structures: Ovaries, Fallopian Tubes, Uterus, and Vagina

Ovaries are critical organs of the female reproductive system that are primarily responsible for the production of oocytes and the secretion of sex hormones, including estrogen and progesterone. They are bilaterally located in the pelvic cavity in the shape of almond-shaped structures. These structures play a crucial role in regulating the menstrual cycle through hormonal feedback mechanisms. Folliculogenesis occurs in the ovaries, where ovarian follicles develop and discharge gametes via ovulation. It is crucial to understand ovarian function not only for the understanding of normal reproductive physiology but also for the management of disorders of infertility and endocrine disturbances. Furthermore, advances in reproductive technologies and hormone therapies have put more focus on the study of ovarian physiology in research and clinical settings, which has continued to highlight the necessity of new approaches in the management of conditions that compromise ovarian function, such as the increasingly prevalent polycystic ovary syndrome (PCOS) in women today (Kim et al., 2025). Extending from the ovaries, the fallopian tubes are tubes along which the oocytes travel towards the uterus and are also the primary site where fertilization takes place. The two fallopian tubes each consist of four distinct components: the infundibulum, ampulla, isthmus, and interstitial component. Together, they transport both the egg and sperm through a complex process of muscle contractions and ciliary motion. The importance of these tubes cannot be overstated, such that any obstruction or malfunction will lead to tubal factor infertility, which ensures that the sperm will never get to the egg. There has been increased research focused on unraveling the cellular and molecular mechanisms that control the functioning of fallopian tubes, with a focus on how they can be affected by various environmental, physiological, and disease-related factors. An investigation of these characteristics is essential for the development of therapeutic interventions aimed at restoring tubal function and improving reproductive outcomes in affected women (Kim et al., 2025). The uterus, or rather a muscular and pear-shaped organ, is an integral part of the female reproductive system. Its critical function is to offer accommodation and nourish the fetus as it grows in gestation, with its structural layering—endometrium, myometrium, and perimetrium—having different roles to play in this function. The endometrium is particularly significant since it undergoes cyclical variation with the hormonal changes and is shed during menstruation if pregnancy does not occur. The uterine environment is most critical for implantation, and conditions such as endometriosis or uterine fibroids can drastically handicap this process and result in infertility. The vagina is also a passageway for menstrual efflux, sexual intercourse, and delivery. It is important to comprehend the intricate interconnections and functions of these internal structures for resolving reproductive health issues and enhancing the treatments for fertility.

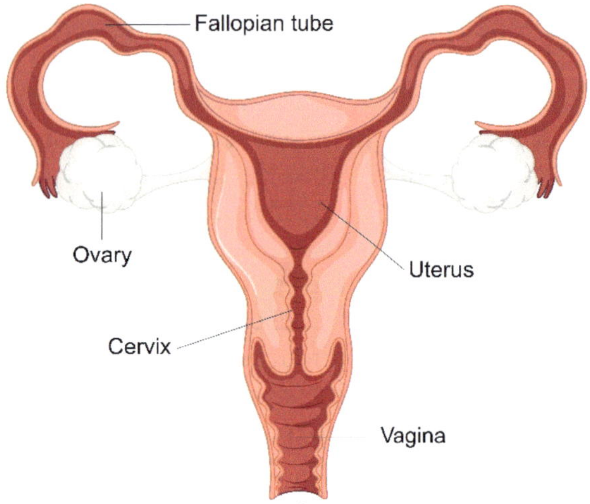

Figure 12.4. Internal reproductive organs in the female.

Source: https://media.healthdirect.org.au/images/inline/original/female-reproductive-system-90e91e.jpg

12.1.3. Role of Ligaments and Supporting Tissues

Within the female reproductive tract, supporting ligaments and tissues are essential components that contribute structural support and function to reproductive organs. The round, broad, and uterosacral ligaments are the major ligaments responsible for providing vital support to the uterus and maintaining its position within the pelvic cavity. Not only do these ligaments allow anchorage, but they also accommodate the variations in changes that occur with pregnancy, including enlargement and relocation. In addition, support tissues surrounding the uterus, including fascia and connective tissues, are also credited with the biomechanical stability of the female reproductive system. Damage or deformation to these ligaments leads to conditions such as pelvic organ prolapse, which markedly affects a woman's quality of life and reproductive health, justifying the need to maintain the integrity of these structures. Besides, supportive tissues and ligaments not only provide structural support but also play an active part in hormonal regulation and reproductive activity. The broad ligament contains blood vessels, nerves, and lymphatics, which are responsible for the crucial vascular and neural supply to the reproductive organs. This is the anatomical setup that allows optimal transportation of hormones necessary for such activities as ovulation, the menstrual cycle, and pregnancy. Moreover, the interactions of the ligaments with other tissues can influence the local hormonal environment and thus affect ovarian function and overall fertility. These complex associations need to be understood in order to diagnose and treat reproductive dysfunction because any changes in the integrity or function of these supporting tissues could lead to problems in fertility. Lastly, the ongoing research on the role of ligaments and supportive tissues of the female reproductive tract underlines the role played by these tissues in health as opposed to disease. Tissue engineering and regenerative medicine research focus on developing therapeutic methods for restoring or repairing impaired ligaments and associated tissues. These findings are most relevant to women with pelvic support disorders or those requiring surgery for reproductive health issues. By examining the biomechanical properties and biological functions of these tissues, researchers can develop innovative solutions that maximize reproductive success and overall health. Thus, the ligaments and supporting tissues do not only constitute an integral component of the physical anatomy of the female reproductive system but also are central to the upkeep of proper hormonal and functional dynamics of the system, leading to a much greater comprehension of women's health.

Test Your Knowledge

1. What is the external female reproductive structures?
2. What is the role of ligaments and supporting tissues?

12.2. Ovarian Function

Learning Outcome

1. Describe the process of oogenesis
2. Understand the hormonal regulation
3. Understand the menstrual cycle phases and their significance

The ovaries are at the core of women's health and reproductive capacity, as the sites of oocyte production and sex hormone secretion. With women's different phases of reproduction, ovarian function falls off in a natural process, culminating in menopause. This reduction is marked by precipitous changes in hormones, i.e., declines in estradiol and progesterone, which are pivotal in the regulation of the menstrual cycle and pregnancy. Consequently, this hormonal shift affects not only fertility but also various physiological systems, including the musculoskeletal system. A cross-sectional study has detected a correlation between ovarian function and health-related quality of life (HRQoL), indicating that alterations in ovarian status can have adverse effects on physical strength and general well-being, particularly with advancing age, highlighting the necessity to understand ovarian function in the context of global health assessment (Luo et al., 2025). In addition, the reduction in ovarian function is associated with multifarious clinical conditions, particularly autoimmune diseases. Research has indicated that autoimmune diseases like rheumatoid arthritis have the potential to exacerbate ovarian dysfunction, especially in young women. Women with such illnesses have the risk of fertility impairment and hormonal imbalance due to systemic inflammation and drug side effects, such as the use of methotrexate. Although some studies indicate a correlation of cumulative doses of methotrexate with impaired ovarian function, additional research would need to be done to clarify these interactions. Additionally, the prevalence of autoimmune ovarian failure among women of childbearing age emphasizes awareness and interdisciplinarity in treating reproductive health against the backdrop of autoimmune diseases (Kazakova et al., 2024).

Ovarian function is also realized in terms of understanding the role that lifestyle choices and exposure to the environment play on reproductive health. Diet, exercise, and endocrine disruptors may all play a very significant role in ovarian function. For instance, studies have indicated that frequent exercise can exert a positive effect on the hormonal balance and ovarian reserve, further solidifying the notion of women's health as a holistic factor. Furthermore, women's psychological state cannot be ruled out since stress is proven to impact the hormone levels and hence ovarian function. This interconnectedness of lifestyle habits, environmental factors, and ovarian function underscores the need for multidisciplinary health education and special interventions that promote good reproductive health throughout a woman's life. Women can be empowered with holistic measures to make self-directed decisions that contribute to their ovarian function and reproductive health.

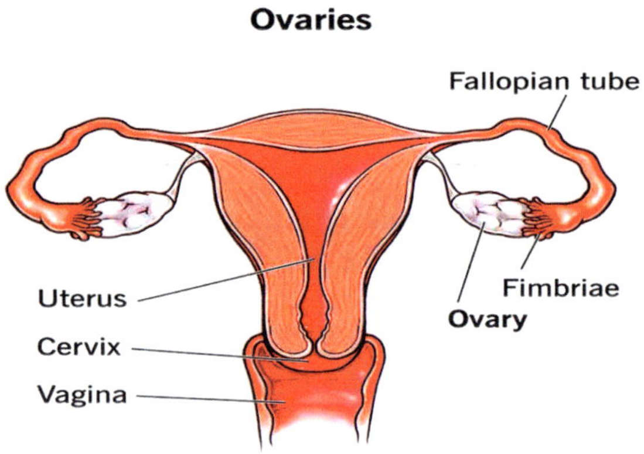

Figure 12.5. The ovaries are small glands located on either side of your uterus. They produce eggs and hormones for menstruation and pregnancy.

Source: https://my.clevelandclinic.org/-/scassets/images/org/health/articles/22999-ovaries

12.2.1. Oogenesis: The Process of Egg Development

The process of oogenesis is a critical aspect of female reproductive biology because it significantly contributes to fertility and the whole reproductive system. Oogenesis begins in the fetal stage, where primordial germ cells proliferate and ultimately provide primary oocytes following a sequence of mitotic division processes. The primary oocyte then enters prophase I of meiosis, remaining dormant until puberty. With the onset of hormonal signals regulated by the menstrual cycle, a few of the oocytes resume meiosis and complete the first meiotic division to give rise to a secondary oocyte and a polar body. Such sophisticated coordination between cellular and endocrine signals guarantees human oocyte maturation into fertile gametes capable of effectively participating in fertilization, upholding the reproductive capability of the female reproductive tract. Besides, oocyte maturation is regulated by intricate biochemical processes and hormonal controls that direct the developmental trajectory of the oocyte. FSH and LH are only a few among numerous hormones that have vital functions in the induction of ovarian follicle growth and maturation. The activity of ecdysteroids, whose function in insect development is well documented, has also been shown to be involved in the oogenesis process in certain model organisms. For example, experiments on the depletion of Halloween gene products, including SchgrSpo, SchgrSad, and SchgrShd, exhibited major changes in oocyte shape and viability, highlighting their critical role during oocyte development (Schellens et al., 2022). These observations not only display the multi-dimensional nature of oogenesis but also open up the scope for understanding the hormonal regulation of female fecundity. In addition to hormonal regulation, the molecular and genetic nature of oogenesis has deep implications for reproductive health. Recent studies of organisms like Ascaris lumbricoides have revealed insights into the transcriptomic patterns that regulate reproductive processes, such as oogenesis. These profiles identified the function of specific genes and regulatory pathways involved in cell signaling, cytoskeleton organization, and embryogenesis, which was found to take a central role in regulating reproductive outcomes (Phuphisut et al., 2022). Investigation into these molecular pathways not only deepens our insight into oocyte development but also offers windows for therapeutic interventions against reproductive disorders. As researchers keep delving deeper into the mechanisms of oogenesis, their work might lead to significant advances in fertility treatment and reproductive health.

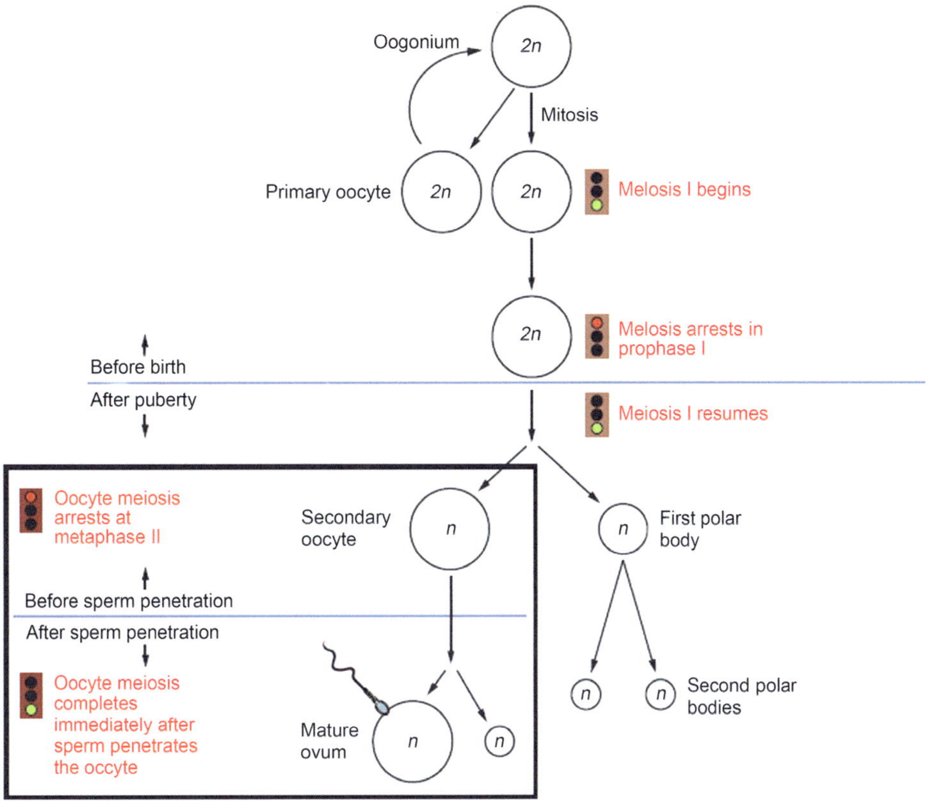

Figure 12.6. The unequal cell division of oogenesis produces one to three polar bodies that later degrade, as well as a single haploid ovum, which is produced only if there is penetration of the secondary oocyte by a sperm cell.

Source: https://s3-us-west-2.amazonaws.com/courses-images-archive-read-only/wp-content/uploads/sites/403/2015/04/21031924/Figure_28_02_03.jpg

12.2.2. Hormonal Regulation: Estrogen and Progesterone

The specific balance of estrogen and progesterone is a crucial modulator of the female reproductive system, overseeing several physiological processes essential to reproductive health. Estrogen, produced primarily by the ovaries, is critical to secondary sexual development and the maintenance of female secondary sexual characteristics as well as to the regulation of the menstrual cycle. Throughout the menstrual cycle, estrogen peaks and dips, stimulating follicular growth and thickening the endometrial lining in preparation for potential implantation. Progesterone, which is produced by the corpus luteum, on the other hand, is instrumental in maintaining the endometrium following ovulation. This coordination between estrogen and progesterone makes for the most ideal environment for fertilization and implantation, testifying to their synergistic functions in the reproductive system. Research has shown that estrogen and progesterone hormonal imbalances can cause significant reproductive issues, thereby emphasizing the need for their regulation. For instance, PCOS and endometriosis have been reported to be linked to aberrant estrogen and progesterone signaling, which leads to ovarian and endometrial biology malfunction. PCOS generally encompasses hyperandrogenism accompanied by concomitant deranged estrogen and progesterone production, which results in irregular menses and infertility. Similarly, in endometriosis, deranged hormonal milieus in turn exacerbate the ectopic growth of the endometrial tissue and result in pain and issues. All these conditions emphasize the significance of understanding hormonal interaction and signal transduction mechanisms to determine effective treatment regimens for women's reproductive health. Combining data from androgen interactions makes the details of hormonal regulation in the female reproductive tract more apparent. Discovery of androgen action, in association with estrogen and progesterone, addresses reproductive physiology and disease. Noted in current research, androgen receptor expression in endometrial and ovarian tissue varies with the menstrual cycle, suggesting a mild regulatory role in association with estrogen and progesterone signaling. For instance, evidence suggests that androgens can regulate estrogen action, affecting follicular kinetics and endometrial receptivity. This intricate interplay of hormones demands an integrated approach within endocrinology since understanding the interrelation is capable of offering more competent clinical intervention in the regulation of hormonal imbalance, hence promoting enhanced reproductive health and outcomes among women (Abbey C Lissaman et al., 2023) (Bedoor A Salim et al., 2023).

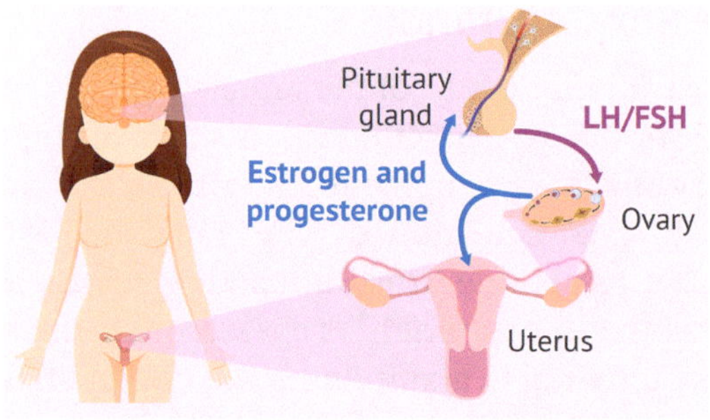

Figure 12.7. Hormonal regulation of the menstrual cycle.

Source: https://www.invitra.com/en/wp-content/uploads/2019/01/hormonal-regulation-of-the-menstrual-cycle.png.webp

12.2.3. Menstrual Cycle Phases and Their Significance

It is important to understand the menstrual cycle in order to understand the female reproductive system. The menstrual cycle itself usually takes between 21 and 35 days and has four phases: menstrual phase, follicular phase, ovulation, and luteal phase. Each of the phases plays an important role in preparing the body for possible pregnancy. The menstrual phase, which begins the cycle, is characterized by the uterine lining breaking up, indicating the hormonal changes that govern this physiological process. In this instance, a decline in estrogen and progesterone causes endometrial tissue breakdown, which signals the beginning of a new cycle. This recidivous shedding, together with unutilized tissue shedding, recycles the hormonal environment to be used for future cycles and thereby provides a physiological rationale for ovulation and potential conception. The follicular phase follows the menstrual phase and is characterized by the growth of ovarian follicles due to stimulation caused by the follicle-stimulating hormone (FSH). At this point, the ovaries now release increasingly more estrogen, which enables these follicles to mature and grow. This is an extremely significant step in that the dominant follicle grows, typically leading one oocyte to be released. The significance of this step lies not only in the development of the follicles, since rising levels of estrogen also prepare the uterine lining for possible implantation of a fertilized egg. Moreover, identification of the variability in this phase, which is environmental- and health-oriented, indicates the vulnerability of reproductive health and calls for hormonal homeostasis during the cycle. The luteal phase terminates the menstrual cycle in preparation for implantation in the event of fertilization. After or with ovulation, the broken follicle transforms into the corpus luteum, which secretes the progesterone required to ensure the endometrium. The only function of this hormone is to prepare the uterine lining for a fertilized egg. In case the fertilization fails, the corpus luteum will dissolve, and the progesterone levels will fall with the onset of the menstrual cycle. A clearer comprehension of the luteal phase is particularly significant in cases such as reproductive health, as interference with this phase will affect fertility and menstruation. Furthermore, recent research shows that illnesses like COVID-19 can affect hormonal levels and menstrual cycle regularity, revealing the interdependency between general health and the reproductive system (Pourmasumi et al., 2023; Gorbacheva et al., 2023). It raises the awareness of reproductive health and suggests the necessity of an integral approach in women's medicine.

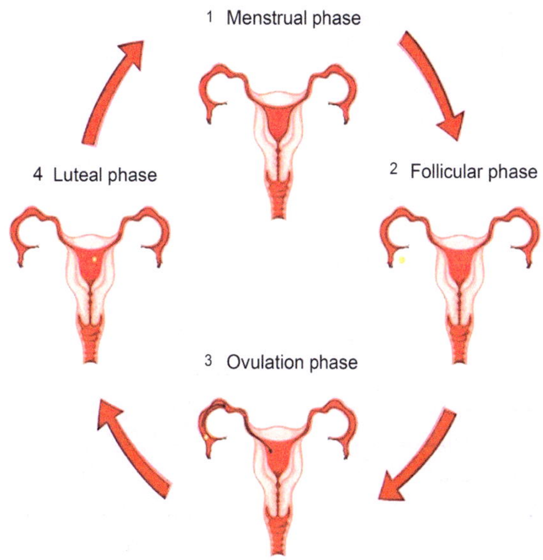

Figure 12.8. Phases of the menstrual cycle.

Source: https://happyhealthyyou.com.au/cdn/shop/articles/4_phases_1200x1200.jpg?v=1695885955

Test Your Knowledge

1. What is the process of oogenesis?
2. What is the significance of the menstrual cycle?

12.3. Fertilization and Early Development

Learning Outcome

1. Describe the process of fertilization in the fallopian tubes
2. Understand the formation of the zygote and early cell division
3. Describe the process of implantation in the uterine lining

Fertilization is a seminal first stage of the female reproductive system that leads to the formation of a zygote. It begins when a sperm fertilizes the egg, thus forming the combination of parental genetic material. The zygote will undergo a series of rapid, successive cell divisions known as cleavage, which will grow into a multicellular organism after fertilization. This phase is pivotal in the sense that it sets in motion the genetic and developmental blueprint of the whole organism, the ability to influence everything from physical traits to biological processes. Developments in reproductive health technology enhance our understanding of this primary phase of development and identify and eliminate myths regarding reproductive health. Advanced case-based expert systems, such as those developed at Utama General Hospital, demonstrate promise for faster and better diagnosis, thus greater access to important reproductive health information and services (Lestari et al., 2024). Following fertilization, the presumptively developing embryo is guided through a critical phase marked by implantation. Here, the embryo travels along the fallopian tubes and settles on the uterine wall, where it will continue to develop and grow. The uterine lining is tasked with providing the necessary nutrients and hormonal nurturing that are crucial to the successful fulfillment of the pregnancy. Development in the female reproductive system is astounding here; the endometrium becomes thicker to provide the developing embryo with the necessary nutrients. Besides, the bodily changes start to develop in the mother's body, which are meant to support the developing fetus. The intimacy of the relationship between fetal development and the mother's health during this period is obvious as the nutritional intake of the mother will affect embryonic development, as well as the overall health of the child in the long run. Improvements in the knowledge regarding the biomechanics of reproduction, and especially that concerning fluid dynamics, shed light on the forces that are felt during implantation (Leftwich and Baumer, 2023). The developing embryo passes through several major milestones that set the stage for future growth and development. This includes the creation of major organs such as the placenta, which is crucial in facilitating nutrient and waste transfer between the mother and the developing fetus. The mother also experiences a series of physiological changes in order to provide space for the developing fetus during pregnancy. This is crucial in maintaining adequate oxygenation and nutrient provision. The complexity of early development illustrates the interaction of the various body systems and alludes to the importance of an optimal reproductive environment. With increasing research on reproductive biomechanics, such as the fluid dynamics of labor and implantation, it is increasingly evident how these mechanical forces overlap and give rise to reproductive success (Leftwich et al., 2023).

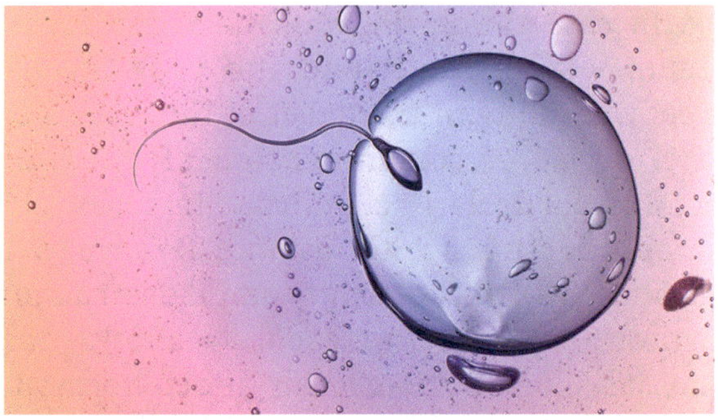

Source: https://images.agoramedia.com/wte3.0/gcms/How-Fertilization-Happens-722x406.jpg

12.3.1. Process of Fertilization in the Fallopian Tubes

Fertilization is a key component of reproduction, occurring primarily in the fallopian tubes, which serve as conduits between the ovaries and uterus. When an ovary releases a mature egg during ovulation, the egg is captured by the fimbriae, finger-like appendages at the end of the fallopian tubes. The movement produced by ciliary action along the tube's inner surface aids in directing the egg towards the ampulla, the region most conducive to fertilization. Sperm, typically inserted in the vagina during sexual intercourse, travel through the cervix and uterus to reach the fallopian tubes.

This is achieved due to muscular contractions and sperm motility, and it emphasizes the function of different female reproductive system anatomical formations in effective fertilization (Snigireva et al., 2024). When the egg is in the ampullary region of the fallopian tube, it reaches a critical period for fertilization. At the same time, functional sperm must pass through the hostile environment of the female reproductive tract with varying pH and immune responses intended to ward off pathogens. Proximity of the sperm to the egg triggers capacitation, during which the sperm undergo physiological changes that enable them to penetrate the egg's protective coverings more effectively. When sperm reach the zona pellucida of the egg, they degrade this layer using enzymes until ultimately the sperm and egg membranes become joined. This sophisticated interaction triggers extensive changes that occur following fertilization, indicating the onset of embryonic development (Snigireva et al., 2024). Following successful fertilization, there is a cascade of developmental landmarks that take place in a short interval within the fallopian tube. The resultant zygote is cleaved, a cell division process that transforms it into a multicellular entity referred to as a blastocyst. Along the journey of the blastocyst through the fallopian tube to the uterus, differentiation also occurs in which the cells specialize for future growth. This is a crucial process toward eventual implantation in the uterine lining in order that the embryo may be supplied with the correct nutrition and support in development. The fallopian tubes, thus, have not just a functional role in gamete movement but also have a critical role to play in the earliest stages of embryonic development, which highlights their significance within the female reproductive system (Septadina, 2023).

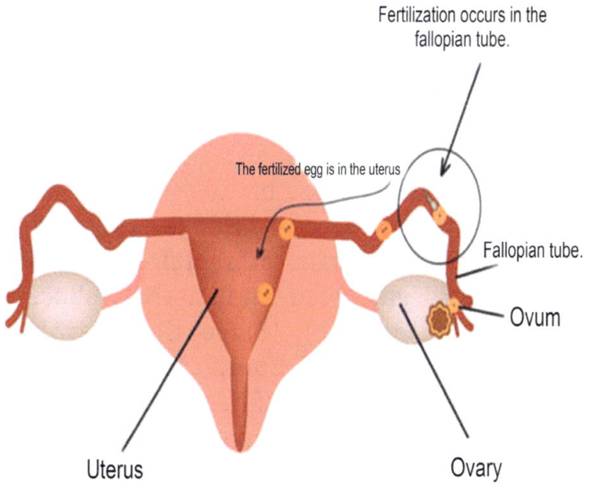

Figure 12.9. Fertilization occurs in the fallopian tube.

Source: https://biologydictionary.net/wp-content/uploads/2020/07/fertilization-optimized.jpg

12.3.2. Formation of the Zygote and Early Cell Division

The formation of the zygote is a milestone in the cycle of the female reproductive system, occurring following fertilization when sperm penetrate the oocyte. The union forms a diploid cell containing genetic material from both parents, thereby laying the foundation for embryonic development. The resulting oocyte then undergoes a wave of remarkable changes, such as sudden cellular movements as the zygote prepares for its first cellular divisions. The integrity of this process is fundamental because any error could lead to developmental disease or implantation failure. The complexity of zygote formation, such as the fusion of genetic material and initiation of key developmental pathways, underscores its significance in reproductive biology. This observation illuminates not only the basics of fertilization but also the nuances of early embryonic development. Following the zygote formation, cleavage, an early cell division commonly referred to, initiates the start of a highly significant period of embryogenesis. During this period, the one-cell zygote undergoes a series of mitotic divisions that ultimately give rise to an increasing number of cells, which are referred to as the blastomeres. The divisions are followed by intense cellular proliferation but without significant growth, thus maintaining the zygote's overall size constant but increasing the number of cells. This is a crucial process since it forms the basis for subsequent differentiation processes, which will lead to the varied cell types and ultimately, the entire organism. The success of this stage of cleavage is also crucial in order to achieve proper gene expression and cellular organization, having relevance to the future viability of the embryo. The intricacy of these early partitions demonstrates the delicate interplay between cell processes and genetics in the production of a successful pregnancy. With continued cell division, the process of morphological alteration moves center stage as the blastomeres reformulate into the morula, ultimately forming the blastocyst. This is not merely a physical transformation; it is intricate signaling pathways and gene control that orchestrate developmental events. The change from the morula to the blastocyst is especially important, as it marks the beginning of differentiation in which cells start to assign unique functions. The outer cell layer will be responsible for the formation of the placenta, and the inner cell mass will form the embryo. The importance of such differentiation and organization cannot be overstressed, as it is determinative of the subsequent implantation within the uterine wall and formation of a healthy pregnancy. Having an understanding of such early stages of zygotic development, shielded by processes of cleavage and differentiation, constitutes a sound basis to address challenges of reproductive health in various environments, like those outlined in Ocañas et al. (2024) and Ilyasova et al. (2024).

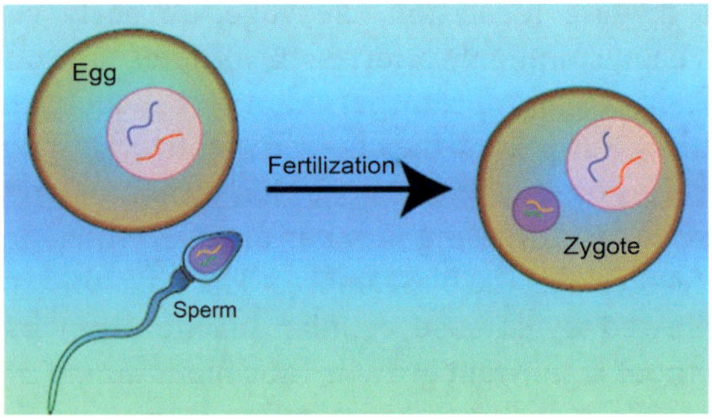

Figure 12.10. Zygote formation.

Source: https://www.stemcellcareindia.com/wp-content/uploads/2023/10/Zygote-Formation-in-Humans-768x432.jpg

12.3.3. Implantation in the Uterine Lining

Implantation of the uterine blastocyst into the uterine lining represents the highlight of human reproduction, signaling the commencement of the transition from pre-embryonic growth to early pregnancy. Once the ovum has been fertilized, the formed blastocyst starts its passage through the fallopian tube into the uterus. The uterine lining or the endometrium also experiences dramatic morphological changes under hormonal influence in the form of progesterone and estrogen. Receptivity during the window of implantation is initiated by these changes, which promote vascularization and cell-to-cell communication between the blastocyst and the uterine endometrium. This multifaceted interaction is crucial, as not only does it permit exchange of nutrients and support of the developing embryo, but also initiates the initial immunological microenvironment that permits successful pregnancy, illustrating the sophisticated interplay of cellular and hormonal factors that modulate implantation. The relationship between gut microbiota and reproductive health is increasingly becoming the focus of studies in the dynamics of implantation. The gut flora was found to have incredible effects on endometrial function, which is extremely significant during implantation. Some of the microbial-metabolites such as short-chain fatty acids, play a critical role in immune system regulation and epithelial integrity at the uterine level. Dysbiosis—imbalance of gut microbiota—has also been demonstrated to play a role in many gynaecological syndromes, including repeated implantation failure and preeclampsia, demonstrating the systemic impact that the health of the gut may have on reproductive success. Hence, knowledge of the gut–endometrial axis illuminates new insights into enhanced implantation success and fertility generally, since the microbial community structure could directly affect hormonal regulation and site-specific immune tolerance for successful embryo attachment to the uterine lining (Mora et al., 2025). In addition, ion channels in the process of implantation are an intriguing area of investigation in reproductive physiology. Current research has confirmed the physiologic presence of certain ion channels, like ASIC2 and PIEZO2, in the reproductive tract tissue, including the uterine lining. They are thought to play a role in many physiologic functions, including the movement of ions and molecules important to cellular functions. Their presence in endometrial tissues suggests they may play a role in maintaining tissue health and enabling embryo implantation. Because these pathways potentially impact vascular regulation and uterine contractility, their proper mechanisms potentially offer new targets for optimizing implantation rates as well as for treating reproductive disease. Research in this field in the future can ideally continue to shed light on the mechanism by which these molecular players regulate the delicate processes of implantation within the female reproductive tract (Mhalhel et al., 2025).

Test Your Knowledge

1. What is the process of fertilization in the fallopian tubes?
2. What is the formation of the zygote?

12.4. Pregnancy and Fetal Development

Learning Outcome

1. Describe the stages of pregnancy
2. Understand the role of the placenta in nutrient and waste exchange
3. Describe the common complications during pregnancy

Pregnancy is a complex and multifaceted process that is the culmination of the female reproductive system. Throughout the process from conception to giving birth, there are varied physiological processes that occur within the female body in order to aid in the development of the fetus. Initially, the fertilized egg or zygote is transported to the uterus, and it implants itself into the endometrium. Development of the care-conditioned environment within which embryonic growth occurs is crucial and is significantly reliant on hormone changes that enable the uptake and metabolism of nutrients. These biochemical changes are critical to the continued growth of the developing embryo and are influenced by many factors, including maternal health and environmental toxins. This intricate interaction between the maternal systems and the embryo during development encapsulates the importance of a healthy functioning reproductive system and how interference may lead to complications during pregnancy, as noted in other studies on reproductive health (Liu et al., 2025). Following implantation, fetal development is one of several phases that is marked by significant change. The embryonic phase begins shortly after implantation, when the basic organ systems begin to form. Cell differentiation occurs as the embryo matures into different structures, laying the groundwork for fundamental physiological functions. Eight weeks from the time of fertilization is when an embryo is developed, which is referred to as a fetus, and with more organ development, neural growth, and overall development. It is during this stage of development that epigenetic elements are able to influence fetal outcomes, and m6A marks play an important role in regulation and development. These marks influence mRNA dynamics essential to the development of the fetus, information important to understanding the nuances of developmental biology within the context of the female reproductive system (Liu et al., 2025). Of growing significance with progressive pregnancy is the necessity to maintain maternal-fetal immune homeostasis. Immune machinery is in place for the accommodation of the expanding fetus, genetically alien to the mother.

The immune response must be optimal to prevent AFD, a remorseful syndrome related to most maternal pathologies. Studies have demonstrated that pathologies of the endometrium, including inflammatory reaction, may predispose to AFD and thus warrant extensive pre-pregnancy evaluations. The state of the maternal immune system and infectious status at conception can play a significant role in influencing pregnancy outcomes. As more and more scientists discover that fetal development and maternal health are interrelated, the application of immunologic assessment in family planning holds strong potential for reducing reproductive losses.

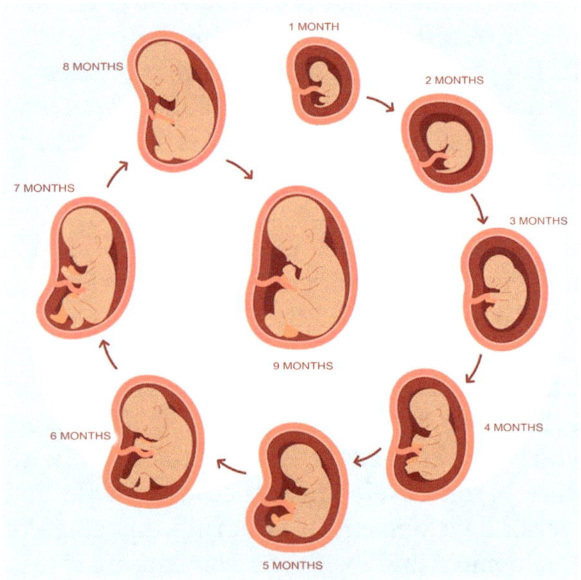

Figure 12.11. Fetal development.

Source: https://www.jeevanwomencareclinic.com/wp-content/uploads/2024/01/Fetal-Development-Week-by-Week.jpg

12.4.1. Stages of Pregnancy: Trimesters and Key Developments

The pregnancy periods are generally divided into three trimesters, each of which has distinctive developmental milestones and bodily changes in the female. The first trimester, lasting from conception until week 12, is when the fetus's fundamental structures are established. During this period, the main organs begin to form, and by the end of the first trimester, the embryo becomes a fetus, with the primary heart, brain, and spinal cord development. Along with these developments, the mother also experiences radical changes in hormone levels, with a rise in hCG (human chorionic gonadotropin) and progesterone, which are crucial for supporting the pregnancy and growth of the baby. Information about these early stages is important for monitoring the mother's and fetus's well-being, as any issue can have long-term effects on both. Early visits by a healthcare provider are essential during this trimester. The second trimester, from week 13 to week 26, is generally characterized by a decrease in symptoms of pregnancy and increased visibility of the growth of the fetus. At this stage, fetal movement is perceived, and the developing body begins to take on more characteristics of a human, including limb and face development. In addition, significant advances in neurological development occur, laying the groundwork for sensory input. Most importantly, this trimester opens the window for critical screening methods, such as ultrasounds and blood tests, to assess maternal and fetal health. Notably, research indicates that health interactions are affected by factors such as hormonal change and microbiome changes in pregnancy, reinforcing the significance of the microenvironment to fetal development, as seen in studies using stressors affecting subjects with prediabetes and pregnancy (Lita M Proctor et al., 2019). The third trimester, week 27 to birth, involves extensive fetal growth and development. Key events during this period include the deposition of body fat, lung development, and brain development, setting the stage for the fetus to be able to survive outside the womb. The mother must also endure significant physical alterations to facilitate the growth of the fetus, including changes in posture and increased weight, which may result in discomfort or issues. Additionally, the fetus has become more sensitive to external stimuli, such as sound and light, which shows active sensory and neurological development. Both fetal and maternal signs need to be monitored around the clock in this last phase to expect potential complications. Recognition of the interface between pregnancy outcome and biological sex further highlights the sophistication of reproductive health and that clinicians need to integrate sex and gender considerations into practice to enhance fetal and maternal health (Mauvais F-Jarvis et al., 2020).

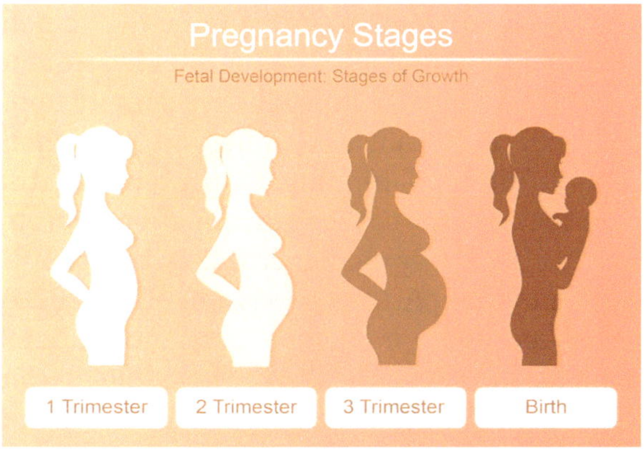

Figure 12.12. Stages of the pregnancy.

Source: https://healthbanks.us/wp-content/uploads/2022/03/Pregnancy-Stages-Infographic-copy.jpg

12.4.2. Role of the Placenta in Nutrient and Waste Exchange

The placenta provides a crucial interface between mother and developing fetus and is chargeable with very efficient transport of nutrients and waste products. The organ is specifically adapted to provide a large surface area for transfer as chorionic villi that penetrate the mother's endometrium. These villi contain numerous microvilli, which facilitate optimal absorption of nutrients such as glucose, amino acids, and fatty acids, all of which are critical for fetal development. In addition, the placenta actively transfers these nutrients through unique transport mechanisms that supply the embryo with the required resources to grow and develop healthily. This active nutrient exchange is essential because deficiencies lead to complications such as intrauterine growth restriction. Therefore, awareness of mechanisms involved in such transfer brings to perspective the placenta's significant role in the grand plan of the female reproductive system. Another important function of the placenta's is the clearing of metabolic products of waste. During growth, the fetus produces waste, which needs to be effectively removed in order for the intrauterine environment to be maintained in a steady state. The placental structure is able to filter and transfer waste products such as carbon dioxide and urea from fetal circulation to the maternal blood for excretion. The transfer occurs by diffusion, with concentration gradients determining the movement of these waste products away from the fetus. The efficacy of this process is of the highest significance, as the accumulation of this waste may lead to fetal distress or even compromised fetal health. The placenta also regulates maternal and fetal blood flow, aiding waste removal. This intricate balancing process confirms the placenta's instrumental role in aiding fetal homeostasis in the female reproductive system paradigm. Besides nutrient and waste exchange, the placenta also has other significant roles, such as the secretion of hormones and immunomodulation. It secretes critical hormones, i.e., human chorionic gonadotropin (hCG) and progesterone, which are vital in maintaining pregnancy and fetal development. They also play a role in modulating maternal physiological adaptations necessary to carry the growing fetus to term. In addition, the placenta has a significant role in modulating maternal immunity. It creates a barrier that protects the mother's immune system from rejecting the semi-allogenic fetus but still allows it to trade immune factors. This immunological tolerance is important for fetal survival and development. But if this functional interaction is dysfunctional, where immune responses are compromised, it can lead to complications that can result in adverse pregnancy outcomes. Thus, the intricate roles of the placenta form part of the normal function of the female reproductive system and observe their importance beyond mere nutrient and waste transfer.

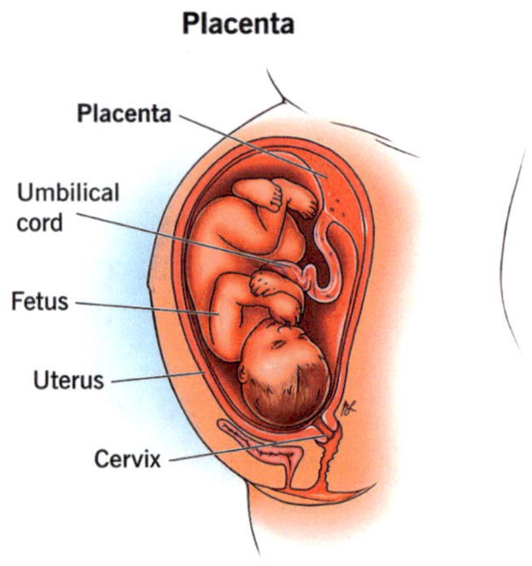

Figure 12.13. The placenta is an organ that develops in the uterus during pregnancy. It provides food and oxygen to the fetus.

Source: https://my.clevelandclinic.org/-/scassets/images/org/health/articles/22337-placenta

12.4.3. Common Complications During Pregnancy

Pregnancy is a complex physiological condition that can result in many health complications and exert a massive effect on both fetal and maternal health. Among the most common complications are hypertension disorders like preeclampsia and gestational hypertension. These have severe negative consequences, including organ dysfunctions and impairment of fetal growth. Preeclampsia usually presents after the 20th week of pregnancy and is accompanied by hypertension and evidence of damage to other organs, specifically the kidneys. These must be watched very closely and controlled to keep factors at bay, which is why prenatal vitamins are required. Gestational diabetes mellitus also has major challenges; it may affect metabolic functions and result in complications during delivery. Awareness of these complications underscores the need for specialized clinical guidelines and research to improve pregnancy outcomes. Complications of pregnancy also result from related medical illnesses that can aggravate prevailing or induce new health issues. For instance, thyroid disease has been linked with infertility and increased risks of pregnancy complications even in euthyroid women. The current research shows that the expression of thyroid antigens in the female reproductive tract can be implicated in the disruption of normal reproductive activity upon exposure to certain antibodies. In particular, thyroid antibody binding to proteins in the reproductive tract causes inflammation, thereby inhibiting fertility and increasing the risk of pregnancy complications (Aissiou et al., 2024). This endocrine-reproductive correlation calls for a holistic style of prenatal care, including thyroid status screening and regulation of hormonal imbalance to reduce the incidence of pregnancy complications. Pregnancy complications are also shaped significantly by the socio-political context, as can be seen in recent work within war zones like Kharkiv. The routine trauma and stress of war here have increased the incidence of various medical complications in pregnant women. In this context, specifically, an increase in endocrine pathology, i.e., thyroid disease, has been recorded, and an increase in urinary tract infection, which is significant in cases of maternal trauma during childbirth (Victorovich I. Lakhno, 2024). The findings indicate that while certain complications remain unchanged, others, particularly those related to infection, have increased significantly and need more intense preventive interventions. The interaction among environmental stressors and pregnancy complications makes it imperative that pregnancy complications should be managed by integrated prenatal care encompassing mental health interventions and effective infection control to promote outcomes for women in crisis situations.

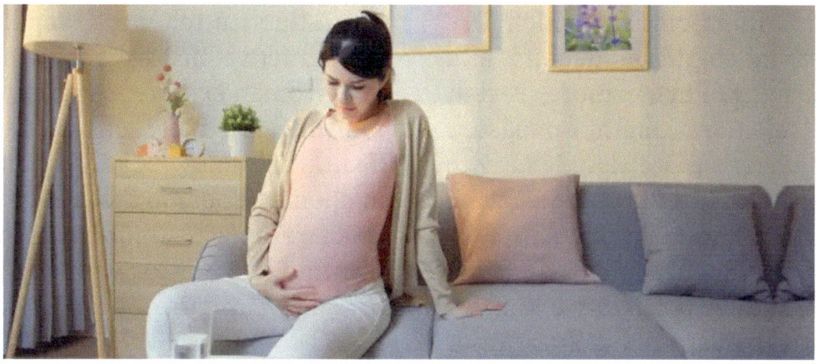

Figure 12.14. Common complications during pregnancy.

Source: https://www.careinsurance.com/upload_master/media/posts/September2023/complications-of-pregnancy.webp

Test Your Knowledge

1. What are the 3 trimesters of pregnancy?
2. What is the role of the placenta in nutrient and waste exchange?

12.5. Menopause and Aging

Learning Outcome

1. Describe the physiological changes during menopause
2. Learn about symptoms and health implications of menopause
3. Describe the impact of aging on reproductive health

Menopause is a major milestone in a woman's life where she completes her childbearing age. It usually happens as one experiences some physical and mental symptoms that can affect the overall health and well-being of the individual. Menopause has been found to cause hormonal imbalances, resulting in a decrease in estrogen levels, which is responsible for vital body functions, such as maintaining bone density and supporting healthy cardiovascular function. Lack of estrogen not only intensifies symptoms such as hot flashes and mood swings but also accelerates the process of aging, with particular relevance to skin elasticity, muscle strength, and general health. Understanding the relationship between menopause and aging is crucial in the development of effective interventions that can make this transition easier and promote healthier aging for women, and thereby a potential role for more integrated healthcare interventions for this group. The aging process, particularly in women during menopause, is closely linked with changes of a biological nature that may occur in the physical as well as cognitive dimensions. Studies have pointed out that the decline in estrogen at this stage can also lead to neurodegenerative changes, as evident in diseases such as Alzheimers disease. Particularly, estrogen deficiency has been associated with increased neuroinflammation and mitochondrial impairment, which are factors implicated in cognitive decline and accelerated brain aging. Furthermore, recent data indicate that telomere length, a measure of cellular aging, shortens more significantly in women during menopause, reflecting the stress and biological changes they endure. This way, understanding how menopause influences aging can contribute to healthier behaviors and drive research on potential therapies that may buffer against these adverse effects, thereby enhancing the health-related quality of life in aging women. Menopause, aging, and overall well-being also interact with individual characteristics such as chronic stress and comorbidities.

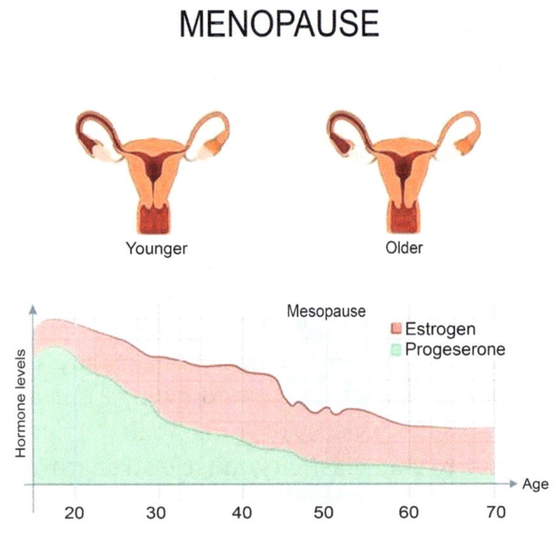

Figure 12.15. Menopause.

Source: https://www.practostatic.com/health-wiki/images/0aed5c19acbb67cbcd52d1760cba0779.jpg

Women with elevated stress levels are more likely to experience poor menopausal symptoms, and this can hasten the aging process. For instance, chronically stressed persons have been linked to shorter telomere length, a marker of accelerated cellular aging. Such correlations underscore the need for an integrated treatment approach in clinical practice. Additionally, factors such as parity and age at menopause can influence telomere length, suggesting that reproductive history may also play a role in how women experience aging. It speaks to these multifaceted interactions both in additional healthcare knowledge of women's health and in opening doors to the creation of interventions that are able to improve mental and physical health outcomes for women at menopause and in aging (Ghimire et al., 2019; Gredilla et al., 2017).

12.5.1. Definition and Physiological Changes During Menopause

Menopause is a normal event that indicates the cessation of the reproductive life of the woman when menstruation ceases, and the secretion of hormones such as estrogen and progesterone is significantly reduced. It takes place between the age group of 45 to 55 years, but the person feels its onset and duration may vary. The endocrine shifts experienced during menopause bring several changes in physiology that influence numerous systems within the body, namely, the reproductive, endocrine, and cardiovascular systems. It is crucial to comprehend these changes so that one may recognize the physical and emotional challenges that women experience during this period in their lives, thus empowering healthcare professionals with the potential to guide and advise based on individual requirements. Possibly the most significant physiological alteration during menopause is thermoregulation, which most commonly presents as hot flashes. These short periods of warmth may be preceded by sweating, increased heart rate, and flushing, and happen in approximately 50-80% of women going through menopause. Pathophysiology is expressed as dysregulation of the hypothalamic thermoregulatory centers through reduced estrogen levels that affect the kisspeptin-neurokinin B-dynorphin (KNDy) neuron complex. As estradiol levels decrease, these KNDy neurons are made hyperactive and produce the physiologic effects of hot flushes to induce cutaneous vasodilation and increased sweating.

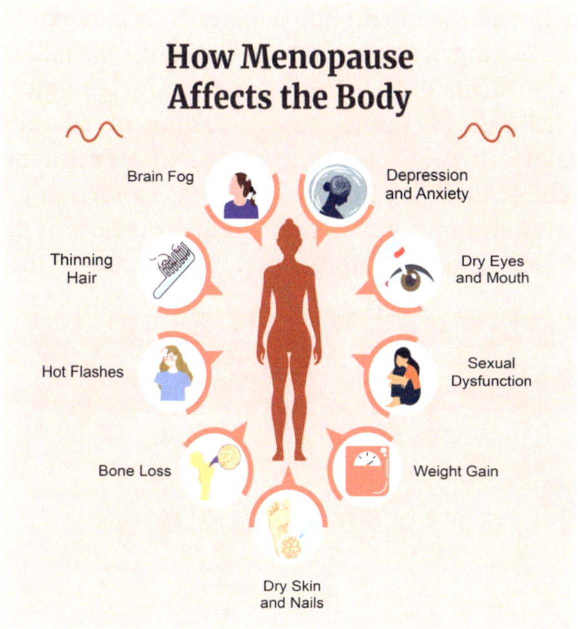

Figure 12.16. How-menopause-affects-the-body.

Source: https://menomartha.com/wp-content/uploads/2024/07/how-menopause-affects-the-body-1030x1030.png

The frequency and severity of these symptoms can have a tremendous impact on the quality of life of a woman and thus warrant rigorous probing of their etiology and potential interventions (Gombert-Labedens et al., 2025). In addition to the thermoregulatory adaptations, menopause influences various parameters of the woman's reproductive system, its structural and functional conduct. Ayurvedic medicine provides a model to comprehend the changes on the basis of the *Artavavaha Srotas* theory that encompasses the organs of menstruation, fertilization, and fetal growth. With menopause, women are likely to show such symptoms as atrophy of the vagina, reduced libido, and positional changes in the uterus on the basis of hormonal imbalance, more specifically, the imbalance in terms of the Vata dosha. Conditions such as uterine prolapse can also result from this, demonstrating the interplay of hormonal transformation and structural integrity of the female reproductive system. Manifestation of such change emphasizes a holistic approach to menopause treatment and the establishment of a general condition of well-being for this period (Pillewan, 2023).

12.5.2. Symptoms and Health Implications of Menopause

Menopause is a significant event in a woman's life when menstruation ceases, typically between the ages of 45 and 55. The hormonal shift that follows results in decreased estrogen and progesterone, which in turn causes a chain of physical and mental symptoms. They typically have hot flushes, night sweats, and dryness in the vagina, all of which can significantly impact everyday functioning. Beyond these short-term symptoms, menopause may also cause long-term health effects, including cardiovascular disease and threats to bone loss. Hormonal changes might influence overall metabolism and fat distribution, threatening weight gain and metabolic syndrome. Understanding these symptoms allows for better management, enabling women to survive this phase of their life with appropriate expectations and interventions to maintain overall health. Besides the immediate physical symptoms, menopause is also likely to create psychological consequences no less important. Mood swings, anxiety, and depression have been reported by most women during this time. These psychological symptoms, along with physical discomfort, are likely to affect interpersonal relationships, work ability, and quality of life adversely. Apart from that, the hormonal imbalances could result in cognitive changes, such as memory loss and concentration issues. This psychosocial aspect of menopause stresses the necessity for an overall approach towards menopause management, encompassing not only the physical health but also the mental health implications. Ongoing research in this respect underscores the critical role of comprehending the multifaceted implications of menopause, prompting healthcare professionals to provide holistic care that suits each individual's needs. Further, current medical studies have started investigating the impact of environmental factors on menopausal symptoms and health consequences. For instance, exposure to certain environmental toxins, such as pesticides, can exacerbate reproductive states or augment the severity of symptoms when undergoing menopause. The toxins have been linked to hormonal deficiencies that could augment typical menopausal experiences, proving an interesting interplay between external variables and the female reproductive system. It proves the significance of including not only biological but also environmental variables when conducting studies on menopause. Reading of current literature, for example, studies of mitochondrial toxicity in relation to chemicals like graphene oxide and the impact of pesticides (Alawiyah et al., 2024; Li et al., 2025), is critical to forming a greater understanding of menopause. A multi-dimensional approach to menopause research will ultimately determine more effective health strategies for women going through this phase of life.

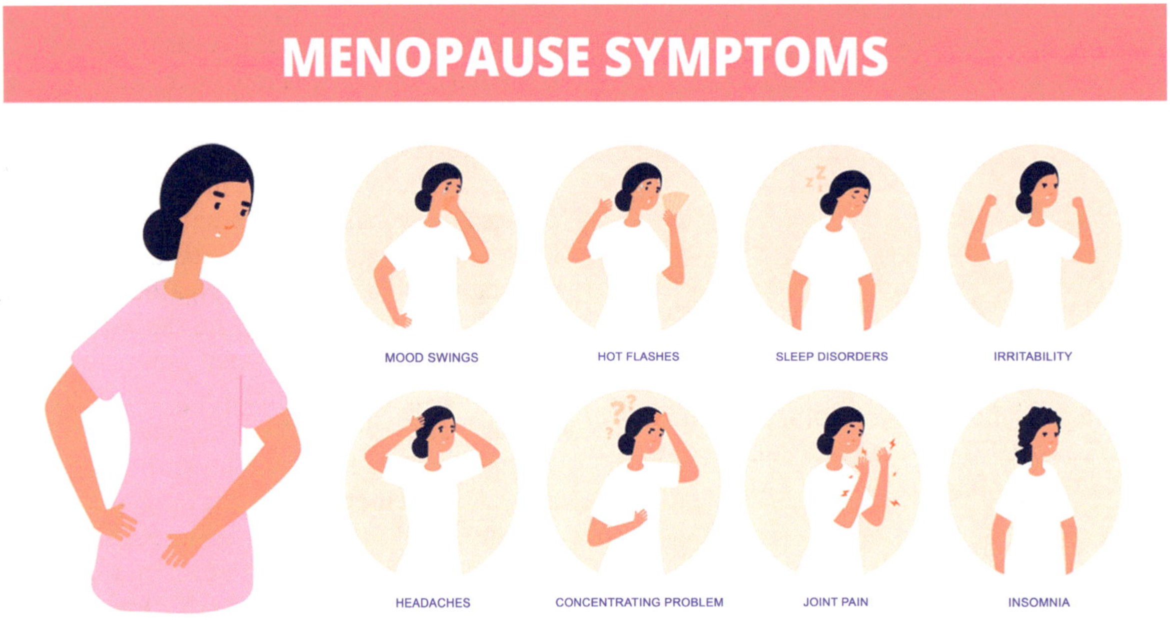

Figure 12.17. Menopause symptoms.

Source: https://www.yatharthhospitals.com/assets/images/menopause-symptoms.jpeg

12.5.3. Impact of Aging on Reproductive Health

The complex interplay between aging and reproductive well-being is highlighted by several biological transformations that occur as females move from the reproductive phase into menopause. With increasing age in women, hormonal imbalances become significant, with the major one being the decrease in estrogen levels, which is the core of most reproductive processes. The menopausal stage has a significant impact on overall reproductive health, for it is also linked with alterations in ovarian activity, leading to irregular menstrual cycles and eventual cessation of menstruation. Not only does this stage have fertility implications, but it also has general health implications for women, impacting conditions such as osteoporosis and cardiovascular disease. Understanding the hormonal and physiological changes that accompany aging is important in comprehending the cumulative effect of such age-related changes on the female reproductive system. Aging is also suspected to play a role in some of the reproductive health disorders, including polycystic ovarian syndrome and endometriosis, that aggravate fertility issues. It has been shown in research that oxidative stress plays a pivotal role in the deterioration of ovarian function with age in females and is a contributor to compromised oocyte viability and quality. Studies reveal that an imbalance between oxidative and antioxidant components leads to reproductive complications, including increased spontaneous abortion rates and infertility. The focus on the role of food antioxidants as therapeutic interventions captures the imperative of an integrated approach in securing reproductive health with aging. By mitigating oxidative stress, women can maximize their chances of fertility and even counteract some of the adverse effects of aging on reproductive health, as a further inducement towards outcomes that support their overall reproductive well-being (Dhiman et al., 2025). Furthermore, newer research identifies the robust connections between ovarian aging and other areas of physiological well-being, such as muscle power and quality of life. Exploration in the correlation of ovarian function with handgrip strength shows that with increasing reproductive aging in women, potential sarcopenia grows, which is indicative of broader systemic impacts that aging has on functioning and HRQoL. The study emphasizes the multiple connotations of hormonal aging, going beyond reproductive function into physical health, and therefore raising the significance of integrative strategies of care that target reproductive and systemic determinants of health. The interconnectedness of aging, reproductive health, and overall well-being is thus crucial to recognizing in an attempt to design targeted interventions that empower women as they undergo the aging process (Luo et al., 2025).

Test Your Knowledge

1. What are the physiological changes during menopause?
2. What is the biggest symptom of menopause?

12.6. Common Disorders of the Female Reproductive System

Learning Outcome

1. Understand the polycystic ovary syndrome (PCOS)
2. Describe the endometriosis and its effects
3. Describe the uterine fibroids and treatment options

The female reproductive system is plagued by a variety of disorders that can have a significant impact on health and quality of life. One of the most dreaded disorders is ovarian cancer, which ranks as the sixth most common cancer among women globally. It is a severe health hazard because it has a high fatality rate, wherein by the time it is diagnosed, it already comes to an advanced stage where treatment is highly constrained. The lack of proper screening mechanisms worsens the situation, and therefore, healthcare providers must counsel patients regarding risk factors and early symptoms. The available treatment options are cytoreductive surgery and platinum-based chemotherapy. Research continues to refine detection methods and develop new therapeutic methods, including the exploration of nanotechnology for drug delivery, which holds the promise to bring new hope to the use of improved outcomes in the treatment of ovarian cancer while fulfilling the critical necessity of early detection (Ramani et al., 2024). Another frequent disorder of the female reproductive tract is endometriosis, which entails the growth of endometrial tissue outside the uterus. It results in chronic pain, particularly during menses, and can lead to infertility in the majority of women. Understanding the pathophysiology of endometriosis highlights the complex interactions between hormonal fluctuations and immune responses within the body. Endometriosis is managed normally by a group of specialists, comprising pain management, hormonal treatment, and, in some cases, surgery. How much cannot be overemphasized, especially with the emotional and physical burden that the disorder places. Practitioners are now focusing on delivering women-centered care that consists of comprehensive assessment and personalized treatment plans, which is required to address both the physiological and psychologic aspects of this disorder (Ford, 2023). Fibroids of the uterus are another common disorder of the female reproductive system, found in a significant percentage of women in the reproductive years. These benign tumors can vary in size and location, often leading to symptoms such as menorrhagia, pelvic pressure or pain, as well as urinary and bowel pressure symptoms. While fibroids are not typically related to an increased risk of cancer, they can nonetheless have a big impact on quality of life and may lead to complications if not managed properly. They can be managed from watchful waiting to medical treatments specifically for symptom relief, and in some cases, the fibroid needs to be removed surgically. Because fibroid experience is so diverse from one woman to another, both intensive education and open communication between patients and health providers are key to establishing a management plan that is tailored to each patient's unique circumstances and needs (Ford, 2023).

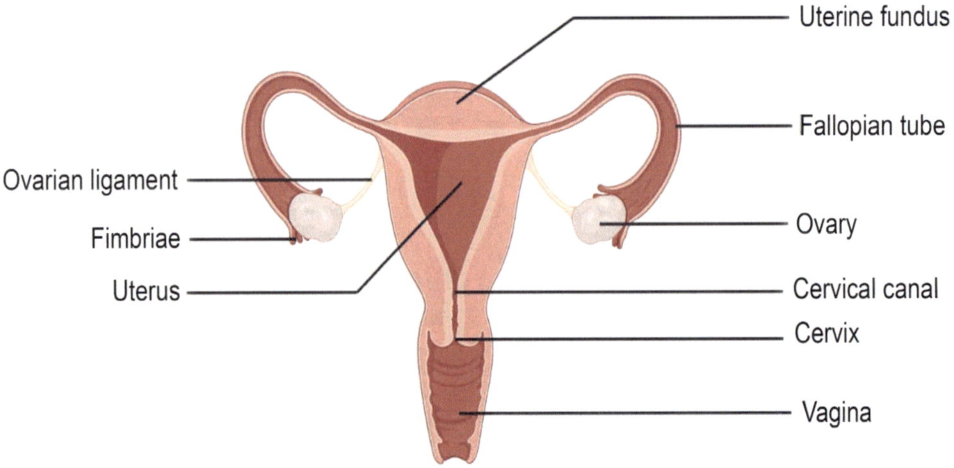

Figure 12.18. Diseases and Disorders of the female reproductive system.

Source: https://microbenotes.com/wp-content/uploads/2020/11/Diseases-and-Disorders-of-the-female-reproductive-system.jpeg

12.6.1. Polycystic Ovary Syndrome (PCOS)

Polycystic Ovary Syndrome (PCOS) is gaining popularity as a multifactorial endocrine disorder that affects a significant proportion of women in the reproductive age range. It is characterized by ovarian cysts, disrupted menstrual activity, and hyperandrogenism. PCOS can result in a host of complications beyond reproduction. These include endocrine dysfunction in metabolism in the form of insulin resistance and dyslipidemia, among others.

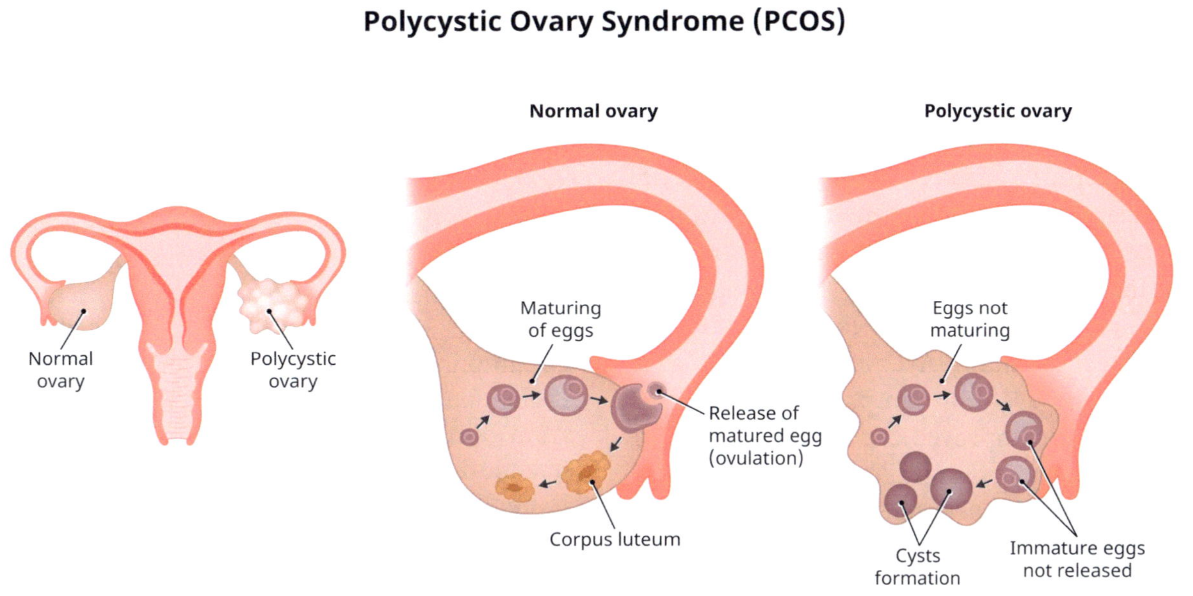

Figure 12.19. Polycystic ovary syndrome (PCOS).

Source: https://cdn-assets-eu.frontify.com/s3/frontify-enterprise-files-eu/eyJwYXRoIjoiaWhoLWhlYWx0aGNhcmUtYmVyaGFkXC9maWxlXC96aEdCUm1VcXBCdHp4QUVZYnFiMi5qcGcifQ:ihh-healthcare-berhad:4Sd7u2CPOmdM7rtQYwsRuB6J_WcMj2S2sMcW_F3B9cE?format=webp

Emotional disturbances such as anxiety and depression may also be present. Research still unveils the inflammation and clinical manifestation of PCOS symptoms, and it is of great significance to obtain a proper etiology and course of this condition. Cooperation between endocrinology, gynecology, and biochemistry as part of an interdisciplinary approach can yield valuable insights leading to productive research into the creation of specific therapeutic protocols, as well as prevention, to alleviate the heavy burden caused by PCOS on women suffering from the condition and the healthcare systems (Gusain et al., 2025). One of the most astounding characteristics of PCOS is that it has long-term health risks, including a higher risk of developing type 2 diabetes, cardiovascular disease, and endometrial cancer. The built-in endocrine imbalance caused by PCOS can lead to chronic anovulation and, in turn, a deranged menstrual cycle. For this reason, the condition seriously impairs fertility, an extremely significant aspect for the majority of women wishing to conceive. Besides, the psychological impact of PCOS cannot be overstated; women experience body image and self-esteem alteration following symptoms like weight gain and hirsutism. The appreciation of

PCOS implications on every health parameter is fundamental in developing efficient interventions and care strategies that not only address the physical symptoms but as well the emotional condition of the concerned persons (Pardhekar et al., 2024). Treatment for managing PCOS ranges from lifestyle modification to medication. Lifestyle modification, including improved diet and exercise, is routinely recommended as a first-line approach to controlling weight and insulin resistance. In addition to lifestyle modifications, drugs such as hormonal contraceptives or insulin-sensitizing agents can also be employed to regulate menstrual cycles and minimize hyperandrogenic symptoms. Furthermore, unconventional treatment modalities, including Ayurvedic therapy, have proved to be useful in symptom augmentation and metabolic improvement for some patients. The combination of several treatment modalities is a promising avenue for the enhancement of the quality of life of women with PCOS. As this study continues to explore the etiology of PCOS, there are hopes of more individualized treatments that are effective both in the physiological and psychosocial dimensions of this multifactorial condition (Gusain et al., 2025).

12.6.2. Endometriosis and Its Effects

Endometriosis is a recurring and often crippling disease affecting a significant proportion of the female population that is caused by abnormal proliferation of endometrial tissue outside uterine locations. The ectopic growth can result in a variety of symptoms, ranging from incapacitating pelvic pain to dysmenorrhea and infertility. Research indicates that around 10% of reproductive-aged women have been diagnosed with endometriosis, but that some undetermined percentage are undiagnosed due to a lack of awareness or misdiagnosis with symptoms. Endometriosis has a profound negative effect on quality of life, both physically and emotionally, in terms of pain and abnormalities. Besides, the condition has also been discovered to interfere with the normal functioning of the female reproductive system, further complicating fertility and hormonal regulation issues. The control of endometriosis in the form of early detection and prolonged treatment options continues to be a very critical area in the aspect of reproductive health. Apart from the physical symptoms, endometriosis also presents inherent psychological and emotional defects for women with the condition. The increased chronic pain can lead to severe mental issues like depression, anxiety, and poor self-esteem. Patients with endometriosis are frustrated and isolated because their symptoms are not appreciated or comprehended by physicians. The following emotional suffering can prolong the physical conditions, and it becomes difficult to break the cycle. The expense of endometriosis treatment, from pills to potential surgery, serves only to put more pressure on the women. That is why it becomes an absolute imperative to design therapeutic environments wherein knowledge and empathy are paramount so that patients receive not just the correct medical treatment but emotional nourishment as well in the bargain. Even more so, the correlation between endometriosis and environmental factors, i.e., exposure to pesticides, has been in the spotlight in recent years as a priority concern. It has been proven by science that certain pesticides have the ability to contribute to the causation of endometriosis by triggering hormonal imbalance and heightened oxidative stress in the body. Such imbalances are actualized through dysfunctional ovaries and heightened vulnerability to the development of the condition. The possible place of environmental toxins supports the necessity to be better aware of how lifestyle factors affect women's health. Both contemporary agricultural production and the chemicals used are vital issues to be taken into account when reproductive health is being considered. Consequently, a review of the role exposure plays in affecting endocrine disease within the environment will be significant to inform future prevention strategies and health generally among women with endometriosis (Panth, 2025; Alawiyah et al., 2024).

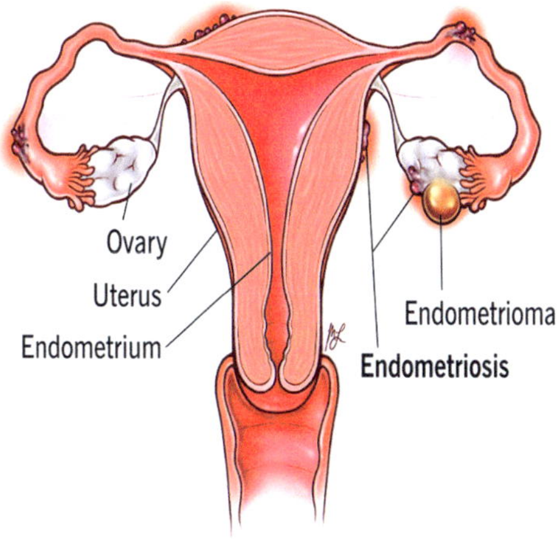

Figure 12.20. Endometriosis.

Source: https://my.clevelandclinic.org/-/scassets/images/org/health/articles/10857-endometriosis

12.6.3. Uterine Fibroids and Treatment Options

Uterine fibroids are benign tumors common to the female reproductive system and have a significant impact on it, occurring in a very high percentage of women throughout their reproductive years. The tumors can cause many symptoms, including heavy menstrual bleeding, pelvic pain, and even infertility issues. Today, research indicates that 70% to 80% of women develop uterine fibroids by the time they reach age 50, pointing to the need for proper treatment. Early detection remains a problem with the widespread asymptomatic presentation of fibroids. Yet, advances in imaging technology, such as ultrasound and magnetic resonance imaging (MRI), have allowed more accurate diagnoses to be made, so early treatment may be undertaken to alleviate symptoms and improve patient quality of life (Chao et al., 2025). Symptomatic uterine fibroids are managed by a variety of different therapeutic modalities, ranging from medical therapy to surgery. Drug treatments typically include hormonal treatments to regulate menstrual cycles and reduce fibroid size. These are not permanent, however.

Myomectomy or hysterectomy is usually reserved for women with bad symptoms or fertility problems. Uterine artery embolization (UAE) is also an option that has been found to be very effective. UAE would be stopping the blood supply to the fibroids, which makes them decrease in size and the symptoms subside. Existing evidence recognizes new access methods for the UAE, i.e., the transradial approach (TRA) and distal transradial artery approach (dTRA), which offer promising fronts for improving surgical success and reducing complications without compromising effectiveness (Chao et al., 2025).

In contrast to the many treatment alternatives, ongoing research into the genetic and molecular determinants of fibroid pathogenesis could introduce new therapeutic options. Genetic studies have revealed mutations associated with fibroid development and shed light on potential biomarkers that may further enhance diagnostic and treatment regimens. Technologies such as gene therapy hold promise to treat fibroids at the molecular level, creating a new field of therapeutic intervention. Further understanding of fibroid biology can lead to the creation of targeted therapies that not just control symptoms but also the causes of fibroid formation. Hence, the integration of biomarker-based diagnostics and genetic profiling into clinical practice is a necessity to optimize the management of uterine fibroids, and consequently, patient outcomes will be enhanced while reducing the dependency on invasive methods (Mukherjee, 2025).

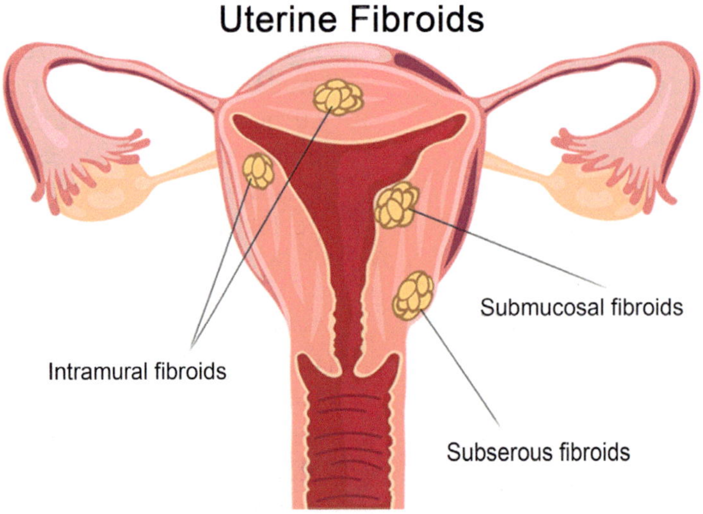

Figure 12.21. Uterine fibroids.

Source: https://preferredvasculargroup.com/wp-content/uploads/2020/01/Preferred-Vascular_Uterine-Fibroids-1024x536.png

Test Your Knowledge

1. What is polycystic ovarian syndrome?
2. What is endometriosis?

SUMMARY

Overall, the intricate processes of the female reproductive system involve several biological and physiological structures that take part in reproduction and overall health. Understanding the variables is integral to creating the science of medicine and the art of women's health management. As evident from recent studies, the intricacy of reproductive mechanisms extends beyond anatomical research, requiring evidence to inform interdisciplinary insights into hormone interactions, genetic mechanisms, and epigenetic impacts. For instance, sexual dimorphism among schistosomes is accentuated by the intersection of genetic influences and host interaction, again emphasizing that such processes have a major implication in our understanding of reproductive physiology and specific therapy (Picard et al., 2016). Also, beyond this, the place of pharmacologic medication, specifically mentioning nonsteroidal anti-inflammatory drugs, on the female reproductive system cannot be avoided. Research on the impact of such medication has provided significant findings into the activity of COX enzymes and prostaglandins in regulating reproductive mechanisms. More specifically, drug use with diminished sperm count and motility depicts the significance of more sophisticated studies exploring how drug use impacts women's reproductive health. As evidence for results from current studies, the role of hormone balance and potential induction of oxidative stress demonstrates the widespread impact of external agents on reproduction efficacy and overall wellness (Bünyamin Uzun et al., 2014). By and large, collectively, the researchers gave us greater insight into the extremely intricate nature of the female reproductive system and its necessity to keep investigating. The significance implied by these studies is amazing, extending into areas as diverse as reproductive health management, contraceptive development, and therapy protocols for reproductive pathology. By bridging an understanding of biological processes and the effect of pharmaceutical interventions, clinical practitioners and researchers can modify their interventions to enhance outcomes within reproductive health. Information gained from observation of normal physiological processes and disease states forms a foundation for further research that aims to reduce reproductive health disparities and maximize women's care interventions in different populations.

The female reproductive system is a human biological system that is intricate and fundamental, characterized by intricate structures and functions. The most critical discussion of all, of all discussions possible, is the management of unexplained infertility (UI), a diagnosis after both the female and male reproductive tests are normal after routine checks. 52 recommendations are retrieved based on a guideline that was proposed by the European Society of Human Reproduction and Embryology (ESHRE), ranging from diagnostic testing to first-line therapeutic interventions such as intrauterine insemination (IUI), and whether or not further testing is indicated. But one has to note that the majority of these suggestions are supported by evidence of widely fluctuating quality, largely of low or very low, and this calls for additional research to support pillars of treatment protocols. This has to concern patients and healthcare workers alike because it reflects the essence of the complexities of female reproductive health and idiopathic infertility (Romualdi et al., 2023). Apart from infertility issues, the importance of knowledge about the female reproductive system is also underscored by ovarian cancer itself. Advanced ovarian cancer is among the most frequent causes of mortality due to gynecologic malignancy and has a high rate of recurrence that warrants seeking novel therapeutic modalities. HIPEC has emerged as a promising therapeutic strategy, said to significantly enhance the overall survival of well-selected patients. Even though there is evidence from the clinic for HIPEC, its mechanism of action is not defined and requires additional research. Emphasized in recent research, the treatment is associated with interaction with other factors, like the timing of operation and the tumor nature of the patient, demonstrating the need for a multidimensional approach towards ovarian cancer pathology and treatment response (Olivia G Huffman et al., 2023). These debates encapsulate the level of issues and developments in women's reproductive health. Essentially, successful understanding of the female reproductive system entails fixing both reproductive health and the issues posed by diseases such as ovarian cancer. The developments in diagnostic tests and treatments, as may be exemplified through ESHRE guidelines and studies on HIPEC, demonstrates to be indicative of ongoing improvement in managing conditions in women's reproduction. But they are a revealing reminder of the huge gaps in high-quality evidence driving much mundane practice, and set doctors and patients in a situation where they need more solid data on which to make clinical decisions. As research is continually evolving, it is therefore important that healthcare practitioners are keen and responsive to emerging evidence that is more forthcoming about the female reproductive system and optimizes treatment outcomes. These emerging studies will ultimately improve patient outcomes, along with further explaining the intricacies of women's reproductive health (Romualdi et al., 2023; Olivia G Huffman et al., 2023).

KEY TERMS FROM THIS CHAPTER

- Antenatal fetal death
- Clitoris
- Estrogen
- Fertilization
- Menstrual cycle
- Oogenesis
- Polycystic ovary syndrome
- Vulva
- Blastomeres
- Endometriosis
- Fallopian tubes
- Maternal nutrition
- Musculoskeletal system
- Ovaries
- Progesterone

CRITICAL THINKING QUESTIONS

1. **The primary female reproductive organs that produce eggs and hormones are the:**
   a. Uterus
   b. Ovaries
   c. Fallopian tubes
   d. Vagina
2. **The tube that carries the ovum from the ovary to the uterus is called the:**
   a. Cervix
   b. Urethra
   c. Fallopian tube (oviduct)
   d. Vagina
3. **The muscular organ where a fertilized egg implants and develops is the:**
   a. Ovary
   b. Vagina
   c. Uterus
   d. Cervix
4. **The external female genitalia are collectively known as the:**
   a. Labia
   b. Vulva
   c. Clitoris
   d. Hymen
5. **The opening of the uterus into the vagina is called the:**
   a. Cervix
   b. Fundus
   c. Endometrium
   d. Perineum

Short Answer Questions

1. What is the female reproductive system?
2. What are the parts of the female reproductive system?
3. What is the main function of the ovaries?
4. What is the process of fertilization in the female reproductive system?
5. What are the common disorders of the female reproductive system?

Answer to Critical Thinking Questions

1. (b) 2. (c) 3. (c) 4. (b) 5. (a)

REFERENCES

1. Aissiou, S., Boucekkine, N., Cunnane, E., Gashti, N. G., Oumeziane, A., & Kaci, N. (2024). Expression of thyroid antigens in the female reproductive system. *African Journal of Reproductive Health, 28*(9), 145–152. https://www.semanticscholar.org/paper/db5f054e47e471edd9701c6217992dabd4b6d4ed (accessed on 15th June 2025).
2. Alawiyah, K., Anggraini, D., Mubarok, W., & Hardestyariki, D. (2024). Molecular and epigenetic impacts of pesticides on the female reproductive system: A review. *BIOVALENTIA: Biological Research Journal.* https://www.semanticscholar.org/paper/997d14689ae842710571daeb43518f2e12f6b03f (accessed on 15th June 2025).
3. Alengebawy, A., Abdelkhalek, S. T., Qureshi, S. R., & Wang, M. Q. (2021). Heavy metals and pesticides toxicity in agricultural soil and plants: Ecological risks and human health implications. *Toxics, 9*, 42–42. https://doi.org/10.3390/toxics9030042 (accessed on 15th June 2025).
4. Baskin, L. S., Cao, M., Cunha, G. R., et al. (2019). Reproductive tract biology: Of mice and men. https://core.ac.uk/download/323311356.pdf (accessed on 15th June 2025).
5. Baumgartner, H., De Backer, J., Babu-Narayan, S. V., Budts, W., Chessa, M., Diller, G.-P., Lung, B., et al. (2020). 2020 ESC Guidelines for the management of adult congenital heart disease. *European Heart Journal, 42*, 563–645. https://doi.org/10.1093/eurheartj/ehaa554 (accessed on 15th June 2025).
6. Chao, H., Xu, Q., Shen, T., Xu, Y., Zhou, Y., Xie, J., Xia, Z., et al. (2025). Efficacy of uterine artery embolization through a distal radial artery approach for treatment of uterine fibroids. *American Journal of Translational Research, 17*(2), 1277–1289. https://www.semanticscholar.org/paper/dfad1e499c7bcc5a46f3c365589a86a9e594ae4d (accessed on 15th June 2025).
7. Deng, Z., Dai, F.-F., Wang, R. Q., Deng, H. B., Yin, T. L., Cheng, Y. X., & Chen, G. T. (2024). Organ-on-a-chip: Future of female reproductive pathophysiological models. *Journal of Nanobiotechnology, 22*. https://www.semanticscholar.org/paper/88bcdba5dc20c153bfad2305ef8c5600927167bd (accessed on 15th June 2025).
8. Dhiman, N. K., & Saini, R. (2025). Natural antioxidants and their impact on female reproductive health. *Journal of Reproductive Healthcare and Medicine.* https://www.semanticscholar.org/paper/3a97885f04e6a5c77f3bb3322c3bc740708e399b (accessed on 15th June 2025).
9. Escorcia Mora, P., Valbuena, D., & Diez-Juan, A. (2025). The role of the gut microbiota in female reproductive and gynecological health: Insights into endometrial signaling pathways. *Life.* https://www.semanticscholar.org/paper/f8fd9183379e8e9acadc8a0611ffb245d3fbaa14 (accessed on 15th June 2025).
10. Ford, C. (2023). An overview of the female reproductive system. *British Journal of Nursing, 32*(9), 420–426. https://www.semanticscholar.org/paper/1e9ffa9c8b9038c5c44464da11c0f96833494dd4 (accessed on 15th June 2025).
11. Ghimire, S., Hill, C. V., Rodriguez, R., et al. (2019). Decline in telomere length by age and effect modification by gender, allostatic load and comorbidities in National Health and Nutrition Examination Survey (1999–2002). https://core.ac.uk/download/250588012.pdf (accessed on 15th June 2025).

12. Gombert-Labedens, M., Vesterdorf, K., Fuller, A., Maloney, S. K., & Baker, F. C. (2025). Effects of menopause on temperature regulation. *Temperature: Multidisciplinary Biomedical Journal, 12*, 92–132. https://www.semanticscholar.org/paper/e806d3504b513e7aeca2bd57260228b3bbe397ef (accessed on 15th June 2025).

13. Gorbacheva, E. Y., Toniyan, K. A., Biriukova, Y. A., Lukicheva, N. A., Orlov, O., Boyarintsev, V. V., & Ogneva, I. V. (2023). The state of the organs of the female reproductive system after a 5-day "dry" immersion. *International Journal of Molecular Sciences, 24*. https://www.semanticscholar.org/paper/091988d07c4f83bcb44fbef32754c543aeb810be (accessed on 15th June 2025).

14. Gredilla, R., Stevnsner, T., & Zarate, S. C. (2017). Role of estrogen and other sex hormones in brain aging: Neuroprotection and DNA repair. https://core.ac.uk/download/159300108.pdf (accessed on 15th June 2025).

15. Gusain, N., Anjankar, A. P., Ambad, R., Jha, R., & Jha, R. (2025). Study the correlation between serum caspase-1, IL-10, HOMA-IR, FAI, dyslipidemia, and oxidative stress status in women with polycystic ovary syndrome (PCOS). *Journal of Pharmacy and Bioallied Sciences*. https://www.semanticscholar.org/paper/84e41e9e0c78fac664a67fdf7c929c53ae96de99 (accessed on 15th June 2025).

16. Huffman, O. G., Chau, D., Dinicu, A. I., Debernardo, R., & Reizes, O. (2023). Mechanistic insights on hyperthermic intraperitoneal chemotherapy in ovarian cancer. *Cancers, 15*. https://www.semanticscholar.org/paper/47b970ab571ffcda8c0d94cf7cd8bb73f84aafae (accessed on 15th June 2025).

17. Ilyasova, V., Melchenkov, E., Vorob'yov, A. P., Archibasov, A. A., Kalmykova, V., & Antipina, Y. A. (2024). Effect of parental ploidy on reproductive system development in sturgeon hybrids in the second year of life. *Rybovodstvo i Rybnoe Hozjajstvo (Fish Breeding and Fisheries)*. https://www.semanticscholar.org/paper/47cf41f885caba49202e6a083f0269b697e6c283 (accessed on 15th June 2025).

18. Kazakova, A., Santalova, G., Kartashova, P. V., Poretskova, G., & Dufinets, I. (2024). Features of the reproductive function of girls and women with rheumatoid arthritis: A review. *Gynecology*. https://www.semanticscholar.org/paper/8984a9460b3545edfee60a776c240cd2eba7fd84 (accessed on 15th June 2025).

19. Kim, Y. H., Kim, H.-S., & Hong, I.-S. (2025). Advances in biomaterials-based tissue engineering for regeneration of female reproductive tissues. *Bio Fabrication, 17*. https://www.semanticscholar.org/paper/33b5c858a6abbf245eb142f5b3d00f0d4c6b5f3c (accessed on 15th June 2025).

20. Lakhno, I. V. (2024). The level of pregnancy and childbirth complications among the residents of front-line city of Kharkiv. *The Journal of V. N. Karazin Kharkiv National University, Series "Medicine."* https://www.semanticscholar.org/paper/66a4b83910a4ed51b9c07487bb0601f446b1d0e6 (accessed on 15th June 2025).

21. Leftwich, M., & Baumer, A. (2023). The fluid mechanics of female reproduction: A review of the biofluid mechanics of pregnancy and delivery. *Annual Review of Fluid Mechanics*. https://www.semanticscholar.org/paper/a770dfd17b21a575c56d02e32d2dbe1eb056ae7b (accessed on 15th June 2025).

22. Lestari, A. D., Siregar, I. K., & Santoso, S. (2024). CBR method expert system for female reproductive health problem detection. *JURTEKSI (Journal Technology dan System Informs)*.

https://www.semanticscholar.org/paper/09f3a8af18c1c310929d7bcbc8501337ec945045 (accessed on 15th June 2025).

23. Li, M., Lu, H., Ye, C., Wang, X., Ji, D., Zhang, Z., Cao, Y., et al. (2025). Graphene oxide nanosheets induce mitochondrial toxicity in human ovarian granulosa cells: Implications for female reproductive health. *International Journal of Nanomedicine, 20*, 4461–4479. https://www.semanticscholar.org/paper/e42528da630f00a5ee3f45717804244c21b6d384 (accessed on 15th June 2025).

24. Lissaman, A. C., Girling, J., Cree, L. M., Campbell, R., & Ponnampalam, A. (2023). Androgen signaling in the ovaries and endometrium. *Molecular Human Reproduction, 29*. https://www.semanticscholar.org/paper/1ad450d167d89fa1d90216ce85d2f049ac1de301 (accessed on 15th June 2025).

25. Liu, L., Ge, D., Lin, Y., Han, Z., Zhao, H., Cao, L., Wu, X., et al. (2025). Epigenetic regulation in oogenesis and fetal development: Insights into m6A modifications. *Frontiers in Immunology, 16*. https://www.semanticscholar.org/paper/6701c08d855b3b28832566355bf72aecbd78cfd7 (accessed on 15th June 2025).

26. Luo, A., Li, H., Lv, X., Zheng, P., Lin, K., Liang, A., & Yang, S. (2025). The impact of ovarian aging on muscle strength and life quality in various reproductive aging stages. *Climacteric: The Journal of the International Menopause Society*. https://www.semanticscholar.org/paper/47f4c5f4e794734519aecddb118da4a7bb432e3d (accessed on 15th June 2025).

27. Mauvais-Jarvis, F., Bairey Merz, C. N., Barnes, P. J., Díaz Brinton, R., Carrero, J. J., DeMeo, D. L., De Vries, G. J., et al. (2020). Sex and gender: Modifiers of health, disease, and medicine. *The Lancet, 396*, 565–582. https://doi.org/10.1016/s0140-6736(20)31561-0 (accessed on 15th June 2025).

28. Mhalhel, K., Cavallaro, M., Pansera, L., Franco, G. A., Montalbano, G., Laurá, R., Abbate, F., et al. (2025). Ion-channel proteins in the prepubertal bitch reproductive system: The immunolocalization of ASIC2, ASIC4, and PIEZO2. *International Journal of Molecular Sciences*. https://www.semanticscholar.org/paper/375c9a8082c4e54de1696081995f7491fab35418 (accessed on 15th June 2025).

29. Migda, M., Migda, M., Słapa, R., Mlosek, R., & Migda, B. (2019). The use of high-frequency ultrasonography in the assessment of selected female reproductive structures: The vulva, vagina and cervix. *Journal of Ultrasonography, 19*, 261–268. https://www.semanticscholar.org/paper/45ef3c584b0f46fd28ac3cb5fadf1084dfecba68 (accessed on 15th June 2025).

30. Mukherjee, P. (2025). Genetic and biomarker approaches to uterine fibroids: Toward precision medicine. *Frontiers in Global Women's Health, 6*. https://www.semanticscholar.org/paper/355105db7f75e42aa32b4f6b47ca46a579cdd850 (accessed on 15th June 2025).

31. Ocañas, S. R., Poljanska, E., Isola, J., Hubbart, C. R., & Stout, M. B. (2024). Changes in resident ovarian macrophages during female reproductive aging. *Innovation in Aging, 8*, 613–613. https://www.semanticscholar.org/paper/be5bd680e8018b396d8a30729709f1228f2046d4 (accessed on 15th June 2025).

32. Pai, M., Mangala, D., Prabhu, V., Latha, D., Shetty, D., & Prakash, D. (2006). Effect of estradiol on mouse vaginal epithelium. https://core.ac.uk/download/pdf/86527.pdf (accessed on 15th June 2025).

33. Panth, P. (2025). Nature to nurture: Herbal approaches to addressing female infertility. *International Journal of Research Publication and Reviews*. https://www.semanticscholar.org/paper/615b94b765b6fb409559bcb595fe9a82fb7901c7 (accessed on 15th June 2025).

34. Pardhekar, A., Waskar, R., Pardhekar, A., & Deshpande, M. (2024). Ayurvedic approaches to holistic management of polycystic ovary syndrome (PCOS). *Journal of Pharmacy & Bioallied Sciences, 16*, S4179–S4181. https://www.semanticscholar.org/paper/c7a635e9ca4e01a92ac6e50217ad16456879e440 (accessed on 15th June 2025).

35. Phuphisut, O., Poodeepiyasawat, A., Yoonuan, T., Watthanakulpanich, D., Chotsiri, P., Reamtong, O., Mousley, A., et al. (2022). Transcriptome profiling of male and female *Ascaris lumbricoides* reproductive tissues. *Parasites & Vectors, 15*. https://www.semanticscholar.org/paper/efb1bf0236c7d8d77d469e87864fd8d82c790956 (accessed on 15th June 2025).

36. Picard, M., Boissier, J., Roquis, D., Grunau, C., Allienne, J. F., Duval, D., Toulza, È., et al. (2016). Sex-biased transcriptome of *Schistosoma mansoni*: Host-parasite interaction, genetic determinants and epigenetic regulators are associated with sexual differentiation. *PLoS Neglected Tropical Diseases, 10*, e0004930–e0004930. https://doi.org/10.1371/journal.pntd.0004930 (accessed on 15th June 2025).

37. Pillewan, S. (2023). Female reproductive system in terms of Artavaha Srotas and changes seen in uterovaginal prolapse. *International Journal of Indian Medicine*. https://www.semanticscholar.org/paper/df8db479b268d09eed64d2a09cb4a6b04160ca17 (accessed on 15th June 2025).

38. Pourmasumi, S., Kounis, N., Naderi, M., Hosseinisadat, R., Khoradmehr, A., Fagheirelahee, N., Kouni, S., et al. (2023). Effects of COVID-19 infection and vaccination on the female reproductive system: A narrative review. *Balkan Medical Journal, 40*, 153–164. https://www.semanticscholar.org/paper/50a68475b632e782afe5d4a7dfc2eedc17fd1216 (accessed on 15th June 2025).

39. Proctor, L. M., Creasy, H. H., Fettweis, J. M., Lloyd-Price, J., Mahurkar, A., Zhou, W., Buck, G. A., et al. (2019). The Integrative Human Microbiome Project. *Nature, 569*, 641–648. https://doi.org/10.1038/s41586-019-1238-8 (accessed on 15th June 2025).

40. Ramani, S. M., Josthna, P., & Padma, K. R. (2024). Emerging updates on tracking new landscapes in nanotechnology for the diagnosis and ovarian cancer therapy. *Journal of Associated Medical Sciences*. https://www.semanticscholar.org/paper/ad318736b7613a98f4543e301d3dc5ef254addfc (accessed on 15th June 2025).

41. Romualdi, D., Ata, B., Bhattacharya, S., Bosch, E., Costello, M., Gersak, K., Homburg, R., et al. (2023). Evidence-based guideline: Unexplained infertility. *Human Reproduction (Oxford, England), 38*, 1881–1890. https://www.semanticscholar.org/paper/c8b7df7d150024eaf1373bef7d2664ac4434c817 (accessed on 15th June 2025).

42. Schellens, S., Lenaerts, C., Pérez Baca, M. D. R., Cools, D., Peeters, P., Marchal, E., & Vanden Broeck, J. (2022). Knockdown of the Halloween genes *spook*, *shadow* and *shade* influences oocyte development, egg shape, oviposition and hatching in the desert locust. *International Journal of Molecular Sciences, 23*. https://www.semanticscholar.org/paper/8dde832708986f38917cd9c776d89857c4cb16ba (accessed on 15th June 2025).

43. Septadina, I. S. (2023). An overview of the female reproductive system: A narrative literature review. *Sriwijaya Journal of Obstetrics and Gynecology*. https://www.semanticscholar.org/paper/7292eefde2faa45043dfb6c624cacdd09d8f1071 (accessed on 15th June 2025).

44. Simawy, M., AL-Khakani, S. S., Fadhil, M., Jawad, A. I., Al-Janabi, S. M., Al-Rubaie, D. M., & Hamad, R. S. (2024). Anatomical and histological study of the female reproductive system of green freshwater turtle (*Chelonia mydas*) during breeding season in Iraq. *World's Veterinary Journal*. https://www.semanticscholar.org/paper/3d41b18bb6badc59f337ef09d2f110f7bb1b4dcf (accessed on 15th June 2025).

45. Snigireva, S. V., Balandina, I., Balandin, A. A., Borodulin, D. V., & Nekrasova, A. M. (2024). Comparative analysis of the parameters of the external diameter of the isthmus, ampulla and funnel of the fallopian tubes in women giving birth in the first and second periods of adulthood. *Astrakhan Medical Journal*. https://www.semanticscholar.org/paper/b4a3596cd4d08c49b9e59fd46ca1a4db4b980e24 (accessed on 15th June 2025).

46. Teleanu, R. I., Chircov, C., Grumezescu, A. M., & Teleanu, D. M. (2019). Tumor angiogenesis and anti-angiogenic strategies for cancer treatment. *Journal of Clinical Medicine, 9*, 84–84. https://doi.org/10.3390/jcm9010084 (accessed on 15th June 2025).

47. Uzun, B., Atlı, Ö., Perk, B. O., Burukoğlu, D., & Ilgın, S. (2014). Evaluation of the reproductive toxicity of naproxen sodium and meloxicam in male rats. *Human & Experimental Toxicology, 34*, 415–429. https://doi.org/10.1177/0960327114542886 (accessed on 15th June 2025).

48. Zhelavskyi, M., Kernychnyi, S., Dmytriv, O., & Betlinska, T. (2025). The role of melatonin in the regulation of the immune system and reproductive health: Mechanisms and prospects for clinical application. *Ukrainian Journal of Veterinary and Agricultural Sciences*. https://www.semanticscholar.org/paper/eb5b4c54c37cbaf8dba876a6aaa8e10195d98f41 (accessed on 15th June 2025).

ENDOCRINE SYSTEM

13

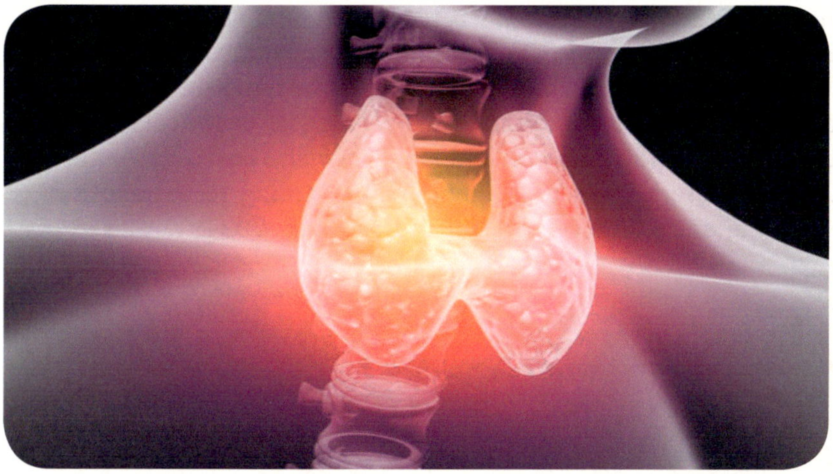

LEARNING OBJECTIVES

After studying this chapter, you will be able to:

1. Describe the major glands of the endocrine system
2. Describe the hormones and their functions
3. Understand the role of the hypothalamus
4. Explain the endocrine disorders
5. Discuss the endocrine system and growth
6. Describe the endocrine system and reproduction

Introduction

The endocrine system is an endocrine system that is very important to the human body, controlling a huge number of physiological occurrences using hormones secreted. The complex network of glands like the pituitary gland, thyroid gland, and adrenal glands are always interacting with other bodily systems in a bid to achieve homeostasis. Hormones are chemical messengers of growth, metabolism, and mood, and any disruption to them can have disastrous health results. Studying the endocrine system is not only requisite for an understanding of basic human biology but also to investigate contemporary health issues that all too often have endocrine effects. Due to the increased exposure to environmental endocrine disruptors, like micro-sized particles, there is a need to study the physiological role of the hormones as well as the environmental stimuli that compromise endocrine health (Zaitseva et al., 2024; Kodila et al., 2023). The above research has demonstrated the role of environmental pollutants, like micro-sized particles and endocrine disruptors, in the functioning of the endocrine system.

For instance, suspended particles in the air have been associated with other diseases in medicine, including endocrine disease (Zaitseva et al., 2024). Similarly, BPA and its substitutes have gained more prominence as they can mimic or interfere with hormone action, which can lead to hormonal and immune system alterations (Kodila et al., 2023). Their existence draws attention to the need for stringent control and public education because they can impact susceptible populations along the life course. Detailed information on these environmental exposures will not only enhance the scientific literature but also inform public health interventions for the minimization of exposure and prevention of hazards related to endocrine disruption. In addition, the impact of disruption of the endocrine system reaches across numerous chronic conditions as well as developmental disorders. Interference may also be described in a variety of different forms, such as metabolic, reproductive, and immune abnormalities, exemplifying the interrelatedness of hormonal health and general overall well-being. Understanding the endocrine system's role in such complex pathways accentuates the need for progress toward the eradication of environmental substances affecting endocrine function. In an era where lifestyle and environmental influences become decisive in determining health conditions, scientific research needs to know how synthetic chemicals and pollutants influence endocrine systems. Closing the gap between endocrinology and environmental science, doctors can better understand the inherent risks of modern living, leading to enhanced and safer living standards that enable optimal endocrine function (Zaitseva et al., 2024; Kodila et al., 2023).

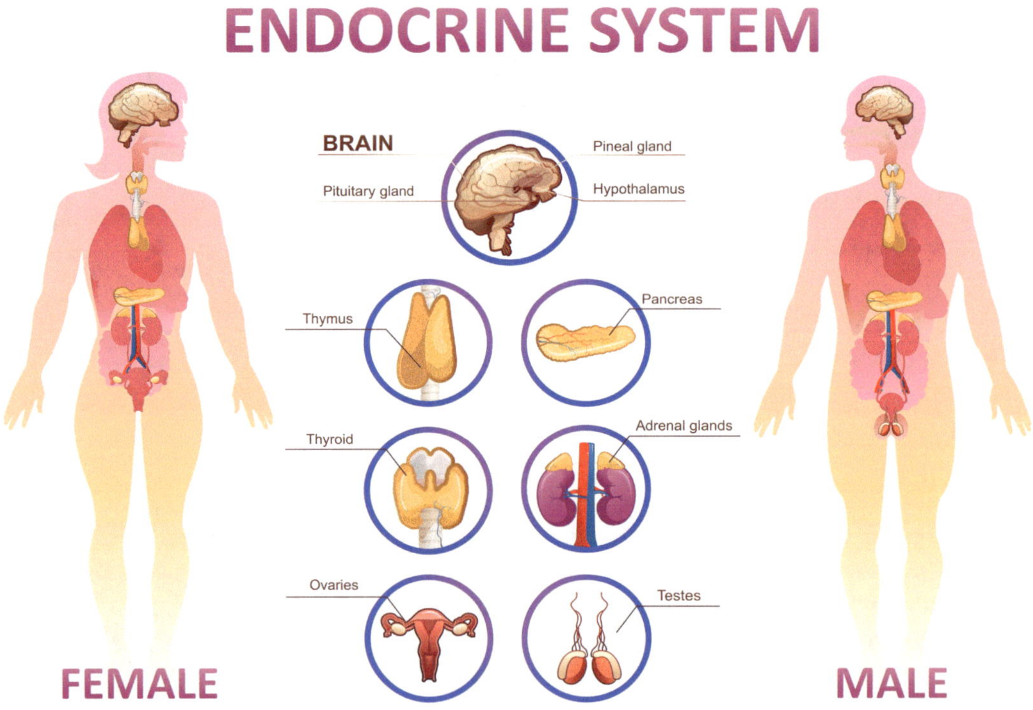

Figure 13.1. Endocrine System.

Source: https://mepss.vbatraining.org/file/29/endocrine-system.jpeg

13.1. Major Glands of the Endocrine System

Learning Outcome

1. Describe the pituitary gland and its functions
2. Understand the thyroid gland and its role in metabolism
3. Describe the adrenal glands and their response to stress

The endocrine system comprises numerous significant glands that regulate many physiological processes through hormone secretion. The pituitary gland, also referred to as the master gland, is significant in coordinating other endocrine organs' function, such as the thyroid, adrenal glands, and gonads. The pituitary gland secretes hormones like growth hormone and adrenocorticotropic hormone, influencing growth, metabolism, and stress response. The hypothalamus, which is connected to the pituitary gland, regulates many functions, including the regulation of body temperature, hunger, and body rhythms. It also plays a significant function in triggering the body's response to stress through hormonal stimulation, thus the regulation of homeostasis after environmental change.

The second major gland is the thyroid, whose hormones, such as thyroxine and triiodothyronine, regulate the rate of metabolism, heart rate, and body temperature. The endocrine function of the thyroid is essential during early development, especially in controlling metabolic processes influencing body growth and energy levels. The gland's output is controlled mainly by pituitary thyroid-stimulating hormone (TSH). In addition, thyroid hormone synthesis relies on iodine, which underlines the necessity of dietary sources. Thyroidal diseases, such as hypothyroidism and hyperthyroidism, can create deep disturbances of metabolism and should be treated by experienced medical therapy in order to restore hormonal homeostasis and prevent complications of metabolic derangement. The adrenal glands, placed above the kidneys, also play an important role in the endocrine system. They consist of two parts: the outer adrenal cortex and the inner adrenal medulla, each secreting characteristic hormones. The adrenal cortex synthesizes corticosteroids like cortisol, involved in stress management and the upkeep of metabolism. The adrenal medulla releases catecholamines like adrenaline, which activate the body for a fight-or-flight response in stressful situations. The coordination of the endocrine system between the adrenal glands and other components is typical of the intricacy of human hormonal regulation. Interestingly, cross-talk between disparate glands through feedback controls ensures optimal operation of functions like mineral and stress hormone homeostasis, which is vital for maintenance of overall health and wellness in varying situations of life (Latic et al., 2022; Szu-Chang et al., 2019).

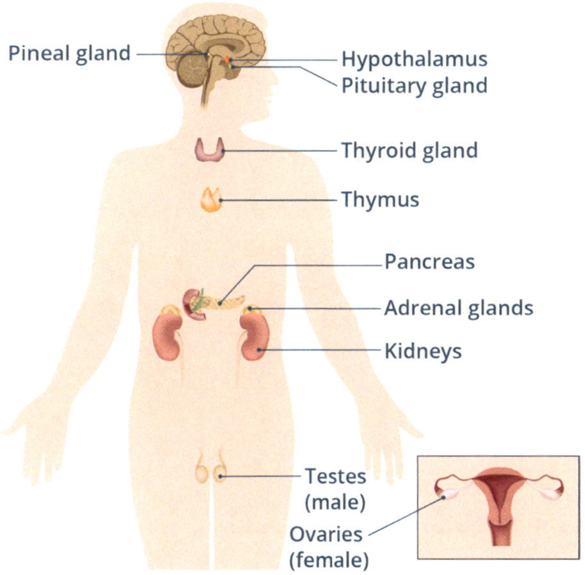

Figure 13.2. The endocrine (hormonal) system.

Source: https://media.healthdirect.org.au/images/inline/original/endocrine-glands-and-their-hormones-85e01a.png

13.1.1. Pituitary Gland and Its Functions

The master gland, the pituitary gland, is an essential body organ that regulates various hormones in controlling the various physiological processes. Located at the base of the brain, this small and complex gland functions as the center for the regulation of the other endocrine glands, including the thyroid gland, adrenal glands, and reproductive organs. The organ releases a host of hormones influencing growth, metabolism, and reproductive function.

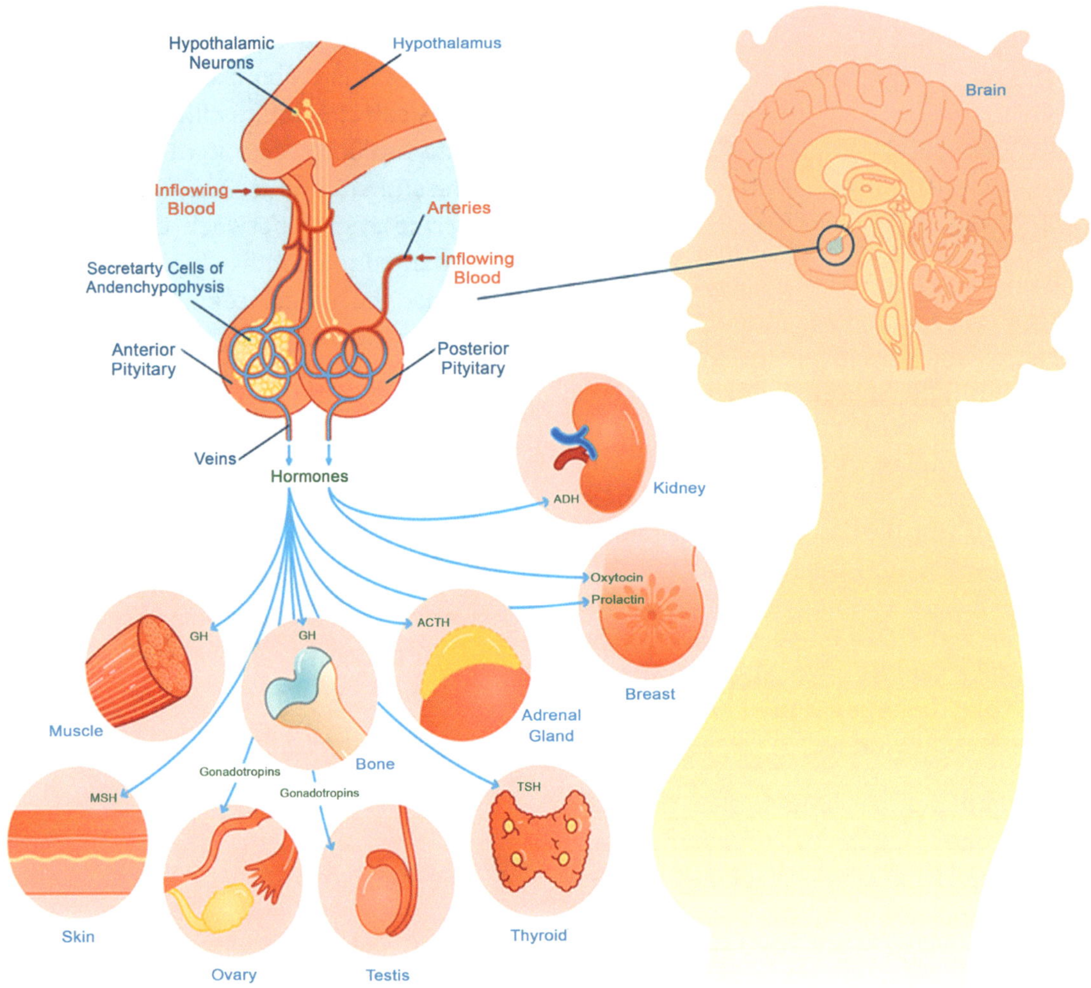

Figure 13.3. Pituitary gland.

Source: https://s3.us-east-2.amazonaws.com/medictests/app/public/ckeditor_assets/pictures/325/content_Pituitary-gland-anatomical-vector-illustration-diagram_-educational-medical-scheme-919611828_1009x1044.jpeg

By responding to signals from the hypothalamus, the pituitary gland maintains a delicately balanced hormonal state, essential for homeostasis. With its central position, any form of pituitary gland dysfunction may cause serious health conditions, such as growth disorders, metabolic disturbances, and reproductive problems, which highlight the need for this gland within the endocrine system as a whole (Khan, 2023). Among the primary characteristics of the pituitary gland function is the intricate interaction between the hypothalamus and the pituitary gland, forming the hypothalamic-pituitary axis. It is important in the regulation of the endocrine response to both internal and external stimuli, where the hypothalamus conveys the neuroendocrine signals to the pituitary, instructing the release of hormones such as growth hormone (GH), prolactin, and adrenocorticotropic hormone (ACTH). Through the assistance of these hormones, the pituitary gland skillfully regulates major physiological functions, including stress response, lactation, and metabolism. The homeostatic feedback loops ensure that the levels of hormones are maintained within optimal limits to prevent the possibility of excess or deficiency, which could lead to pathologies. Thus, the regulatory activities of the pituitary glands not only facilitate normal bodily function but also enable the organism to respond to environmental variations (Borowiec et al., 2018). Besides, environmental factors can interfere with the pituitary gland's normal functioning, leading to various disorders. Plastics and pesticides in everyday commodities have already been shown to disrupt endocrine function and lead to drastic health consequences. These endocrine disruptors will modify the mode of hormone secretion, leading to the genesis of reproductive disturbances, metabolic disorders, and even neurological deviations. The interaction between environmental exposure and pituitary function illustrates the necessity for ongoing research and public health vigilance. As society further becomes aware of these issues, the potential impact of environmental toxins on endocrine health further underscores the necessity to ensure the integrity of the endocrine system, with the pituitary gland as a critical juncture of understanding in both health and disease (Khan, 2023).

13.1.2. Thyroid Gland and Its Role in Metabolism

The thyroid gland is a key feature of the human endocrine system, with its primary function being the regulation of metabolism in the body. By secreting hormones such as thyroxine (T4) and triiodothyronine (T3), the thyroid regulates a wide range of metabolic processes, which regulate the rate at which cells metabolize nutrients to energy. Regulation of these is important not only for the maintenance of basal metabolic rates but also for the maintenance of growth, development, and temperature regulation. Besides this, the sensitive feedback loop between the pituitary gland and hypothalamus also ensures that thyroid hormone levels are kept constant according to the metabolic requirements of the body. Therefore, imbalances in thyroid function are responsible for causing major metabolic disorders, thus bringing into focus the role of this gland in health and metabolic homeostasis. Evidence highlights the various modes of interaction of thyroid hormones with different metabolic pathways, and the gland's function in lipid metabolism is also given much importance. Recent studies have highlighted the direct effects of thyroid hormones on hepatic lipid homeostasis, which are essential for preventing disorders such as fatty liver disease. The pituitary-targeted gland axes (PTGA) network, which is involved in coordinating hormonal regulation across different glands, facilitates the relationship between thyroid function and lipid metabolism. Thyroid hormones regulate gene expression associated with the synthesis of lipids and the oxidation process, thus ensuring balance in lipids within the liver. Identification of these multifaceted relationships is critical, since dysregulation may occur in both metabolic disease and hepatic pathology, and reflects the thyroid gland's broad impact on systemic metabolism and disease evasion (Li et al., 2024). Additionally, with aging comes challenges to thyroid function, and in the majority of instances, leads to decreased metabolic efficiency. Aging can provoke an increased prevalence of subclinical hypothyroidism, which is related to mitochondrial inadequacy and other mechanisms, thus affecting energy metabolism at the cellular level. In recent studies utilizing single-cell RNA sequencing, the specific vulnerabilities of thyroid epithelial cells during aging were elucidated. From this study, it has been demonstrated that there are certain thyroid cell subpopulations that exhibit functional impairment marked by typical gene expression changes. Notably, metallothionein (MT) gene expression has been linked with thyroid losses following aging, a finding indicative of the glands' sensitivity to aging. These findings on aging and thyroid function emphasize the critical need for further insight into the co-operation of endocrine systems throughout life, particularly in terms of metabolic health (Hong et al., 2023).

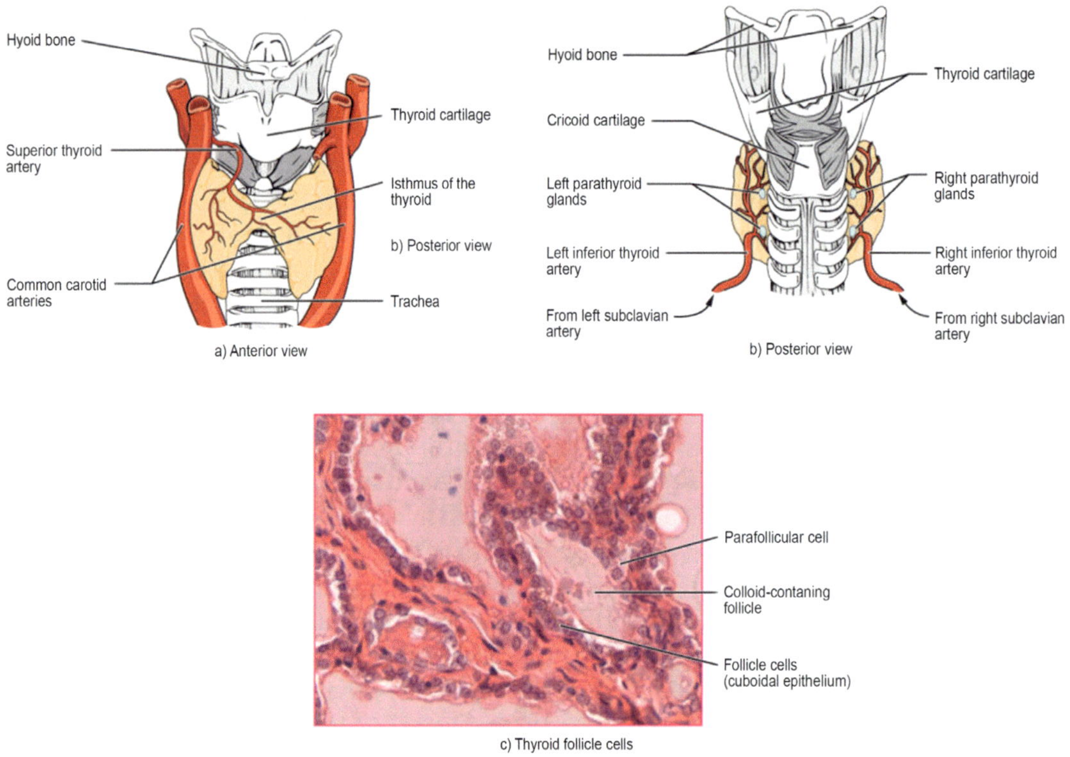

Figure 13.4. The thyroid gland is located in the neck where it wraps around the trachea. (a) Anterior view of the thyroid gland. (b) Posterior view of the thyroid gland. (c) The glandular tissue is composed primarily of thyroid follicles. The larger parafollicular cells often appear within the matrix of follicle cells.

Source: https://s3-us-west-2.amazonaws.com/courses-images/wp-content/uploads/sites/217/2016/10/04213324/1811_The_Thyroid_Gland-1024x704.jpg

13.1.3. Adrenal Glands and Their Response to Stress

The adrenal glands, small but powerful endocrine organs situated above each kidney, are a vital part of the human body's response to stress. Faced with a stressor, be it physical or emotional, the adrenal glands initiate a complicated cascade of hormones primarily involving the secretion of adrenaline and cortisol. These hormones prepare the body for a fight or flight response by increasing heart rate, elevating blood sugar, and increasing metabolic activity. This quick hormonal response is essential for survival as it enables the body to respond instantly to perceived danger. Prolonged or extreme stimulation of the adrenal glands, however, is detrimental to overall health, underscoring the delicate balance required for their functioning. The impact of stress on the adrenal glands is typically exacerbated by environmental stimuli such as exposure to endocrine-disrupting chemicals (EDCs). The chemicals would interfere with the secretion and regulation of adrenal hormones, and this results in adrenal dysfunction. More than 60 EDCs that have been identified through research to cause adrenocortical toxicity have been shown to greatly alter the morphology and function of the glands. Disruption of the steroidogenic pathway is of particular interest as it may affect the synthesis of critical hormones such as cortisol and aldosterone. Although much remains to be understood about the long-term effects of such toxicants on adrenal function, the need for regulatory protocols that encompass testing of adrenal function has become even more imperative with the growing evidence of a potential effect on health based on exposure to EDC (Li et al., 2025). Meanwhile, the intricate interaction between adrenal hormones and oxidative stress cannot be overlooked. Adrenal hormone secretion dysregulation, for instance, glucocorticoids and mineralocorticoids, may lead to excess oxidative stress in the body. The disease is responsible for a variety of hormonal disorders, for instance, adrenal insufficiency and Cushing's syndrome, which also play a role in increasing the risk of health due to stress. Antioxidants such as vitamins C and E have been found to be useful in decreasing oxidative damage related to hormonal imbalance. Through the avoidance of oxidative stress, such dietary molecules may serve as an intervention for enhancing adrenal well-being and health. With continuous studies, it will be essential to understand the dynamic relationship between adrenal glands, stress response, and oxidative stress when planning effective interventions and maintaining hormonal homeostasis in the midst of challenges faced with modern life (Patani et al., 2023).

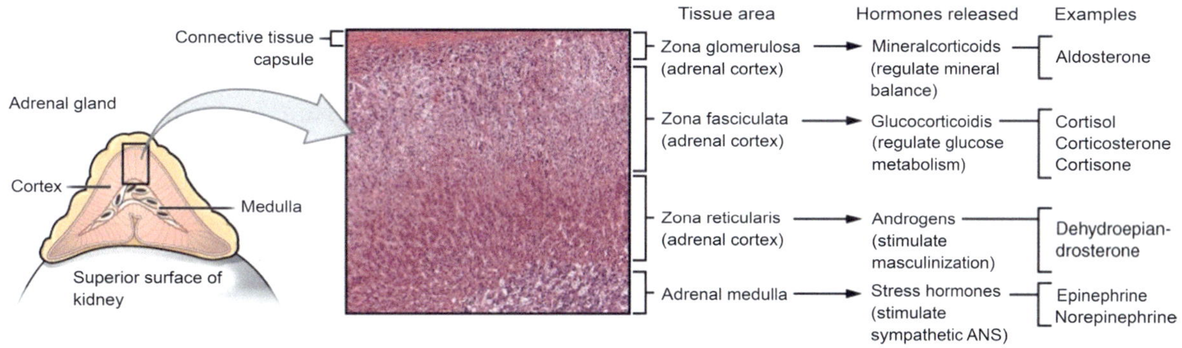

Figure 13.5. Both adrenal glands sit atop the kidneys and are composed of an outer cortex and an inner medulla, all surrounded by a connective tissue capsule. The cortex can be subdivided into additional zones, all of which produce different types of hormones.

Source: https://s3-us-west-2.amazonaws.com/courses-images-archive-read-only/wp-content/uploads/sites/403/2015/04/21031214/1818_The_Adrenal_Glands.jpg

Test Your Knowledge

1. What is the pituitary gland?
2. What is the role of the thyroid gland in metabolism?

13.2. Hormones and Their Functions

Learning Outcome

1. Describe the types of hormones
2. Describe the mechanisms of hormone action on target cells
3. Understand the feedback loops in hormone regulation

The endocrine system regulates and sustains homeostasis by controlling many processes of the body through the release of hormones. Hormones are biochemicals that allow for communication among many organs and systems, coordinating functions of the body such as metabolism, growth, and reproduction. Among the many hormones, peptide hormones are unique; they are released from endocrine and neuroendocrine cells in the central nervous system and peripheral organs. The exact balance of these hormones is required, and their imbalance leads to metabolic diseases, sexual dysfunction, and other associated health problems. For instance, pancreatic imbalance of insulin resulting from it results in diabetes, and sex hormone changes like estrogen and testosterone affect fertility and sexuality, reinforcing the dependence of hormones on the overall well-being of human beings. Experiments increasingly show that several hormone systems have functional homologies in different vertebrate groups, suggesting evolutionary conservation of the mechanisms. This can be best exemplified in the evolution of peptide hormones and their receptors, as recent studies of non-osteichthyan vertebrates clearly show. These analyses reveal the mechanisms by which gene repertoires diverged and evolved, contributing to reproductive and homeostatic functions across a broad spectrum of animals. Uncovering the genetic basis of hormone function has the potential to uncover secrets of endocrine disease and susceptibility. Comparative research also highlights the need to investigate evolutionary adaptations and their implications for the functionality of hormones in humans. An evolutionary understanding allows scientists to form more targeted treatments that undo hormonal imbalance and associated medical conditions. Outside influences, such as chemical exposure, are involved in regulating hormones that cannot be ignored. For instance, pesticides have been known to be endocrine disruptors that can affect or mimic the hormonal messages to generate significant impacts on the well-being. The interferences lead to dysfunction of body systems like the neurological, hepatic, and reproductive systems. In addition, pesticide interference in hormone signaling disruption is bound to lead to decreased fertility and reproductive malfunction through effects on sperm capacitation processes required for successful fertilization. Resolution of these kinds of problems requires a solid understanding of how various variables interact with the endocrine system, calling for ongoing research that bridges the intricate balance of environmental exposure and hormone well-being. By combining hormone function data with environmental toxicology, scientists can better inform public health policy and protective measures. Through this, human health is safeguarded in the current rapidly changing world (Uwamahoro et al., 2024) (Kuraku et al., 2022).

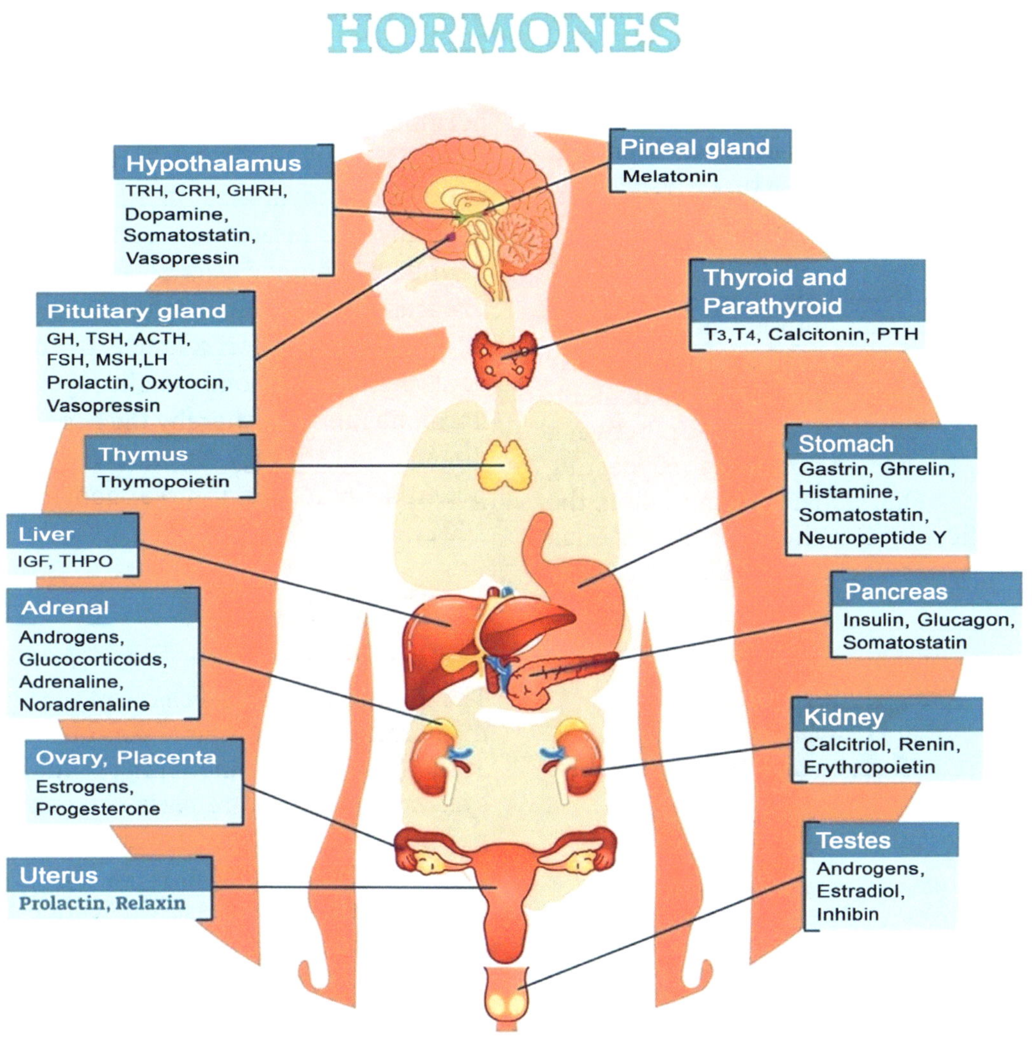

Figure 13.6. Human body hormones.

Source: https://d2jx2rerrg6sh3.cloudfront.net/image-handler/ts/20250319083824/ri/950/src/images/Article_Images/ImageForArticle_793_17424310885043381.jpg

13.2.1. Types of Hormones: Steroid Vs. Peptide Hormones

The endocrine system functions through an enormous array of hormones that can be generally classified into two wide groups: steroid hormones and peptide hormones. Steroid hormones are lipid-soluble, derived from cholesterol, and hence easily diffuse through cell membranes. This facilitates direct action on intracellular receptors, with alterations in gene expression and thus protein synthesis. Some of the steroid hormones include cortisol, estrogen, and testosterone, which all play important functions in stress, reproduction, and metabolism. Their solubility in lipid enables the hormones to act slowly but have a longer duration of action on target cells because changes in protein synthesis take time to appear within the organism. The peptide hormones, however, are amino acid chains and most often hydrophilic. These hormones cannot pass through the lipid bilayer of the cell membrane at random; instead, they exert their effects by binding to cell-surface receptors. This binding leads to a cascade of intracellular signal transduction mechanisms, typically mediated through second messengers, that ultimately lead to rapid-acting physiological effects. Insulin and glucagon are classic examples of such a group, which regulate blood glucose levels by having immediate metabolic effects. Peptide hormones thus address the immediate physiological reaction, which mirrors their primary role in the body's subtle adjustment of functions. Here lies the distinction between these two categories of hormones, suggesting the complexity of hormonal transmission in the body and reflecting the effects of factors such as receptor types and the cellular pathways involved.

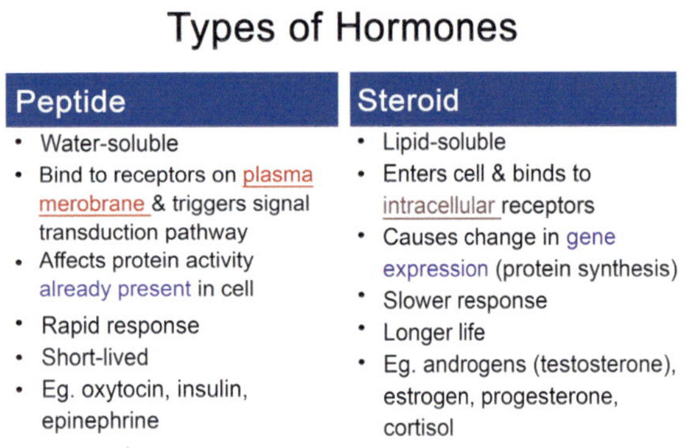

Figure 13.7. Types of hormones.

Source: https://external-content.duckduckgo.com/iu/?u=https%3A%2F%2Fslideplayer.com%2Fslide%2F14869116%2F90%2Fimages%2F7%2FTypes%2Bof%2BHormones%2BPeptide%2BSteroid%2BWater-soluble.jpg&f=1&nofb=1&ipt=f489c686ade3293b216d19deada63cd314fa41b872b62cbe58c465afac93205b

Categorization and functional diversity of hormones are critical in a complete understanding of the endocrine system. Hormones regulate not only metabolic activities, but also growth, development, and homeostasis. One example is a complete study of human hormone classifications that determined 88 types, where the majority of them were peptide hormones and constituted 65 of the determined 88 (Kabir, 2021). This reflects the broad role of peptide hormones in human physiology. Secondly, the interaction between steroid and peptide hormones can be very contributory towards disease and health. As hypothesized in recent studies, for instance, Bandyopadhyay et al., steroid hormones might regulate peptide hormone function, thereby the need for a multi-dimensional strategy for endocrine disease and potential treatment interventions (Raza et al., 2022).

13.2.2. Mechanisms of Hormone Action on Target Cells

The multifunctional mechanism through which the hormones exert their effects on target cells is at the heart of the functioning of the endocrine system. Hormones are classified generally into peptide hormones, steroid hormones, and amine hormones with different mechanisms to influence cellular processes. In peptide hormones such as insulin, the action is primarily through cell surface receptors that lead to a cascade of intracellular signal transduction pathways. This is typically done through second messengers, like cyclic AMP (cAMP) or calcium ions, which subsequently activate various kinases and transcription factors, ultimately modifying gene expression and metabolic processes. Steroid hormones are lipid-soluble and easily diffuse across plasma membranes and bind intracellular receptors. This binding elicits direct modulation of gene expression through modification of the transcription of target genes, thereby underscoring the diverse modalities through which such biological messengers influence their specific cellular targets. Specificity of hormone action is controlled by the availability of specific receptors on target cells. Each hormone binds specifically to its corresponding receptor due to high affinity and induces conformational changes that activate downstream pathways. This specificity is necessary because it enables cells to respond appropriately to hormonal cues, which would regulate an incredibly vast array of biological events from metabolism to growth and reproduction.

Recent developments in our understanding of these mechanisms have further highlighted the ways the spatial organization of receptors and how receptors interact with other molecules of the cell regulate hormone action. For instance, the receptor may function as a complex of other proteins, influencing the signal initiated by the hormone to generate various physiological responses. Such mechanisms are also vital in the development of targeted therapies for endocrine disease (Miki et al., 2024). The function of regulatory mechanisms within hormone signaling is also significant, e.g., processes that control breakdown and turnover of hormone-sensitive elements. Long noncoding RNAs (lncRNAs) are also involved in gene expression regulation that is linked to hormone signaling. LncRNA TERRA, for example, has been reported to be involved in the control of cell cycle and genomic stability of breast cancer.

The exosome complex, members of which are Exosc9, is involved in the degradation of lncRNAs, thus affecting the availability of transcripts involved in responding to hormones. Their regulation is necessary as their dysregulation will lead to hormone signaling aberrations and susceptibility to the causation of diseases such as endocrine therapy-resistant breast cancer. Their multifunctionality and involvement in protein interaction within the telomeres illustrate the multidimensionality of hormone action on cellular targets, revealing novel therapeutic approaches (Quttina et al., 2023).

13.2.3. Feedback Loops Controlling Hormones

The intricate web of feedback loops in hormonal regulation is the essence of the human endocrine system. The feedback loops are predominantly accomplished through a system of a network of messages to ensure homeostasis by modulating the release of the hormones based on the requirements of the body. The feedback loops have been divided into negative and positive feedback mechanisms. Negative feedback is more prevalent and required to stabilize internal states; e.g., an increase in the level of a hormone usually signals inhibition of its further production. Such a control strategy is required in processes such as blood glucose level, where high glucose induces insulin release to lower the level of sugar and, therefore, inhibit insulin secretion. Conversely, whereas positive feedback loops, which occur less often, amplify hormonal responses, such as oxytocin rising to accelerate contractions during delivery, which in turn trigger more oxytocin release. Such active processes are some of the advanced functions of hormones in human biology. Knowledge of specific hormonal interactions also explains the feedback loop mechanism, as in the interaction between fibroblast growth factor 23 (FGF23) and parathyroid hormone (PTH) for regulating vitamin D metabolism. PTH and FGF23 are a complex regulatory system with minerals such as calcium and phosphate that play a crucial role in numerous physiological functions. FGF23, secreted primarily in the bone, inhibits vitamin D production, establishing a negative feedback to the stimulatory effect of PTH on vitamin D production. Vitamin D, having entered the circulation, controls FGF23 secretion in a close feedback loop, maintaining mineral homeostasis and demonstrating how hormonal regulation is interconnected. Such a feedback mechanism not only regulates mineral and vitamin metabolism but also provides the luxury of hormonal control in which a single hormone can stimulate other hormones to activity and thereby provide an adaptive and responsive balance in body functions. The impact of such feedback is greater than regulatory mechanisms because it underlines the physiological significance of the interaction of hormones. For example, the vitamin D signaling pathway goes beyond mineral homeostasis to include cardiovascular disease, and a deficiency in vitamin D is linked to heart disease and hypertension. Research reveals that vitamin D is an inhibitor of the renin-angiotensin-aldosterone system (RAAS) through which blood pressure is maintained. Thus, disruptions to this feedback mechanism will be of grave importance to overall health, demonstrating regulation of hormone function to be vital not only to homeostasis but to more general health situations. This interconnectedness puts focus on holistic research on the endocrine system, particularly because there remain knowledge gaps regarding molecular mechanisms of such sophisticated feedback loops, and there remain avenues to which upcoming research efforts can be directed (Liu et al., 2024) (Latic et al., 2022).

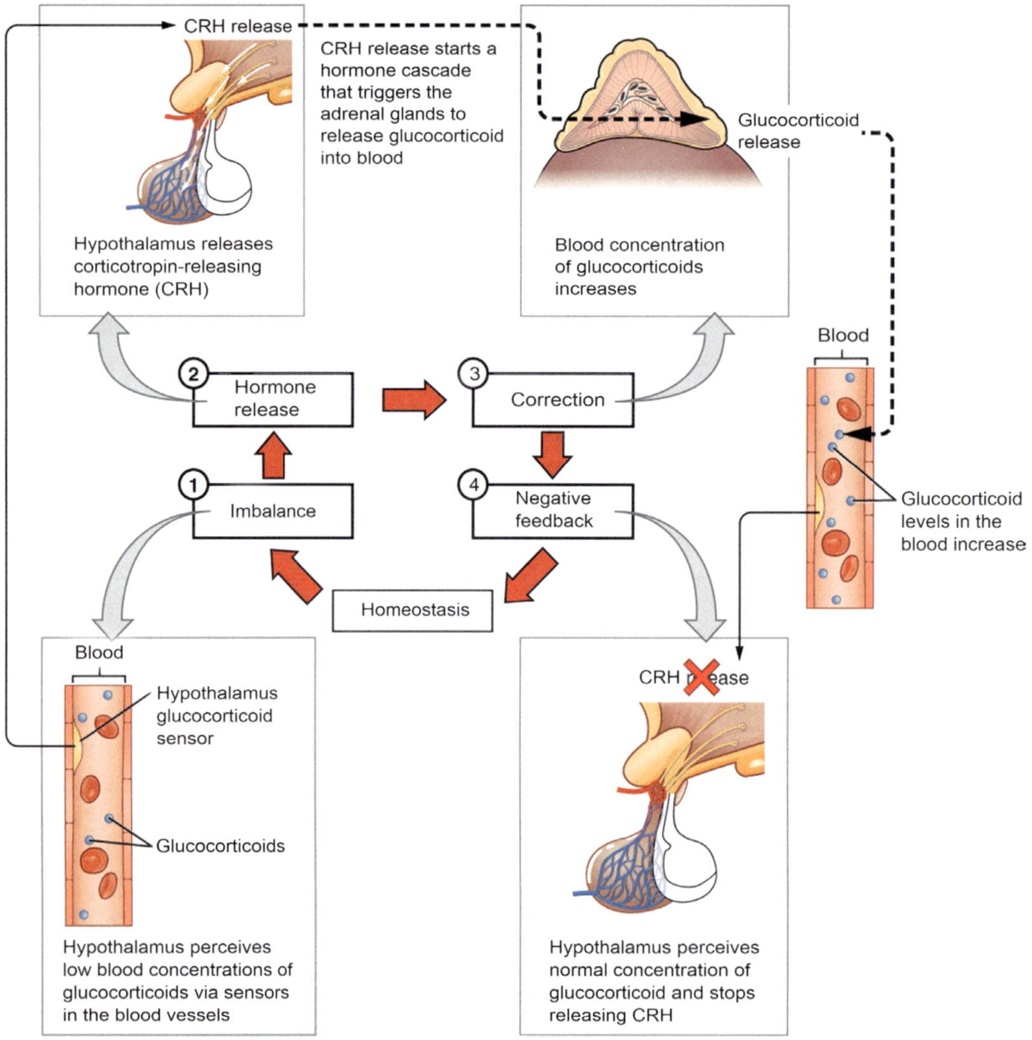

Figure 13.8. Negative Feedback Loop.

Source: https://s3-us-west-2.amazonaws.com/courses-images/wp-content/uploads/sites/3047/2018/03/26184143/1805_Negative_Feedback_Loop.jpg

Test Your Knowledge

1. What are the 2 main types of hormones?
2. What are the feedback loops in hormone regulation?

13.3. The Role of the Hypothalamus

Learning Outcome

1. Know the connection between the hypothalamus and the pituitary gland
2. Understand the regulation of homeostasis through hormonal control
3. Describe the influence of the hypothalamus on the autonomic nervous system

The hypothalamus is an important endocrine structure that serves as a command center by regulating various physiological processes through the virtue of its intricate network of neurons and hormonal signals. As an important part of the secretion of hormones, the hypothalamus communicates with the pituitary gland in order to regulate functions such as growth, metabolism, and reproduction.

Through the release of hormones like gonadotropin-releasing hormone (GnRH), the hypothalamus influences the release of luteinizing hormone (LH) and follicle-stimulating hormone (FSH), which are essential for the normal functioning of reproductive organs. This regulatory action underscores the hypothalamus's role in homeostasis and in responding to internal and external stimuli, thereby mirroring its importance for the overall functioning of the endocrine system and overall wellness (Robert L. Goodman et al., 2022). Apart from this, the role of the hypothalamus is to play a central function in the onset of puberty, which is a multifactorial process with a cascade of hormonal events. Research has pointed to the involvement of the Kisspeptin-Neurokinin-Dynorphin (KNDy) system within the hypothalamus in the pulsatile release of GnRH that is needed to initiate puberty. The kisspeptin, neurokinin B, and dynorphin interaction controls the release of GnRH and thus acts as a hormonal signal that triggers sexual development (Livadas et al., 2019). The intricate balance of stimulatory and inhibitory signals also underscores the central role of the hypothalamus in reacting to countless factors like nutritional well-being and external stimuli to decide on the onset of puberty and reproductive well-being. Besides the reproductive functions, the hypothalamus is important in energy homeostasis and control of metabolism.

Through its association with peripheral signals of energy storage and expenditure, the hypothalamus is involved in the control of body weight and nutritional status. For instance, some hypothalamic neurons respond to adipose tissue signals, such as leptin, to control hunger and energy intake. This regulatory function is not in isolation, as it blends the feedback mechanisms of other systems, including the adrenal glands and the gastrointestinal system. The hypothalamus is therefore a necessary interface between the nervous and endocrine systems that allows energy balance and metabolism to be finely tuned based on the body's requirements in a dynamically changing world (Robert L Goodman et al., 2022).

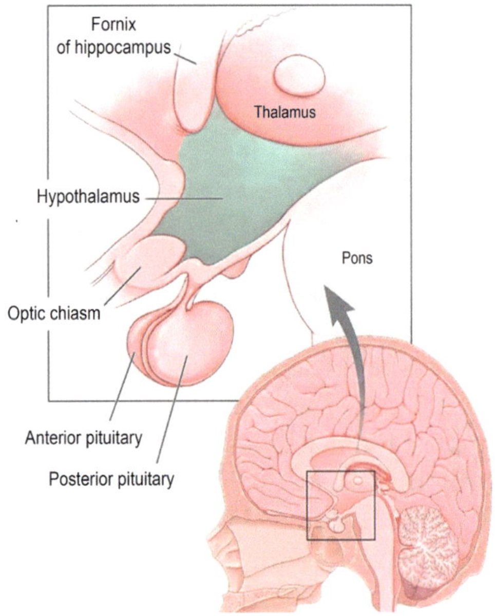

Figure 13.9. Hypothalamus.

Source: https://assets.lybrate.com/imgs/tic/enadp/image-of-the-hypothalamus.jpg

13.3.1. Connection Between the Hypothalamus and the Pituitary Gland

The dialogue between the pituitary gland and the hypothalamus forms the foundation of the human endocrine system's operation. The hypothalamus resides at the brain's base and acts as the essential regulator of numerous body functions by controlling neurological communications and the feedback of hormones. Releasing and inhibiting hormones are released by the hypothalamus, which directly influence the secretion of the pituitary hormones. Specifically, the hypothalamus uses hormones such as corticotropin-releasing hormone (CRH) and gonadotropin-releasing hormone (GnRH) to stimulate the anterior pituitary gland. This intricate system of information enables the body's homeostasis to be maintained appropriately, responding to internal and external stimuli in turn. Without this balancing act, the pituitary gland wouldn't be able to regulate many of the body's functions effectively, a testament to the hypothalamus's central role in endocrine signaling. Further, the communication of the hypothalamus with the pituitary also exemplifies an endocrine system of hierarchical regulation. The anterior pituitary produces and secretes hormones that respond in target organs to control growth, reproduction, and metabolism. Significantly, growth hormone (GH), luteinizing hormone (LH), and follicle-stimulating hormone (FSH) are essential for the growth and operation of the metabolic and reproductive systems. The pituitary similarly reacts to feedback messages from the endocrine organs it regulates, evidence of the subtle operation of hormonal dynamics. Thankfully, disruption of this mechanism can lead to catastrophic hormonal imbalance and disease conditions. For instance, interference of pituitary function after exposure to endocrine-disrupting chemicals (EDCs) during embryogenesis might have lasting consequences for the signaling and secretion of hormones and underscores the value of guarding this critical axis (Ge et al., 2024). Furthermore, hypothalamus-pituitary communication channels are intricate and involve circulatory as well as direct neural mechanisms. The portal system of the hypothalamic-pituitary facilitates the free passage of hypothalamic hormones to the pituitary gland so that the need for the hormones to go into systemic circulation is diminished. This ensures rapid response to the variations in body needs because the pituitary has the capability to respond rapidly to adjust hormone release based on the feedback from the hypothalamus. The inter-acting influence of the pituitary with other organs, such as the adrenal and thyroid glands, serves as another indicator of the cascading nature of the interaction. Moreover, as established in the present literature, discovering how a factor such as pituitary gland hormonal stimuli influences other endocrine organs—such as the prostate—serves as an opportunity for explanation of complex pathophysiological disorders (André Sarmento-Cabral et al., 2025).

This interconnectivity is not merely the significance of the hypothalamus-pituitary axis, but also the broader significance of endocrine regulation for human health.

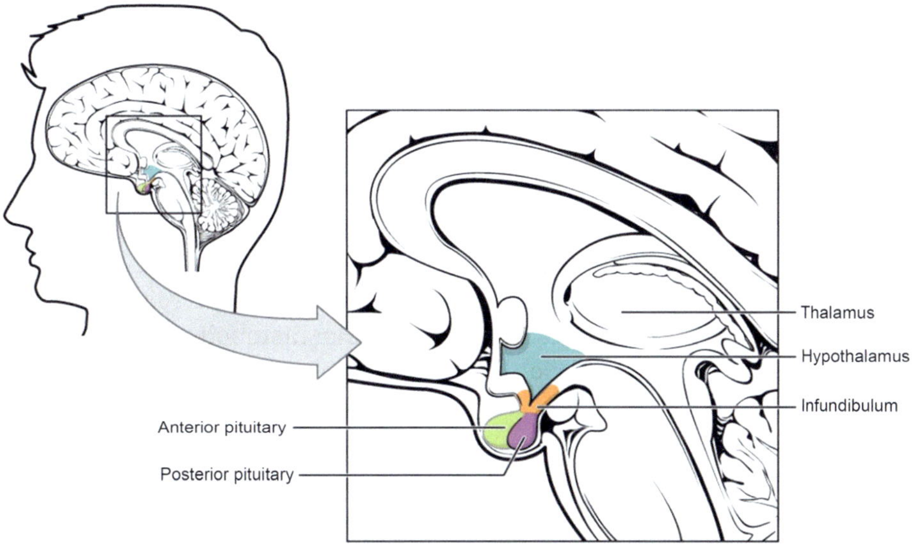

Figure 13.10. The hypothalamus region lies inferior and anterior to the thalamus. It connects to the pituitary gland by the stalk-like infundibulum. The pituitary gland consists of an anterior and posterior lobe, with each lobe secreting different hormones in response to signals from the hypothalamus.

Source: https://s3-us-west-2.amazonaws.com/courses-images-archive-read-only/wp-content/uploads/sites/403/2015/04/21031152/1806_The_Hypothalamus-Pituitary_Complex.jpg

13.3.2. Regulation of Homeostasis Through Hormonal Control

Hormone regulation control of homeostasis is the focus of maintenance of the body's internal balance despite fluctuating external environments. Various endocrine glands release hormones, which act as control messengers to ensure the functioning of vital physiological processes. Insulin and glucagon, released by the pancreas, for instance, are crucial in glucose metabolism. Insulin stimulates the uptake of glucose by cells, i.e., fat and muscle cells, leading to an anabolic condition in which energy is being stored. Glucagon, conversely, triggers the release of stored glucose during periods of low energy. This very fine balance between insulin and glucagon is crucial in order to avoid disease states such as Type 2 diabetes, which occurs due to a breakdown of these hormone mechanisms. By humoral stimuli and neural feedback mechanisms, the endocrine system is dynamically adjusting and managing the amount of hormones to maintain the body in an optimal physiological state (Herold, 2023). The influence of hormonal regulation also extends to glucose homeostasis to regulate a more comprehensive range of body functions, such as growth, metabolism, and sexual health. Foremost among these processes is the intricate function of the hypothalamus, which regulates the release of the pituitary gland's hormones and impacts other endocrine glands. Hormonal communication is not only vital in responding to immediate body change but also to long-term adjustment. For instance, the organism adjusts hormonal outputs as a response to chronic stress, adaptive nutrition, or environmental transition. Such regulatory modifications are required for disease and health resilience building. Besides, existing studies point to the importance of acknowledging pathways through which extrinsic sources, such as endocrine disruptors, could enter regular hormonal signal pathways and thus affect homeostatic control as well as general health (Shepelska et al., 2021). Given the key role hormones play in homeostasis, one should recognize the danger that endocrine disruptors pose to disrupt the sensitive balance that is supplied by the endocrine system. Exposure to endocrine disruptors from pesticides and industrial chemicals, for instance, may cause aberrant hormonal communication that yields adverse impacts on reproductive integrity and metabolic function. Experiments have shown that low doses of such substances have the potential to trigger pathological effects, and this emphasizes the necessity for strict regulatory policy and preventive health practices. Non-monotonic dose responses as a process emphasize how small changes at the hormonal level may have drastic long-term implications on the development and health of the human being. Therefore, the study of endocrine disruptor activities is essential in an attempt to ensure that future generations will be able to maintain hormonal equilibrium effectively and continue homeostatic processes (Shepelska et al., 2021).

13.3.3. Effect Upon the Autonomic Nervous System

The autonomic nervous system (ANS) stands at the forefront of the complex interplay between endocrine and physiological response, particularly stress. Stress hormones, particularly those of the hypothalamic-pituitary-adrenal (HPA) axis, control ANS activation. Catecholamines, such as epinephrine and norepinephrine, are secreted in acute stress, elevating heart rate and shunting blood supply to the life-sustaining organs to allow for immediate response to injury. This conversation addresses how hormonal signaling can affect autonomic control to modulate both behavioral and physiological functions. Additionally, dysregulation of the HPA axis can lead to states of pathophysiology where increased autonomic tone is coupled with gastrointestinal disturbances, highlighting the extensive interaction of these systems in maintaining homeostasis and managing environmental stress. Apart from stress, the gut microbiome significantly impacts the autonomic nervous system, displaying a complex relationship between microbial ecosystems and host physiology. Recent research underscores that microbial metabolites and signaling may impact brain behavior and function through various mechanisms, demonstrating modulation by the gut of autonomic function. For example, gut-derived signals have been shown to modulate neural and hormonal function, influencing mood and resilience to stress. This interaction demonstrates the potential for microbial modulation of the ANS, with modulation of gut flora having the potential to induce quintessential changes in autonomic control. Conversely, ANS changes also affect gut microbial content, with two-way interactive potentialities that have significant implications for the knowledge of disorders in the two systems. To this end, then, therefore, the gut microbiota seems to have a significant effect on autonomic control, particularly during stress and emotional states (Osadchiy et al., 2019). Corticotropin-releasing factor (CRF) is another mediator with significant function linking stress response and the autonomic nervous system. During the state of stress, CRF pathways stimulate not only behavioral but also endocrine and autonomic responses. Intriguingly, CRF receptor signaling controls gastrointestinal dynamics via modulation of gut motility, secretory function, and visceral sensitivity. Stimulation of CRF-R1, for instance, has been shown to enhance colonic secretomotor activity, while antagonists are able to decrease gut dysfunctions elicited by stress. Such complex function displays the complexity of endocrine signaling, i.e., CRF, and its connection to autonomic response in the gut, with likely therapeutic applications for gastrointestinal stress-related disorders. Detection of such interactions is important in establishing strategies for both the endocrine and autonomic systems toward maintaining health in patients with chronic stress or pathologies of the same (Tach Yé et al., 2017).

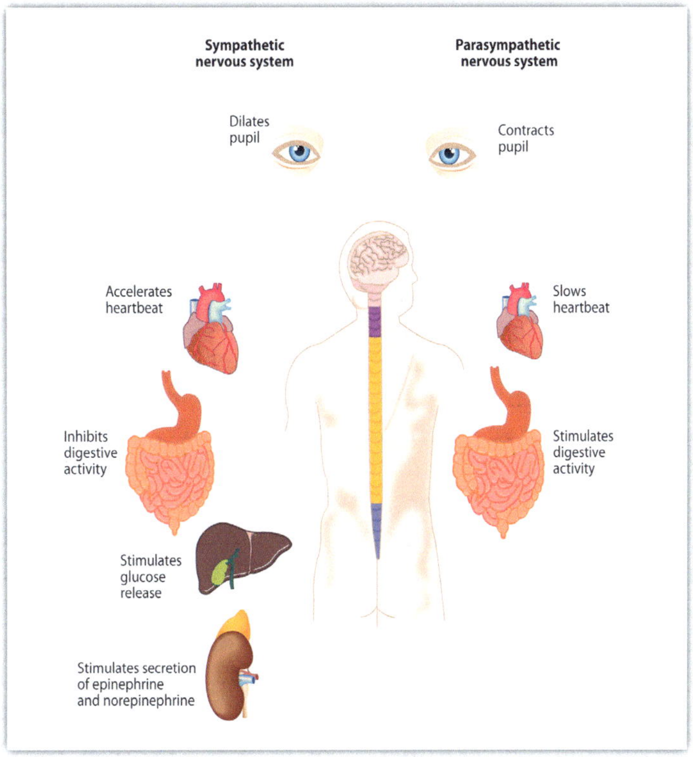

Figure 13.11. The autonomic nervous system. The autonomic nervous system has two divisions: The sympathetic division acts to energize the body, preparing it for action. The parasympathetic division acts to calm the body, allowing it to rest.

Source: https://opentextbc.ca/introductiontopsychology/wp-content/uploads/sites/9/2013/11/0a33a241806f78f7ee50cd1ad1d4bccd.jpg

Test Your Knowledge

1. What is the connection between the hypothalamus and the pituitary gland?
2. How does the hypothalamus influence the autonomic nervous system?

13.4. Endocrine Disorders

Learning Outcome

1. Know diabetes mellitus and its impact on health
2. Describe hyperthyroidism and hypothyroidism
3. Understand Cushing's syndrome and its symptoms

The endocrine system plays a vital role in maintaining homeostasis in the human body, regulating critical physiological processes such as metabolism, growth, and reproduction through the release of hormones. Endocrine disorders, though, have the potentil to wreak havoc on such processes, leading to a wide range of health issues. Diabetes, hyperthyroidism, and polycystic ovary syndrome (PCOS) are some of the endocrine disorders. Diabetes, with its failure to secrete enough insulin or react to the action of insulin, is a case in point illustrating how endocrine imbalance can lead to serious complications like cardiovascular disease and neuropathy. Similarly, hyperthyroidism involves the overproduction of thyroid hormones, which leads to increased metabolic activity resulting in weight loss, anxiety, and heart disease. Knowledge of the mechanisms behind these diseases is critical to good management and treatment, thus the significance of research in this area. Recent research identified how environmental influences, especially endocrine disruptors, disturb hormone balance and lead to endocrine disorders. Chemicals such as phthalates and Bisphenol A, which are commonly found in consumer goods and plastics, have been linked with hormonal disruption and adverse effects on reproductive health and metabolic processes. The widespread nature of these contaminants is concerning owing to their potential to contribute to the heightened incidence of conditions such as obesity and reproductive disorders. Moreover, recent research indicates that exposure to the culprit chemicals may have an interaction with the gut microbiome and add to the complication of the interaction of environmental toxins with endocrine health. Such a complicated relationship illustrates the necessity of a multidisciplinary approach towards public health and environmental policy to minimize exposure to the culprit agent, thus helping to alleviate the burden of the endocrine disorders. In summary, the endocrine health-environment interaction is a critical research field that requires concerted attention. Accumulating data suggest that pollution, particularly from plastics, has an adverse impact on the functioning of the endocrine system, thus causing a variety of disorders. An elaborate understanding of these dynamics will not only inform prevention efforts but also therapy in the affected populace. For instance, addressing the medical costs of endocrine diseases induced by environmental toxins can lead to improved healthcare policy and outcomes. As scientific studies continue to attempt to de-mystify the complexities of the microbiome and its interactions with endocrine functions, it becomes more evident to craft stringent regulations against dangerous chemicals in order to underscore the need for a unified approach towards combatting these ubiquitous health challenges (Philip J Landrigan et al., 2023; Singh et al., 2022).

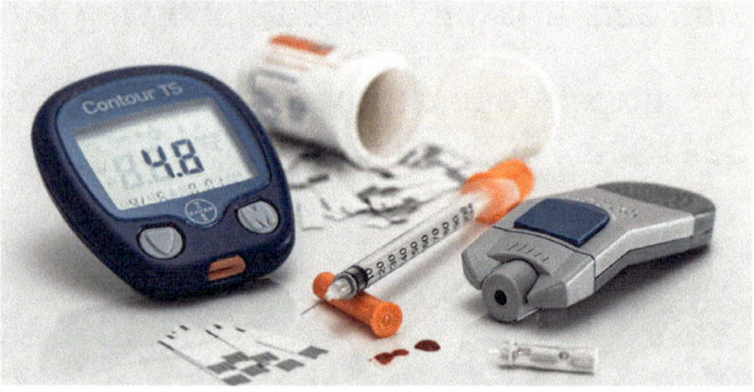

Source: https://northwayclinic.co.uk/wp-content/uploads/2019/06/136.png

13.4.1. Diabetes Mellitus and Its Impact on Health

The impact of diabetes mellitus on health is serious and encompasses multiple physiological and psychological considerations. As a chronic condition with hyperglycemia, diabetes can lead to serious complications in multiple organ systems. For instance, uncontrolled diabetes often leads to cardiovascular diseases, neuropathy, and kidney failure, which seriously affect quality of life. Underlying mechanisms are insulin resistance or inadequate insulin secretion, which affect not only glucose metabolism but also trigger inflammatory responses. These responses can initiate signaling pathways leading to chronic disease states. Diabetes also increases susceptibility to infection because hyperglycemic environments facilitate the growth of pathogens. Thereafter, diabetic patients are prone to developing increased morbidity and mortality, further emphasizing the need for early diagnosis and effective interventions to enhance health status among the affected subjects. Apart from its physiological impact, diabetes mellitus also encompasses extreme psychological and social effects that further reinforce health status challenges. The long-term illness demands ongoing care and lifestyle changes, which may lead to stress and tension among patients. Diabetic patients have been shown to be more at risk for depression because of the day-to-day hassles of managing blood glucose levels, adherence to medications, and coping with dietary controls. This psychological burden can adversely affect adherence to treatment, leading to poor metabolic control and complication development related to diabetes. Furthermore, diabetes is likely to have socio-economic implications by way of the cost of medication, self-monitoring of glucose, and admissions to hospital. Both the psychological and socio-economic aspects of diabetes should be addressed for the successful formulation of multi-faceted care plans that ensure well-being. Understanding its broader effects on health comes from knowledge of the interaction between diabetes mellitus and inflammatory processes. Inflammation, a common occurrence with diabetes, tends to heighten insulin resistance and aid in the development of complications such as atherosclerosis and nephropathy. Elevated levels of inflammatory cytokines and chemokines could disrupt normal endocrine function, which in turn leads to a cycle of violence that further deteriorates health. Additionally, the role of inflammation is far-reaching, including involvement in the immune response, thus predisposing diabetes patients to infections that cause further health emergencies. With diabetes on the rise worldwide, focusing on inflammation pathways is increasingly critical for developing therapies targeting specific targets. These approaches can potentially reverse the multifactorial impact of diabetes and enhance the overall quality of life for patients, which points towards the significance of multifaceted approaches to treatment of the inflammatory and metabolic characteristics of the disorder. (Christopher J L Murray et al., 2022) (Chen et al., 2017).

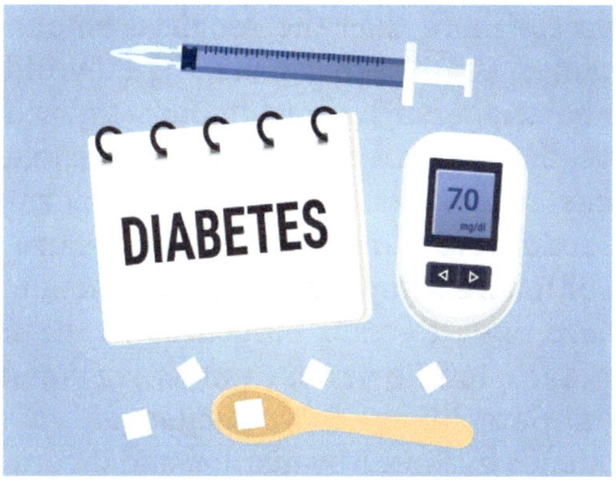

Figure 13.12. Diabetes mellitus.

Source: https://www.omegahospitals.com/blog/storage/2024/09/109c8350-786b-4a71-a406-da787e50cac0-1200x900.jpg

13.4.2. Hyperthyroidism and Hypothyroidism

The endocrine system plays a role in the regulation of several body processes in humans, while thyroid hormones play a crucial role in the maintenance of metabolic homeostasis. Two extremes of thyroid malfunction are hyperthyroidism and hypothyroidism, which can lead to various serious health problems. Hyperthyroidism, when excess thyroid hormone is secreted, usually comes with symptoms from unexplained weight loss, increased heart rate, and heightened anxiety. Conversely, hypothyroidism involves insufficient hormone production, leading to symptoms like fatigue, weight gain, and depression. Both conditions can profoundly affect an individual's quality of life and require careful diagnosis and management to mitigate long-term consequences. Moreover, the impact of such disorders extends beyond metabolic effects to influence psychological health as seen in the relation between thyroid status and behavior expressed in discussions of medical conditions that affect behavioral modifications (Tomàs Camps et al., 2019). Pathogenesis of hyperthyroidism typically occurs through Graves disease, an autoimmune disease where the thyroid gland is stimulated to secrete more than the required amount of hormones. On the other hand, hypothyroidism may be triggered by Hashimoto's thyroiditis, where the body's immune system mistakenly attacks thyroid tissue, weakening hormone production over time. These diseases are not only of inherent thyroid gland malfunction but also are open to extra influences in the form of dietary iodine levels and environmental toxins. Both illnesses are diagnosed using a confluence of clinical evaluation and laboratory tests measuring levels of thyroid-stimulating hormone (TSH) and thyroid hormones (T3 and T4). Understanding the nuances of thyroid disease is crucial as early treatment via medication, dietary modification, or surgery can greatly improve patient outcomes and reduce risk for resultant complications (Puzanov et al., 2017). Apart from that, both hyperthyroidism and hypothyroidism treatment plans involve a number of different treatment modalities that are specialized based on the patients individual requirements. Hyperthyroidism may be treated with antithyroid medications, radioactive iodine, or surgery, while hypothyroidism most often requires a lifetime regimen of thyroid hormone replacement medication. The complexity of these conditions is further amplified by their potential influence on mental well-being, as thyroid abnormality patients can experience disrupted mood and intellectual function. This exchange emphasizes the importance of a multidisciplinary approach, including endocrinologists, family physicians, and mental health professionals, to address patients' overall needs. Lastly, an understanding of the impact of hyperthyroidism and hypothyroidism in the overall context of the endocrine system highlights their importance in health outcomes as well as the need for ongoing research into effective management strategies (Tomàs Camps et al., 2019).

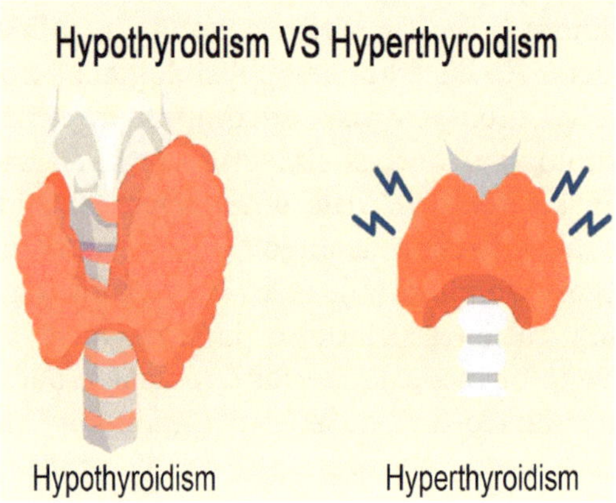

Figure 13.13. Hyperthyroidism and hypothyroidism.

Source: https://knyamed.com/cdn/shop/articles/Hypothyroidism-VS-Hyperthyroidism.jpg?v=1707743997

13.4.3. Cushing's Syndrome and Its Symptoms

Cushing's syndrome is a multifaceted endocrine illness that is primarily induced by overexposure to high cortisol levels, a hormone secreted by the adrenal glands. Cushing's syndrome may result from several sources, including adrenal tumors, pituitary adenomas, or ectopic ACTH secretion from non-endocrine neoplasms. The presentation of Cushing's syndrome is variable, making it hard to diagnose since it is non-specific in nature. Easily observed are signs of rapid weight gain, particularly in the face and abdominal area, fat redistribution, and additional fat deposits on the rear of the neck, or a buffalo hump. Patients are similarly frequently discovered to have muscle weakness, fragile skin that easily bruises, and hypertension. Given the multiaxis nature of the disorder, familiarity with these symptoms is critical for prompt diagnosis and effective treatment of Cushing's syndrome in the context of the broader human endocrine system.

The psychological impact of Cushing's syndrome significantly complicates the clinical presentation as patients also exhibit dramatic mood swings, anxiety, and depression. Researchers have shown a tendency among healthcare workers to overlook psychological symptoms for the treatment of physical presentation linked with weight gain and body image. This is meant to emphasize a common miscommunication in hospitals, whereby patients are made to feel ignored or underestimated, and there is a general overall feeling of isolation and exasperation. Patients have regularly reported difficulty in their encounters with healthcare workers, leading to what has been termed medical gaslighting. The delay in diagnosis is normally exacerbated by the stigmatization of symptoms, particularly where weight gain is a symptom, ultimately impacting the overall quality of care to patients with Cushing's syndrome (Sarah C Jones et al., 2024). With continued advancements in the technological world, bio-nanosensors offer promising tools in cortisol level monitoring, which has the potential to revolutionize Cushing's syndrome care. These sensors are able to dynamically detect hormonal variations and, in the process, enable real-time monitoring, which is important in preventing disease advancement and associated complications. With the integration of nanotechnology into medicine, wearable technologies are able to provide patients with real-time feedback on cortisol levels, thus assisting both patients and medical practitioners in making real-time decisions. Non-invasive monitoring approaches stand to improve patient outcomes by allowing on-time interventions as cortisol levels become erratic. These developments are crucial, as they ensure balanced cortisol levels that are important to maintain overall health and prevent the adverse effects of diseases like Cushing's syndrome (Nibha M Desai et al., 2025). The combination of new technology and endocrinologic insight will play an important role in the future for the treatment of this complex disease.

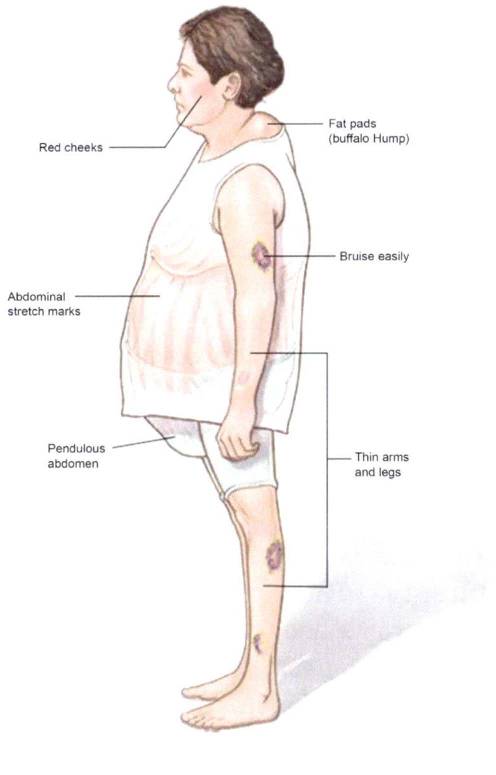

Figure 13.14. Cushing's syndrome.

Source: https://www.mayoclinic.org/-/media/kcms/gbs/patient-consumer/images/2013/08/26/10/11/ds00470_im00313_r7_cushingssyndromethu_jpg.jpg

Test Your Knowledge

1. What is the impact of diabetes mellitus on health?
2. What is Cushing's syndrome?

13.5. The Endocrine System and Growth

Learning Outcome

1. Describe the hormones involved in growth and development
2. Understand the role of growth hormone
3. Describe the effects of endocrine disorders on growth

The relationship between the endocrine system and human growth is fundamental in the regulation of various physiological activities. Hormones secreted by endocrine glands, such as growth hormone (GH), play a critical role in stimulating growth, cell repair, and metabolism. GH, produced by the pituitary gland, influences various tissues such as bone and muscle to control tissue growth and build muscle mass. GH imbalance can also cause growth disorders; e.g., hypersecretion of GH leads to gigantism or acromegaly, and hyposecretion leads to dwarfism.

The crucial functions of GH reflect the significance of the endocrine system in achieving proper body growth and homeostasis, highlighting the need for clear-cut knowledge and research into its mechanisms. Such knowledge is crucial in order to treat endocrine growth disorders appropriately. Aside from GH, other hormones also contribute significantly to growth, particularly during major stages of development. Energy balance and metabolism, which have a direct influence on growth rates, are regulated by thyroid hormones and insulin. Insulin, secreted by the pancreas, regulates blood glucose levels and triggers anabolic processes that are essential to growth. Thyroid hormones, on the other hand, are crucial in maintaining normal growth and development, particularly during early life. They facilitate efficient use of energy, controlling metabolic rate and cellular differentiation. Any discrepancies in the levels of these hormones can lead to dire growth and developmental issues, showing how fine a balancing act the endocrine system performs to allow human growth. Hence, the study of hormones is critical for the investigation of normal growth and for the management of conditions affecting growth patterns. Moreover, extrinsic factors can significantly affect the endocrine system and, by proxy, growth. Chemicals in the environment, referred to as endocrine disruptors, such as bisphenols and phthalates, bind to hormonal pathways and potentially interfere with normal endocrine function. For instance, prenatal exposure to these chemicals can potentially be a cause of adverse effects on fetal development and growth by altering maternal hormone levels and placental activity. These aberrations can be long-lasting, affecting metabolic health and offspring growth. Endocrine stresses, particularly during phases of critical fetal development, emphasize the vulnerability of the endocrine system to environmental factors. Therefore, the studies being conducted now have to focus on the effects of these disruptors on the endocrine processes that are crucial for growth and development, as highlighted in the growing literature on the topic (Karavitaki et al., 2024; Basak et al., 2023).

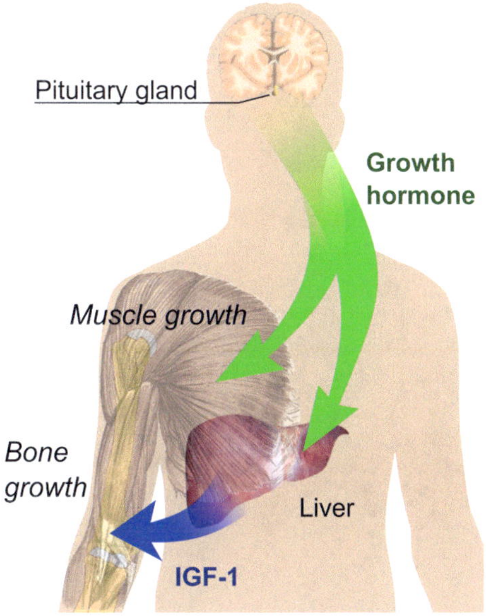

Figure 13.15. Endocrine growth regulation.

Source: https://upload.wikimedia.org/wikipedia/commons/9/99/Endocrine_growth_regulation.svg

13.5.1. Hormones Involved in Growth and Development

Hormones play a key role in regulating growth and development during life. Body messengers, hormones orchestrate a grand symphony of cell processes from childhood growth accelerations to the maintenance of body functions in adulthood. The most important among them are growth hormone (GH), insulin-like growth factors (IGFs), and thyroid hormones. GH is released from the anterior pituitary and induces growth in all tissues, but none, making cells divide and regenerate. IGFs, particularly IGF-1, also perform the majority of the functions of GH, offering a mechanism for muscle and bone growth and regulation of metabolism. These hormones, together, demonstrate the web of endocrine signaling throughout essential periods of growth and development. Thyroid hormones, primarily triiodothyronine (T3) and thyroxine (T4), also illustrate the complexity of the regulation of growth. Both are released by the thyroid gland and are required to control metabolism, energy expenditure, temperature regulation, and the development of the central nervous system. They influence a wide range of aspects of physiological activity, such as lipid metabolism and protein synthesis, and thus indirectly influence growth per se. It should be noted that alterations in thyroid function have the potential to lead to serious medical issues, ranging from stunted growth in children to metabolic disease in adults. Its significance is compounded by the danger of the environmental endocrine-disrupting chemicals, such as plasticizers, that have been found to interfere with thyroid function and undermine growth and development. It is important to understand the role of these hormones to fully understand human development and physiological and environmental processes, particularly during early life. Disruption in hormone signaling can have a profound effect on growth and development. Environmental chemicals that have been termed endocrine-disrupting chemicals (EDCs) have become an issue of concern with possible disruption of hormonal function. EDCs can mimic or compete with endogenous hormones and induce alterations in growth and development patterns, particularly at susceptible stages such as prenatal and pubertal development. The compounds have been shown to produce long-lasting effects on thyroid function, metabolic homeostasis, and reproductive processes. For instance, EDCs have also been shown to cause abnormal growth and development disability patterns, with further research being required into their long-term health effects and mechanisms of action. This implies that ongoing research is required to determine the intricate interaction between hormones and the environment, resulting in better health for future generations as we tackle the common risk imposed by environmental toxins, e.g., EDCs (Predieri et al., 2022) (Bereketoglu et al., 2022).

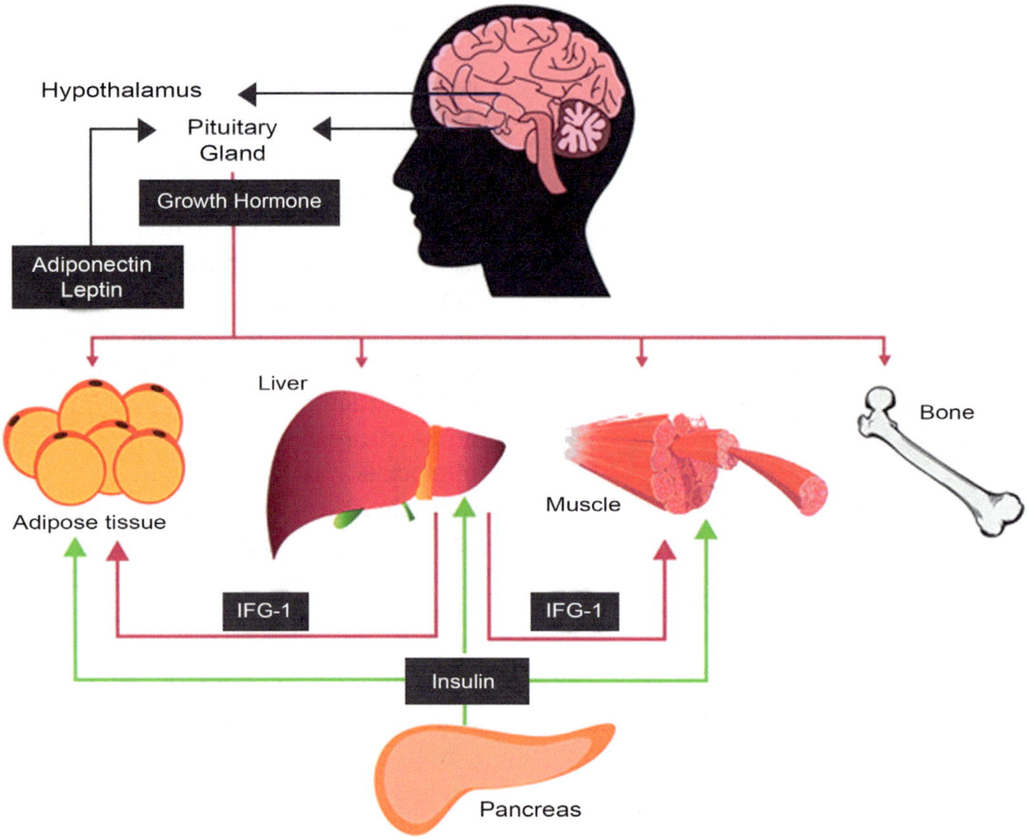

Figure 13.16. Growth hormones.

Source: https://media.geeksforgeeks.org/wp-content/uploads/20220803113318/GrowthHormones.png

13.5.2. The Role of Growth Hormone

Of the many hormones released by the human endocrine system, growth hormone (GH) or somatotropin plays a role in growth, metabolism, and homeostasis. It is released and secreted by the anterior pituitary gland, and it is especially significant during childhood and adolescence, with GH playing a direct role in linear growth and bone and muscle development. Aside from its growth foundation roles, GH plays a critical role in metabolic actions, including the augmentation of protein synthesis, the degradation of fat degradation (lipolysis), and glucose regulation of carbohydrate metabolism. Contrary to popular belief, GH actions are intermediate via insulin-like growth factor 1 (IGF-1), which enhances its anabolic action by promoting cell growth and addition of muscle and bone mass. Therefore, the complex GH signaling pathways need to be explained, especially with its multifunctionality in the endocrine system as depicted in the relevant studies (William J Kraemer et al., 2020). Surprisingly, the regulation of growth hormone release is intricate and well-regulated by various physiological stimuli such as exercise, sleep, and nutrition. For instance, it has been illustrated that exercise increases the levels of GH, which is an ingredient in muscle growth and recovery, a subject deposited during exercise. Sleep, particularly at the deeper non-REM sleep stages, is also a time of GH's essential secretion, setting the hormone's position in restoration processes during sleep. Secondly, nutritional components such as fasting and carbohydrate intake also regulate GH levels and reflect a correlation of diet with endocrine homeostasis. Such utter richness is the underlying reason why treatments for maximizing GH levels or GH disorders have to be approached through a systems approach. The multifaceted interaction of GH with the outside world is employed to demonstrate its utility in the clinic, especially concerning metabolic well-being and bodily function (Fátima Cardoso et al., 2018). In endocrinological well-being, beyond metabolism and growth, growth hormones play a role in influencing aging and regulating other long-term diseases. For instance, the low levels of GH in old age have been implicated in excess obesity, type 2 diabetes, and muscle wasting, and thus indicate potential therapeutic interventions such as replacement therapy of GH. GH therapy of aging and metabolic disease has, however, been at the center of controversy. These moral problems and potential hazards of GH therapy must be resisted, particularly in vulnerable patients, as improper use or misuse can lead to adverse effects such as cardiovascular disorders and musculoskeletal disorders. Thus, research emphasizes the need for appropriate balancing of the benefits of GH in therapeutic application with risks involved, having a radical impact on the regulation and awareness of health with regard to the aging endocrine system and chronic disease (William J Kraemer et al., 2020).

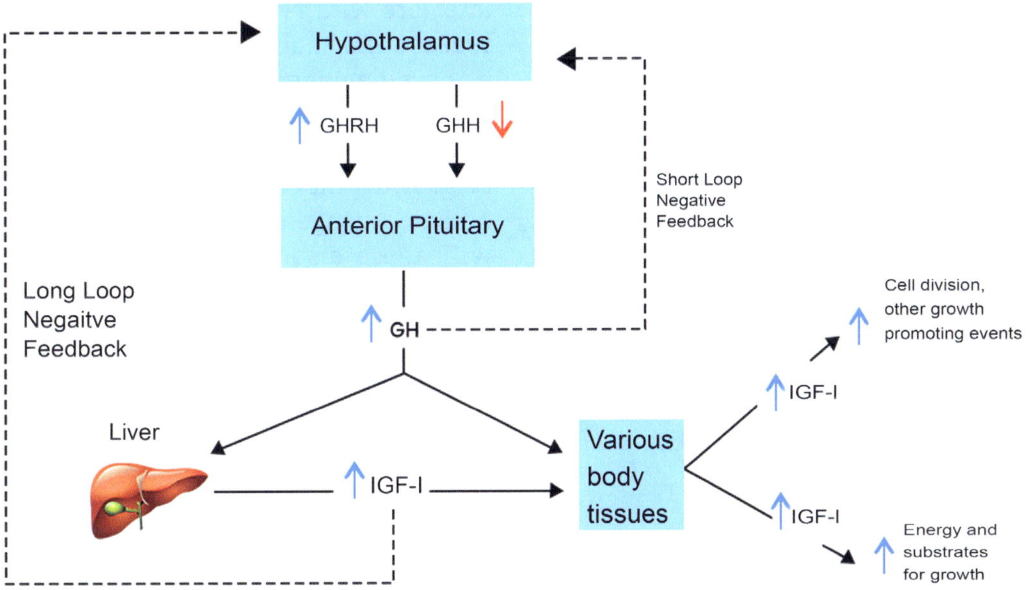

Figure 13.17. Growth hormone mechanism.

Source: https://media.geeksforgeeks.org/wp-content/uploads/20220803113235/GrowthHormoneMechanism.png

13.5.3. Effects of Endocrine Disorders on Growth

The endocrine system regulates growth and development through an interactive set of hormones. Endocrine illnesses, such as GH axis disorders, can impose significant negative effects on human growth. For instance, a deficiency in GH can cause growth delay in children, which results in a condition known as growth hormone deficiency (GHD). This disorder not only affects height but also psychological growth and overall health. Abnormalities during periods of crucial growth, particularly during childhood and adolescence, may result in permanent effects extending beyond height and affecting individuals' self-esteem and social relationships. The implications of these deficiencies underscore the importance of understanding how endocrine dysfunction leads to growth retardation and necessitates immediate identification and treatment (Yang and Ma, 2021). Endocrine disorders, including hypothyroidism and hyperthyroidism, also play important roles in growth patterns. In children, deficient levels of thyroid hormones will lead to delayed growth and maturation of bones, known as juvenile hypothyroidism. Thyroid hormones are also essential for the development of the skeletal system and basal metabolic rate, both of which are vital for normal development. In contrast, excessive production of thyroid hormone can lead to increased growth in infancy and early childhood but eventually results in closure of the growth plates, leading to dwarfism. The subtle balance of thyroid hormones is therefore critical not only for typical growth but also for maintenance of metabolic processes throughout the life span of an individual. Appreciation of these interactions highlights the significance of appropriate management of thyroid diseases for facilitating proper physiological growth (Cunningham et al., 2021). Another point equally significant to consider is the contribution of adrenal diseases, particularly those affecting cortisol levels. Conditions such as Cushing's syndrome, which can be caused by excess cortisol production, can lead to suppression of growth due to its catabolic effect on muscle and bone. Adrenal insufficiency, conversely, can limit cortisol production, leading to hypotension, hypoglycemia, and many other symptoms, indirectly suppressing growth by interfering with appetite and overall levels of energy. These disorders demonstrate the way in which abnormal patterns of hormone secretion interfere with regular patterns of growth, and these abnormalities result in several types of developmental delay and disease. As more and more studies come out on the connections between the endocrine system and processes of growth, they further support the need for holistic management techniques for individuals with these disorders to cushion the effect on growth and development (Yang and Ma, 2021).

Test Your Knowledge

1. What is the role of growth hormone?
2. How does the endocrine system affect growth?

13.6. The Endocrine System and Reproduction

Learning Outcome

1. Understand the hormonal regulation of the menstrual cycle
2. Describe the role of testosterone in male reproductive health
3. Describe the impact of endocrine disruptors on fertility

The endocrine system is crucial to regulating the reproductive processes through intricate hormone balance. The main interest of this system is hormones such as estrogen, progesterone, and testosterone that harmonize the development and maintenance of reproductive health. These hormones oversee varied physiological processes such as the menstrual cycle, spermatogenesis, and sexual differentiation. Critical stages of human development, starting in embryonic development and continuing into adulthood, are set by hormonal signals that are sensitive not only to biological but also to environmental needs. The capacity of the endocrine systems to adapt in response to different conditions is essential for the development of phenotypic traits related to reproduction. It is an understanding of this adaptability that becomes increasingly important with ongoing human activity altering environmental states, potentially disrupting hormone balance and reproductive health (Little et al., 2024).

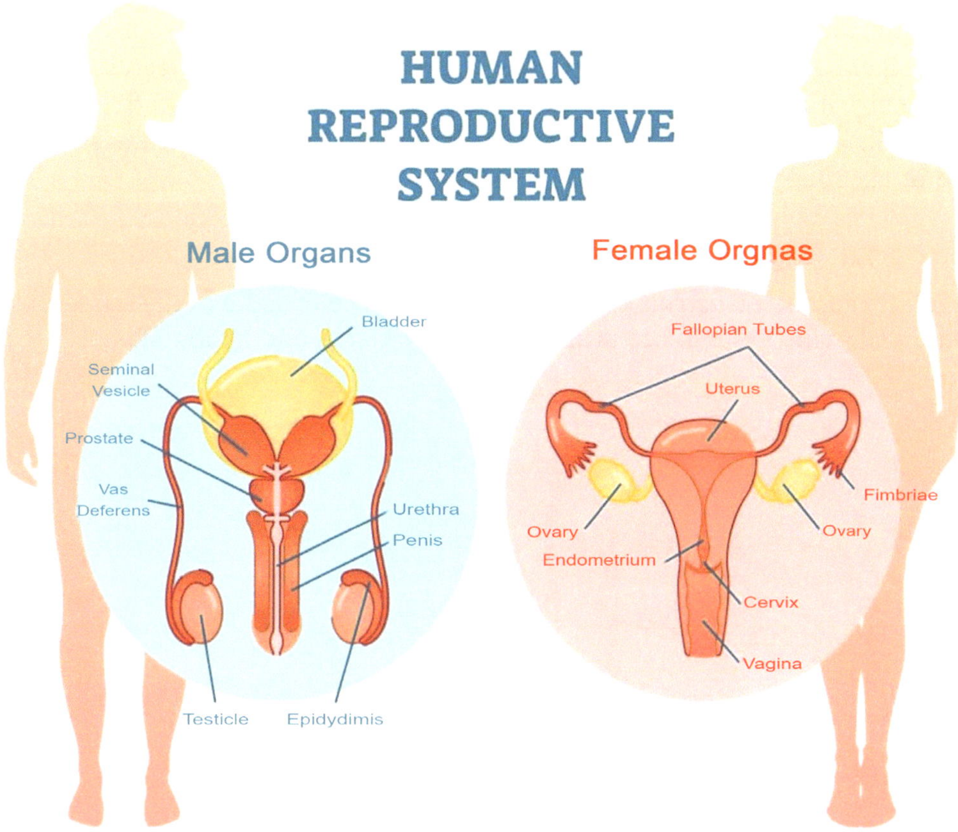

Figure 13.18. Human reproductive system.

Source: https://ngsmagnified.com/wp-content/uploads/humanreprosystem-1024x810.jpg

Endocrine disruptors, and particularly endocrine-disrupting chemicals (EDCs), pose a significant threat to reproductive health by interfering with normal hormonal communication. Among these, estradiol is specifically regarded as one of the most potent EDCs, linked with numerous health implications that can affect growth, metabolism, and the reproductive process. The occurrence of high environmental exposures to estradiol has been identified as related to adverse health implications, such as reproductive disorder and cancer threats. As these chemicals are ubiquitous in everyday products such as food and beverages, there is a critical requirement for strict control and surveillance to offset exposure to them among the human population. New technologies like electrochemical aptasensing contribute to bringing new methods to sense estradiol levels in biological fluids, yielding insights into not only environmental impact but also personal health diagnosis (Waifalkar et al., 2022). Integration of endocrine response research into conservation is critical to the maintenance of reproductive health under intensifying environmental stressors. Endocrine plasticity enables organisms to phenotypically modify their behavior in response to environmental cues, and plasticity is critical to survival and reproduction in changing environments. With the pressures of human forces like climate change, pollution, and habitat fragmentation, this plasticity becomes more critical. By comprehending the interface between endocrine disruption and reproductive health, conservation can better respond to challenges of ongoing environmental change. Effective management and intervention strategies will emanate from an integrated comprehension of how hormone signaling interfaces with ecological systems to ultimately affect populations and ecosystems becoming healthier as we are challenged to understand the complexities of environmental change (Little et al., 2024).

13.6.1. Hormonal Regulation of the Menstrual Cycle

Hormonal regulation of the menstrual cycle is a subtle balance of some of the numerous hormones secreted by the endocrine system, i.e., ovaries, pituitary gland, and hypothalamus.

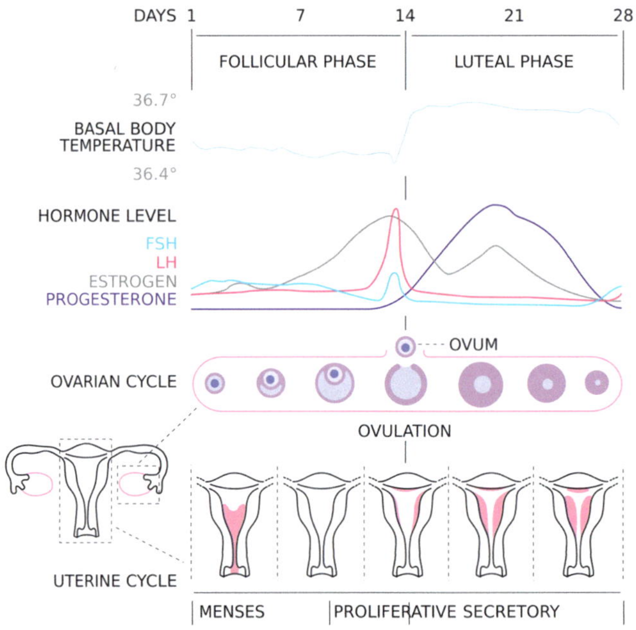

Figure 13.19. Menstrual cycle.

Source: https://upload.wikimedia.org/wikipedia/commons/9/92/Menstrual_cycle.svg

The cycle is usually divided into four phases: menstruation, the follicular phase, ovulation, and the luteal phase. At the start of the cycle, the hypothalamus releases gonadotropin-releasing hormone (GnRH), which stimulates the pituitary gland to secrete luteinizing hormone (LH) and follicle-stimulating hormone (FSH). FSH triggers growth of the ovarian follicles, while LH triggers ovulation and leads to the release of an egg. The timing of the peak hormones is crucial to conception, and disruptions to the cycle can lead to fertility or other endocrine disorders. Following ovulation is the luteal phase, which involves maturation of the corpus luteum, secreting estrogen and progesterone. These are the hormones that prepare the endometrial lining for the potential implantation of an implanted egg. Progesterone plays a significant role in the upkeep of endometrial lining, which supports thickening for the growth of the embryo. If there is non-fertilization, the corpus luteum collapses and progesterone and estrogen levels diminish. Withdrawal of these hormones results in the physiologic changes creating menstruation. The cyclical nature of such hormonal variations underscores the intricacy of menstrual cycle regulation and the necessity of female reproductive health. Such extrinsic influences risk derangement of the hormonal control over the menstrual cycle, indicating environmental sensitivity of the mechanisms. Diet, stress, and exposure to endocrine-disrupting substances can alter normal hormone balance and create a pattern of irregularity like dysmenorrhea or amenorrhea. For example, chemicals like per- and polyfluoroalkyl substances (PFAS) have been demonstrated to influence reproductive hormones, which in turn may be the cause of adverse reproductive outcomes (Suzanne E Fenton et al., 2020). This in turn places emphasis on the importance of comprehending these complexities not merely for the understanding of the menstrual cycle itself but also for resolution of more general public health issues regarding endocrine disruptors. A properly regulated menstrual cycle is one indicator of overall reproductive well-being that underscores the significance of hormonal equilibrium in womens health in the context of the endocrine system.

13.6.2. Role of Testosterone in Male Reproductive Health

Testosterone, the primary male sex hormone, is needed to build and maintain reproductive health integrity in men. It is an important component of the physiological mechanisms that cause sexual differentiation, libido, and spermatogenesis. Testosterone secretion primarily occurs in the testicular Leydig cells under regulation by the luteinizing hormone (LH) of the pituitary gland. There are necessary levels of testosterone required not just for the production of sperm but also for the development of secondary sexual characteristics, such as muscle mass and facial hair. Furthermore, testosterone has impacts on behavioral characteristics, such as aggression and mood, that indirectly affect male reproductive capability. As identified in latest studies, endocrine disruptions in testosterone management may lead to fertility issues, underlining the importance of hormonal balance for optimal reproductive health (Alekseeva et al., 2024). Curiously, environmental reasons for testosterone malfunction, including xenobiotic exposure to chemicals such as bisphenol A (BPA), can seriously undermine testosterone function and, by extension, male reproductive health. BPA as an endocrine disruptor is of concern since it can have the ability to generate free radicals and disrupt the hormonal milieu of the body. There is evidence that exposure to BPA leads to adverse effects on testosterone development through disruption of Leydig cell integrity and spermatogenesis in general. Fueling the fire still more, circadian rhythm disturbances—fueled all too frequently by modern lifestyles—have been linked with low testosterone levels. The interaction between the external environmental influences and the balance of hormones shows that conquering these external influences is crucial to preserve male fertility and reproductive health (Rasool et al., 2024). Further, recent studies have shown potential preventative measures against the adverse effects of endocrine disruptors on testosterone levels. For instance, curcumin, a bioactive compound isolated from turmeric, has been shown to be an antioxidant with a potential to modulate oxidative stress and improve reproductive processes. Administration of curcumin has also been shown to reverse the reduced testosterone levels brought about by BPA, while increasing the levels of other significant hormones such as luteinizing hormone (LH) and follicle-stimulating hormone (FSH). This protective role highlights the potential of nutritional and supplemental therapies in advancing the reproductive health of men. Such findings lend credence to calling for further research into the nexus between lifestyle, environment, and hormonal regulation in a world increasingly filled with contaminants (Rasool et al., 2024).

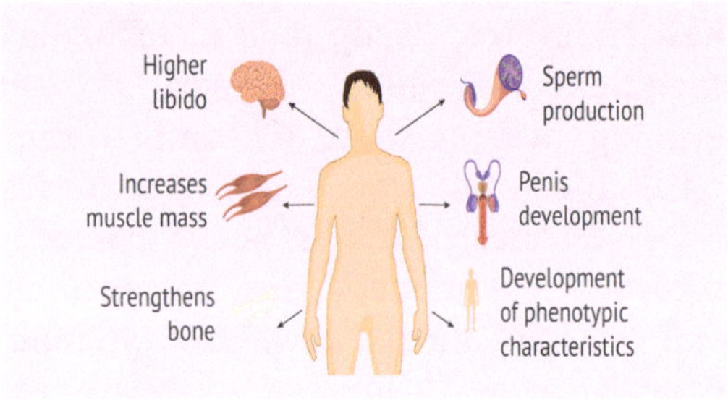

Figure 13.20. Functions of testosterone in men.

Source: https://www.invitra.com/en/wp-content/uploads/2019/12/functions-of-testosterone-in-men.png

13.6.3. Impact of Endocrine Disruptors on Fertility

The presence of endocrine disruptors (EDCs) has raised significant concern regarding their impact on human fertility. These chemical entities found in everyday products such as plastics, cosmetics, and agrochemicals have the ability to disrupt hormone communication and cause improper reproductive mechanisms. There is scientific evidence that exposure to EDCs correlates with various reproductive pathologies. For instance, certain chemicals like phthalates and bisphenol A (BPA) have been reported to have been involved in oocyte maturation as well as competency degradation in women, leading to anovulation and endometriosis. Moreover, the effect of EDCs is even more pronounced in women, who are found to have greater exposures to them due to the utilization of personal care products containing them. The vulnerability of impaired fertility highlights the need for increased vigilance and research on the impact of such ubiquitous pollutants in our world (Tricotteaux-Zarqaoui et al., 2024). Endocrine disruptor effect on fertility is extended to both sexes, but the damaging processes may vary. Toxifying EDC exposure in men has been associated with compromised sperm quality and hormonal imbalance. Research has established that compounds such as dioxins and pesticides disrupt testosterone synthesis and sperm morphology, thus decreasing male reproductive capacity. Such a trend is alarming with the decline in sperm count and quality among most populations, and doubts exist concerning the long-term effects on fertility. Furthermore, synergistic action of EDCs with lifestyle and genetic determinants can enhance these risks, pointing to the complexity of assessing their contribution to male and female fertility. Continuous research is unavoidable in order to completely cover the extent of EDC action on male reproductive health (Tricotteaux-Zarqaoui et al., 2024). Awareness of EDC exposure consequences not only informs public health policy, but it also influences individual-level decision-making in lifestyle and environmental exposures. As evidence has evolved on EDC effects on reproductive health, the stakes have increased for regulatory action to avert toxic chemicals' use in consumer products. More education on potential sources of EDC exposure may give individuals the information they need to make intelligent decisions that safeguard their fertility. Moreover, measures to reduce exposure to EDCs will ease some of the reproductive issues, pushing improved fertility rates. As more research is conducted, there is a necessity to align scientific proof with public campaigns and policy recommendations to ensure the difficulties caused by endocrine disruptors in the area of human reproduction are effectively addressed.

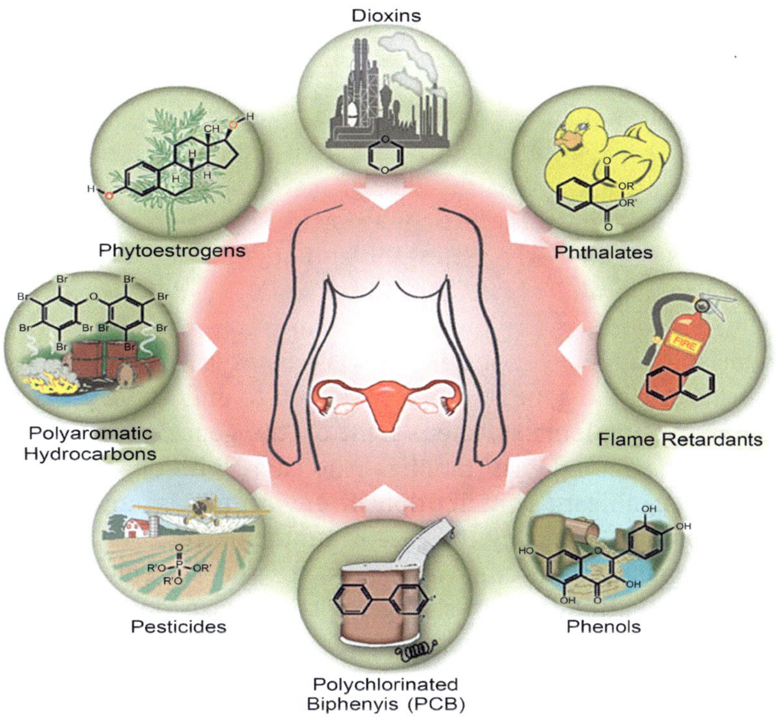

Figure 13.21. Endocrine disruptors and their impact on fertility.

Source: https://www.medlineacademics.com/assets/img/Blog/endocrine-disruptors-and-their-impact-on-fertility.jpg

Test Your Knowledge

1. What are the hormonal regulations of the menstrual cycle?
2. What is the role of testosterone in male reproductive health?

SUMMARY

In brief, the fine balance of the endocrine system is intended to underscore its important role in maintaining homeostasis and adjusting physiological activities throughout the human body. The various glands—i.e., the thyroid, pituitary, and adrenal glands—are hormone-secreting organs that directly influence metabolic activity, growth, and stress reaction. The impact of endocrine disturbances acts to further validate the proclivity of this system, as attested to by the rise in reported adverse reactions, particularly among older patients who receive immune checkpoint agents such as pembrolizumab and nivolumab. Interestingly, endocrine AEs possess the ability to cause significant effects, such as prolonged hospitalization and even mortality, thus precise measurement of endocrine function, especially in risk-exposed individuals (H-Xia et al., 2024), becomes unavoidable. Further, the genetic etiology related to endocrine pathology, particularly in menstrual disease among young females, sheds light on the genetic component of such etiology. Genealogical evaluation done among girls' families who came with oligomenorrhea and abnormal uterine bleeding sets the significant contribution of environmental and family determinants in defining endocrine well-being. Pregnancy lifestyle of mother, stress, and sedentary lifestyle with excessive use of technologies were predictive factors for the aforementioned disorders. These findings are beneficial in identifying high-risk groups and also point towards the function of preventive interventions and early intervention in the management of endocrine conditions (Bagatska, 2024). Ultimately, the complexity of the endocrine system must be addressed by a multidisciplinary approach not only by healthcare interventions but by public health strategies as well with a motive of education and behavior modification. To appreciate the interaction between the genetic, environmental, and behavior variables, endocrine diseases can better be controlled. More work is needed to clarify the sophisticated modes in which these factors interact to allow more effective therapy and patient outcomes. Future healthcare stakeholders will be forced to prioritize endocrine health as the foundation for overall well-being and for diverse groups (H-Xia et al., 2024; Bagatska, 2024).

The endocrine system is a vital regulatory system of the human organism, tasked with the work of maintaining the body in homeostasis by the release and production of hormones. Biochemical messages from the various glands like the pituitary gland, thyroid gland, and adrenal glands circulate in the blood to the target organs. With defective operation of this system, a range of body processes, such as metabolism, growth, and mood, would be compromised. Insulin and cortisol hormones demonstrate the complexity with direct energy and stress response regulation, respectively. Studies on these hormonal pathways provide valuable insight into how the endocrine system controls a wide array of body functions, cementing its place in disease and health (Schedlowski et al., 2024). Besides controlling metabolism and body reactions, the endocrine system also has an important role in the immune response. The relationship between the immune and hormonal systems displays a high level of systemized communications whereby hormones associated with stress, e.g., catecholamines, are able to regulate the immune system. Early research has confirmed that associative learning affects immune processes and that behavioral and psychological states affect physiological processes. This convergence suggests that extrinsic experience, as mediated by the nervous system, can condition immune response, illustrating the endocrine system's complexity. These observations are in support of evidence for the need for consideration of psychological status in immune competence assessment, since the ability to affect health may be great (Schedlowski et al., 2024). Moreover, clinical significance of dysfunctions in the endocrine system is more and more recognized, including the effect of drugs such as opioids on endocrine control. Opioids have further been demonstrated to adversely impact the hypothalamic-pituitary-adrenal (HPA) axis and cause such disorders as hypogonadism and adrenal insufficiency. The interaction between opioid use and endocrine function is an important risk factor within the context of long-term health status, and affects bone mineral content and total metabolic health. Extending the evidence base, filling gaps in what is currently known concerning opioid-induced endocrine effects will be valuable. By studying these associations, healthcare providers are able to design more effective interventions to limit the adverse effect of opioids on hormone homeostasis and enhance outcomes.

KEY TERMS FROM THIS CHAPTER

Adrenal glands
Corticotropin-releasing hormone
Cushing's syndrome
Endocrine disruptors
Endocrine system
Hyperthyroidism
Hypothyroidism
Parabens
Peptide hormones
Pituitary gland
Steroid hormones
Thyroid gland
Thyroid-stimulating hormone
Thyroxine
Triclosan
Triiodothyronine

CRITICAL THINKING QUESTIONS

1. **The endocrine system primarily functions to:**
   a. Transmit nerve impulses
   b. Produce hormones that regulate bodily functions
   c. Provide structural support
   d. Filter blood
2. **Which gland is often referred to as the "master gland"?**
   a. Thyroid gland
   b. Adrenal gland
   c. Pituitary gland
   d. Pineal gland
3. **The anterior pituitary secretes all the following hormones EXCEPT:**
   a. Growth hormone (GH)
   b. Thyroid-stimulating hormone (TSH)
   c. Antidiuretic hormone (ADH)
   d. Adrenocorticotropic hormone (ACTH)
4. **The thyroid gland produces which hormone that regulates metabolism?**
   a. Insulin
   b. Thyroxine (T4)
   c. Cortisol
   d. Glucagon
5. **The adrenal medulla secretes:**
   a. Cortisol
   b. Aldosterone
   c. Epinephrine and norepinephrine
   d. Insulin

Short Answer Questions

1. What is the endocrine system?
2. What are the major glands of the endocrine system?
3. What are the hormones?
4. What is the role of the hypothalamus?
5. What are the most common endocrine disorders?

Answer to Critical Thinking Questions

1. (b)   2. (c)   3. (c)   4. (b)   5. (c)

REFERENCES

1. Alekseeva, M. V., Bykova, O. V., Shaderkina, A., Borisenko, Y. V., Gritskevich, E., & Krasnyak, S. S. (2024). The role of circadian rhythms in the functioning of male reproductive system. *Experimental and Clinical Urology*. https://www.semanticscholar.org/paper/90b9439d54abf13d46cdd92b082da646759096ea (accessed on 15th June 2025).
2. Areta, J., Taylor, H. L., & Koehler, K. (2020). Low energy availability: History, definition and evidence of its endocrine, metabolic and physiological effects in prospective studies in females and males. *European Journal of Applied Physiology, 121*, 1–21. https://www.semanticscholar.org/paper/410069dc6010e80f0acfd1e48bb0fa120eb108e1 (accessed on 15th June 2025).
3. Bagatska, N. (2024). Determination of predictive factors in families of girls with menstrual disorders comorbid with endocrine system pathology. *Ukrainian Journal of Pediatric Endocrinology*. https://www.semanticscholar.org/paper/530488e0f02e11b5be200bc486b1509f5076582b (accessed on 15th June 2025).
4. Basak, S., Varma, S., & Duttaroy, A. (2023). Modulation of fetoplacental growth, development and reproductive function by endocrine disrupters. *Frontiers in Endocrinology, 14*. https://www.semanticscholar.org/paper/3152f17ad53e84d420583efd4191d82538e2cfe0 (accessed on 15th June 2025).
5. Bereketoglu, C., & Pradhan, A. (2022). Plasticizers: Negative impacts on the thyroid hormone system. *Environmental Science and Pollution Research International, 29*, 38912–38927. https://www.semanticscholar.org/paper/a6ff3be8ea1c8787e98f189d740ff97a06686ae3 (accessed on 15th June 2025).
6. Borowiec, B., Popis, M., & Jankowski, M. (2018). Factors involved in the development of pituitary and hypothalamus: A short review. *Medical Journal of Cell Biology, 6*, 150–154. https://www.semanticscholar.org/paper/e8e19e335a23cd8fdcd4e39f29009da017e9b93e (accessed on 15th June 2025).
7. Camps, T., Amat, M., & Manteca, X. (2019). A review of medical conditions and behavioral problems in dogs and cats. *Animals, 9*, 1133–1133. https://doi.org/10.3390/ani9121133 (accessed on 15th June 2025).
8. Cardoso, F., Senkus, E., Costa, A., Papadopoulos, E., Aapro, M., André, F., Harbeck, N., et al. (2018). 4th ESO–ESMO international consensus guidelines for advanced breast cancer (ABC 4). *Annals of Oncology, 29*, 1634–1657. https://doi.org/10.1093/annonc/mdy192 (accessed on 15th June 2025).
9. Chang, S. W., & Lee, H. C. (2019). Vitamin D and health–The missing vitamin in humans. *Pediatrics & Neonatology, 60*, 237–244. https://doi.org/10.1016/j.pedneo.2019.04.007 (accessed on 15th June 2025).
10. Chen, L., Deng, H., Cui, H., Fang, J., Zuo, Z., Deng, J., Li, Y., et al. (2017). Inflammatory responses and inflammation-associated diseases in organs. *Oncotarget, 9*, 7204–7218. https://doi.org/10.18632/oncotarget.23208 (accessed on 15th June 2025).
11. Cunningham, M., Azcárate-Peril, M. A., Barnard, A., Benoit, V., Grimaldi, R., Guyonnet, D., Holscher, H. D., et al. (2021). Shaping the future of probiotics and prebiotics. *Trends in Microbiology, 29*, 667–685. https://doi.org/10.1016/j.tim.2021.01.003 (accessed on 15th June 2025).

12. Desai, N. M., Dwivedi, D. V. J., Upadhyaya, C., & Mehta, M. (2025). Design perspectives of bio nano sensors using nanomaterials for endocrine hormones. *Journal of Information Systems Engineering and Management*. https://www.semanticscholar.org/paper/2fd65733880720141696e0aea92c9d0353f86287 (accessed on 15th June 2025).

13. Fenton, S. E., Ducatman, A., Boobis, A. R., DeWitt, J. C., Lau, C., Ng, C. A., Smith, J. S., et al. (2020). Per- and polyfluoroalkyl substance toxicity and human health review: Current state of knowledge and strategies for informing future research. *Environmental Toxicology and Chemistry, 40*, 606–630. https://doi.org/10.1002/etc.4890 (accessed on 15th June 2025).

14. Ge, X., Weis, K., & Raetzman, L. (2024). Impact of developmental exposures to endocrine disrupting chemicals on pituitary gland reproductive function. *Reproduction*. https://www.semanticscholar.org/paper/05c2aff4dab12f1727a8049868bb7171ae29da72 (accessed on 15th June 2025).

15. Goodman, R. L., Herbison, A. E., Lehman, M. N., & Navarro, V. M. (2022). Neuroendocrine control of gonadotropin-releasing hormone: Pulsatile and surge modes of secretion. *Journal of Neuroendocrinology, 34*. https://doi.org/10.1111/jne.13094 (accessed on 15th June 2025).

16. Herold, K. (2023). Hormones—Modulators of metabolism. *Acta Physiological, 238*. https://www.semanticscholar.org/paper/6013f4c9a7a843e8e3c8985afdec64b5564431e4 (accessed on 15th June 2025).

17. Hong, Y., Kim, H. J., Park, S., Yi, S., Lim, M., Lee, S., Chang, J. W., et al. (2023). Single cell analysis of human thyroid reveals the transcriptional signatures of aging. *Endocrinology*. https://www.semanticscholar.org/paper/4dfdf77e3c63b39803918a06fb58f67f67629d96 (accessed on 15th June 2025).

18. Jones, S. C., Nutter, S., & Saunders, J. F. (2024). "The healthcare system did fail me repeatedly": A qualitative study on experiences of healthcare among Canadian women with Cushing's syndrome. *BMC Primary Care, 25*. https://www.semanticscholar.org/paper/cdb81c230d56b46eba0191b1e07c7d090f809cb2 (accessed on 15th June 2025).

19. Kabir, A. (2021). Latest classification and such functions of human hormones. https://www.semanticscholar.org/paper/544042c7e08ab2ec28782741a0eeb87de8c5dab2 (accessed on 15th June 2025).

20. Karavitaki, N., Bettinger, J. J., Biermasz, N., Christ-Crain, M., Gadelha, M. R., Inder, W., Tsourdi, E., et al. (2024). Exogenous opioids and the human endocrine system: An Endocrine Society Scientific Statement. *Endocrine Reviews*. https://www.semanticscholar.org/paper/5b0e7af69f3f1d154c344be93560eb12f5266091 (accessed on 15th June 2025).

21. Khan, Y. (2023). Chemicals that disrupt the endocrine system and their effects on human health. *Open Access Journal of Endocrinology*. https://www.semanticscholar.org/paper/beed58bc3f6e1f281440f0978afbac8ad071fe53 (accessed on 15th June 2025).

22. Kodila, A., Franko, N., & Sollner Dolenc, M. (2023). A review on immunomodulatory effects of BPA analogues. *Archives of Toxicology, 97*, 1831–1846. https://www.semanticscholar.org/paper/0c50797cdad623ef860fd50ab1307ba0798f2254 (accessed on 15th June 2025).

23. Kraemer, W. J., Ratamess, N. A., Hymer, W. C., Nindl, B. C., & Fragala, M. S. (2020). Growth hormone(s), testosterone, insulin-like growth factors, and cortisol: Roles and integration for cellular development and growth with exercise. *Frontiers in Endocrinology, 11*. https://doi.org/10.3389/fendo.2020.00033 (accessed on 15th June 2025).

24. Kuraku, S., Kaiya, H., Tanaka, T., & Hyodo, S. (2022). Evolution of vertebrate hormones and their receptors: Insights from non-Osteichthyes genomes. *Annual Review of Animal Biosciences*. https://www.semanticscholar.org/paper/ecf32034a8794b0e8508f44a88efc725334e3137 (accessed on 15th June 2025).

25. Labayen, M., Ochoa de Eribe, D., Aramburu, A., Nieto, M., & Aginako, N. (2024). European common data management platform definition for railway AI function development. *Transportation Development Research*. https://www.semanticscholar.org/paper/8cf4fd0285463ee8458d6d1168e3263ceef82d41 (accessed on 15th June 2025).

26. Landrigan, P. J., Raps, H., Cropper, M., Bald, C., Brunner, M., Canonizado, E. M., Charles, D., et al. (2023). The Minderoo-Monaco Commission on plastics and human health. *Annals of Global Health, 89*. https://doi.org/10.5334/aogh.4056 (accessed on 15th June 2025).

27. Li, Y., Zheng, M., Limbara, S., Zhang, S., Yu, Y., Yu, L., & Jiao, J. (2024). Effects of the pituitary-targeted gland axes on hepatic lipid homeostasis in endocrine-associated fatty liver disease—A concept worth revisiting. *Journal of Clinical and Translational Hepatology, 12*, 416–427. https://www.semanticscholar.org/paper/a4fc60a0b0ea85e583bca52a4d3dbf31553ce04a (accessed on 15th June 2025).

28. Li, Z., & Robaire, B. (2025). Effects of endocrine-disrupting chemicals on adrenal function. *Endocrinology, 166*. https://www.semanticscholar.org/paper/b6d42a0487f515be3698aa7b6eb21c7542778c44 (accessed on 15th June 2025).

29. Little, A., & Seebacher, F. (2024). Endocrine responses to environmental variation. *Philosophical Transactions of the Royal Society B: Biological Sciences, 379*. https://www.semanticscholar.org/paper/47c2dee5929c1f692071947c26bf8e7c1788a407 (accessed on 15th June 2025).

30. Liu, S., Ezran, C., Wang, M. F. Z., Li, Z., Awayan, K., Long, J. Z., De Vlaminck, I., et al. (2024). An organism-wide atlas of hormonal signaling based on the mouse lemur single-cell transcriptome. *Nature Communications, 15*. https://www.semanticscholar.org/paper/5235d1b57d33123f37cf349634d49fab065cc46e (accessed on 15th June 2025).

31. Livadas, S., & Chrousos, G. P. (2019). Molecular and environmental mechanisms regulating puberty initiation: An integrated approach. *Frontiers in Endocrinology, 10*. https://doi.org/10.3389/fendo.2019.00828 (accessed on 15th June 2025).

32. Łukasiewicz, S., Czeczelewski, M., Forma, A., Baj, J., Sitarz, R., & Stanisławek, A. (2021). Breast cancer—Epidemiology, risk factors, classification, prognostic markers, and current treatment strategies—An updated review. *Cancers, 13*, 4287–4287. https://doi.org/10.3390/cancers13174287 (accessed on 15th June 2025).

33. Miki, Y., Iwabuchi, E., Inoue, C., Yamazaki, Y., & Suzuki, T. (2024). Histopathological analysis potential for unveiling hormone signaling in endocrine-related tumors. *Endocrine Oncology, 4*. https://www.semanticscholar.org/paper/75b74e5179750b8179711f59eed17a4a3fb5e261 (accessed on 15th June 2025).

34. Murray, C. J. L., Ikuta, K. S., Sharara, F., Swetschinski, L. R., Robles Aguilar, G., Gray, A. P., Han, C., et al. (2022). Global burden of bacterial antimicrobial resistance in 2019: A systematic analysis. *The Lancet, 399*, 629–655. https://doi.org/10.1016/s0140-6736(21)02724-0 (accessed on 15th June 2025).

35. Osadchiy, V., Martin, C. R., & Mayer, E. A. (2019). Gut microbiome and modulation of CNS

function. *Comprehensive Physiology*. https://doi.org/10.1002/cphy.c180031 (accessed on 15th June 2025).

36. Patani, A., Balram, D., Yadav, V. K., Lian, K. Y., Patel, A., & Sahoo, D. (2023). Harnessing the power of nutritional antioxidants against adrenal hormone imbalance-associated oxidative stress. *Frontiers in Endocrinology, 14*. https://www.semanticscholar.org/paper/8532bd64bb8e2166021695d682987e33e80192ac (accessed on 15th June 2025).
37. Predieri, B., Iughetti, L., Bernasconi, S., & Street, M. (2022). Endocrine disrupting chemicals' effects in children: What we know and what we need to learn? *International Journal of Molecular Sciences, 23*. https://www.semanticscholar.org/paper/e9c3ce9ac1f36e857585e4e1717e79451102cf5d (accessed on 15th June 2025).
38. Puzanov, I., Diab, A., Abdallah, K., Bingham, C. O., Brogdon, C. F., Dadu, R., Hamad, L., et al. (2017). Managing toxicities associated with immune checkpoint inhibitors: Consensus recommendations from the Society for Immunotherapy of Cancer (SITC) Toxicity Management Working Group. *Journal for Immunotherapy of Cancer, 5*. https://doi.org/10.1186/s40425-017-0300-z (accessed on 15th June 2025).
39. Quttina, M., Waiters, K. D., Khan, A., Karami, S., Peidl, A. S., Babajide, M. F., Pennington, J., et al. (2023). Exosc9 initiates SUMO-dependent lncRNA TERRA degradation to impact telomeric integrity in endocrine therapy insensitive hormone receptor-positive breast cancer. *Cells, 12*. https://www.semanticscholar.org/paper/acd10a324464558f1fe091910cc8ad5af4bf90ed (accessed on 15th June 2025).
40. Rasool, M. H., Al-Nuaimi, A. J., & Al-Sabbagh, J. (2024). Investigation of the role of curcumin against the toxicity induced by bisphenol A on the reproductive system in male rats. *Journal of Kerbala for Agricultural Sciences*. https://www.semanticscholar.org/paper/007243627f8dbe7de46dbca417d07e28c82dde1e (accessed on 15th June 2025).
41. Raza, G., & Herzig, K. (2022). Hepatic glucose production and storage as a potential strategy for type 2 diabetes treatment–The effect of catestatin– "Just another new kid in town?." *Acta Physiological, 235*. https://www.semanticscholar.org/paper/978c6a0e0b6fc4e4f51800238ba9bc3a086e2714 (accessed on 15th June 2025).
42. Sarmento-Cabral, A., Fuentes-Fayos, A. C., Mata Ordoñez, F., León-González, A. J., Martínez-Fuentes, A., Gahete, M., & Luque, R. M. (2025). From pituitary cells to prostate gland in health and disease: Direct and indirect endocrine connections. *Reviews in Endocrine & Metabolic Disorders, 26*, 187–203. https://www.semanticscholar.org/paper/677997f69f290fcf26df8da3d1e3fcbee6ed7675 (accessed on 15th June 2025).
43. Schedlowski, M., & Hadamitzky, M. (2024). Behaviorally conditioned immune responses: "To learn new things, read old books and papers." *Neuroimmunomodulation, 31*, 102–113. https://www.semanticscholar.org/paper/b96192a485d2620e7f556ce4b3ab9c5191767278 (accessed on 15th June 2025).
44. Shepelska, N., Prodanchuk, M., & Kolianchuk, Y. (2021). Pesticides as endocrine disruptors of the reproductive system (literature review and own research). *Journal of the National Academy of Medical Sciences of Ukraine*. https://www.semanticscholar.org/paper/7b6807ada6e54c0c59188dc13f4a3b5e0a0737de (accessed on 15th June 2025).
45. Shi, H. X., He, Y., Dan, S. Y., Yang, L., Wang, J., Chen, L., & Chen, Z. L. (2024). Endocrine system-related adverse events associated with PD-1/PD-L1 inhibitors: Data mining from the FDA

adverse event reporting system. *Frontiers in Medicine, 11*. https://www.semanticscholar.org/paper/941f7cbd665d5da4613afcd41eb9aba99b9207f6 (accessed on 15th June 2025).

46. Singh, S., Sharma, P., Pal, N., Kumawat, M., Shubham, S., Sarma, D. K., Tiwari, R., et al. (2022). Impact of environmental pollutants on gut microbiome and mental health via the gut–brain axis. *Microorganisms, 10*, 1457–1457. https://doi.org/10.3390/microorganisms10071457 (accessed on 15th June 2025).

47. Taché, Y., Larauche, M., Yuan, P. Q., & Million, M. (2017). Brain and gut CRF signaling: Biological actions and role in the gastrointestinal tract. *Current Molecular Pharmacology, 11*. https://doi.org/10.2174/1874467210666170224095741 (accessed on 15th June 2025).

48. Tricotteaux-Zarqaoui, S., Lahimer, M., Abou Diwan, M., Corona, A., Candela, P., Cabry, R., Bach, V., et al. (2024). Endocrine disruptor chemicals exposure and female fertility declining: From pathophysiology to epigenetic risks. *Frontiers in Public Health, 12*. https://www.semanticscholar.org/paper/311b17dfec77e652206b35b4d8e2600c48d30571 (accessed on 15th June 2025).

49. Uwamahoro, C., Jo, J. H., Jang, S. I., Jung, E., Lee, W. J., Bae, J. W., & Kwon, W. S. (2024). Assessing the risks of pesticide exposure: Implications for endocrine disruption and male fertility. *International Journal of Molecular Sciences, 25*. https://www.semanticscholar.org/paper/7d77fd2fcde6222ff561c999bcfe0a76366467ac (accessed on 15th June 2025).

50. Waifalkar, P. P., Noh, D., Derashri, P., Barage, S., & Oh, E. H. (2022). Role of estradiol hormone in human life and electrochemical aptasensing of 17β-estradiol: A review. *Biosensors, 12*. https://www.semanticscholar.org/paper/8d7437459c5e67ca0a61b3e77cd6ada4fcea84d4 (accessed on 15th June 2025).

51. Yang, J., & Ma, Z. (2021). Research progress on the effects of nickel on hormone secretion in the endocrine axis and on target organs. *Ecotoxicology and Environmental Safety, 213*, 112034–112034. https://doi.org/10.1016/j.ecoenv.2021.112034 (accessed on 15th June 2025).

52. Zaitseva, N., Kleyn, S. S., Chetverkina, K. V., Andrishunas, A. M., & Tsinker, M. J. (2024). On the safe levels of micro-sized particles PM1.0 in ambient air. *Hygiene and Sanitation*. https://www.semanticscholar.org/paper/07796028d4d75eec19049c4aa2846561f9cdac7a (accessed on 15th June 2025).

53. Zhang, Y., Tu, L., Chen, J., & Zhou, L. (2024). Interference mechanisms of endocrine system and other systems of endocrine-disrupting chemicals in cosmetics—*In vitro* studies. *International Journal of Endocrinology, 2024*. https://www.semanticscholar.org/paper/d6eff96663f5d432cb382150520f877093c7e83a (accessed on 15th June 2025).

INDEX

U

V

W